T0252620

Valvular
Heart Disease

FUNDAMENTAL AND CLINICAL CARDIOLOGY

Editor-in-Chief

Samuel Z. Goldhaber, M.D.

Harvard Medical School
and Brigham and Women's Hospital
Boston, Massachusetts

Associate Editor, Europe

Henri Bounameaux, M.D.

University Hospital of Geneva
Geneva, Switzerland

Valvular Heart Disease

edited by

Muayed Al Zaibag

Armed Forces Hospital
Riyadh, Saudi Arabia
and Loma Linda University Medical Center
Loma Linda, California

Carlos M. G. Duran

King Faisal Specialist Hospital
Riyadh, Saudi Arabia

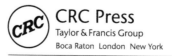

CRC Press
Taylor & Francis Group
Boca Raton London New York

CRC Press is an imprint of the
Taylor & Francis Group, an **informa** business

CRC Press
Taylor & Francis Group
6000 Broken Sound Parkway NW, Suite 300
Boca Raton, FL 33487-2742

© 1994 by Taylor & Francis Group, LLC
CRC Press is an imprint of Taylor & Francis Group, an Informa business

No claim to original U.S. Government works

Visit the Taylor & Francis Web site at
http://www.taylorandfrancis.com

and the CRC Press Web site at
http://www.crcpress.com

Series Introduction

When I visited the teaching hospitals in Riyadh in 1990, it was immediately apparent that the scope of valvular heart disease surpassed greatly what could be experienced in any academic center in North America. Transesophageal echocardiography was routinely scheduled on an hourly basis every day. Balloon valvuloplasty was undertaken daily to treat young adults who had disabling valvular stenoses. In the midst of all the action, Dr. Al Zaibag has played a central and prominent role in spearheading the cardiologic research and advances in valvular heart disease. Dr. Al Zaibag is an internationally known and respected expert in interventional cardiology, with a subspecialty in balloon valvuloplasty. Therefore, it was a personal privilege when this busy academic cardiologist accepted my suggestion of editing a book in the Fundamental and Clinical Cardiology Series published by Marcel Dekker, Inc.

This book, which Drs. Al Zaibag and Duran have assembled, relies upon world-renowned experts in all aspects of valvular heart disease. The first section deals with pathology, echo Doppler, and radiologic examination among patients with valvular heart disease, and provides an overview of acute rheumatic fever. The second part has specific chapters dealing with the most vexing and common problems that one confronts in managing specific valvular heart disease conditions of the mitral, aortic, and tricuspid valves. This second section also includes a rather controversial chapter on management of pregnancy and valvular heart disease. Finally, the concluding part of the book deals with treatment and emphasizes the role of valvular surgery. With Dr. Duran as coeditor, it is no surprise that one can learn about the latest available techniques in conservative valve surgery he has pioneered.

In summary, I am particularly proud of this book. *Valvular Heart Disease* fits beautifully in the series of books we have assembled on fundamental and clinical cardiology. I have been impressed with the care and individualized attention the publisher has devoted to the authors and editors in this series. I am certain that this particular book will help to define the broad scope of the overall series and will provide a practical tool for physicians and other health care professionals dealing with valvular heart disease patients.

Samuel Z. Goldhaber

Preface

The unique combination of the high prevalence of rheumatic cardiac pathology in developing countries and the state-of-the-art medical treatment at the Riyadh Armed Forces Hospital (personally supported by H.R.H. Prince Sultan bin Abdul Aziz) was the driving force behind the scientific advances in the treatment of stenotic cardiac valves using balloon catheters. This original work on valvular diseases, carried out in the Arabian peninsula, led Marcel Dekker, Inc., to invite us to edit this major work on valvular heart diseases which brings together the world's experts in this field. The application, at King Faisal Specialist Hospital and Research Centre, of the modern techniques of valve repair to the more complex valve pathology caused by rheumatic heart disease has led to new knowledge and has modified the surgical therapeutic approach for these disorders.

Progress in the field of diagnosis and management of valvular heart diseases was formerly restricted to the industrialized (Western) countries because of the lack of resources in the developing world. Now some of the latter have acquired advanced and sophisticated cardiac services and will continue to increase their already significant contribution to the development of methods of diagnosis and treatment of these disorders (1).

Today's diagnostic tools have uncovered pathology and pathophysiology that formerly were unknown or dismissed. This information, together with the range of therapeutic modalities available to the surgeon and intervention cardiologist, allows more appropriate therapy for patients suffering from valvular heart disease.

Embracing new methods with enthusiasm must be tempered with pragmatic considerations of availability, cost, and safety. Therefore, although this book includes discussion of the technological advances available today, it also emphasizes the importance of clinical features. Let there be no mistake that the overall tenets of the best medical practice still apply: the diagnosis of valvular heart disease still requires the skills of a highly trained clinician.

It is interesting to note that the principles of organized clinical description were founded by the Muslims, Nestorian Christians, and Jews, working together in what were the first organized hospitals, with pharmacies and structured methods for clinical description and treatment of disease. Some of the textbooks of that era, such as *The Cannon*, by Avicenna, 980–1037 *(ibn-Sina)*, formed the basis of the early medical curriculum in the Western universities, including those in the British Isles, even into the 1700s (2). No developments since that time have displaced the patient's clinical presentation as the single most significant element in directing patient care, but we have expanded our clinical descriptions beyond the six clinical features they described!

Recent improvements in diagnosis and interventional procedures have also resulted in radical changes in our approach to the management of acutely ill patients. For example, pregnant women with mitral stenosis and pulmonary edema can now be treated by a simple and safe percutaneous balloon intervention. Other examples include surgical repair of valvular lesions, low-dose anticoagulation therapy for patients with prosthetic valves, and earlier surgery in patients with bacterial endocarditis.

Echocardiography has transformed the management of patients with valvular heart disease, and it provides a clear and objective basis for the timing of interventions and assessment of outcome. In the area of therapeutic guidance, biplane transesophageal echocardiography provides the surgeon precise intraoperative evaluation of valve performance following repair.

Parallel with the advances, it must be acknowledged, we have created a new class of disorders as the sequelae of prosthetic valve implantation and other procedures, whether surgical or interventional, in the catheter laboratory. Risks and benefits for alternative choices are evaluated, and management of related iatrogenic problems is addressed. Reviews of long-term outcome incorporate these concerns.

In the following chapters the more well-known aspects of the management of valvular heart disease have been updated, but we have also included topics and approaches that are not normally encountered between book covers.

Our primary objective was to produce a volume that would make a substantial contribution to the knowledge of valvular heart disease, to be read by practicing clinicians working in this field. We are aware that much more could have been written, but we have been rigorous in selection of the material to maintain practical dimensions. After all, the book is meant to be accessible in day-to-day encounters with the patients whose problems are addressed, as a practical guide to a better outcome of modern management of valvular heart disease.

We were overwhelmed by the enthusiastic response of our contributing authors, whose commitment needs no other advocate than their chapters. Working with them has been both stimulating and rewarding. Our sincerest thanks to them all for their effective participation in producing such impressive contributions despite their exceedingly busy schedules.

Muayed Al Zaibag
Carlos M. G. Duran

REFERENCES

1. Roberts WC. Editor in chief. The Kingdom of Saudi Arabia, oil, money and cardiology (editorial). Am J Cardiol 1988, 61:410–412.
2. Lyons AS. Medicine, an illustrated history, Lyons AS, Petrucelli RJ, eds. New York: Harry N Abrams, 1978; 295–317.

Contents

Contributors

Mario Albertucci, M.D. Assistant Professor, Department of Cardiothoracic Surgery, Albany Medical College, Albany, New York

Muayed Al Zaibag, M.B.Ch.B., F.R.C.P., F.A.C.C. Head, Department of Adult Cardiology, Riyadh Cardiac Centre, Armed Forces Hospital, Riyadh, Saudi Aradia, and Associate Professor of Medicine, Department of Medicine, Loma Linda University Medical Center, Loma Linda, California

Elia M. Ayoub, M.D. Professor, Department of Pediatrics, University of Florida, Gainesville, Florida

Ramesh C. Bansal, M.D., F.A.C.C. Director, Echocardiography Laboratory, and Professor, Department of Medicine, Loma Linda University Medical Center, Loma Linda, California

K. Chandrasekaran, M.D. Associate Professor, Division of Cardiology, Department of Medicine, and Director, Echocardiography Laboratory, Hahnemann University Hospital, Philadelphia, Pennsylvania

Richard Coulden, M.D. Visiting Research Fellow, Department of Radiology, University of Chicago, Chicago, Illinois

Adnan S. Dajani, M.D. Professor, Department of Pediatrics, Wayne State University, and Chief, Division of Infectious Diseases, Children's Hospital of Michigan, Detroit, Michigan

Carlos M. G. Duran, M.D., Ph.D. Professor and Chairman, Department of Cardiovascular Diseases, King Faisal Specialist Hospital, Riyadh, Saudi Arabia

L. Henry Edmunds, Jr., M.D.   Julian Johnson Professor of Cardiothoracic Surgery, Department of Surgery, University of Pennsylvania, Philadelphia, Pennsylvania

Nabil El-Sherif, M.D., F.A.C.C.   Head, Division of Electrophysiology, Department of Cardiology, State University of New York—Health Science Center, Brooklyn, New York

Begonia Gometza, M.D., Pharm.D.   Cardiology Division, Department of Cardiovascular Diseases, King Faisal Specialist Hospital, Riyadh, Saudi Arabia

Moh'd Ali Habbab, M.D., F.A.C.P., F.A.C.C., F.C.C.P., F.A.C.A.   Head, Division of Electrophysiology and Pacing, Department of Adult Cardiology, Riyadh Cardiac Centre, Armed Forces Hospital, Riyadh, Saudi Arabia

Murtada A. Halim, M.D., F.R.C.P.   Consultant Cardiologist, Department of Adult Cardiology, Riyadh Cardiac Centre, Armed Forces Hospital, Riyadh, Saudi Arabia

Jeffrey M. Isner, M.D.   Professor, Departments of Medicine and Pathology, Tufts University School of Medicine, and Chief, Cardiovascular Research, St. Elizabeth's Medical Center, Boston, Massachusetts

Kenneth R. Jutzy, M.D., F.A.C.C.   Head, Section of Cardiology, and Associate Professor, Department of Medicine, Loma Linda University Medical School, Loma Linda, California

Robert B. Karp, M.D.   Professor and Chief, Department of Cardiac Surgery, University of Chicago Hospitals, Chicago, Illinois

Daniel L. Kulick, M.D.   Division of Cardiology, Department of Medicine, University of Southern California, Los Angeles, California

Martin J. Lipton, M.D.   Professor and Chairman, Division of Radiology, and Professor, Department of Medicine, University of Chicago, Chicago, Illinois

Anilkumar Mehra, M.D.   Cardiology Fellow, Division of Cardiology, Department of Medicine, University of Southern California, Los Angeles, California

Charles E. Mullins, M.D.   Professor, Department of Pediatrics, Baylor College of Medicine, Houston, Texas

Celia M. Oakley, M.D., F.R.C.P., F.A.C.P. Professor and Head, Division of Cardiology, and Professor, Department of Medicine, Hammersmith Hospital, The Royal Postgraduate Medical School, London, England

John A. Odell*, M.D., Ch.B., F.R.C.S. (ed). Chris Barnard Professor of Cardiothoracic Surgery and Head, Department of Cardiothoracic Surgery, University of Cape Town Medical School, and Surgeon, Groote Schuur and Red Cross Children's Hospital, Cape Town, South Africa

Dennis F. Pupello, M.D., F.A.C.C. Chief, Department of Cardiac Surgery, St. Joseph's Heart Institute, Tampa, Florida

Shahbudin H. Rahimtoola, M.D. George C. Griffith Professor of Cardiology and Professor, Division of Cardiology, Department of Medicine, University of Southern California, Los Angeles, California

Paulo A. Ribeiro, M.D., Ph.D., F.A.C.C. Associate Professor, Section of Cardiology, Department of Medicine, Loma Linda University Medical Center, Loma Linda, California

William C. Roberts, M.D. Executive Director, Baylor Cardiovascular Institute, Baylor University Medical Center, Dallas, Texas

Elias Saad, M.D. Assistant Cardiologist, Department of Cardiovascular Diseases, King Faisal Specialist Hospital, Riyadh, Saudi Arabia

Pravin M. Shah, M.D., F.A.C.C. Director, Academic Program in Cardiology, and Professor, Department of Medicine, Loma Linda University Medical Center, Loma Linda, California

Maie S. Shahed, M.B.B.S., M.R.C.P.(U.K.) Consultant Cardiologist, Department of Adult Cardiology, Riyadh Cardiac Centre, Armed Forces Hospital, Riyadh, Saudi Arabia

A. Jamil Tajik, M.D. Thomas J. Watson Jr. Professor, Professor of Medicine and Pediatrics, and Chairman, Division of Cardiovascular Diseases, Mayo Clinic, Rochester, Minnesota

Susan M. Vosloo, M.D. Surgeon, Groote Schuur and Red Cross Children's Hospital, Cape Town, South Africa

---

* Present affiliation: Division of Thoracic and Cardiovascular Surgery, Mayo Clinic, Rochester, Minnesota.

Valvular
Heart Disease

Part I

Morphological Aspects of Cardiac Valve Dysfunction

William C. Roberts
Baylor Cardiovascular Institute
Baylor University Medical Center
Dallas, Texas

This chapter focuses on congenital and acquired conditions affecting one or more cardiac valves and causing valvular dysfunction. The emphasis is on the mitral and aortic valves.

I. MITRAL REGURGITATION

A. Mitral Valve Prolapse

Although it was recognized earlier (1–4), delineation of the click-late systolic murmur syndrome as a consequence of mitral valve prolapse was not appreciated until the 1960s (5–9). It is now apparent that the click-late systolic murmur is common, probably occurring in 5% or more of persons >15 years of age (10–12). Although it is generally not considered as such, the click-systolic murmur syndrome, is in most persons probably a form of congenital heart disease, and therefore is the most common congenital heart disease (13). The auscultatory manifestations, however, are usually not evident until adulthood.

The click-murmur syndrome may be viewed from both auscultatory and morphologic standpoints as manifesting three stages: (1) systolic click(s) only, (2) click(s) plus a mid to late systolic murmur, and (3) pansystolic murmur only. Although progression from stage 1 to 3 has been documented in relatively few patients, it appears likely that this is the natural sequence of events in some patients. In others there may be no progression from stage 1, patients in stage 2 may revert to stage 1, patients in stage 1 may lose their click(s) altogether, and patients appearing in stage 3 (pansystolic murmur) may have had no documentation of stages 1 and 2. With rare exceptions, stages 1 and 2 are not associated with symptomatic evidence of cardiac dysfunction. The exceptions include patients with arrhythmias and/or chest pain. Patients in stage 3 have congestive heart failure because of the associated severe mitral regurgitation. The stage 3 floppy mitral valve is the major cause of *pure* (no element of stenosis) *severe, isolated* (aortic valve normal anatomically and functionally) mitral regurgitation requiring valve replacement or repair (14). As a consequence, there is considerable anatomic information available on the floppy mitral valve that produces a pansystolic murmur (stage 3) and causes severe mitral regurgitation (15). In contrast, there is less anatomic information available in patients with only a systolic click(s) (stage 1) or those with both a click(s) and a late systolic murmur (stage 2) (16).

Several names applied to this syndrome describe to some extent what the valve looks like anatomically, thus the names "prolapsing posterior mitral leaflet," "prolapsing mitral valve," "billowing or ballooning mitral leaflet syndrome" "overshooting or hooded mitral valve," "floppy mitral valve," and "myxomatous or mucinous degeneration of the mitral valve." I prefer the term "mitral valve prolapse."

Defining mitral valve prolapse morphologically has not been easy. Pomerance (17) defined the entity as a ballooning deformity of the mitral leaflets, the affected portions of which were increased in area and protruded into the left atrium in ventricular systole. Waller and associates (14) also utilized either a focal or a diffuse increase in mitral area as a criterion but also required an increased length, either focal or diffuse, from basal attachment of the leaflet to its distal margin. Lucas and Edwards (18) listed the following features for diagnosis: (1) interchordal hooding involving both the rough and the clear zones of the involved leaflet or leaflets, (2) height of the interchordal hooding >4 mm, (3) interchordal hooding involving >50% of the anterior leaflet of >67% of the posterior leaflet. Dollar and Roberts (16) used two criteria for mitral valve prolapse: (1) elongation of a portion of posterior mitral leaflet such that the distance from distal margin to its attachment at the mitral anulus was >1.5 cm; or (2) presence of mitral leaflet protrusion toward the left atrium, usually also associated with missing chordae tendineae, and the prolapsed portion of the leaflet involving >50% of the anterior leaflet and >33% of the posterior leaflet. Others have referred to this leaflet prolapse as "interchordal hooding."

Other useful anatomic findings in identifying mitral valve prolapse include the following.

1. *An increase in the transverse dimension of the leaflets such that the length of the mitral circumference measured on a line corresponding to the distal margin of the posterior leaflet is much larger than the circumference measured at the level of the mitral anulus.* In the normal valve, the two are the same. The result is analogous to an accordion that is not fully extended or, better, a skirt that is gathered at the waist. The leaflets of the opened mitral valve are flat or smooth (like the mucosa of the ileum), whereas those of the opened floppy mitral valve are undulating (like those of the duodenum or jejunum).

2. *Excessive thinning and lengthening of chordae tendineae.* Chordal elongation, however, is rare without concomitant leaflet elongation. The chordae also occasionally may be shorter than normal.

3. *Dilatation of the mitral anulus.* This does not occur to any significant degree in the absence of the mitral valve prolapse (19). Anular dilatation is the major cause of development of severe mitral regurgitation in the presence of mitral valve prolapse (The other is rupture of chordae tendineae.) (15). Normally, the mitral anulus in adults averages about 9 cm in circumference. In patients with left ventricular dilatation from any cause, with or without mitral regurgitation, the circumference of the mitral anulus usually dilates slightly, usually to about 11 cm or <25% above normal. Among patients with mitral valve prolapse associated with severe mitral regurgitation, the circumference of the mitral anulus generally increases >50% above normal or to circumferences of 14 to 18 cm. When the anulus dilates to this extent, the leaflets may "stretch" or flatten transversely, and this stretching diminishes the amount of scalloping. In addition, the left ventricular dilatation may cause longitudinal stretching of the leaflets. The amount of scalloping in the stage 3 valves, therefore, appears to be less than that observed in the stage 2 valves. Roberts (15) examined operatively excised mitral valve in 83 patients [aged 26–79 years (mean 60); 26 women (31%) and 57 men (69%)] with mitral valve prolapse and mitral regurgitation severe enough to warrant mitral valve replacement. All 83 operatively excised valves were examined by the same person, and all excised valves had been purely regurgitant (no element of stenosis). No patients had hemodynamic evidence of dysfunction of the aortic valve. In each valve a portion of the posterior mitral leaflet was elongated such that the distance from the distal margin to basal attachment of this leaflet was similar to the distance from the distal margin of the anterior leaflet to its basal attachment to the left atrial wall. Two major mechanisms for the severe mitral regurgitation were found: (1) dilatation of the mitral anulus with or without rupture of chordae tendineae and (2) rupture of chordae tendineae with or without dilatation of the mitral anulus. Of the

83 patients, 48 (58%) had both dilated anuli (>11 cm in circumference) and ruptured chordae tendineae; 16 (19%) had dilated anuli without ruptured chordae; and 16 (19%) had ruptured chordae without significant anular dilatation. In 3 patients the anulus was not dilated, nor were chordae ruptured, and therefore the mechanism of the mitral regurgitation is uncertain. Mitral chordal rupture was nearly as frequent in the 64 patients with clearly dilated anular circumferences as in the 19 patients with normal or insignificantly dilated anular circumferences (≤ 11 cm).

4. *Focal thickening of mural endocardium of left ventricle behind the posterior mitral leaflet and the mitral chordae tendineae.* Salazar and Edwards (20) called these fibrous thickenings "friction lesions" to indicate that they are believed to result from friction between the overlying leaflets and chordae and the underlying left ventricular wall. Of the 102 necropsy cases with mitral valve prolapse studied by Lucas and Edwards (18), 77 (75%) had these friction lesions, and in 3 (3%) the mural endocardial friction lesions had entrapped the overlying chordae. Dollar and Roberts (16) observed these friction lesions in 23 (68%) of 34 patients with mitral valve prolapse in whom each heart was examined specifically for these lesions. The friction lesions, therefore, are common in patients with mitral valve prolapse, and their presence strongly suggests the presence of mitral valve prolapse.

5. *Fibrinous deposits on the atrial surface of the prolapsed portion of mitral leaflet and particularly at the angle formed between prolapsed leaflet and left atrial wall* (mitral valve-left atrial angle). These deposits in the angle may be a source of emboli.

Microscopically, the prolapsed mitral leaflet may or may not contain an excessive amount of acid mucopolysaccharide material. Both the normal and the prolapsed mitral leaflets consist of two elements, the fibrosa and the spongiosa. The *fibrosa* consists of fibrous tissue (collagen), and the *spongiosa*, of mucoid or myxomatous material high in acid mucopolysaccharide material. In most valve diseases the fibrosa element is increased; it may entirely replace the spongiosa element. In the prolapsed mitral leaflet, the spongiosa element, the more central portion of the leaflet, may increase to a greater extent than the fibrosa element. The resulting increased myxoid or myxomatous stroma, however, does not appear abnormal—that is, degenerated. Thus the term myxoid or myxomatous "degeneration" for this condition is not appropriate. The amount of fibrous tissue in the mitral leaflets in mitral valve prolapse also is usually increased, but its increase may be a secondary phenomenon. The fibrosa element may be subdivided into two components, the *auricularis*, which normally is a thin layer forming the atrial or contact aspect of the leaflet, and the *ventricularis*, which normally is a relatively thick layer that covers the ventricular aspect of the leaflet. The atrial aspect of the prolapsed mitral leaflet often is focally thickened. This change probably is secondary to abnormal friction from contact between the prolapsed segment of the leaflet and its "opposite number," that is, the other leaflet, or between two prolapsed segments of the same leaflet (21,22). The changes on the ventricular surface of the leaflet consist of connective tissue "pads" forming primarily in the interchordal segments, and this proliferation of fibrous tissue may extend into adjacent chordae tendineae and onto ventricular endocardium behind the posterior mitral leaflet (20,22). The interchordal collections of fibrous tissue are considered responses to the tension and stretching that occur at the undersurface of a prolapsed leaflet or segment of leaflet (22). This increase in fibrous tissue, particularly on the ventricular surface of the leaflet, has caused, I suspect, the floppy valve in years past to be considered rheumatic in origin. Fibrin deposits also may occur on the atrial aspects of the prolapsed mitral leaflet, and they may not be found on gross examination (17).

Ultrastructural studies of floppy mitral valves have disclosed alterations of the collagen fibers in the leaflets and in the chordae tendineae (23). These changes have included fragmentation, splitting, swelling, and coarse granularity of the individual collagen fibers, and, in addition, spiraling and twisting of the fibers. Also, some elastic fibers are fragmented and contain cystic spaces. These alterations in the structure of the collagen may be more important than the accumulation of the acid mucopolysaccharide material in that they lead to focal weaknesses in the leaflets. The left ventricular systolic pressure exerted against these weakened areas may lead to prolapse or focal interchordal hooding. Although the actual prolapse of the mitral valve may be acquired and a consequence of the left ventricular systolic (closing) pressure, the focally weak areas of the leaflets are probably most often congenital in origin, and the later bulging with or without rupture is acquired as a consequence of the high intraarterial pressure. The frequency of mitral valve prolapse also may be higher in persons with elevated left ventricular systolic pressures compared with persons in whom this pressure is at normal levels (24).

Opportunities for structural study of a mitral valve associated with only a click(s) have been rare. I have studied one such valve. (The child had been examined by John Barlow, M.D., of Johannesburg, South Africa.) The child, who had no symptoms of cardiac dysfunction, died of leukemia and at necropsy had a perfectly competent mitral valve but three distinct foci where leaflet overlapped adjacent leaflet. The leaflets otherwise were smooth and, specifically, devoid of so-called scallops. There are no reported anatomic descriptions, to my knowledge, of mitral valves producing one or more systolic clicks without an associated precordial systolic murmur. Examination at necropsy of mitral valves of patients who during life had documentation of systolic click(s) plus a mid-late systolic murmur (Barlow syndrome) also are infrequent. Death in stage 2, as in stage 1, is usually from a noncardiac cause. In this stage, the most characteristic feature is leaflet scalloping, which represents excessive leaflet owing to an increase in the transverse or commissure-to-commissure dimension of the leaflet (16). The mitral anulus, as in stage 1, is not dilated. The chordae tendineae may or may not be elongated.

Just as the frequency of mitral valve prolapse varies clinically depending on the age and sex group being examined and in the clinical criteria employed for diagnosis (ausculatory, echocardiographic, angiographic), its frequency at necropsy is quite variable and the variation is determined by several factors: (1) age and sex group of population being examined; (2) type of institution where necropsy is performed [general hospital, referral hospital for cardiovascular disease, or medical examiner's (coroner's) office]; (3) expertise in cardiovascular disease of the physician performing the necropsy or reporting the findings; (4) percent of total deaths having autopsies at the particular hospital; (5) presence or absence of evidence of cardiac disease before death; (6) whether the patient underwent mitral valve replacement or repair; and (7) whether the percentage of patients being examined had a high frequency of the Marfan syndrome, infective endocarditis, atrial septal defect, and so on. No study shows better how bias alters the findings in necropsy studies than the one performed by Lucas and Edwards (18). These investigators, in one portion of their study, determined the frequency of and complications of floppy mitral valves observed at necropsy in one community (nonreferral) hospital for adults. Of 1376 autopsies performed, 7.4% or 102 patients had morphologically floppy mitral valves at necropsy. Their mean age at death was 69 ± 12 years; 62 (61%) were men and 40 (39%) were women. Of the 102 patients, mitral valve prolapse was the cause of death in only 2. Of the 102 patients, one leaflet had prolapsed in 34 patients, and two leaflets in 68. Only 18 had anatomic evidence of previous mitral regurgitation; 7 had infective endocarditis; 7 had ruptured chordae tendineae (without infection); 1 had the Marfan syndrome; and 3 had secundum atrial septal defect. No patient died suddenly. In contrast, in the other portion of their study, these authors described complications in 69 necropsy patients whose hearts had been sent to Edwards for his opinion and interest. Among these 69 patients, 16 (23%) had died suddenly and unexpectedly; 19 (28%) had ruptured chordae tendineae (without infection); 7 (10%) had infective endocarditis; 20 (29%) had the Marfan syndrome; and 9 (13%) had secundum-type atrial septal defect. Thus, in contrast to their infrequency in their community hospital series, most cases submitted to their cardiovascular registry from other institutions had ruptured chordae, infective endocarditis, sudden unexpected and unexplained death, or the Marfan syndrome.

Two other necropsy studies can be compared with the community hospital series collected by Lucas and Edwards. Pomerance (17) collected from one general hospital 35 cases at necropsy of "ballooning deformity" of the mitral valve: 23 (66%) were men and 12 (34%) were women; their ages ranged from 51 to 98 years (mean 74). Death was attributed to mitral valve prolapse in only 4 patients (11%). One leaflet only had prolapsed in 12 patients, and two leaflets in 23 (6%). Eight patients had anatomic evidence of mitral regurgitation, only 1 had atrial septal defect, 9 (26%) had anatomic evidence of tricuspid valve prolapse, 9 (26%) had mitral anular calcific deposits, and 13 (37%) had hearts of increased weight. Davies and associates (25) gathered 90 necropsy cases of the floppy mitral valve from four general hospitals. This number represented 4.5% of autopsies at the four hospitals during the time. Of the 90 patients, 44 (49%) were men and 46 (51%) were women; they ranged in age from <40 to 100 years. Death in 15 was attributed to mitral valve prolapse (the number dying suddenly was not mentioned). The prolapse involved one leaflet in 69 patients (77%) and both mitral leaflets in 21 (23%); 63 (70%) also had anatomic evidence of tricuspid valve prolapse. Only 6 (7%) had patients dilated mitral anuli; only 3 (3%) had mitral anular calcium, and 8 had hearts weighing >300 g.

Dollar and Roberts (16) studied at necropsy 56 patients aged 16 to 70 years (mean 48), with mitral prolapse: Fifteen patients, aged 16 to 69 years (mean 39), died suddenly, and mitral valve prolapse was the only cardiac condition found at necropsy (hereafter called isolated mitral valve prolapse); the remaining 41 patients had other conditions that were capable of being fatal. Of the latter 41 patients, 7, aged 17 to 59 years (mean 45), had associated congenital heart disease, and 34 patients, aged 17 to 70 years (mean 52), had no associated congenital cardiac abnormalities. Compared with the 34 patients without associated congenital heart disease and with nonmitral valve prolapse conditions capable in themselves of being fatal, the 15 patients who died suddenly with isolated mitral valve prolapse were younger (mean age 39 ± 17 versus 52 ± 15 years; $p = 0.01$), more often women (67% versus 26%; $p = 0.008$) and had a lower frequency of mitral regurgitation (7% versus 38%; $p = 0.02$). The 15 patients dying suddenly with isolated mitral valve prolapse also were less likely to have evidence of ruptured chordae tendineae (29% versus 67%; $p = 0.04$). The frequency of increased heart weight (67% versus 59%), a dilated mitral valve anulus (80% versus 81%), a dilated tricuspid valve anulus (17% versus 17%), an elongated anterior mitral leaflet (86% versus 54%), and

formed in 23; only 3 (13%) had significant coronary arterial narrowing, limited in each to one coronary artery. Auscultation and hemodynamic data at cardiac catheterization were not helpful in delineating the origin of the mitral regurgitation. None of the 97 patients—including the 60 classified as having mitral valve prolapse—had systolic clicks, and the systolic precordial murmurs in all 97 patients were holosystolic. The average pulmonary arterial, left atrial (or pulmonary arterial wedge), and left ventricular pressures were similar in the 97 patients, regardless of the origin of the mitrál regurgitation. The systolic systemic arterial pressures, however, were significantly higher in the patients with mitral valve prolapse and ruptured chordae tendineae than in those with mitral valve prolapse and intact chordae tendineae.

Mitral valve prolapse appears now to be a more common cause of rupture of mitral chordae tendineae than does infective endocarditis. Among 25 patients having mitral valve replacement for pure mitral regurgitation associated with rupture of chordae tendineae, Jeresaty and associates (27) found mitral valve prolapse (based on "redundancy and marked hooding of the mitral leaflets") to be the cause of the chordal rupture in 23 (92%), only 1 of whom had had infective endocarditis. Four of the 25 patients had auscultatory and angiographic or echocardiographic evidence of mitral valve prolapse before the chordal rupture. Among patients with ruptured chordae tendineae associated with mitral valve prolapse, sometimes it is actually difficult to identify ruptured chords. The term "rupture," however, is commonly applied to those leaflets where chordal insertions are no longer present but clearly chordae should be attached (15).

In addition to mitral regurgitation, rupture of chordae tendineae, and infective endocarditis, other complications of mitral valve prolapse include *mitral anular calcium*. Pomerance (17) observed mitral anular calcium in 9 (26%) of her 35 necropsy patients with mitral valve prolapse. The cause of the *arrhythmias* and *chest pain* is unclear (28). There is no evidence of a myocardial or coronary arterial factor. Shrivastava and associates (22) have suggested that the friction between mitral chordae tendineae and the underlying left ventricular mural endocardium may be an arrhythmic stimulus. The cause of the *acute strokes* or *transient cerebral ischemic attacks* that occur in an occasional patient with mitral valve prolapse also is unclear. It has been suggested that the small fibrin-platelet thrombi occasionally seen at the mitral valve-left atrial angle are sources of emboli for either cerebral or myocardial ischemia (18).

The cause of mitral valve prolapse, as alluded to earlier, almost certainly is congenital in origin in most patients, or at least the connective tissue of the mitral leaflets, chordae, and anulus appears to be congenitally defective. The finding of classic mitral valve prolapse at birth is evidence for the congenital thesis. The occurrence of mitral valve prolapse in certain clearly hereditary conditions—for example, the Marfan syndrome— is evidence of congenitally defective mitral tissue. Its association with aneurysm of the fossa ovale membrane or atrial septal defect and Ebstein's anomaly of the tricuspid valve also may support this thesis (29–31).

B. Cleft Anterior Mitral Leaflet

Partial atrioventricular "defect" includes a spectrum of five anatomic anomalies (32,33). Some patients have all five and others have only one or two. The five are the following: (1) defect in the lower portion of the atrial septum, so-called primum atrial septal defect; (2) defect in, or absence of, the posterobasal portion of ventricular septum; (3) cleft, anterior mitral leaflet; (4) anomalous chordae tendineae from the anterior mitral leaflet to the crest of the ventricular septum; and (5) partial or complete absence of the septal tricupsid valve leaflet. There are at least four potential functional consequences of these five anatomic anomalies: (1) shunt at the atrial level, (2) shunt at the ventricular level, (3) mitral regurgitation, and (4) obstruction to left ventricular outflow. Well over 95% of patients with partial atrioventricular defect have a primum-type atrial septal defect, and most of those without a primum defect have a shunt at the ventricular level. The occurrence of mitral regurgitation from a cleft in the anterior mitral leaflet unassociated with a defect in either atrial or ventricular septa is rare, but such has been the case in several reported patients (34–36). Indeed, at least 10 patients have been reported at necropsy to have a cleft in the anterior mitral leaflet unassociated with a defect in either the atrial or ventricular septum (36). Only 5 were over 10 years of age. Nine of the 10 patients had mitral regurgitation.

C. Left-Sided Atrioventricular Valve Regurgitation Associated with Corrected Transposition of the Great Arteries

Corrected transposition is an entity that has produced much confusion (37). Corrected transposition and complete transposition are quite different; the only thing they have in common is the word "transposition." Complete transposition is essentially one defect: The great arteries are transposed, so that the aorta arises from the right ventricle and the pulmonary trunk from the left ventricle. In corrected transposition, the great arteries also are transposed, but, in addition, the ventricles, atrioventricular valves, coronary arteries, and conduction system are inverted. Patients with complete transposition die because they have inadequate communications between the two circuits. Patients with corrected transposition theoretically should be able to live a full lifespan, but usually this is not the case because associated defects—namely, ventricular septal defect or regurgitation of the left-sided atrioventricular valve, or both—cause the heart to function abnormally. Abnormalities of the left-sided atrioventricular valve, a systemic valve but anatomically a tricupsid valve, are the most common associated anomalies in correct transposition (37,38). Of the anomalies, the most frequent is the Ebstein-type malformation. These valves are intrinsically regurgitant because the chordae are short and the leaflets are closely adherent to the ventricular endocardium.

Most patients with corrected transposition have a defect in the ventricular septum which is associated with a left-to-right shunt (37). Thus, most patients with corrected transposition present with evidence of excessive pulmonary blood flow. An occasional patient with corrected transposition, however, may have no defects in the cardiac septa and no ductus (38). These individuals may present with evidence of pure mitral regurgitation, and some of these patients during life have been considered to have rheumatic mitral regurgitation (38).

II. MITRAL STENOSIS

The essential hemodynamic fault caused by mitral stenosis is the inability to the left atrium to empty normally. In sinus rhythm, left atrial contraction serves to augment its emptying, but atrial contraction is lost in atrial fibrillation. The obstruction, represented by a pressure gradient across the valve, results in pulmonary venous obstruction which may lead to pulmonary arterial hypertension.

Of the single or combined cardiac valve lesions severe enough to be fatal, mitral stenosis, in my experience, ranks second (33). Of 1010 patients >14 years of age with functionally severe (class III or IV, New York Heart Association) valvular cardiac disease whom I had studied at necropsy up to 1980, 434 (44%) had mitral stenosis. Only aortic valve stenosis was more common. Mitral stenosis occurred alone in 189 (44%) patients and in combination with other functional valvular lesions in the other 245 (56%) patients. Mitral stenosis was rheumatic in origin in all 434 patients.

Although a functional classification of valvular heart disease is most useful from physiological and therapeutic standpoints, an anatomic classification is helpful from an etiological standpoint (39). Five anatomic categories have proved useful; isolated mitral, isolated aortic, combined mitral and aortic, combined tricupsid and mitral with or without aortic, and both tricuspid and mitral. Anatomically isolated aortic valve disease is never rheumatic in origin. Isolated mitral disease causing mitral stenosis is, with rare exception, rheumatic in origin, but isolated mitral disease causing pure regurgitation is usually nonrheumatic in origin. Anatomic valve disease involving more than one cardiac valve is usually rheumatic in origin. Isolated anatomic disease of the tricupsid or pulmonic valves, or both, is usually congenital or infectious in origin or is associated with the carcinoid syndrome (40,41).

A valve may function normally and yet be anatomically abnormal. Only 62% of the 189 patients with isolated mitral stenosis (with or without mitral regurgitation) had anatomic involvement limited to the mitral valve (33). In contrast, 88% of the 292 patients with clinically isolated aortic valve stenosis (with or without regurgitation) had anatomic disease limited to the aortic valve only.

Rheumatic heart disease may be viewed as a disease of the mitral valve; other valves also may be involved both anatomically and functionally, but anatomically the mitral valve is always involved (39). To my knowledge, *Aschoff bodies* have never been found in hearts without anatomic disease of the mitral valve (42). Of the first 543 patients with severe valvular heart disease whom I studied at necropsy, 11 (27%) had Aschoff bodies, and all had anatomic mitral valve disease (39). The ages of the 11 patients with Aschoff bodies ranged from 18 to 68 years (mean 38), and 9 had a history of acute rheumatic fever earlier in life (42). Clinical study revealed that 9 of the 11 patients had mitral stenosis with or without dysfunction of one or more other cardiac valves, 1 had isolated pure aortic regurgitation, and 1 had both mitral and aortic regurgitation. All 11 patients had diffuse fibrous thickening of the mitral valve leaflets, and all but 1 had diffuse anatomic lesions of at least two other cardiac valves. No patient with anatomic lesions limited to the aortic valve had Aschoff bodies. Thus, among patients with chronic valvular heart disease, Aschoff bodies, the only anatomic lesion pathognomonic of rheumatic heart disease, usually indicate diffuse anatomic lesions of one or more other cardiac valves. The functional mitral lesion is usually stenosis.

Although they are rare at necropsy in patients with fatal chronic valvular heart disease, Aschoff bodies are fairly common in the heart in patients having mitral valve commissurotomy for mitral stenosis (43). Among 481 patients undergoing various mitral valve operations, Aschoff bodies were found in 40 (21%) of 191 operatively excised left atrial appendages, in 4 (2%) of 273 operatively excised left ventricular papillary muscles (one per patient), and in 1 (6%) of 17 patients with both left atrial appendage and papillary muscle operatively excised. Of the 45 patients with Aschoff bodies, 44 had mitral stenosis preoperatively, and only 1, a 10-year-old boy, had pure mitral regurgitation. Sinus rhythm was present in 38 (84%), and atrial fibrillation in 7 (16%). Perioperatively, only 1 of the 45 patients with Aschoff bodies had clinical or laboratory stigmata compatible with acute rheumatic fever, and 58% had an illness compatible with acute rheumatic fever at any time.

Not only is rheumatic heart disease a disorder of the cardiac valves, it also affects mural endocardium, pericardium, and myocardium. On histological study, the atrial walls virtually always have increased amounts of fibrous tissue in both myocardial interstitium and in the mural endocardium, atrophy of some and hypertrophy of other myocardial cells, and hypertrophy of smooth muscle cells of the mural endocardium. In all patients with rheumatic mitral stenosis, the leaflets are diffusely thickened, either by fibrous tissue or calcific deposits or both; the commissures are usually fused, and the chordae tendineae are shortened and usually fused to some degree. The great obstruction to this funnel-shaped valve occurs at its apex, which is within the left ventricular cavity. The primary orifice, located at the level of the anulus, is far less narrowed. Fusion may involve one or both commissures. When only one is fused or one is fused more than the other, the stenotic orifice is eccentrically located. A centrally located orifice indicates symmetrical commissural fusion. In rheumatic mitral stenosis, the chordae tendineae are occasionally so retracted that the leaflets appear to insert directly into the papillary muscles. When this occurs, the mitral stenosis is always severe, because the interchordal spaces are almost entirely obliterated. Sometimes chordae inserting into one papillary muscle are well preserved, whereas those inserting into the other papillary muscle are partially or completely fused. Mitral commissurotomy on a valve in which the leaflets insert almost directly into the papillary muscle(s) usually must include a splitting of the papillary muscle(s) as well as the commissure(s). If there are normally about 120 third-order chordae and about 24 first-order chordae, in mitral stenosis these numbers are usually halved and, on occasion, even reduced to just 1 (33).

The amount of *calcium* in the leaflets of stenotic mitral valves varies considerably (44). Generally, calcium is more frequent and occurs in larger quantities in men than in women, in older than in younger patients, and in patients with higher compared with those with lower pressure gradients between left atrium and left ventricle (44). The rapidity with which calcium develops also varies considerably; it is present at a younger age in men than in women. Lachman and I (44) determined the presence or absence and the extent of calcific deposits in operatively excised stenotic mitral valves by radiography of the excised valve in 164 patients aged 26 to 72 years. The extent of the mitral calcific deposits was determined by the percentage of the valvular circumference containing the deposits: grade 0 (14 patients); grade I = 1–25% (43 patients); grade II = 26–50% (34 patients); grade III = 51–75% (39 patients); and grade IV = 76–100% (34 patients). The amount of calcific deposits in the stenotic mitral valves correlated with *sex* and with the *mean diastolic pressure gradient across the mitral valve*, but it did not correlate with the patient's age (after age

25 years), cardiac rhythm, pulmonary arterial or pulmonary arterial wedge pressure, previous mitral commissurotomy, presence of thrombus in the body of left atrium, or the presence of disease of one or more other cardiac valves.

Among the 164 patients with mitral stenosis having mitral valve replacement and roentgenography of the excised mitral valve, 14 had no mitral calcium and 43 had only trace or minimal mitral calcific deposits (45). Thus we wondered why these 57 patients had mitral replacement rather than mitral commissurotomy. Of the 57 patients, 37 had moderate to severe mitral regurgitation, and therefore they clearly deserved mitral valve replacement. The remaining 20 had absent or minimal calcific deposits, but nevertheless, they too had mitral replacement. Although in the prevalve replacement era all 20 patients almost surely would have been considered good or ideal candidates for mitral commissurotomy, other factors swung the surgeon to valve replacement rather than commissurotomy. These factors included the need to replace one or more other cardiac valves (13 patients), the utilization of cardiopulmonary bypass allowing visual inspection rather than simple palpation of the diseased mitral valve (all 20 patients), relatively little experience with mitral commissurotomy in four of the five surgeons (17 patients), displeasure with attempted commissurotomy (3 patients), previous mitral commissurotomy (11 patients), and incorrect identification of mitral calcific deposits (2 patients). Even though mitral commissurotomy has been in use for 30 years, the mere alternative of valve replacement may have altered the definition of the stenotic mitral valve previously considered ideal for mitral commissurotomy.

A major complication of mitral stenosis is *thrombus formation in the left atrial cavity*. The thrombus may be limited to atrial appendage (most common) or be located in both the left atrial appendage and body. The latter group hereafter will be referred to as "left atrial body thrombus." Left atrial body thrombus was observed in 5% of 1010 personally studied necropsy patients with fatal valvular heart disease; all had severe mitral stenosis (33). Left atrial body thrombus was not observed in any of the 165 patients with pure mitral regurgitation with or without aortic valve dysfunction. All patients with left atrial body thrombi had atrial fibrillation. Comparison of these necropsy patients with 46 patients with mitral stenosis operated upon at the National Heart, Lung, and Blood Institute and in whom thrombus was found at operation in the left atrial body disclosed that 42 (91%) patients had atrial fibrillation. In contrast, of 40 living patients undergoing mitral valve replacement for pure mitral regurgitation and operated upon at the National Heart, Lung, and Blood Institute, none had thrombus in the body of the left atrium, although 75% had atrial fibrillation. *Thrombus appears to occur in the body of the left atrium only in patients with mitral stenosis, and atrial fibrillation without mitral stenosis is incapable of forming a thrombus in the left atrial body.*

Calcific deposits on the mural endocardium of the left atrium are indicative of previous organization with calcification of left atrial thrombi (46,47). Histologically, the "calcific thrombi" also contain cholesterol clefts and are identical to atherosclerotic plaques. The observation that left atrial thrombi can organize into lesions identical to atherosclerotic plaques supports the view that atherosclerotic plaques may be the result of organization of thrombi. If calcific deposits form on left atrial body endocardium before the left atrial cavity has had time to dilate, this cavity may be prevented thereafter from dilating (48). The elevated left atrial pressure may lead more rapidly to pulmonary venous, pulmonary arterial, and right ventricular dilatation with subsequent tricuspid regurgitation and development of huge right atrial dilatation.

Nonrheumatic causes of mitral stenosis include *congenital anomalies, neoplasms* (particularly myxoma) protruding through the mitral orifice from the left atrium [but malignant neoplasms primary or secondary in the lung may grow in the mitral orifice by way of the pulmonary veins (49)]; *large vegetations from active infective endocarditis* (50); and *massive mitral anular calcific deposits* (51), particularly when associated with small-sized left ventricular cavities and left ventricular outflow tract obstruction. A relatively new, acquired cause of mitral stenosis is a *mechanical prosthetic or bioprosthetic cardiac valve* (52–54). Since the native mitral valve is within the left ventricle, a prosthetic mitral valve also is located within this cavity. The prosthesis must be small enough for the contracting left ventricular wall not to interfere with movement of the prosthetic poppet or disk. When the prosthesis is too large for the cavity into which it was inserted, the poppet may be prevented from moving adequately and may therefore obstruct left atrial emptying. The latter state is far more common than obstruction to left ventricular emptying by the prosthesis. Thrombus formation on a mitral prosthesis also may obstruct left atrial emptying.

III. AORTIC VALVE STENOSIS

If papillary muscle dysfunction is excluded, valvular aortic stenosis is the most common fatal cardiac valve lesion, comprising 49% of 1010 personally studied necropsy patients >15 years of age with valvular heart disease (33). Of the 495 necropsy patients with aortic stenosis (with or without aortic regurgitation), the lesion was isolated in 59%, and in the other 41% the mitral valve was stenotic or regurgitant or both. The evidence is substantial that the cause of aortic stenosis, when associated with mitral valve disease, is rheumatic (39). In contrast, the evidence is substantial that isolated (mitral valve anatomically normal) aortic stenosis (with or without associated aortic regurgitation) is nonrheumatic origin (39). This section focuses on patients with isolated aortic stenosis.

In contrast to what was generally believed 30 or so years ago (55), at least three factors indicate that anatomically isolated aortic valve disease (actually either stenosis or pure regurgitation) is nonrheumatic in origin (39): (1) the low frequency (about 10%) of a positive history of acute rheumatic fever; (2) the absence of Aschoff bodies; and, most important, (3) the frequency of an underlying congenital malformation of the aortic valve.

The structure of the aortic valve in aortic stenosis can be correlated to some extent with the age of the patient (56). In patients <15 years old, the aortic valve most commonly (60%) is congenitally unicuspid and unicommissural (57,58); in patients 16 to 65 years of age, the valve is most commonly (60%) congenitally bicuspid; and in patients age >65 years, the valve is most commonly (90%) tricuspid (39). the stenosis is either due to, or superimposed on, the congenitally malformed aortic valve in virtually all patients <15 years of age, and in about 70% of patients aged 16 to 65 years. A congenitally malformed, in this case congenitally bicuspid, valve appears to be the underlying condition in about 10% of patients >65 years with aortic stenosis.

The unicommissural valve, the only type of unicuspid valve observed in the aortic valve position, was described initially by Edwards in 1958 (59). Although this valve, like all other congenitally malformed aortic valves, tends to get progressively more stenotic with time, the unicuspid aortic valve is almost certainly stenotic from the time of birth, whereas this usually is not the case with the congenitally bicuspid valve. Actually, the fewer the number of aortic valve cusps and commissures, the greater is the likelihood that the valve is stenotic from birth.

Next to the floppy mitral valve, the congenitally bicuspid aortic valve is the most frequent major congenital malformation of the heart or great vessels (60–62). Although its exact frequency is uncertain, this malformation appears to occur in about 1% of human births. Osler (63) found 10 apparently normally functioning congenitally bicuspid aortic valves in 800 autopsies (750 of which were performed by him), a frequency of 1%. Eight additional patients had infective endocarditis involving congenitally bicuspid aortic valves. Thus, 18 (2%) of 800 had either normally functioning or infected congenitally bicuspid aortic valves. Grant and associates (64) found apparently normally functioning congenitally bicuspid aortic valves in 12 (1%) of 1350 necropsy patients. Osler (63), Lewis and Grant

(65), and Grant and co-workers (64) do not appear to have appreciated that the bicuspid condition of this valve may underlie severe stenosis at this site. Thus, if congenitally bicuspid aortic valves that develop complications (stenosis or regurgitation with or without infection) are added to those that function normally during the entire lifetime, the frequency of congenitally bicuspid aortic valves may exceed 1% of the population.

Among the complications of the bicuspid condition of the aortic valve, stenosis is by far the most frequent (60,62); pure regurgitation is next (61), and the latter lesion is most frequently the result of its being the site of infective endocarditis (66). Among 200 patients (75% male) with congenitally bicuspid aortic valves studied personally *at necropsy*, 157 (79%) had aortic stenosis, 22 (11%) had pure aortic regurgitation (in 19 from infective endocarditis), and 21 (10%) had normally functioning bicuspid valves (62). The latter 21 patients died of noncardiac causes, and the presence of the congenitally bicuspid aortic valve was a surprise finding at necropsy. Of the 157 patients with aortic stenosis, calcific deposits were present on both aortic valve cusps in 155 (99%); the 2 patients without calcific deposits were <30 years of age. Calcific deposits, in contrast, were rare in the patients with pure aortic regurgitation. Infective endocarditis occurred in 14 (9%) of the 157 patients with aortic stenosis and in 19 (86%) of the 22 with pure aortic regurgitation, and the infection was the prime cause of the regurgitation in all 19 patients. Infective endocarditis usually affects the normally functioning or only mildly dysfunctioning bicuspid aortic valve (66). It infrequently affects a significantly stenotic aortic valve. The infection usually causes considerable destruction of one or both aortic valve cusps, leading to severe aortic regurgitation. Rarely, perforation of a cusp may occur without superimposed infective endocarditis (67). The presence of a bicuspid aortic valve in an intravenous drug user is particularly devastating (68).

Congenitally bicuspid aortic valves also are observed commonly in patients having aortic valve replacement for *isolated* (mitral valve function normal) aortic stenosis with or without associated aortic regurgitation (61). Among 393 patients aged 17 to 74 years with aortic stenosis with or without aortic regurgitation having aortic valve replacement at the National Heart, Lung, and Blood Institute from 1962 to 1982, 28 (7%) had unicommissural, unicuspid aortic valves; 203 (52%) had congenitally bicuspid aortic valves; 101 (26%) had three-cuspid aortic valves; and in 61 (15%) the number of cusps could not be determined by examination of the operatively excised valve. Subramanian and associates (69) determined the number of aortic valve cusps present in 338 patients (most aged 50 to 70 years) undergoing aortic valve replacement for isolated (I excluded their 36 patients with associated mitral stenosis or regurgitation) "pure" aortic stenosis during four different years (1965, 1970, 1975, and 1980). Of the 338 patients, 21 (6%) had unicommissural, unicuspid valves; 171 (51%) had congenitally bicuspid valves; 94 (28%) had tricuspid aortic valves; and in 14 patients (4%), the number of cusps present was not discernible.

Congenitally bicuspid aortic valves also are found commonly among patients undergoing aortic valve replacement for *isolated* (normal mitral valve function), pure (no element of stenosis) aortic regurgitation. Of 190 patients having aortic valve replacement for pure, chronic aortic regurgitation (mitral valve normal) at the National Heart, Lung, and Blood Institute, 21 (11%) had congenitally bicuspid aortic valves (62). Of the 21 patients, 14 (67%) never had infective endocarditis, and therefore the regurgitation was on the basis of the congenital malformation only; the other 7 (33%) had infective endocarditis superimposed on the bicuspid condition, and severe aortic regurgitation in each resulted primarily from the infection, which in each was healed by antibiotics. Olson and associates (70) also determined the frequency of bicuspid aortic valves in 145 patients having isolated aortic valve replacement for pure aortic regurgitation or severe regurgitation associated with only mild aortic stenosis. (The basis of the presence or absence of associated aortic stenosis was by "clinical" means, which apparently did not mean hemodynamic studies.) Of the 145 patients, 49 (34%) had congenitally bicuspid aortic valves. Of these 49 patients, 41 (84%) apparently never had infective endocarditis, and the regurgitation was primarily on the basis of the bicuspid state of the valve; the other 8 (16%) had had infective endocarditis, which was the major cause of the regurgitation. Of the remaining 96 patients (66%), 94 (65% of total) had three-cuspid aortic valves, and 2 (1% of total) had quadricuspid valves. Of the 94 patients with three-cuspid aortic valves, the cause of the aortic regurgitation in 34 (36%) was "postinflammatory" (presumably rheumatic in at least 31–each of the aortic valve cusps in these patients was diffusely fibrotic, with or without cuspal retraction and/ or commissural fusion); associated with aortic root dilatation in 44 (47%) [idiopathic in 43 (98%) and syphilitic in 1 (2%)]; associated with infective endocarditis in 12 (13%); and associated with ventricular septal defect in 4 (4%).

The reason that one congenitally bicuspid aortic valve becomes stenotic, another purely regurgitant, and another the site of infective endocarditis is unknown. It is clear, however, that stenosis, regurgitation, and infection are complications of the bicuspid condition of the aortic valve, and none of them is present at birth. It appears likely that a congenitally bicuspid aortic valve becomes stenotic only as its cusps become fibrotic and calcified; neither cusp of a congenitally bicuspid aortic valve is severely thickened by fibrous tissue or calcific deposits at time of birth.

The frequency of development of stenosis or pure regurgitation at the site of a congenitally bicuspid aortic valve also is unknown. Lewis and Grant (65) concluded that vegetations develop at these sites in about 23% of adults (16 of 69) with congenitally bicuspid valves. Of 31 patients with "subacute infective endocarditis" studied at necropsy by Lewis and Grant (65), 8 (26%) had congenitally bicuspid aortic valves. Two (9%) of 22 patients studied at necropsy by Fulton and Levine (71) had congenitally bicuspid aortic valves. None of these investigators apparently was aware that congenitally bicuspid aortic valves also could become stenotic.

The mechanism by which a congenitally bicuspid aortic valve becomes stenotic or purely regurgitant is uncertain. There is no evidence that the valve is stenotic or regurgitant at birth. Likewise, there is no evidence that superimposed rheumatic fever or rheumatic heart disease is the cause of the stenosis or pure regurgitation. The explanation advanced by Edwards (72) is attractive. He proposed that it is not mechanically possible for a congenitally bicuspid aortic valve to open and close properly. The distances between the lateral attachments of normal aortic valvular cusps along their free margins are curved lines. The extra length allows the cusps to move freely during opening and closing of the orifice. In contrast, the distances between the lateral attachments of congenitally bicuspid aortic valves along their free margins approach straight lines. If these distances were exactly straight lines, the valve could not open during ventricular systole. Consequently, at least one cusp is larger than the other. But the excessive length of one or both cusps of a congenitally bicuspid aortic valve produces abnormal contact between the cusps. This abnormal contact, in turn, causes focal fibrous thickening that with time becomes diffuse, and dystrophic calcification occurs thereafter. Thus, stenosis of a congenitally bicuspid aortic valve may be the result of trauma to these cusps produced by their abnormal contact with each other. Although this explanation is appealing, it does not explain why one congenitally bicuspid aortic valve becomes stenotic, another becomes entirely regurgitant with or without infection, and another remains free of complications.

It is well recognized that patients with aortic isthmic coarctation often have congenitally bicuspid aortic valves. Of 200 patients with aortic ischemic coarctation studied at necropsy by Abbott (73), 27% had congenitally bicuspid aortic valves. Of 104 patients with aortic isthmic coarctation studied at necropsy by Reifenstein and associates (74), 62% had congenitally bicuspid aortic valves. These authors also pointed out that ascending aortic tears with or without dissection also were common (about 20%) in patients with aortic isthmic coarctation, but similar aortic lesions have an increased frequency among patients with congenitally bicuspid aortic valves unassociated with aortic isthmic coarctation. It is less well appreciated that an occasional patient may present with clinical features of aortic stenosis but by aortogram be found to have aortic isthmic coarctation. Among 157 personally studied necropsy patients with stenotic congenitally bicuspid aortic valves, 7 (4%) had aortic isthmic coarctation (62).

Patients with bicuspid aortic valves have an increased frequency of aortic dissection compared to persons with a tricuspid aortic valve. A bicuspid aortic valve was found in 11 (13%) of 85 patients with aortic dissection reported by Gore and Seiwert (75), in 11 (9%) of 119 cases reported by Edwards et al (76), and in 14 (7.5%) of 186 necropsy patients with aortic dissection reported by Roberts and Roberts (77). Aortic dissection was found in 8 (5%) of 152 necropsy patients ≥20 years of age with a bicuspid aortic valve by Fenoglio et al (78). Larson and Edwards (79) observed aortic dissection in 18 (6%) of 293 necropsy patients with a bicuspid aortic valve, and in 141 (0.67%) of 21,105 persons with a tricuspid aortic valve, a ninefold difference. Roberts and Roberts (77) found aortic dissection in 14 (4%) of 328 patients studied at necropsy with a congenitally bicuspid aortic valve. Of the 16 patients with congenitally malformed aortic valves (14 bicuspid and 2 unicuspid) studied by Roberts and Roberts (77), the entrance tear was in the ascending aorta in all 16. The aortic valve was stenotic in 6, and 2 had associated aortic isthmic coarctation. Histological sections of aorta disclosed severe degeneration of the elastic fibers of aortic media in 90% of the patients studied. Thus a congenitally malformed aortic valve appears to be present at least five times more frequently in adults with than in those without aortic dissection.

The use of echocardiography and magnetic resonance imaging allows detection of the presence of a bicuspid aortic valve before symptoms or signs of cardiac dysfunction appear (80,81). In a person found to have a bicuspid valve, the following advice may be useful in preventing the development of complications (82).

1. *Avoid infection.* Prophylactic antibiotics obviously are required during dental and other operative procedures. Sir William Osler was the one who pointed out in 1885 the extreme propensity of the bicuspid aortic valve to be the site of infective endocarditis (83). Certainly one with a bicuspid aortic valve should not use illicit drugs intravenously (84).

2. *Maintain a normal systemic blood pressure.* Although the bicuspid aortic valve probably is not affected adversely by the left ventricular systolic pressure regardless of its level, the level of the valve's closing pressure, that is, the aortic diastolic pressure, probably plays a prominent role in determining whether the bicuspid valve becomes stenotic, or purely regurgitant (without superimposed infective endocarditis), or functions normally throughout life.

3. *Keep the heart rate relatively slow.* It is reasonable to believe that if the aortic valve closes only 55 times a minute rather than 75 times a minute (a 27% heart rate reduction), the wear and tear received by the aortic valve from the aorta's closing pressure would be reduced. The best way to produce a relatively slow heart rate is by various aerobic exercises. Although the heart rate increases during exercise, the total 24-hour heart beats probably would be reduced substantially. Beta-blocker therapy could be useful to achieve this objective.

4. *Keep the serum total cholesterol level relatively low.* The major reason a bicuspid aortic valve becomes stenotic is because large calcific deposits develop on the aortic aspects of the cusps and the large deposits impart an immobility to the cusps which prevent their opening adequately during ventricular systole. Thus, prevention of calcific deposits is essential for prevention of stenosis. In older persons in the Western world it is common to develop calcific deposits on the aortic aspects of the aortic valve cusps, on the ventricular aspects of the posterior mitral leaflet (mitral "anular" calcium), and in atherosclerotic plaques in the coronary arteries (as well as in plaques in other arteries). The development of calcific deposits on the aortic valve, mitral anulus, and coronary arteries with age occurs only in those populations with serum total cholesterol levels >150 mg/dL and usually in those persons with levels >200 mg/dL. Thus, maintaining a low serum total cholesterol level prevents calcific deposits on a normally formed aortic valve, and therefore it is reasonable to believe that maintaining a low level would have similar effect on a bicuspid aortic valve. Calcific deposits are never present on the aortic valve at birth; they are always acquired. Calcific deposits are less common on stenotic mitral valves (rheumatic origin) in persons residing in the undeveloped nations of the world (where the serum total cholesterol levels often are <150 mg/dL) than in persons in the Western world these levels are usually >150 mg/dL. Thus, maintaining a relatively low serum total cholesterol level might deter calcific deposition on a bicuspid aortic valve, and if no calcium usually no stenosis. Preventing calcific deposits, however, would not prevent the development of pure aortic regurgitation or infective endocarditis.

Try to forget that the aortic valve is bicuspid. As long as the bicuspid valve functions normally, there is nothing to worry about, and no one can predict which bicuspid aortic valve will function normally for a full lifetime and which one will become stenotic, purely regurgitant (without superimposed infective endocarditis), or infected. In other words, the natural history of a congenitally bicuspid aortic valve is unknown. It appears that about 1% of live births have a congenitally bicuspid valve. If that is the

case, about 50 million (of 5 billion) persons on planet Earth have a congenitally bicuspid aortic valve, and about 2.5 million persons in the United
States have a bicuspid aortic valve. What percentage of them will develop
stenosis, pure regurgitation, infection, or no complications in a lifetime
is unknown. Thus, life must continue, and the focus must be on things
other than the bicuspid aortic valve. Even with the worst scenario, aortic
valve replacement is usually highly successful.

In contrast to the congenitally bicuspid aortic valve, the congenitally
unicuspid aortic valve is far less common (about 15 times less common).
At least two varieties of the unicuspid aortic valve exist. In one, the orifice
is located in the center of the cusp and there are no attachments or only
rudimentary ones to the wall of the aorta. Edwards (59) referred to this
valve as the *simple-dome* type. Another name might be *acommissural*
valve. This type of valve is commonly found in patients with congenital
pulmonic stenosis—indeed, it is the most frequent type of valve seen in
that setting—but it is exceedingly uncommon in the aortic valve position.
A second type of unicuspid valve is the *unicommissural* one. This valve,
described by Edwards in 1958 (59), is characterized by an eccentrically
located orifice and only one lateral attachment to the aortic wall and that
at the level of the orifice. From above, this valve has the appearance of
an exclamation mark. In contrast to the bicuspid aortic valve, the unicuspid valve is nearly always stenotic from the time of birth.

Tricuspid aortic valves rarely appear to be stenotic at birth. If stenosis
is present at birth and the aortic valve has three cusps, the stenosis is
usually the result of a very small aortic "anulus" rather than the result
of fusion of the cusps. Acquired stenosis of a three-cuspid aortic valve,
in contrast, is common. Of necropsy patients aged 16 to 65 years studied
personally with clinically isolated aortic stenosis (with or without regurgitation), 25% had tricuspid valves, and among those aged >65 years of
age, 90% had tricuspid valves (56). In the age group 16 to 65 years, about
50% of these patients with clinically isolated aortic stenosis and three-
cuspid aortic valves also had diffuse fibrous thickening of the mitral leaflets. The associated diffuse mitral leaflet thickening is strong evidence
that the etiology of the aortic stenosis in this group is rheumatic (39).
Also, nearly 75% of this group had positive histories of acute rheumatic
fever, whereas 10% of the other group—that is, those with anatomically
normal mitral valves with aortic stenosis—had positive histories (39). The
etiology of the aortic stenosis in patients ≤65 years with three-cuspid
aortic valves and anatomically normal mitral valves is unsolved. Possibly,
minor abnormalities in the sizes of the aortic valve cusps from birth set
the stage for abnormal contact of the cusps with one another with resultant
fibrosis and finally stenosis (85).

Stenosis of the aortic valve in patients over age 65 years is usually characteristic (86–88). The valves are tricuspid; calcific deposits are distributed rather uniformly on the aortic aspects of the cusps; and the commissures are not fused. Obstruction is due entirely to the presence of large calcific deposits, which prevent the cusps from retracting adequately during ventricular systole. Because the commissures are usually not fused, associated aortic regurgitation is infrequent.

Clinically, aortic stenosis in the elderly is characterized by several features which are either absent or more prominent than in younger subject with this valvular lesion (86): (1) The systemic arterial pulse pressure may be increased due to a systolic hypertension; (2) a harsh right basal systolic murmur may be relatively inconspicuous, while a pure musical systolic murmur may be prominent at the apex; (3) a coexisting apical systolic murmur of mitral regurgitation may be related to mitral anular calcium and not to left ventricular failure; and (4) systemic systolic hypertension can result in a comparatively small pressure gradient despite severe left ventricular outflow obstruction.

Ausculatory signs that accompany aortic stenosis in the elderly may differ from those in younger subjects. Ejection sounds are characteristically absent, since the cusps are rigid and ejection sounds depend on abrupt movement of mobile valves. Atrial sounds (fourth heart sounds) are useful signs for judging the severity of aortic stenosis in the younger adult but are of little help in the elderly patient, since they may occur normally in the older age group. Ordinarily, the systolic murmur of valvular aortic stenosis is harsh, rough, grunting, and loudest at the right base, with radiation upward and to the right. In elderly patients with aortic stenosis, the harsh murmur at the right base may persist but be of less intensity, and auscultation may be dominated instead by a loud, pure-frequency, musical systolic murmur maximal at or near the cardiac apex. At least three reasons account for these patterns. First, older persons tend to have increased upper thoracic chest dimensions, which soften the basal murmurs. Second is the effect of the morphology of the stenotic aortic valve. A rigid, calcified valve with commissural fusion provides a suitable mechanism for a high-velocity jet into the ascending aorta; the noisy murmur at the right base appears to originate within the ascending aorta because of turbulence caused by the high-velocity jet. A calcified, stenotic, trileaflet aortic valve without commissural fusion, the most common type in the elderly, behaves differently. Ejection into the ascending aorta may take the form of a "spray" instead of a jet, so that the harsh murmur at the right base may be comparatively inconspicuous. Since the cusps are not fused, they may vibrate during ventricular ejection and the latter may account for the pure-frequency, musical, cooing murmur recordable within the left ventricle. Third, calcium in the mitral anulus, itself a producer of precordial murmurs, frequently accompanies calcium of the aortic valve in elderly patients. Mitral regurgitation can result from inability of the calcified anulus to decrease its circumference during ventricular contraction. Accordingly, the holosystolic murmur of mitral regurgitation may be present at the apex and may be difficult to distinguish from the coexisting pure-frequency aortic stenotic apical murmur. Although mitral anular calcium tends to complicate the ausculatory diagnosis of aortic stenosis, the radiological identification of these calcific deposits implies that coexisting aortic stenosis is likely to be caused by calcific deposits on a trileaflet valve without commissural fusion.

The degree of left ventricular systolic hypertension in elderly patients may be considerably higher than that occurring in younger subjects with similar degrees of aortic stenosis, since the peripheral systolic systemic pressure usually rises with age. The degree of systolic hypertension which the elderly left ventricle is capable of achieving can be astonishingly high, particularly since this chamber seldom maintains a systolic pressure in excess of 250 mmHg even in younger subjects. Systemic hypertension may reduce the aortic gradient, and the degree of obstruction may be underestimated in elderly patients if the peak systolic pressure difference is taken as the only index of severity. As the gradient diminishes in the presence of systemic systolic hypertension, the murmur at the right base may soften and shorten. Even if this auscultatory change does not occur with systemic hypertension, the modification of the systemic arterial pulse may be misleading, since the rate of rise can be relatively normal and the pulse pressure increased despite severe obstruction to the left ventricular outflow.

The frequency of atrial fibrillation is higher in older compared to younger patients with aortic stenosis. This arrhythmia, however, is common in elderly persons without valvular cardiac disease. The left atrial cavities are dilated in patients with aortic stenosis, but left atrial dilatation commonly accompanies old age in the absence of functionally significant valvular lesions. The left ventricular wall becomes less compliant with age, and the superimposed left ventricular hypertrophy (without left ventricular dilatation) of aortic stenosis may further impede left atrial emptying. The only common anatomic feature in elderly patients with atrial fibrillation is left atrial dilatation. The combination of atrial fibrillation, a long apical systolic murmur, and left atrial dilatation can obscure the diagnosis of aortic stenosis and lead to a mistaken diagnosis of isolated mitral regurgitation. Atrial fibrillation is especially undesirable in aortic stenosis, since the left ventricle requires the help of augmented left atrial contraction, which increases end-diastolic fiber length and permits the left ventricle to contract with greater force.

The cause of the aortic stenosis in elderly patients has been considered "wear and tear" of aging. My own view is that the calcific deposits are a form of atherosclerosis because they occur only in societies where the serum total cholesterol level is >150 mg/dL (89). Most patients >65 years of age with aortic stenosis also have calcific deposits in the mitral anular region, and virtually 100% have calcific deposits in the coronary arteries (within plaques). The latter lesions of course are the result of atherosclerosis, a fact which suggests that calcific deposits in both aortic valve cusps and mitral anular region are atherosclerotic in nature.

Although relatively few patients with valvular aortic stenosis have positive histories of acute rheumatic fever, the occurrence of a positive history in a patient presenting clinically with apparently pure aortic stenosis (with or without regurgitation) should caution the examining physician to the possibility of accompanying mitral valvular disease. Usually in this situation the mitral leaflets are diffusely, although mildly, thickened, but mitral valvular function is normal. On rare occasions, however, mitral stenosis may be an accompanying lesion and of such severity that it is clinically silent. Mitral stenosis should be ruled out, however, before operative therapy is undertaken in any patient presenting with apparently isolated valvular aortic stenosis (with or without regurgitation) and a positive history of acute rheumatic fever.

IV. AORTIC REGURGITATION

In contrast to valvular aortic stenosis, which basically has only three etiologies (congenital, atherosclerotic, and rheumatic), there are numerous causes of pure aortic regurgitation (88). The causes may be subdivided into those resulting from conditions affecting primarily the valvular cusps and those affecting primarily the aorta. This discussion will include only the major causes of fatal aortic regurgitation. Those affecting primarily the cusps include rheumatic disease, infective endocarditis, and congenital malformations. Those causing aortic regurgitation primarily by affecting the aorta include syphilis, the Marfan syndrome and its forme fruste varieties, and ankylosing spondylitis.

A. Rheumatic Heart Disease

Rheumatic heart disease is primarily a disease of the mitral valve (33). Other valves may be affected, but the mitral valve is always involved anatomically, although it may function normally. Rheumatic heart disease never affects only the aortic valve, and if this valve is the only one involved anatomically, the cause is a condition other than rheumatic. The aortic valve, however, may be made seriously incompetent (or stenotic) by rheumatic involvement and yet the mitral valve show only mild fibrous scarring but no dysfunction. Most patients with serious rheumatic aortic valve disease have some aortic stenosis as well as incompetency. Less frequently is the aortic valve made purely incompetent by rheumatic involvement unless the mitral valve also is made to function improperly by this condition.

Among the causes of pure aortic regurgitation, rheumatic disease is still an important one. Clinically, the clue to a rheumatic etiology is a positive history of acute rheumatic fever, which was present in 8 of the 10 necropsy patients studied personally. The purely incompetent rheumatic aortic valve is diffusely thickened by fibrous tissue, and one or more of the three cusps is severely retracted. A cusp may be so contracted by the rheumatic process that only a small residue of the original cusp is identifiable. The commissures are only mildly fused if at all. Most valves associated with significant commissural fusion have elements of stenosis and therefore are not purely regurgitant. Calcific deposits are either absent or present in small amounts. The major feature of the rheumatic process therefore is diffuse fibrous thickening of the three cusps with retraction of one or more of them. The ascending aorta may be dilated, but it is of normal thickness and the intima is not affected. The mitral valve cusps are diffusely thickened by fibrous tissue.

B. Infective Endocarditis

Infective endocarditis is the most common cause of fatal isolated pure aortic regurgitation, and the aortic valve is the valve most commonly affected by fatal infective endocarditis (66). Not all patients with active infective endocarditis involving the aortic valve, however, develop aortic regurgitation. The aortic regurgitation results from perforations or tears of one or more of the cusps. Usually vegetations are present on each aortic valve cusps when the valve is regurgitant. Although it is well appreciated that the congenitally bicuspid aortic valve has a particular propensity to become the site of vegetations, the aortic valve in most patients with infective endocarditis consists of three cusps.

Fatal infective endocarditis is more often observed when the infection involves a previously normal rather than a previously abnormal aortic valve (66). Because infection of previously anatomically normal valves is nearly always by virulent organisms, and because the infective process can more easily destroy a thin, delicate (normal) valve as opposed to a thick, tough (abnormal) valve, the frequency of involvement by infective endocarditis of previously anatomically normal valves in a necropsy study might be abnormally high. The frequency of infective endocarditis is clearly higher in persons with underlying cardiac disease than in persons with previously normal hearts. Among cases of infective endocarditis, however, there is more involvement of previously normal than previously abnormal valves. This fact may be explained simply by the larger number of normal than abnormal valves.

An unfortunate consequence of infective endocarditis affecting the aortic valve is the frequency with which ring abscesses develop. Ring abscesses of the mitral valve, in contrast, occur infrequently. Ring abscesses are due to the spreading of the infective process from the valve cusps into the adjacent tissue. Although the material within the abscess can be made sterile by antibiotics, the presence of a ring abscess can prevent successful valve replacement were this procedure necessary during the period of activity.

Considerable destruction to an aortic valve by active infective endocarditis does not prevent healing of the infective process. Relatively little information, however, is available on the morphological aspects of healed infective endocarditis. The only anatomic abnormality definitely indicative of healed infective endocarditis of the aortic valve is the presence of cuspal perforations (90).

C. Congenital Malformations

Aortic regurgitation commonly occurs in patients with *congenitally malformed aortic valves*, particularly those that are bicuspid. The aortic regurgitation may be severe and unassociated with any element of stenosis or any signs of previous infective endocarditis (61).

D. Syphilis

Syphilis remains an important cause of severe aortic regurgitation (87,88). The luetic process causes the aortic wall to be as much as four times thicker than normal. The thickening is due to both intimal and adventitial scarring. The aortic media, in contrast, is not thickened, and many of its elastic fibers are replaced by scar tissue. The walls of the vasa vasora are thickened and their lumens are narrowed. Collections of lymphocytes and plasma cells surround many vasa vasora. Arteriosclerotic plaques are superimposed on the diseased aorta in all patients. No spirochetes are found on special stains of aorta. The aortic "anulae" are dilated, and this root dilatation may prevent coaptation of the aortic valve cusps. The distal margins of the aortic cusps are thickened, but the cusps are freely mobile and otherwise grossly and histologically normal. The commissures are usually not "widened."

Aortic regurgitation occurs in about 30% of patients with cardiovascular syphilis. The aortic regurgitation is due primarily to aortic root dilatation, the result of the destructive aortitis. Stretched by the dilated aortic root, the cusps are unable to meet in ventricular diastole, and a central regurgitant stream results. The fibrosis of the rolled free margins of the aortic valve cusps appears to be secondary to the aortic regurgitation and not due to valvulitis per se. Syphilitic aortitis may involve the entire ascending aorta, or some portions may be spared. The site of disease in the aorta is the major determinant of valvular dysfunction. Extensive destruction of the ascending aorta, even with aneurysm, may occur in the absence of aortic regurgitation if the aortic wall immediately behind the sinuses is spared. Thus the aortic root is the important determinant of aortic valve function, and involvement of it by the luetic process usually prevents valve closure during ventricular diastole.

E. Ankylosing Spondylitis

Bulkley and Roberts (91) studied at necropsy 8 patients with *ankylosing spondylitis* and aortic regurgitation. All were men aged 34 to 55 years. All had severe congestive cardiac failure and signs and symptoms of joint involvement consistent with ankylosing spondylitis. In all 8 patients, the joint symptoms antedated those of congestive cardiac failure, in 7 of them by 10 to 20 years. In 5 of the 8 patients, however, precordial murmurs of aortic regurgitation were noted at the same time or within one year of the onset of joint symptoms. Serologic tests (VDRL) for syphilis were negative in all patients. Conduction disturbances were present in 6 patients. At catheterization, the left ventricular and systemic arterial diastolic pressures were equal in 5 of 7 patients studied. Aortic valve replacement was carried out in 5 patients. Death in 7 patients was related directly to the aortic valvular disease and occurred at an average of 6 years from the onset of congestive cardiac failure.

At necropsy, the hearts weighed 520 to 1100 g (average 756). The aortic valve cusps were shortened and always thickened at their basal attachments and distal margins, and frequently in between. Focal calcific deposits were present along the bases of the cusps in 4 patients, and in one it extended to the anterior mitral leaflet and membraneous septum. The ascending aorta was diffusely dilated in all 8 patients. The thickening was limited to the most caudal 3 cm of the ascending aorta, and the wall behind the sinuses of Valsalva was always involved. The thickening resulted from dense connective tissue in the adventitia of the aorta. The adventitial scarring was continuous, with similar scarring in the groove between the anterior mitral leaflet and the aortic valve cusps, producing a fibrous ridge between the base of the aortic valve cusps and the anterior mitral leaflet. In 4 patients the fibrous tissue also infiltrated the membraneous ventricular septum. A few mononuclear cells were present in the adventitia of the aorta, and the lumens of the vasa vasorum were narrowed by extensive intimal fibrous proliferation and medial hypertrophy (just as in syphilis). The media of the aorta behind the sinuses showed evidence of severe degeneration, and the overlying intima was thickened by proliferated fibrous tissue.

Although aortic regurgitation had been described previously in ankylosing spondylitis, the distinctive morphological features of the cardiovascular lesion were described by Bulkley and Roberts. The aortic valve cusps, particularly their basal attachments and margins, are thickened by fibrous tissue. The extension of the dense adventitial fibrosis below the attachments of the aortic valve cusps to the anterior mitral leaflet and the membraneous ventricular septum distinguished these patients morphologically from those with aortic regurgitation of other etiologies. The extension of the scarring process below the aortic valve also explains the frequency of conduction disturbances in ankylosing spondylitis and their infrequency in patients with syphilis.

Although the aortic valve cusps are abnormal in as high as 20%, aortic regurgitation is said to occur clinically in only about 3% of patients with ankylosing spondylitis. Symptoms of arthritis usually antedate the cardiac disease by 10 to 20 years. In 5 of the 8 patients studied by Bulkley and me (91) and in patients described by others, precordial murmurs were noted within 2 years of the onset of joint symptoms. Symptoms of cardiac dysfunction, however, developed much later. This observation suggests that the joints and the aortic root area may be attacked at the same time, but that it takes many years for the sclerosing process to produce aortic regurgitation.

Ankylosing spondylitis has been described as a benign disease. Seven of the 8 patients studied by Bulkley and Roberts, however, died of consequences of aortic regurgitation at a mean age of 46 years, with death occurring within 6 years of the first symptoms of cardiac disease. The age at death in the 16 patients with ankylosing spondylitis and aortic regurgitation reported by Clark et al. (92) was 45 years, and the interval from the onset of symptomatic heart disease to death also was 6 years. In contrast, the overall mortality of patients with ankylosing spondylitis has been reported to be similar to that of the general population. Thus the presence of aortic regurgitation appears to be a prime determinant of whether or not ankylosing spondylitis shortens life.

F. The Marfan Syndrome

The Marfan syndrome generally involves the bones, joints, eyes, heart, and blood vessels. The extremities are long and thin (dolichostenomelia), the ligaments and joint capsules are redundant, the lenses are dislocated (ectopia lentis), the ascending aorta often is dilated, and one or both left-sided cardiac valves frequently are regurgitant. Cardiovascular disease is by far the most common cause of death in patients with the Marfan syndrome. Of 18 personally studied necropsy patients fulfilling McKusick's criteria for this syndrome, all died from cardiovascular disease, and death in each was premature [mean age = 34 years (range 15 to 52)] (93). Of 56 deceased patients with this syndrome studied during life by Murdoch and associates (94), cardiovascular disease was the cause of death in 52 (93%), and the mean age at death was 32 years. Of the 151 previously reported necropsy patients with the Marfan syndrome, the mean age at death was 23 years and range from stillbirth to 65 years. [The 91 articles in which these 151 patients were described are listed in the article by Roberts and Honig (93)].

A variety of cardiovascular lesions has been observed in the great arteries and hearts of patients with the Marfan syndrome. The personally studied 18 necropsy patients with this syndrome readily separated into three groups on the basis of their cardiovascular lesions. Group I included 13 patients with *fusiform aneurysms of the ascending aorta*. All 13 patients had aortic regurgitation, and 6 also had associated mitral regurgitation. In each, the aneurysm involved the sinus and the proximal tubular portions of ascending aorta; 2 also had fusiform aneurysms in the descending thoracic aorta. Histological study of the wall of the ascending aorta disclosed the typical lesion of this syndrome, that is, massive loss of elastic fibers and increased amounts of mucoid material in the media. Group II included 3 patients with *dissection* of the entire aorta. Before dissection, the aorta in each was of normal size, and, histologically, the wall of the aorta was normal. None of these 3 patients had either aortic or mitral regurgitation before the aortic dissection. Two, however, had had systemic hypertension. Group III included 2 patients with isolated mitral regurgitation with floppy mitral leaflets and markedly dilated mitral anuli. In each, the aortic lumen was of normal size and its wall was normal histologically.

In contrast to the predominant occurrence of fusiform ascending aortic aneurysm in the personally studied patients (13 of 18) and the relatively infrequent occurrence of aortic dissection (3 of 18), aortic dissection was the most frequent gross cardiovascular abnormality observed in the previously reported necropsy patients with the Marfan syndrome [57 (38%) of 151 patients], followed by aortic root aneurysm without dissection [53 (38%) patients], then mitral regurgitation without aortic root aneurysm or dissection [33 (22%) patients]; and finally, 8 patients (5%) did not have aortic dissection or root aneurysm or mitral regurgitation and were placed in a miscellaneous group. Analysis of the previously reported necropsy patients disclosed that those with either fusiform ascending aortic aneurysm or aortic dissection had similar mean ages (28 and 27 years), males were slightly more frequent in both groups (3:2), and only 10% of the 110 patients were aged ≤15 years (nearly 70%). Sisk and associates (95) observed similar findings in 15 patients with the Marfan syndrome diagnosed <15 years of age.

As in all my 13 patients with fusiform ascending aortic aneurysms (or "anulaortic ectasia"), evidence of aortic regurgitation was present in almost all (95%) of the previously reported necropsy patients with fusiform ascending aortic aneurysm. As an indication of the severity of the aortic regurgitation in the reported patients with fusiform ascending aortic aneurysm, the average indirect peak systolic systemic arterial pressure in the 29 (of the 53) patients in whom this information was available was 146 mmHg (range 100 to 195), and the average end-diastolic systemic arterial pressure was 43 mmHg (range 0 to 90), yielding an average pulse pressure of just over 100 mmHg (range 40 to 170). Of the 29 patients with fusiform root aneurysm and reported blood pressure measurements, 18 (62%) had systemic arterial systolic pressures <140 mmHg, 26 (90%) had systemic diastolic pressures <60 mmHg, and 23 (79%) had pulse pressures >60 mmHg.

In contrast to their frequent recording in the reported necropsy patients with fusiform ascending aortic aneurysms, blood pressure values *before the dissection occurred* were virtually unreported in the 57 previously reported necropsy patients with aortic dissection [see Roberts and Honig (93)]. Nevertheless, evidence of the presence of aortic regurgitation before the aortic dissection was rare. The reason that aortic regurgitation before dissection is rare in the patient with aortic dissection is because dissection is infrequent in the patients with fusiform ascending aortic aneurysm, and it is the latter which is primarily responsible for the severe aortic regurgitation (in the absence of healed dissection). With few exceptions, aortic dissection in patients wit the Marfan syndrome tends to affect the previously normal-sized aorta or the aorta only slightly dilated. None of 13 personally studied necropsy patients with fusiform ascending aortic aneurysm had aortic dissection, and none of 3 personally studied patients with dissection of the entire aorta had evidence of fusiform ascending aortic aneurysm of aortic regurgitation before the dissection. Of the reported patients with aortic dissection, those with dilated ascending aortas over a long period of time usually had healed dissections, and the dilatation in them appeared to be the result of aneurysm of the false channel. In at least 14 of the 57 previously reported patients with aortic dissection, the dissection had healed [see Roberts and Honig (93)].

The reason that fusiform ascending aortic aneurysm occurs in some patients with the Marfan syndrome and aortic dissection in others appears to lie in the status of the aortic media. In each of the 13 personally studied necropsy patients with fusiform aneurysm of the ascending aorta, histologic study of the wall of the aorta disclosed severe degrees of "cystic medial necrosis." In contrast, none of 3 patients with dissection involving the entire aorta had cystic medial necrosis by histologic examination. Furthermore, in 44 of the 53 previously reported necropsy patients with fusiform ascending aortic aneurysm, cystic medial necrosis was described, and in the other 9 patients its presence or absence was simply not mentioned. It was not mentioned as being absent in any patient, and in those in whom photomicrographs were illustrated, the degree of cystic medial necrosis was nearly always severe. Among the 57 previously reported necropsy patients with aortic dissection, cystic medial necrosis was described as being present in 35 and as being absent in 7. In the patients, however, in whom photomicrographs of aorta were illustrated, the degree of cystic medial necrosis was usually minimal or mild, and rarely was the degree of cystic medial necrosis as severe as that observed routinely in the patients with fusiform ascending aortic aneurysm.

Thus the aortic media appears to be quite different in the patient with fusiform ascending aortic aneurysm and in those with aortic dissection, particularly when the latter involves the entire aorta. In the patients with fusiform ascending aortic aneurysm, there are usually "massive" degeneration or loss of the elastic fibers of the media and increased quantities of collagen and mucoid material. The increased quantities of collagen would appear to prevent longitudinal aortic dissection. The aortic media in the patients with aortic dissection, in contrast, tends to be normal or to have only a mild degree of cystic medial necrosis, just as in patients with aortic dissection and systemic hypertension who do not have the Marfan syndrome (96). Two of the 3 personally studied patients with aortic dissection had evidence of diastolic systemic hypertension, whereas none of the other 16 patients had diastolic hypertension.

In none of the previous reports describing necropsy patients with the Marfan syndrome was the degree of cystic medial necrosis graded. In 1970, however, Carlson and associates (96) graded the severity of cystic medial necrosis from 1 to 4 among patients with systemic hypertension and among others with normotension. They found that the frequency of cystic medial necrosis increased progressively from 10% in the first two decades of life to 60% and 64% in the seventh and eighth decades, respectively. The frequency and extent of cystic medial necrosis were higher in the hypertensive than in the normotensive patients of similar age. Schlatmann and Becker (97) confirmed the observation that certain degrees of cystic medial necrosis are observed in the normal aorta and that the degrees of cystic medial necrosis increase with age. Schlatmann and Becker (98) also compared the ascending aortic media in patients with dilated aortas with those in patients with complete or incomplete dissection and found only quantitative differences between the normal aging aorta and the overtly abnormal aorta. Thus, these newer observations regarding the frequency, extent, and significance of cystic medial necrosis must be taken into account when evaluating its presence in patients with the Marfan syndrome. Probably many of the Marfan patients with aortic dissection have no more cystic medial necrosis than might be expected for the patient's age or level of systemic arterial pressure.

The term "cystic medial necrosis," incidentally, has certain defects, because "cysts" are relatively infrequent and "necrosis" is difficult to identify. Furthermore, the striking histological aortic lesion, when full blown, is massive degeneration of elastic fibers, and this feature is ignored by the term "cystic medial necrosis." When Gsell (99) in 1928 first used the term "medionecrosis" and a year later Erdheim (100,101), the term "cystic medial necrosis," stains for elastic fibers were apparently infrequently employed and loss or degeneration of elastic fibers may be difficult to appreciate on hematoxylin-eosin-stained sections.

When elastic fibers disappear from the aortic wall in this condition, the space previously occupied by them appears to be replaced by collagen fibrils and mucoid material. Although the increased acid mucopolysaccharide material has been considered an inherent defect in this condition, it is just as reasonable to believe that this material serves simply as "a filler" for the lost elastic fibers. Normally, the media of aorta in the ascending portion contains approximately 58 elastic lamellae (102). It is not clear whether or not the numbers of the elastic lamellae are normal or decreased at the time of birth in the patients with the Marfan syndrome. Whether normal or decreased, however, fusiform ascending aortic aneurysm, with or without tears, has not been described in newborns with this syndrome. Thus it appears that although the composition of the aortic media may be defective at birth, the aneurysms form later, presumably the consequence of the intraaortic pressure's effect on an inherently weak wall.

Although most fusiform aneurysms in the Marfan syndrome involve the ascending aorta (both sinus and tubular portions), aneurysm also may involve the descending thoracic aorta (as it did in 2 personally studied patients) and, as reported by others, the abdominal aorta. Because the numbers of elastic fibers in the abdominal aorta are only about half of those present in the ascending aorta with intermediate numbers in between (102), and because the major histologic finding in the medial portion of the aneurysmal wall is massive loss of elastic fibers, it is logical, of course, that the ascending aorta is the most common location of fusiform aneurysm in the Marfan syndrome. The ascending portion also moves ("stretches") the most with each heart beat ("hypermobile aorta"), and this factor also may play a role in this preferential location of aneurysms in this syndrome (103).

Although the major consequence of fusiform ascending aortic aneurysm in the Marfan syndrome is aortic regurgitation (100% of 13 personally studied patients and 95% of 42 previously reported patients where this information was recorded), rupture of the aneurysm, of course, is also a danger. This event occurred in 2 of 13 personally studied patients and in at least 14 (25%) of the 57 previously reported necropsy patients with aortic dissection. Thus treatment of Marfan patients with fusiform ascending aortic aneurysms must be directed at elimination or prevention of aortic regurgitation and at prevention of aneurysmal rupture, not at prevention of dissection, because the latter is an infrequent complication in such patients.

Mitral regurgitation also is frequent in patients with the Marfan syndrome. At least six factors may be important in causing the mitral regurgitation: (1) *dilatation of mitral anuli*; (2) *floppiness or prolapse of mitral leaflets and/or elongation of chordae tendineae*; (3) *calcification of mitral anuli*; (4) *rupture of mitral chordae tendineae*; (5) *infective endocarditis*; (6) *papillary muscle dysfunction*. Of these six factors, numbers 1, 2, 3, and 5 appear most important in causing severe degrees of mitral regurgitation. Of the 18 personally studied necropsy patients, 9 had mitral regurgitation, isolated in 2 and combined with aortic regurgitation in 7. Of these 9 patients, 4 had floppy mitral valves, whereas none of the 9 patients without mitral regurgitation had floppy valves. The "floppiness" involved the posterior mitral leaflet in all 4 patients. Of the 9 patients with mitral regurgitation, the circumference of the mitral anulus ranged from 10 to 17 cm (mean = 15; normal = 9); and of the 9 patients without mitral regurgitation, the circumference ranged from 9 to 13 cm (mean 11). Thus, the mean circumference of the mitral anulus in the 9 patients with mitral regurgitation was dilated 67% over normal (15 compared with 9), and that in the 9 patients without mitral regurgitation, only 22% over normal (12 compared with 9). Thus, both mitral leaflet prolapse and anular dilatation play significant roles in causing mitral regurgitation in these patients.

Calcification of the mitral anulus is known to cause or at least to be associated with mitral regurgitation. The degree of regurgitation produced by this mechanism alone, however, is nearly always mild or minimal, and, in addition, the mitral anuli in non-Marfan patients with mitral anular calcium are nearly always of normal or near-normal circumference. Of the 18 personally studied necropsy patients, 5 had mitral anular calcific deposits; all 5 had associated mitral regurgitation, but, in addition, 4 had prolapsing mitral leaflets and in 4 the circumference of the mitral anulus was quite dilated [range 13 to 17 cm (mean = 15)]. Evidence for rupture of mitral chordae tendineae was found in 5 of 9 personally studied patients with, and in none of the 9 patients without mitral regurgitation. Two of these 5 patients had histories of infective endocarditis that had healed. All 5 patients with evidence of mitral chordal rupture had prolapsing mitral leaflets, and 4 had dilated mitral anuli [range 15 to 17 cm (mean = 16)].

The role played by *"papillary muscle dysfunction"* in causing mitral regurgitation in these patients is less clear. Among the 18 personally studied patients, the left ventricle was dilated in each and the left ventricular mass was increased in each. The hearts of the 18 patients ranged in weight from 375 to 850 g (mean = 654). In 13 of the 18 patients, the mitral leaflets were increased in length from their basal attachments to their distal margins. This "stretching" probably in part was the result of the elongation (apex to base) of the left ventricular cavities, resulting primarily from the associated aortic regurgitation. The resulting left ventricular dilatation may have altered the normal angulation between the papillary muscles and mitral leaflets. Whether or not mitral regurgitation was increased in any patient by this mechanism, however, is uncertain.

In contrast to fusiform ascending aortic aneurysm and dissection, which generally become manifest after childhood, mitral valve abnormalities in the Marfan syndrome may be present at birth. I have studied at necropsy the heart of a 2-day-old child who at birth was found to have a loud murmur typical of mitral regurgitation and, at necropsy, floppy mitral and tricuspid valve leaflets. Although this child had the typical musculoskeletal features of the Marfan syndrome, the eyes were not examined and there was no history of the Marfan syndrome in other family members; therefore this child was not included among the 18 personally studied necropsy patients because the definition of the syndrome was not fulfilled. Nevertheless, it is likely that the child did have the Marfan syndrome. Others also have described abnormalities of the mitral or tricuspid valves in patients <1 year of age with the Marfan syndrome.

Although most reports describing necropsy observations in patients with the Marfan syndrome have not mentioned the status of the mitral or tricuspid valves, it must be recalled that the floppy or prolapsing mitral valve was not recognized clinically until 1963 (5) and at necropsy not until a year or so later. Thus, morphologic descriptions of floppy or prolapsing mitral or tricuspid valves would not be expected in the Marfan patients until about 1965, and most of the detailed reported necropsy descriptions were before that date. Nevertheless, it is now clear that prolapse of one or both mitral leaflets is common at necropsy in the Marfan syndrome and that clicks, late systolic murmurs, and echocardiographic evidence of prolapse are common in these patients. Spangler and associates (104) found mitral valvular abnormalities by echocardiogram in 16 (62%) of 26 patients with the Marfan syndrome, and late or pansystolic apical murmurs and/or clicks or both in 16 (62%). Of 50 consecutive patients with the Marfan syndrome examined and reported by Pyeritz and McKusick (105), 24 (48%) had mid-systolic clicks with or without late systolic murmurs, and 29 (58%) had echocardiographic evidence of mitral valve prolapse. Although necropsy studies demonstrate abnormalities of the aorta with or without aortic regurgitation to be the most frequent cardiovascular abnormality in the Marfan syndrome, recent clinical and echocardiographic studies show that mitral valve dysfunction is even more common. Even among the previously reported necropsy patients aged ≤15 years, however, mitral regurgitation was the most frequent type of cardiovascular dysfunction.

Relatively little information on the circumference of the mitral and tricuspid valve anuli has been provided in the previously reported necropsy patients with the Marfan syndrome with or without mitral regurgitation. Of the reported patients with mitral regurgitation, the mitral or tricuspid anular circumference was described as "increased" in several patients. In the 21-year-old man with severe mitral regurgitation reported by Van Buchem (106), the mitral anulus was reported to be 18 cm and the tricuspid anulus 23 cm in circumference. These are the largest anular circumferences encountered.

Marfan patients with fusiform ascending aortic aneurysms also may have mitral valvular abnormalities with or without mitral regurgitation. Seven of 13 personally studied patients with fusiform ascending aortic aneurysms had mitral regurgitation, but none of the 3 patients with aortic dissection had mitral regurgitation. Of the 53 previously reported necropsy patients with fusiform ascending aortic root aneurysms, at least 9 (17%) had anatomic mitral valve abnormalities, but only 1 definitely had evidence of mitral regurgitation and that patient was only 7 months old, by far the youngest of any of the reported patients with aortic root aneurysm and the Marfan syndrome (see Ref. 79). Of the 57 reported necropsy patients with aortic dissection, 9 (16%) had anatomic abnormalities of the mitral valve with mitral regurgitation in at least 3.

The Marfan syndrome may be associated with mitral anular calcium at a young age. Mitral anular calcific deposits were described in 5 of the 151 previously reported necropsy patients with the Marfan syndrome, and their ages ranged from 15 to 35 years (mean 27) (102); 3 were female and 2 were male; only 2 definitely had evidence of mitral regurgitation.

Infective endocarditis involving the mitral valve was described in 6 and possibly 7 of the 151 previously reported necropsy patients with the Marfan syndrome. Five of the 6 definite cases were among the 33 patients in the mitral regurgitation group. In all 7 patients, the infection involved the mitral valve, and in 1, also the aortic valve. Thus the mitral valve is the usual site of vegetations when infective endocarditis occurs in patients with the Marfan syndrome. The floppy or prolapsing valve is the one most likely to be the site of infection. Because rupture of chordae tendineae is a frequent complication of infection involving the mitral valve, the degree of mitral regurgitation resulting from the infection can be severe (107).

Although the heretofore discussion concerned only patients with typical features of the Marfan syndrome, the cardiovascular features described in them also occur in patients without skeletal or ocular features of this syndrome or histories of this syndrome in other family members (108). In addition, the characteristic histologic features in the wall of ascending aorta also have been observed in the aorta of patients with congenitally malformed aortic valves, particularly the bicuspid condition, and in patients with aortic stenosis superimposed on a congenitally malformed valve (109,110).

REFERENCES

1. Griffith JP. Mid-systolic and late systolic mitral murmurs. Am J Med Sci 1892; 104:285.
2. Levine SA, Thompson WP. Systolic gallop rhythm. A clinical study. N Engl J Med 1935; 213:1021–5.
3. Brigden W, Leatham A. Mitral incompetence. Br Heart J 1953; 15:55.
4. Reid JVO. Mid-systolic clicks. S Afr Med J 1961; 35:353.
5. Barlow JB, Pocock WA, Marchand P, Denny M. The significance of late systolic murmurs. Am Heart J 1963; 66:443–52.
6. Segal BL, Likoff W. Late systolic murmur of mitral regurgitation. Am Heart J 1964; 67:757–63.
7. Barlow JB, Bosman CK. Aneurysmal protrusion of the posterior leaflet of the mitral valve. An ausculatory-electrocardiographic syndrome. Am Heart J 1965; 71:166–78.

8. Criley JM, Lewis KB, Humphries JO, Ross RS. Prolapse of the mitral valve: clinical and cine-angiocardiographic findings. Br Heart J 1966; 28:488–96.

9. Barlow JB, Bosman CK, Pocock WA, Marchand P. Late systolic murmurs and non-ejection ("mid-late") systolic clicks. An analysis of 90 patients. Br Heart J 1968; 30:203–18.

10. Markiewicz W, Stoner J, London E, Hunt SA, Popp RL. Mitral valve prolapse in one hundred presumably healthy young females. Circulation 1976; 53:464–73.

11. Procacci PM, Savarn SV, Schreiter SL, Bryson AL. Prevalence of clinical mitral-valve prolapse in 1169 young women. N Engl J Med 1976; 294:1086–8.

12. Savage DD, Garrison RJ, Devereux RB, Castelli WP, Anderson SJ, Levy D, McNamara PM, Stokes J III, Kannel WB, Feinleib M. Mitral valve prolapse in the general population. I. Epidemiologic features. The Framingham study. Am Heart J 1983; 106:571–6.

13. Roberts WC. The 2 most common congenital heart diseases. Am J Cardiol 1984; 53:1198.

14. Waller BF, Morrow AG, Maron BJ, Del Negro AA, Kent KM, McGrath FJ, Wallace RB, McIntosh CL, Roberts WC. Etiology of clinically isolated severe, chronic, pure mitral regurgitation: analysis of 97 patients over 30 years of age having mitral valve replacement. Am Heart J 1982; 104:276–88.

15. Roberts WC, McIntosh CL, Wallace RB. Mechanisms of severe mitral regurgitation in mitral valve prolapse determined from analysis of operatively excised valves. Am Heart J 1987; 113:1316–23.

16. Dollar AL, Roberts WC. Morphologic comparison of patients with mitral valve prolapse who died suddenly with patients who died from severe valvular dysfunction or other conditions. J Am Coll Cardiol 1991; 17:921–31.

17. Pomerance A. Ballooning deformity (mucoid degeneration) of atrio-ventricular valves. Br Heart J 1969; 31:343–51.

18. Lucas RV Jr, Edwards JE. The floppy mitral valve. Current Probl Cardiol 1982; 7(#4):1–48.

19. Bulkley BH, Roberts WC. Dilatation of the mitral anulus. A rare cause of mitral regurgitation. Am J Med 1975; 59:457–63.

20. Salazar AE, Edwards JE. Friction lesions of ventricular endocardium. Relation to chordae tendineae of mitral valve. Arch Pathol 1970; 90:364–76.

21. Guthrie RB, Edwards JE. Pathology of the myxomatous mitral valve: nature, secondary changes and complications. Minn Med 1976; 59:637–47.

22. Shirvastava S, Guthrie RB, Edwards JE. Prolapse of the mitral valve. Modern Concepts Cardiovasc Dis 1977; 46:57–61.

23. Renteria VG, Ferrans VJ, Jones M, Roberts WC. Intracellular collagen fibrils in prolapsed ("floppy") human atrioventricular valves. Lab Invest 1976; 35:439–43.

24. Roberts WC. Mitral valve prolapse and systemic hypertension. Am J Cardiol 1985; 56:703.

25. Davies MJ, Moore BP, Baimbridge MV. The floppy mitral valve. Study of

nosis resulting from unicommissural valve. Clinical and anatomic features in twenty-one adult patients. Circulation 1971; 44:272–80.

59. Edwards JE. Pathologic aspects of cardiac valvular insufficiencies. Arch Surg 1958; 77:634.

60. Roberts WC. The congenitally bicuspid aortic valve. A study of 85 autopsy cases. Am J Cardiol 1970; 26:72–83.

61. Roberts WC, Morrow AG, McIntosh CL, Jones M, Epstein SE. Congenitally bicuspid aortic valve causing severe, pure aortic regurgitation without superimposed infective endocarditis. Analysis of 13 patients requiring aortic valve replacement. Am J Cardiol 1981; 47:206–9.

62. Roberts WC. Congenital Cardiovascular Abnormalities Usually Silent Until Adulthood. Adult Congenital Heart Disease, Philadelphia: FA Davis, 1987: 631–91.

63. Osler W. The bicuspid condition of the aortic valves. Trans Assoc Am Physicians 1886; 2:185–92.

64. Grant RT, Wood JE, Jones TD. Heart valve irregularities in relation to subacute bacterial endocarditis. Heart 1928; 14:247–61.

65. Lewis T, Grant RT. Observations relating to subacute infective endocarditis. Part 1. Notes on the normal structure of the aortic valve. Part 2. Bicuspid aortic valves of congenital origin. Part 3. Bicuspid aortic valves in subacute infective endocarditis. Heart 1923; 10:21–99.

66. Arnett EN, Roberts WC. Active infective endocarditis: a clinico-pathologic analysis of 137 patients. Current Problems Cardiol 1976; 1:1–76.

67. Roberts WC, McIntosh CL, Wallace RB. Aortic valve perforation with calcific aortic valve stenosis and without infective endocarditis or significant regurgitation. Am J Cardiol 1987; 59:476–8.

68. Dressler FA, Roberts WC. Infective endocarditis in opiate addicts: analysis of 80 cases studied at necropsy. Am J Cardiol 1989; 63:1240–57.

69. Subramanian R, Olson LJ, Edwards WD. Surgical pathology of pure aortic stenosis: a study of 374 cases. Mayo Clin Proc 1984; 59:683–90.

70. Olson JJ, Subramanian R, Edwards WD. Surgical pathology of pure aortic insufficiency: a study of 225 cases. Mayo Clin Proc 1984; 59:835–41.

71. Fulton MN, Levine SA. Subacute bacterial endocarditis, with special reference to the valvular lesions and previous history. Am J Med Sci 1932; 183: 60–77.

72. Edwards JE. The congenital bicuspid aortic valve. Circulation 1961; 23: 485–8.

73. Abbott ME. Coarctation of the aorta of the adult type. II. A statistical study and historical retrospect of 200 recorded cases, with autopsy, of stenosis or obliteration of the descending arch in subjects above the age of two years. Am Heart J 1928; 3:392–574.

74. Reifenstein GH, Levine SA, Gross RE. Coarctation of the aorta. A review of 104 autopsied cases of "adult type," 2 years of age or older. Am Heart J 1947; 33:146.

75. Gore I, Seiwert VJ. Dissecting aneurysm of the aorta: pathologic aspects. An analysis of eighty-five fatal cases. Arch Pathol 1952; 53:121–41.

76. Edwards WD, Leaf DS, Edwards JE. Dissecting aortic aneurysm associated with congenital bicuspid aortic valve. Circulation 1978; 57:1022–5.
77. Roberts CS, Roberts WC. Dissection of the aorta associated with congenital malformation of the aortic valve. J Am Coll Cardiol 1991; 17:712–6.
78. Fenoglio JJ Jr, McAllister HA Jr, DeCastro CM, Davia JE, Cheitlin MD. Congenital bicuspid aortic valve after age 20. Am J Cardiol 1977; 39:164–9.
79. Larson EW, Edwards WD. Risk factors for aortic dissection: a necropsy study of 161 cases. Am J Cardiol 1984; 53:849–55.
80. Brandenburg RO Jr, Tajik AJ, Edwards WD, Reeder GS, Shub C, Seward JB. Accuracy of 2-dimensional echocardiographic diagnosis of congenitally bicuspid aortic valve. Echocardiographic-anatomic correlation in 115 patients. Am J Cardiol 1983; 51:1469–73.
81. Stewart WJ, King ME, Gillam LD, Guyer DE, Weyman AE. Prevalence of aortic valve prolapse with bicuspid aortic valve and its relation to aortic regurgitation: a cross-sectional echocardiographic study. Am J Cardiol 1984; 54:1277–82.
82. Roberts WC. Living with a congenitally bicuspid aortic valve. Am J Cardiol 1989; 64:1408–9.
83. Osler W. Malignant endocarditis. Lancet 1885; 1:415, 459, 505.
84. Dressler FA, Roberts WC. Modes of death and types of cardiac diseases in opiate addicts: analysis of 168 necropsy cases. Am J Cardiol 1989; 64: 909–20.
85. Silver MA, Roberts WC. Detailed anatomy of the normally functioning aortic valve in hearts of normal and increased weights. Am J Cardiol 1985; 55:454–61.
86. Roberts WC, Perloff JK, Costantino T. Severe valvular aortic stenosis in patients over 65 years of age. A clinicopathologic study. Am J Cardiol 1971; 27:497–506.
87. Roberts WC, Dangel JC, Bulkley BH. Non-rheumatic valvular cardiac disease. A clinicopathologic survey of 27 different conditions causing valvular dysfunction. Cardiovasc Clin 1973; 5:333–446.
88. Roberts WC. Left ventricular outflow tract obstruction and aortic regurgitation. In: Edwards JE, Lev M, Abell MR, eds. The Heart. Baltimore: Williams & Wilkins, 1974: 110–75.
89. Roberts WC. The senile cardiac calcification syndrome. Am J Cardiol 1986; 58:572–4.
90. Roberts WC, Buchbinger NA. Healed left-sided infective endocarditis: a clinico-pathologic study of 59 patients. Am J Cardiol 1977; 40:876–88.
91. Bulkley BH, Roberts WC. Ankylosing spondylitis and aortic regurgitation. Description of the characteristic cardiovascular lesion from study of eight necropsy patients. Circulation 1973; 48:1014–27.
92. Clark WS, Kulka P, Bauer W. Rheumatoid aortitis with aortic regurgitation. An unusual manifestation of rheumatoid arthritis (including spondylitis). Am J Med 1957; 22:580–90.
93. Roberts WC, Honig MS. The spectrum of cardiovascular disease in the Marfan syndrome: a clinico-morphologic study of 18 necropsy patients and

comparison of 151 previously reported necropsy patients. Am Heart J 1982; 104:115–35.

94. Murdoch JL, Walker BA, Halpern BL, Kuzma JW, McKusick VA. Life expectancy and causes of death in the Marfan syndrome. N Engl J Med 1972; 286:804–8.

95. Sisk ME, Zahka KG, Pyeritz RE, with the technical assistance of Cathy Hensley. The Marfan syndrome in early childhood: analysis of 15 patients diagnosed at less than 4 years of age. Am J Cardiol 1983; 52:353–8.

96. Carlson RG, Lillehei CW, Edwards JE. Cystic medial necrosis of the ascending aorta in relation to age and hypertension. Am J Cardiol 1970; 25: 411–5.

97. Schlatmann TJM, Becker AE. Histologic changes in the normal aging aorta: implications for dissecting aortic aneurysm. Am J Cardiol 1977; 39:13–20.

98. Schlatmann TJM, Becker AE. Pathogenesis of dissecting aneurysm of aorta. Comparative histopathologic study of significance of medial changes. Am J Cardiol 1977; 39:21–6.

99. Gsell O. Wandnekrosen der aorta als selbständige Erkrankung und ihre Beziehung zur spontanruptur. Virchows Arch Path Anat Physiol 1928; 270: 1–36.

100. Erdheim J. Medionecrosis aortae idiopathica. Virchows Arch Path Anat Physiol 1929; 273:454–79.

101. Erdheim J. Medionecrosis aortae idiopathica cystica. Virchows Arch Path Anat Physiol 1930; 276:187–229.

102. Wolinsky H, Glagov S. A lamellar unit of aortic medial structure and function in mammals. Circ Res 1967; 20:99.

103. Benchimol A, Dresser KB, Neese TC. Hypermobility of the aorta in Marfan's syndrome. Angiology 1972; 23:103–4.

104. Spangler RD, Nora JJ, Lorfscher RH, Wolfe RR, Okin JT. Echocardiography in Marfan's syndrome. Chest 1976; 69:72–8.

105. Pyeritz RE, McKusick VA. The Marfan syndrome: diagnosis and management. N Engl J Med 1979; 300:772–7.

106. Van Buchem FSP. Cardiovascular disease in arachnodactyly. Acta Med Scand 1958; 161:197–205.

107. Roberts WC, Braunwald E, Morrow AG. Acute severe mitral regurgitation secondary to ruptured chordae tendineae. Clinical, hemodynamic, and pathologic considerations. Circulation 1966; 33:58–70.

108. Waller BF, Reis RL, McIntosh CL, Epstein SE, Roberts WC. Marfan cardiovascular disease without the Marfan syndrome. Fusiform ascending aortic aneurysm with aortic and mitral valve regurgitation. Chest 1980; 77:533–40.

109. Fukuda T, Tadavarthy SM, Edwards JE. Dissecting aneurysm of aorta complicating aortic valvular stenosis. Circulation 1976; 53:169–75.

110. Roberts CS, Roberts WC. Dissection of the aorta associated with congenital malformation of the aortic valve. J Am Coll Cardiol 1991; 17:712–6.

2

Acute Rheumatic Fever

Elia M. Ayoub
University of Florida
Gainesville, Florida

Adnan S. Dajani
Wayne State University
and Children's Hospital of Michigan
Detroit, Michigan

I. INTRODUCTION

Rheumatic fever is a member of a group of diseases known as collagen-vascular diseases. Like other members of this group of diseases, rheumatic fever is characterized pathologically by inflammation of the connective and vascular tissue. This inflammatory process leads clinically to involvement of multiple organs; the major organs involved include the heart, the joints, and the central nervous system. Of these, cardiac involvement is potentially the most serious.

II. EPIDEMIOLOGY

Rheumatic fever was once considered to be primarily a disease of temperate climates, but it is now encountered worldwide. A marked decline in the incidence of rheumatic fever—which started in the early part of this century—has been documented in many Western countries; the factors responsible for this decline have not been identified. It is important to note that the decrease in incidence in Western countries preceded the advent of antibiotics and has occurred despite the fact that the incidence of streptococcal pharyngitis has remained relatively constant in these countries.

A transient resurgence of rheumatic fever, limited to some areas of the United States, has been noted over the past 5 years (1-7). The number of cases involved in this resurgence is relatively miniscule compared to the large numbers of patients with rheumatic fever that continue to be encountered worldwide. The incidence of rheumatic fever in developing countries is estimated at 100 to 150 cases per 100,000, which is 200- to 300-fold greater than the incidence of the disease in industrialized countries. Factors that may contribute to the higher incidence of rheumatic fever in nonindustrialized countries include crowded living conditions and poor access to medical care.

A decline in the prevalence of rheumatic heart disease has also been observed in industrialized countries. However, the prevalence of rheumatic heart disease in nonindustrialized countries remains quite high (8) (Table 1). Reports from India indicate that rheumatic heart disease is responsible for 30% to 50% of cardiac disease in children (9).

Because streptococcal pharyngitis occurs most frequently between the ages of 5 and 15 years, it follows that the peak incidence of rheumatic fever is seen in this age group. There is no difference in susceptibility to rheumatic fever between males and females. Racial or ethnic differences in prevalence of rheumatic fever have been documented; for example, the disease is more common in the Maori population in New Zealand and in Samoan children in Hawaii. In the United States, blacks, Hispanics, and Native Americans have a higher incidence of rheumatic fever and more severe heart disease (10). While the increased incidence of rheumatic fever in the Maoris is not related to socioeconomic factors (11), the higher incidence of rheumatic fever in the other ethnic groups does appear to be related to these factors.

Table 1 Prevalence of Rheumatic Heart Disease in Children in Different Geographic Areas[a]

Area	Prevalence per 1000 (range)
North America	0.6
South America	5.3 (1.0–17)
Africa	6.7 (0.3–15)
Asia	6.0 (1.2–21)
Pacific (excluding Japan)	8.7 (1.0–18.6)
Japan	0.7

[a] Adapted from WHO Study Group (8).

III. PATHOGENESIS

A. Etiological Agent

Early observations suggested an association between rheumatic fever and streptococcal pharyngitis or scarlet fever. Work by Rebecca Lancefield established that the group A streptococcus, also known as *Streptococcus pyogenes*, was responsible for these infectious illnesses. The group A streptococcus belongs to the family of β-hemolytic streptococci. These organisms are gram-positive cocci that grow in chains and produce complete hemolysis (β-hemolysis) of the red cells when cultured on agar medium containing 5% blood. These organisms differ from other streptococci which produce partial or green hemolysis (α streptococci) and from nonhemolytic streptococci (γ streptococci).

β-Hemolytic streptococci have been divided into 20 serologically identifiable groups, groups A to T. This separate identity is based on differences in the chemical structure and composition of the cell wall polysaccharide, also known as the group-specific carbohydrate. As pointed out above, the group A streptococcus is the only serogroup responsible for inducing rheumatic fever. Other groups have been associated with human infection but not with rheumatic fever. In addition to the group-specific carbohydrate, the cell wall of the group A streptococcus contains three protein structures, the M, T, and R proteins. The M protein is an α-helical coiled coil structure whose carboxyl terminal is anchored in the cell wall, while the amino terminal occurs at the free end (12). The M protein is seen on electron microscopy as free fimbriae on the cell surface. Variations in the amino acid composition of the M protein do occur, leading to a number of different M proteins among group A streptococci. To date, a large number of proteins with differing structures, and hence with different antigenic specificities, have been described. Although the total number of different M proteins is said to be about 150, only 80 have been identified so far. Based on this, group A streptococci have been divided into 80 serotypes, each designated with an Arabic numeral.

A major function of the M protein is its capacity to retard phagocytosis. Antibody to the M protein neutralizes this antiphagocytic activity. It is now well established that immunity to infection by the group A streptococcus is serotype specific and is dependent on the presence of antibody to the specific M protein, or type-specific antibody.

Early observations indicated that outbreaks of poststreptococcal glomerulonephritis tended to be associated with certain M serotypes. These serotypes, which include M 1, 4, 12, 25, and 49, were described as nephritogenic, since they appeared to have the potential of inducing glomerulonephritis (13). This contrasted with the concept that all group A streptococci were capable of inducing rheumatic fever. However, during the recent resurgence of rheumatic fever in the United States, it was noted that certain mucoid strains belonging to M serotypes 1, 3, 5, 6, 18, 19, and 24 were prevalent in association with these outbreaks (14). This observation has led current investigators to suggest that these strains may be rheumatogenic.

In addition to the above cellular antigens, a number of extracellular antigens produced by the group A streptococcus have been identified. These include the following enzymes: streptolysin O and streptolysin S, streptokinase, hyaluronidase, several deoxyribonucleases (A, B, C, and D)—of which deoxyribonuclease B is most commonly produced—nicotinamide adenine dinucleotidase, protease, and amylase. Because of their antigenic specificity, these products are used in various antibody tests for the serological diagnosis of group A streptococcal infection.

B. Streptococcal Antibody Tests

The antistreptolysin O (ASO) test was the first streptococcal antibody test described. It is still the most commonly employed and best standardized test. Devised by Todd in 1932 (15), this test measures the level of neutralizing antibody to streptolysin O in human serum. The antibody titer is the reciprocal of the serum dilution that inhibits the hemolytic activity of purified streptolysin O on red blood cells. The antibody response to streptolysin O and to most streptococcal antigens, peaks at about 3 weeks after the acute infection, persists at an elevated level for 4 to 6 months and then declines to normal levels.

Because of past infections by the group A streptococcus, normal individuals may have low levels of ASO in their blood. An "upper limit of normal" level is determined by assaying the ASO on a sample of normal individuals from a local population (16). Any titer that exceeds that normal level by two dilutions is considered as abnormally elevated and is indicative of an antecedent streptococcal infection. Another means for providing evidence for streptococcal infection is by obtaining serial bleedings, one during the acute infection and another 3 to 4 weeks thereafter. A significant rise of two dilutions or greater in the antibody titers between the acute and convalescent sera would also be evidence for an antecedent streptococcal infection. The latter method is used to confirm a streptococcal etiology for acute purulent infections, particularly when a culture is negative. However, in patients with rheumatic fever, the onset of the clinical manifestations corresponds to the peak of the antibody response.

Hence, performance of an antibody test at the onset of acute rheumatic fever should yield a maximal titer in most cases.

Following the description of the ASO test, several other streptococcal antibody tests were described. These tests included the anti-streptokinase, the antihyaluronidase, anti-deoxyribonuclease B (anti-DNase B), and antinicotinamide adenine dinucleotidase (Anti-NADase). Like the ASO, the tests measure neutralizing antibody to these streptococcal products. Because only about 85% of all individuals respond to any of the above antigens, and because patients with impetigo have a feeble ASO response, these tests are useful adjuncts to the ASO when the latter is negative in a patient suspected of having a streptococcal infection or its nonpurulent complication (16–19).

An additional test that may be useful in patients with rheumatic heart disease is the antibody test to the streptococcal group A carbohydrate. Studies have revealed that this antibody persists for several years in most patients with rheumatic mitral valve disease. The unique persistence of this antibody may help the differentiation of rheumatic from nonrheumatic mitral valve disease if a patient presents with mitral insufficiency without a prior history of a rheumatic episode (19–21).

The streptozyme test assays simultaneously for agglutinating antibodies to several antigens. It is not as specific or as reproducible as the above tests. While it can be used as an initial screening test, concrete evidence for antecedent streptococcal infection should be confirmed with other tests (22).

It should be emphasized that the above antibody tests serve to present evidence for an antecedent streptococcal infection only. None is diagnostic of rheumatic fever by itself, but they complement the clinical manifestations of the Jones criteria for the diagnosis of acute rheumatic fever. These antibodies, except for the antibody to the A carbohydrate, are usually not elevated in patients with chronic rheumatic heart disease.

C. Mechanisms of Tissue Injury

The onset of the clinical manifestations of rheumatic fever is preceded by a latency period of about 3 weeks. During this period, which follows the streptococcal pharyngitis, the patient is asymptomatic. This period of latency underlies our current thinking regarding the pathogenic mechanism responsible for tissue injury in rheumatic fever. Previous suggestions, that tissue injury in rheumatic fever is due to either invasion of the tissue by the streptococcal organism or by some of its toxins, could not be confirmed. These two possibilities were discarded in favor of the current theory, which proposes that an immune mechanism is operative in producing the inflammation and tissue damage seen in rheumatic fever. This concept, which is in line with the observed period of latency following the inciting throat infection, was supported by studies showing the presence of common or cross-reactive antigens between the group A streptococcus and human tissues. The presence of shared antigenic determinants between the M protein and myocardial tissue was first described by Kaplan (23). Subsequently, other investigators described similar immunological cross-reactivity between structures present in the streptococcal protoplast membrane and myocardial tissue as well as neuronal tissue of the caudate and subthalamic nuclei (24–26).

The above observations suggested that "antigenic mimicry" plays a role in the pathogenesis of rheumatic fever. Additional evidence for this mechanism and the role of cross-reactive antibodies was encountered when antibodies to these common antigens were found in the serum of patients with rheumatic fever. However, other individuals, such as patients with poststreptococcal glomerulonephritis, were also found to have these cross-reactive antibodies in their blood (23). This finding raised the possibility that other immunologic mechanisms, such as cell-mediated immunity, may be involved. Data that support the role of cell-mediated cytotoxicity as a mediator of injury to cardiac cells have been provided by subsequent studies (27).

D. Susceptibility to Rheumatic Fever

The low frequency (2–3%) with which rheumatic fever follows untreated streptococcal pharyngitis in previously normal individuals contrasts with the very high frequency (30–80%) with which rheumatic fever recurrences occur following streptococcal pharyngitis in patients who have rheumatic fever. This observation has suggested that certain individuals have an inherent susceptibility to this disease. Several epidemiological studies have provided support for this concept, suggesting that susceptibility to rheumatic fever is genetically controlled by a single recessive gene (28). Recent studies by Zabriskie have described the presence of an allotypic marker on B lymphocytes, recognized by a monoclonal antibody (D8/17), which is found in almost all patients with rheumatic fever (29).

Additional evidence supporting genetic susceptibility to this disease is found in studies that show a relationship between the inheritance of certain HLA-DR antigens and rheumatic fever. To date, susceptibility to rheumatic fever has been linked with HLA-DR 1, 2, 3, and 4 haplotypes in various ethnic groups (30–33). More recent findings show an even strong association between susceptibility to rheumatic heart disease and inheritance of Dw/10, a subtype of HLA-DR 4 (34). An important aspect of the above association is the established role of HLA-DR molecules in antigen processing and in modulating the immune response. The possibility that susceptibility to rheumatic fever may be due to a state of hyperimmune responsiveness to streptococcal antigens has been entertained by several investigators. The observations described above which suggest that an immunological mechanism may be responsible for tissue injury in rheumatic fever, provide a link for the potential mechanism that may be responsible for the pathogenesis of this disease.

IV. CLINICAL MANIFESTATIONS

The clinical manifestations of rheumatic fever can be divided into two categories. The major manifestations reflect involvement of various organs and tissues in the acute inflammatory process of rheumatic fever. They include arthritis, carditis, Sydenham's chorea, erythema marginatum, and subcutaneous nodules. These clinical manifestations are more specific for rheumatic fever and, except for arthritis, do not overlap with clinical presentation of other collagen-vascular diseases. The minor manifestations are less specific for rheumatic fever and are encountered commonly in patients presenting with a variety of rheumatological diseases. The major and minor manifestations constitute the premise for the Jones criteria that are used for the diagnosis of acute rheumatic fever.

Arthritis, although the least specific of the major manifestations, is by far the most frequent. Arthritis, alone or in conjunction with other symptoms, occurs in about 70% of patients with acute rheumatic fever. Large joints are most commonly involved. Affected joints are painful, red, swollen, and warm. The arthritis is characteristically migratory and rarely symmetrical. The inflammation in a joint may subside spontaneously in a few hours, only to appear in a different joint. Arthritis in rheumatic fever is exquisitely responsive to aspirin and rarely persists for more than a few days.

Carditis, the most serious and most specific of the clinical findings, occurs in about 50% of patients. Like arthritis, it may present alone or with other manifestations during acute rheumatic fever. Efforts should be made to exclude the presence of carditis in any patient presenting primarily with the other manifestations, as cardiac involvement may be either subtle or delayed. In a patient with acute arthritis, the clinical appearance of carditis may be delayed for 10 days after the onset of arthritis, rarely later. Carditis in patients presenting with Sydenham's chorea is notoriously subtle. Studies to exclude carditis should include an electrocardiogram, an echocardiogram, or Doppler ultrasonography.

During the acute stage, myocardial inflammation is the most serious component of carditis. It is usually associated with endocardial inflammation involving the valves. Less commonly, pericarditis may be present in conjunction with endocardial and myocardial disease. The finding of pericarditis under these circumstances should raise serious concern, since it usually signals the presence of pancarditis, a major cause of severe morbidity and mortality in acute rheumatic fever. Tachycardia when the patient is afebrile and asleep is the most reliable clinical sign of myocarditis. Arrhythmia and varying degrees of heart block can be associated with myocarditis; the latter is evidenced by a prolonged P-R interval on ECG. Cardiac dilatation and heart failure are often associated with severe myocarditis.

Valvular inflammation is highly specific for rheumatic heart disease. Mitral valve involvement occurs in 75% of cases, while involvement of the aortic valve alone occurs in only 13% of patients; inflammation of the tricuspid valve alone is rare in rheumatic fever. The simultaneous presence of mitral and aortic insufficiency should suggest a rheumatic etiology in almost all cases.

Acute valvular inflammation is clinically manifested by incompetence of the valve with signs of regurgitation. The presence of a holosystolic murmur, loudest at the apex and radiating to the axilla, is a sign of mitral incompetence and the most common feature of rheumatic carditis. Although "relative" mitral stenosis may be present during the acute stage, due to severe dilatation of the mitral annulus, true mitral stenosis or aortic stenosis are seen only in chronic rheumatic heart disease. Residual inflammation of the valve leaflets and chordae tendinae manifests as persistent insufficiency. This occurs after the acute stage and may progress to stenosis or resolve after several years if recurrence of rheumatic fever is prevented (35).

Sydenham's chorea, also known as St. Vitus' dance, occurs in about 15% of patients with acute rheumatic fever. This involvement of the central nervous system during acute rheumatic fever manifests by choreiform activity consisting of involuntary, purposeless movements of the upper extremities and muscular incoordination. The characteristic signs include gross fasciculations in the tongue known as "wormian movements," spooning of the hands when the arms are extended, pronation of the hands when raised above the head, and irregular contractions of the hand muscles that are felt when the patients grips the fingers of the examiner, known as "milkmaid's grip." Phonation cannot be sustained at the same level. When the patient is asked to draw a vertical line, the upstroke is irregular. Some of the patients will have emotional lability with tendency to easy frustration and crying. Unlike arthritis and carditis, Sydenham's chorea tends to manifest after a much longer period of latency following the inciting pharyngitis, usually 3 to 6 months. Choreiform manifestations vary in their severity. They are usually self-limited, with resolution in 2 to 4 weeks, although in some cases they may recur at intervals or persist for several months.

Erythema marginatum occurs in about 5% of patients. The lesions consist of circular serpentigenous erythematous lines with a pale center; they are nonpruritic. The rash is usually found in the trunk and proximal parts of both extremities, very rarely on the face. Application of warmth to a suspicious area makes the rash more prominent. Erythema marginatum rash is fairly specific for rheumatic fever and is rarely seen in other diseases.

Subcutaneous nodules are seen occasionally, particularly in patients with chronic rheumatic heart disease. Only 2% to 3% of patients present with nodules located on the extensor surfaces of joints, mainly in the elbows, knuckles, and ankles. The nodules are painless, freely moveable, and measure about 1 cm in diameter.

The minor manifestations consist of nonspecific clinical or laboratory features. They may occur in numerous other diseases, and their diagnostic value is limited to support of the diagnosis of rheumatic fever when only one major manifestation is present. They include the clinical manifestations of fever, arthralgia (joint ache with no objective joint findings), and past history of rheumatic fever. The two laboratory features include abnormality of an acute-phase reactant test (leukocytosis, elevated ESR, and abnormal C-reactive protein) or a prolonged P-R interval on ECG.

V. DIAGNOSIS

There is no single symptom, sign, or laboratory test that is pathognomonic of acute rheumatic fever. The Jones criteria (Table 2) are the most widely accepted guidelines for arriving at a diagnosis. These guidelines were originally established to minimize the overdiagnosis of rheumatic fever. They are to guide physicians in making the diagnosis but are not to be substitutes for clinical judgment and careful follow-up. The presence of two major, or of one major and two minor, criteria indicates a high probability of rheumatic fever, if there is also evidence of preceding group A streptococcal infection.

Because rheumatic fever is a consequence of group A streptococcal tonsillopharyngitis, supporting evidence for a preceding streptococcal infection is a *sine qua non* for establishing the diagnosis of acute rheumatic fever. A positive throat culture for group A streptococcus at the time of diagnosis is not commonly found for several reasons: (1) long latent period

Table 2 Guidelines for the Diagnosis of Initial Attack of Rheumatic Fever
(Jones Criteria, Updated 1992)[a]

Major manifestations	Minor manifestations
Carditis	Clinical
Polyarthritis	Arthralgia
Erythema marginatum	Fever
Subcutaneous Nodules	Laboratory
Chorea	Elevated acute phase reactants
	Erythrocyte sedimentation rate
	C-reactive protein
	Prolonged P-R interval

Supporting evidence of antecedent group A streptococcal infection

Positive throat culture or rapid streptococcal antigen test.
Elevated or rising streptococcal antibody titer.

If supported by evidence of preceding group A streptococcal infection, the presence of two major manifestations or of one major and two minor manifestations indicates a high probability of acute rheumatic fever.

[a] Adapted from Dajani et al. (36).

between infection and the subsequent development of rheumatic fever symptoms; (2) delay in consideration of the diagnosis; and (3) frequent administration of antibiotics for sore throats without the benefit of a throat culture. Furthermore, many children harbor group A streptococci as part of their normal flora, and the mere presence of the organisms in a throat culture may not be of significance.

The most reliable evidence of antecedent group A streptococcal infection in acute rheumatic fever is an elevated streptococcal antibody titer. Because the onset of the clinical manifestations of acute rheumatic fever corresponds to the peak of the antibody response to the streptococcal antigens, a blood sample obtained at the time of presentation with acute rheumatic fever should determine the presence of an elevated streptococcal antibody titer. However, as pointed out above, an elevated titer to one of the streptococcal antigens (ASO) is encountered in about 85% of patients. The presence of a normal ASO, in the face of strong clinical suspicion of acute rheumatic fever, should prompt the performance of another test, anti-DNAse B or anti-streptokinase. If these antibody tests then do not indicate the occurrence of an antecedent group A streptococcal infection, the diagnosis of acute rheumatic fever should be questioned. In many situations, the diagnosis of rheumatic fever cannot be easily made at the time of presentation. Questionable cases should be followed up very carefully and for an extended period to ascertain the exact nature of the presenting illness.

VI. THERAPY

A. General

Whenever possible, the patient should be admitted to a hospital for close observation and appropriate workup. This is particularly important in patients with carditis. Laboratory evaluations should include a throat culture, blood count, erythrocyte sedimentation rate, streptococcal antibody titers, chest roentgenogram, electrocardiogram, and echocardiogram.

Bed rest is generally considered important, because it tends to reduce physical activity and may lessen joint pain. The duration of bed rest may be variable and individually determined. Ambulation may be attempted once fever abates and acute-phase reactants return to normal; the patient should be allowed to return to a reasonably active life with normal physical activity. Strenuous physical exercise should be avoided, however, particularly if carditis was present.

Although throat cultures are rarely positive for group A streptococcus at the time of onset of rheumatic fever, the patient should receive a course of penicillin therapy, either as an injection of benzathine penicillin or as a 10-day course of oral penicillin. Systemic therapy is preferable to oral therapy in patients with cardiac involvement. Patients who are allergic to penicillin should be treated with oral erythromycin (Table 3).

If heart failure is present, the patient should receive diuretics, oxygen, and digitalis and be on a restricted salt intake. Digitalis preparations should be used cautiously, because cardiac toxicity may occur with conventional dosages.

B. Antirheumatic Therapy

There is no specific treatment for inflammatory reactions initiated by rheumatic fever. Supportive therapy is aimed at reducing constitutional symptoms, controlling toxic manifestations, and ameliorating cardiac function.

Patients with mild or no carditis usually respond well to salicylates. Salicylates are particularly effective in relieving joint pain; such pain usually abates within 24 hours of starting salicylates. Indeed, if joint pain persists for several days after starting salicylate treatment, the diagnosis

Table 3 Primary Prevention of Rheumatic Fever (Treatment of Streptococcal
Tonsillopharyngitis)[a]

Agent	Dose	Mode	Duration
Benzathine penicillin G	600,000 units for patients <30 kg 1,200,000 units for patients >60 kg	Intramuscular	Once
	or		
Penicillin V (phenoxymethyl penicillin)	250 mg 3 times daily	Oral	10 days
	For Individuals Allergic to Penicillin:		
Erythromycin estolate	20–40 mg/kg/day 2–4 times daily (maximum 1 g/day)	Oral	10 days
	or		
Ethylsuccinate	40 mg/kg/day 2–4 times daily (maximum 1 g/day	Oral	10 days

The following agents are acceptable but usually not recommended: amoxicillin,
   dicloxacillin, oral cephalosporins, and clindamycin.
The following are *not* acceptable: sulfonamides, trimethoprim, tetracyclines, and
   chloramphenicol.

[a] Adapted from Ref. 37.

of rheumatic fever may be questionable and the patient should be reevaluated. Because no specific diagnostic tests for rheumatic fever exist, antiinflammatory therapy should be withheld until the clinical picture has become sufficiently clear to allow for a diagnosis. Early administration of antiinflammatory agents may suppress clinical manifestations and prevent appropriate diagnosis.

For optimal antiinflammatory effect, serum salicylate levels around 20 mg are required. Aspirin, in a dose of 100 mg/kg per day, given 4 to 5 times daily, usually results in adequate serum levels to achieve a clinical response. Optimal salicylate therapy must be individualized, however, to assure adequate response and avoid toxicity. Tinnitus, nausea, vomiting, anorexia, and hepatitis are common dose-related toxicities associated with salicylism. Side effects may subside after a few days of treatment despite continuation of the medication.

Children with significant cardiac involvement, particularly those with pericarditis or congestive heart failure, are believed to respond more promptly to corticosteroids. Also, an occasional patient who does not respond to adequate doses of salicylates may benefit from a trial course of corticosteroids. Prednisone, 1 to 2 mg/kg per day, is the usual dose.

There is no evidence that salicylate or corticosteroid therapy affects the course of carditis, diminishes the incidence of residual heart disease, or shortens the duration of the illness. Therefore, the duration of therapy with antiinflammatory agents is arbitrarily based on an estimate of the severity of the episode and the promptness of the clinical response.

Mild attacks with little or no cardiac involvement may be treated with salicylates for about one month, or until there is sufficient clinical and laboratory evidence of subsidence of inflammatory activity. In more severe cases, therapy with corticosteroids may be continued for 2 to 3 months. The medication is then gradually reduced over 2 weeks. Even with prolonged therapy some patients (approximately 5%) will continue to demonstrate evidence of rheumatic activity for 7 months or more. A "rebound," manifested by the reappearance of mild symptoms or of abnormal acute-phase reactants, may occur in some patients after antiinflammatory medications have been discontinued, usually within 2 weeks. Modest symptoms usually subside without treatment; more severe symptoms may require treatment with salicylates. To reduce the likelihood of a rebound, it is recommended that salicylates (aspirin, 75 mg/kg per day) be administered when corticosteroids are tapered.

Information about the use of salicylates other than aspirin is very limited. There is no evidence that other nonsteroidal antiinflammatory agents are more effective than aspirin. In children who cannot tolerate aspirin or who are allergic to it, a trial of the nonsteroidal agents may be warranted. Aspirin preparations that are coated, or that contain alkali or buffers, may also be tried; however, there is little evidence that such preparations are better tolerated, and some may have undesirable side effects.

VII. PREVENTION

A. Primary Prevention

Prevention of primary attacks of rheumatic fever depends on the prompt recognition and proper treatment of group A streptococcal tonsillo-pharyngitis. Eradication of group A streptococci from the throat is essential. Although appropriate antimicrobial therapy started several days after the onset of acute streptococcal pharyngitis is effective in preventing primary attacks of rheumatic fever, early therapy is advisable because it reduces both morbidity and the period of infectivity. Usually, patients are considered noncontagious after 24 hours of therapy.

Table 3 outlines the current recommendation for the primary prevention of rheumatic fever as established by the Committee on Rheumatic Fever, Endocarditis, and Kawasaki Disease of the Council on Cardiovascular Disease in the Young, the American Heart Association. Penicillin remains the agent of choice, except in individuals who are allergic to it.

B. Secondary Prevention

Continuous antimicrobial prophylaxis provides the most effective protection from rheumatic fever recurrences. A patient who has an attack of rheumatic fever is inordinately susceptible to recurrent attacks following subsequent group A streptococcal infections of the upper respiratory tract. Such infections need not be symptomatic to cause a recurrence.

The risk of recurrences depends on several factors. The risk decreases as the interval from the most recent attack increases. Risk increases with multiple previous attacks. The risk increases in individuals who are more likely to be exposed to group A streptococci, such as school teachers, parents of young children, physicians, nurses, military recruits, and other individuals living in crowded conditions. The risk of recurrent carditis is particularly high in individuals who have had rheumatic carditis; each recurrence is likely to sustain further cardiac involvement and damage.

The American Heart Association regimens for prophylaxis are listed in Table 4. Injectable penicillin has an advantage because it does not depend on the patient's compliance, but it is painful. Oral sulfadiazine is comparable to oral penicillin as a prophylactic agent. Sulfadiazines should be used for prophylaxis only; they should *not* be used for the treatment of group A streptococcal infection. Other sulfonamides may also be acceptable as prophylactic agents, but little information is available about their efficacy.

Patients who develop rheumatic carditis should receive long-term antibiotic prophylaxis well into adulthood and perhaps for life. Prophylaxis in the form of monthly injections of benzathine penicillin G is advisable in patients with cardiac involvement, particularly during the 5 years following the onset of the disease. Prophylaxis should continue even after valve surgery or valve replacement, because the risk of rheumatic fever recurrence persists. Patients who do not develop carditis should receive prophylaxis for at least 5 years after the last attack of rheumatic fever and until they are 20 years old. Prophylaxis beyond that period should be determined on an individual basis and after assessing the various factors

Table 4   Secondary Prevention of Rheumatic Fever (Prevention of Recurrent Attacks)[a]

Agent	Dose/frequency	Mode
Benzathine penicillin G	1,200,000 units every 4 weeks[b]	Intramuscular
	or	
Penicillin V (phenoxymethyl penicillin)	250 mg twice daily	Oral
	or	
Sulfadiazine	0.5 g once daily for patients <30 kg 1.0 g once daily for patients >30 kg	Oral
For Individuals Allergic to Penicillin and Sulfadiazine:		
Erythromycin	250 mg twice daily	Oral

[a] Adapted from A. S. Dajani et al. (37).
[b] In high-risk situations, administration every 3 weeks is advised.

listed above. No single regimen is totally effective in either eradicating streptococci from the tonsillopharynx or in preventing recurrent attacks of rheumatic fever.

REFERENCES

1. Veasy LG, Wiedmeier SE, Orsmond GS, et al. Resurgence of acute rheumatic fever in the intermountain area of the United States. N Engl J Med 1987; 316:421–7.
2. Wald ER, Dashefsky B, Feidt C, et al. Acute rheumatic fever in Western Pennsylvania and the tristate area. Pediatrics 1987; 80:371–4.
3. Hosier DM, Craenen JM, Teske DW, et al. Resurgence of rheumatic fever. Am J Dis Child 1987; 141:730–3.
4. Congeni B, Rizzo C, Congeni J, et al. Outbreak of acute rheumatic fever in northeast Ohio. J Pediatr 1987; 111:176–9.
5. Papdinos T, Escanmilla J, Garst P, et al. Acute rheumatic fever at a Navy training center-San Diego, California. MMWR 1988; 37:101–4.
6. Sampson GL, Williams RG, House MD, et al. Acute rheumatic fever among Army trainees-Fort Leonard Wood, Missouri, 1987–1988. MMWR 1988; 37: 519–22.
7. Westlake RM, Graham TP, Edwards KM. An outbreak of acute rheumatic fever in Tennessee. Pediatr Infect Dis J 1990; 9:97–100.
8. WHO Study Group. Rheumatic fever and rheumatic heart disease. WHO Tech Rep Ser 1988; 764:21–5.

9. Agarwal BL. Rheumatic heart disease unabated in developing countries. Lancet 1981; 11:910–1.

10. Pope RM. Rheumatic fever in the 1980's. Bull Rheum Dis 1989; 38:1.

11. Wannamaker LW. Changes and changing concepts in the biology of Group A streptococci and in the epidemiology of streptococcal infections. Rev Infect Dis 1979; 1:967–75.

12. Fischetti VA, Parry DAD, Trus BL, Hollingshead SK, Scott JR, Manjula BN. Conformational characteristics of the complete sequence of Group A streptococcal M6 protein. PROTEINS: Structure, Function, and Genetics 1988; 3:60–9.

13. Dillon HC. Streptococcal skin infections and glomerulonephritis. In: Hoeprich PD, Jordan MC. Infectious Diseases: A Treatise of Infectious Processes. 4th ed. Philadelphia: Lippincott, 1989: 995–1000.

14. Kaplan EL, Johnson DR, Cleary PP. Group A streptococcal serotypes isolated from patient and sibling contacts during the resurgence of rheumatic fever in the United States in the mid-1980s. J Infect Dis 1989; 159:101–3.

15. Todd EW. Antihaemolysin titers in haemolytic streptococcal infections and their significance in rheumatic fever. Br J Exp Pathol 1932; 13:248–59.

16. Ayoub EM, Wannamaker LW. Evaluation of the streptococcal desoxyribonuclease B and diphosphopyridine nucleotidase antibody tests in acute rheumatic fever and acute glomerulonephritis. Pediatrics 1962; 29:527–38.

17. Wannamaker LW. Differences between streptococcal infections of the throat and of the skin. N Engl J Med 1970; 282:23–31.

18. Wannamaker LW. Differences between streptococcal infections of the throat and of the skin. N Engl J Med 1970; 282:78–85.

19. Ayoub EM. Streptococcal antibody tests in rheumatic fever. Clin Immunol News 1982; 3:107–11.

20. Dudding BA, Ayoub EM. Persistence of streptococcal Group A antibody in patients with rheumatic valvular disease. J Exp Med 1968; 128:1081–98.

21. Appleton RS, Victorica BE, Tamer D, et al. Specificity of antibody to the streptococcal Group A carbohydrate in rheumatic valvular disease. J Lab Clin Med 1985; 105:114–9.

22. Gerber MA, Wright LL, Randolph MF. Streptozyme test for antibodies to Group A streptococcal antigens. Pediatr Infect Dis J 1987; 6:36–40.

23. Kaplan MH. Rheumatic fever, rheumatic heart disease, and the streptococcal connection: the role of streptococcal antigens cross reactive with heart tissue. Rev Infect Dis 1979; 1:988–96.

24. Zabriskie JB, Freimer EH. An immunological relationship between group A streptococci and mammalian muscle. J Exp Med 1966; 124:661–8.

25. Dale JB, Beachey EH. Multiple, heart-cross-reactive epitopes of streptococcal M proteins. J Exp Med 1985; 161:113–22.

26. Husby G, Van de Rijn I, Zabriskie JB, et al. Antibodies reacting with cytoplasm of subthalamic and caudate nuclei neurons in chorea and acute rheumatic fever. J Exp Med 1976; 144:1094–110.

27. Hutto J, Ayoub EM. Cytotoxicity of lymphocytes from patients with rheumatic carditis to cardiac cells in vitro. In: Read SE, Zabriskie JB, eds. Strep-

tococcal Disease and the Immune Response. New York: Academic Press, 1980: 733–8.

28. Ayoub EM. The search for host determinants of susceptibility to rheumatic fever: the missing link. Circulation 9184; 69:197–201.
29. Khanna AK, Buskirk DR, Williams RC, et al. Presence of a non-HLA B cell antigen in rheumatic fever patients and their families as defined by a monoclonal antibody. J Clin Invest 1989; 83:1710–6.
30. Ayoub EM, Barrett DJ, Maclaren NK, et al. Association of class II human histocompatibility leukocyte antigens with rheumatic fever. J Clin Invest 1986; 77:2219–26.
31. Anastasiou-Nana MI, Anaderson JL, Carquist JF, et al. HLA-DR typing and lymphocyte subset evaluation in rheumatic heart disease: a search for immune response factors. Am Heart J 1986; 112:992–7.
32. Jhingham B, Mehra NK, Reddy KS, et al. HLA, blood groups and secretor status in patients with established rheumatic fever and rheumatic heart disease. Tissue Antigens 1986; 27:172–8.
33. Maharaj B, Hammond MG, Appadoo B, et al. HLA-A, B, DR, and DQ antigens in black patients with severe chronic rheumatic heart disease. Circulation 1987; 76:259–61.
34. Alsaeid KA, Schiffenbaur J, Atkinson MA, Ayoub EM. Association of HLA-DR4 subtype Dw10 with rheumatic fever. Pediatr Res 1991; abstract.
35. Thompson DG, Boxerbaum B, Liebman J. Long-term prognosis of rheumatic fever patients receiving regular intramuscular benzathine penicillin. Circulation 1972; 45:543–51.
36. Dajani AS, Ayoub E, Bierman FZ, Bisno AL, Denny FW, Durack DT, Ferrieri P, Freed M, Gerber M, Kaplan EL, Karchmer AW, Markowitz M, Rahimtoola SH, Shulman ST, Stollerman G, Takahashi M, Taranta A, Taubert KA, Wilson W. Special report. Guidelines for the Diagnosis of Rheumatic Fever: Jones Criteria, Updated 1992. Special writing Group of the Committee on Rheumatic Fever, Endocarditis, and Kawasaki Disease of the Council on Cardiovascular Disease in the Young, Amercian Heart Association. Circulation 1993; 87:302–7.
37. Dajani AS, Bisno AL, Chung KJ, Durack DT, Gerber MA, Kaplan EL, Millard D, Randolph MF, Shulman ST, Watanakunakorn C. Special report. Prevention of rheumatic fever. A statement of health professionals by the Committee on Rheumatic Fever, Endocarditis and Kawasaki Disease of the Council on Cardiovascular Disease in the Young. Circulation 1988; 78: 1082–6.

3

Echocardiography in Valvular Heart Disease

Maie S. Shahed
Armed Forces Hospital
Riyadh, Saudi Arabia

A. Jamil Tajik
Mayo Clinic
Rochester, Minnesota

Transthoracic echocardiography has become the most widely used noninvasive cardiac diagnostic tool that provides accurate, reproducible information in valvular heart disease. In this chapter, a summary of its basic principles will be discussed before we proceed to discuss its use in specific valvular lesions. For more detailed discussion, the reader should refer to one of the standard references or textbooks (1–8).

I. BASIC PHYSICS AND PRINCIPLES

The basic principle behind all modes of echocardiography is the use of sound waves of high frequency (2.0–7.5 mHz), generated by piezoelectric crystals contained within a transducer, which are transmitted in short pulses through the heart and received back after being reflected. These waves are reflected either by an interface between two tissues of different acoustic properties, such as myocardium and valves [the basis for two-dimensional or cross-sectional echocardiography (2-DE), which provides real-time information about structural anatomy and morphology], or by moving blood, with resultant change or shift in frequency (the basis for

Doppler echocardiography, which gives information about blood flow and pressure differences). The reflected waves are received and processed to give the required information. The time elapsed from when the sound waves are transmitted to when they are received is converted into a display of distances, and a real-time, two-dimensional image of the heart is thus created at 30 frames per second.

Doppler echocardiography compliments 2-DE by offering noninvasive information on blood flow velocity within heart chambers and the great vessels. The Doppler effect was described by the Austrian physicist Christian Doppler, who published his observation in 1862 while observing moving stars (9). The Doppler principle states that when sound waves of a known frequency encounter a moving object, the reflected waves have a different frequency which is in proportion to the velocity of the object. In Doppler echocardiography, the sound waves of known frequency generated by the elements in the transducer are reflected by moving red blood cells with a frequency which will be higher or lower according to whether the blood flow is moving toward or away from the transducer. The difference in frequencies, referred to as the *Doppler shift*, can be measured and is directly proportional to the velocity of red blood cells (V) through the Doppler equation: $V = \Delta F \times C/2F_0 \times \cos \theta$, where ΔF is the detected frequency shift, C is the velocity of sound in blood (1540 m/s), F_0 is the frequency of the transmitted sound, and $\cos \theta$ is cosine of the angle of incidence between the sound beam and the direction of blood flow. This is why when performing Doppler examination, every effort is made to align the sound beam as parallel to blood flow as possible in order to minimize the angle θ, bringing its cosine as near to unity as possible. By convention, the Doppler spectral signal is displayed with velocity along the y axis, while time is displayed along the x axis. Positive velocities (flow directed toward the transducer) are depicted above the baseline, while negative velocities (flow moving away from the transducer) are depicted below the baseline.

A. Doppler Modalities

Two modes for Doppler echocardiographic examination are available: continuous- and pulsed-wave Doppler. In the continuous-wave Doppler mode (CWD), two adjacently positioned transducer elements are utilized: One as a continuous transmitter, while the other continuously receives the reflected signals. CWD can measure high-velocity jets and is quite useful with stenotic, regurgitant, and shunt jets.

With the second mode of Doppler echocardiography, pulsed-wave Doppler (PWD), single transducer elements act as both the transmitter and the receiver of the sound waves. Intermittent pulses are transmitted and the reflected signals are received after a specific time delay. This time delay can be adjusted so that a specific "sample volume" can be interrogated to the exclusion of others along the sound beam. This is referred to as *range gating*. The rate at which the pulses are generated is termed the *pulse repetition frequency* (PRF). It is related to the depth of the interrogated sample volume. It must be at least twice the highest expected Doppler frequency shift (corresponding to highest flow velocity) for accurate determination of peak velocity. The maximal Doppler frequency shift accurately recorded by PWD is termed the *Niquist limit*. If the velocity of flow and the corresponding frequency shift is high, exceeding the Niquist limit, aliasing of the signal occurs. This leads to display of signal both above and below the baseline, leading to ambiguity of analysis.

The more recently employed technique of Doppler color flow imaging (CFI) has greatly improved the clinical application of echocardiography. It allows simultaneous two-dimensional imaging of intracardiac structures and flow patterns by superimposing color-coded PWD flow information on the two-dimensional image. Hundreds of points along the image will act as sample volumes whose frequency shifts, and corresponding mean velocities, are calculated by the use of an autocorrelator and color encoded to provide information about direction, velocity, and turbulence. Direction is displayed conventionally as either red (blood flow toward the transducer) or blue (blood flow away from the transducer). Velocities are displayed as different shades of either red or blue: Higher velocities are coded in brighter shades, and lower velocities are coded in darker shades. When turbulent flow is present, it is recognized as a marked variation in velocities, and various shades of green are added to the primary colors of red and blue, resulting in a mosaic color pattern.

As CFI is an application of PWD, it has the same limitations pertaining to the maximum velocity that can be measured. Aliasing is depicted as a reversal of color (red to blue or vice versa).

B. Bernoulli Equation

The velocities measured by the Doppler technique can be converted into pressure gradients across orifices by applying the modified Bernoulli equation:

$$\text{Pressure gradient} = 4(V_2{}^2 - V_1{}^2)$$

where V_2 and V_1 are velocities in meters per second of the blood flow after and before the orifice, respectively. In practice, V_1 is usually less than 1 m/s, and V_1^2 is thus negligible and can be ignored. The simplified formula

$$\text{Pressure gradient} = 4V_2^2$$

is applied to measure gradients.

With this introduction, we will now proceed to discuss the 2-D/Doppler assessment of various valve lesions.

II. ECHOCARDIOGRAPHY IN MITRAL STENOSIS

Mitral stenosis (MS) is most commonly a late sequelae of rheumatic carditis, although rarely it may be congenital or associated with other diseases (10–12). Progressive symptomatic deterioration in rheumatic MS is the result of the haemodynamic changes that occur secondary to the reduction in the effective mitral orifice area, which becomes severe at an area below 1 cm². Optimal timing of intervention to relieve symptoms, whether through surgery or, more recently, percutaneous balloon mitral valvuloplasty (PBMV) (13–16), depends on accurate measurements of the valve area. This was formerly achieved using hemodynamic data obtained by cardiac catheterization (17), which was limited by the need to perform an invasive examination and by the limitations inherent in the method itself, such as coexistent mitral regurgitation or low cardiac output status. Echocardiography, however, has come to play a crucial role in the diagnosis of MS and in assessing its severity: Two-dimensional echocardiography (2-DE) permits estimation of mitral valve area (MVA) by planimetry, and Doppler echocardiography allows for measurement of transmitral flow velocity, pressure gradient, and the mitral pressure half-time ($t^{1/2}$), from which MVA can be calculated.

A. M-Mode and Two-Dimensional Echocardiography

The typical two-dimensional echo-guided M-mode echocardiogram of MS, usually obtained from the parasternal long axis view, is characterized by thickened leaflets, with diminished separation, abnormal motion of the posterior leaflet which tends to move anteriorly during diastole, and diminished EF slope (18–20) (Fig. 1). However, except for the abnormal motion of the posterior leaflet, none of these other features is specific for MS.

2-DE imaging of the mitral leaflets and support apparatus should be undertaken from the parasternal long- (LAX) and short-axis (SAX) views and the apical two- and four-chamber views to allow for detailed assessment of the morphology. It is imperative to characterize leaflet texture,

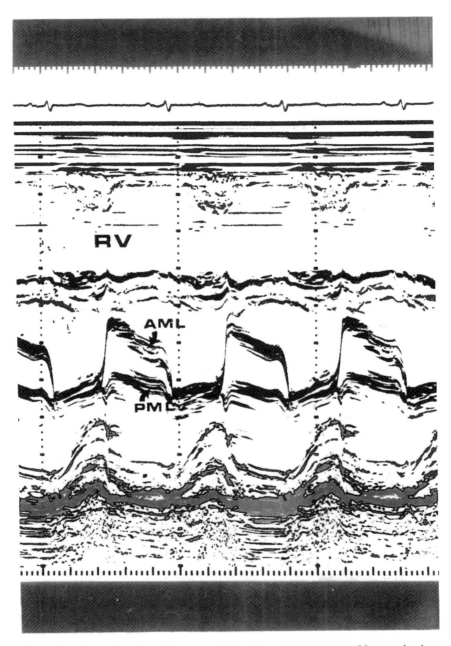

Figure 1 M-mode echocardiogram obtained from the parasternal long-axis view in a patient with severe mitral stenosis. Note the thickened anterior (AML) and posterior (PML) mitral valve leaflets, with the anterior movement of PML due to commissural fusion. Note also the slow closing velocity. RV = right ventricle.

pliability, and mobility, and to assess the degree of calcification. Characteristically, the leaflets are thickened, with restricted mobility (diastolic doming) due to commissural fusion (Fig. 2). The parasternal SAX view allows for measurement of MV orifice area by planimetry, with good correlation to MVA measured directly at the time of surgery (21) or during catheterization using the Gorlin formula (22–24). However, adequate views for planimetry are unavailable in up to 17% of cases (22), and the method tends to underestimate MVA when the valve is heavily calcified (25) and is not very reliable post-surgical mitral commissurotomy (26). What is more, the method depends heavily on operator skill in optimizing the picture with proper gain setting, proper alignment of the beam perpendicular to the valve leaflet plane, and proper localization of the minimal orifice to the tip of the leaflet and not to a more proximal, more pliable level which will lead to overestimation of the valve area (23, 25). Standard and modified parasternal LAX and the apical views allow for careful assessment of the MV annulus and the subvalvular apparatus, determining the degree of annular calcification and the extent of chordal thickening, shortening, or calcification, which is helpful in planning surgery or balloon

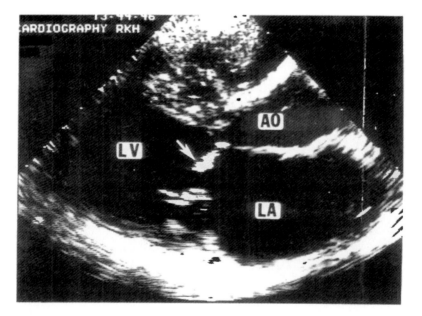

Figure 2 Two-dimensional echocardiogram of a rheumatically stenosed mitral valve (arrow) in the parasternal long-axis view. Note the thickened, doming leaflets and the dilated left atrium (LA). AO = aorta, LV = left ventricle.

valvotomy (27–31). With respect to mitral balloon valvotomy, an echocardiographic scoring system of 1 to 4 (from mild to severe) had been devised in relation to four morphological features of the valve apparatus: leaflet thickening, leaflet mobility, subvalvular thickening, and calcification. A high score (≥ 10), implying advanced leaflet/chordal deformity, is associated with a suboptimal outcome. 2-DE is also useful in screening other valves for coexisting involvement, evaluating the degree of left atrial (LA) enlargement, and excluding the presence of LA thrombi (32, 33) (Fig. 3). Transesophageal echocardiography (TEE) has emerged as an excellent means of diagnosing or excluding LA and LA appendage thrombi (34–36) (Fig. 4).

B. Doppler Echocardiography

Doppler echocardiography is now in wide clinical use for estimating the severity of MS. The Doppler examination of the MV flow is best performed from the apical or para-apical position, since the stenotic jet is frequently directed to the apex. The flow velocity signal is characteristic: There is increased early diastolic velocity, which tends to persist until the

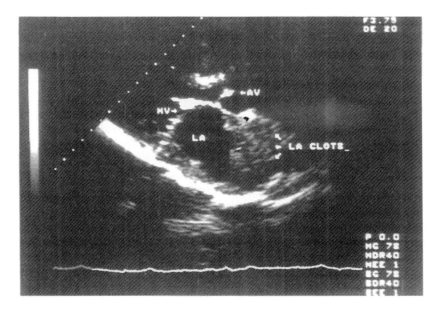

Figure 3 Two-dimensional echocardiogram in the parasternal long-axis view, showing a severely calcific, stenosed, restricted mitral valve (MV), a dilated left atrium (LA), and a huge clot (arrows) in the roof of the LA. AV = aortic valve.

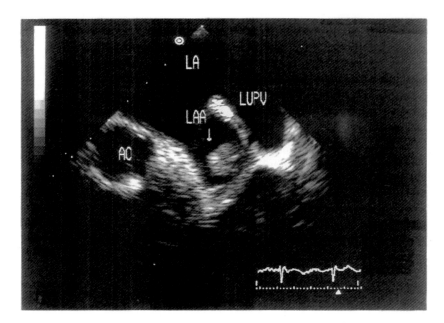

Figure 4 Transesophageal two-dimensional echocardiogram of the left atrium (LA) and left atrial appendage (LAA) in a patient with mitral stenosis showing a thrombus in the LAA. AO = aorta, LUPV = left upper pulmonary vein.

end of diastole (Fig. 5). Color flow imaging (CFI), by demonstrating the direction of the typical jet (37), will facilitate the positioning of the CWD parallel to the jet to obtain the optimal flow velocity signal (Fig. 6, see color plate). CFI is also helpful in quantifying coexisting mitral regurgitation. The width of the color stenotic jet at the mitral orifice was found to correlate reasonably well with MVA obtained by 2-DE (38), but more validated methods of estimating MS severity exist, such as pressure half-time and the continuity equation.

In 1976, Holen et al. (39) were the first to use the Doppler effect to determine pressure gradient in mitral stenosis. The simplified version of the Bernoulli equation, $\Delta P = 4V^2$, where ΔP is the transmitral pressure gradient (in mmHg) and V is the maximal transmitral velocity (in m/s), is now a widely accepted and applied method to measure gradient across MV and thus assess MS severity. Mean pressure gradient can also be calculated by equipment software and has been found to correlate well with mean gradient measured at cardiac catheterization (40, 41).

Libanoff and Rudband (42) described the concept of pressure half-time

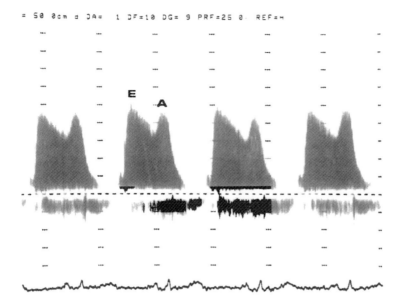

Figure 5 Continuous-wave Doppler signal from a patient with severe mitral stenosis in sinus rhythm. Peak velocity (point E) is 2.5 m/s, corresponding to a peak gradient of 25 mmHg across the mitral valve in diastole (the distance between the calibration dots corresponds to a velocity of 0.5 m/s). Note the slow deceleration of the velocity signal with further increase in velocity (point A) with atrial contraction.

($t^{1/2}$) obtained at cardiac catheterization to assess MS severity and found it to be independent of cardiac output and insignificantly affected by heart rate. Hatle and associates (43) later applied this concept to Doppler echocardiography. Pressure half-time is the time required for the pressure gradient to fall to half of its original value. As the severity of MS increases, the diastolic gradient between LA and left ventricle (LV) is maintained for a longer time, resulting in longer $t^{1/2}$. Pressure half-time longer than 220 ms is indicative of severe MS. A pressure half-time of 220 ms correlates with MVA of 1.0 cm^2, therefore, MVA can be determined by dividing the empiric constant of 220 by the Doppler $t^{1/2}$ (Fig. 7). This concept has been validated by several studies (26,44,45), and is reproducible and independent of cardiac output, the presence of mitral regurgitation (MR), or presence of atrial fibrillation (43,46). It is negligibly affected by exercise (47,48), but tends to overestimate MVA in the presence of aortic regurgita-

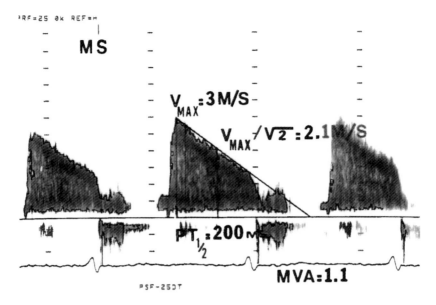

Figure 7 Continuous-wave Doppler signal of mitral inflow velocity obtained from apical position in a patient with severe mitral stenosis and atrial fibrillation. The maximum velocity (V_{max}) of the signal is 3 m/s, corresponding to a gradient across the mitral valve of 36 mmHg. The pressure half-time ($PT_{1/2}$) of 200 ms is calculated as the time interval over which V_{max} falls to a value equal to V_{max} divided by the square root of 2. This corresponds to a mitral valve orifice area (MVA) of 1.1 cm^2 calculated as 220/pressure half-time.

tion (49–52). It may also be affected by acute changes in LA and left ventricular compliance (50), as occurs immediately post-PBMV (53,54).

C. Continuity Principle for Measuring Mitral Valve Area

MVA can also be calculated by applying the continuity principle (49,55), which states that the volume of flow per unit time through the MV is equal to the volume of flow per unit time through the aortic valve (AV), provided there are no left-side regurgitant lesions or shunts. Flow is calculated by multiplying the flow velocity integral (FVI) measured by Doppler at each valve by the valve cross-sectional area (CSA). Thus:

$$CSA_{(MV)} \times FVI_{(MV)} = CSA_{(AV)} \times FVI_{(AV)}$$

and

$$CSA_{(MV)} = \frac{CSA_{(AV)} \times FVI_{(AV)}}{FVI_{(MV)}}$$

The limitations of this method lie in obtaining accurate diameter measurements to calculate area and in measuring the flow velocity integral.

More recently, a method has been described for measuring MVA that depends entirely on factors inherent in the MS CFI jet, utilizing the proximal isovelocity surface area (PISA) of the jet (56). However, this method still needs to be validated.

D. Role of Transesophageal Echocardiography

Transesophageal examination is performed to exclude the presence of left atrial thrombus in patients in whom percutaneous balloon valvuloplasty is anticipated. TEE is also useful in the evaluation of the morphology of mitral leaflets and the subvalvular apparatus, as well as in detection and grading of any associated mitral regurgitation.

E. Role of Cardiac Cathetherization

With all the above-mentioned modalities to assess severity of MS, the role of cardiac catheterization is changing to one of therapeutic rather than diagnostic value. Echocardiography is becoming the current "gold standard" in mitral stenosis for complete assessment of severity and characterization of the valvular and subvalvular apparatus. Rarely is cardiac catheterization indicated for assessment of severity of mitral stenosis.

F. Summary

In summary, echocardiography is an excellent tool for the noninvasive diagnosis of MS and for assessing its severity. It is also a reliable noninvasive tool for following patients and documenting the degree of progression of their disease. Cardiac catheterization will be indicated diagnostically only in patients for whom marked discrepancy exists between symptoms and 2-D/Doppler findings, or in patients who are suspected to have associated coronary artery disease.

III. ECHOCARDIOGRAPHY IN AORTIC STENOSIS

Aortic stenosis (AS), whether of congenital origin or acquired, is a common form of valvular disease, particularly in the older population (57–59). An accurate assessment of hemodynamic severity may be difficult to determine solely on the basis of clinical examination, especially in the older age group, who also have increased incidence of associated hypertension and coronary artery disease (60–63). Several studies have been reported evaluating AS severity utilizing electrocardiography (61–64), phonocardiography and external carotid pulse recordings (61, 64–66), the presence of calcification on chest roentgenography (61,62), and treadmill exercise testing (61,67,68). These different diagnostic modalities can separate normal individuals from those with AS, but are not sensitive enough to assess hemodynamic severity reliably. This is why, until recently, cardiac catheterization offered the only definite means of determining the hemodynamic severity of AS and its progression (63,69–71). However, the application of echocardiography and especially Doppler echocardiography for the diagnosis and evaluation of AS has markedly modified our understanding of its natural history and our management of individual patients. Besides providing essential data with respect to severity, it offers a reproducable, reliable method for following the hemodynamic progression of the disease (72,73), with a frequency that would have not been accepted if only invasive measures were available.

A. Two-Dimensional Echocardiography

The anatomic hallmark of AS is reduced orifice dimension with or without associated calcification (60,74,75). Two-dimensional echocardiography is sensitive in detecting valvular thickening, calcification, and decreased leaflet excursion (76,77) (Fig. 8). In addition, it can delineate the structural morphology of the valve, identify the number of cusps (78,79), identify commissural fusion associated with rheumatic heart disease, and distinguish calcific from noncalcific valves. It can identify other associated anatomic abnormalities, such as poststenotic aortic root dilatation left ventricular wall thickness, systolic function, chamber size, and involvement of other valves. Several studies to assess AS severity were reported, utilizing M-mode or 2-DE measured cusp separation, and direct measurement of aortic valve cross-sectional area (AVA) in the parasternal short-axis view, correlating these measurements with catheter-estimated AVA and/or aortic gradient (76,77,80–82). However, Doppler echocardiography, with its capabilities of measuring transvalvular velocity and pressure gradient directly, and AVA, have rendered most of these methods obsolete.

B. Doppler Echocardiography

Blood flow proximal to a stenotic AV is laminar, usually with a velocity of 0.8–1.2 m/s. As blood passes through a stenosed valve, its velocity will increase depending on severity of obstruction (typically 2–6 m/s). Continuous-wave Doppler echocardiography is capable of measuring such high velocities. The direction of the stenotic jet is unpredictable and is almost always eccentric. An optimal recording of this jet velocity is usually obtained when the Doppler beam is as parallel to the jet as possible. To achieve this, recordings should be attempted from multiple windows, with

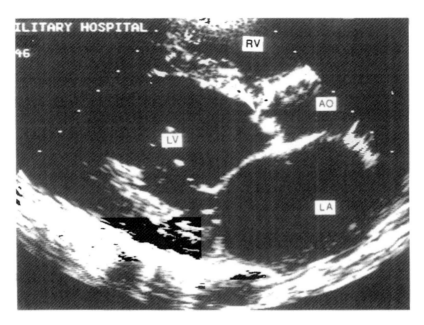

Figure 8 Two-dimensional echocardiogram in the parasternal long-axis view showing a heavily calcified aortic valve, hardly opening in systole (note closed position of mitral valve). The left ventricle (LV) is hypertrophied. AO = aorta, LA = left atrium, RV = right ventricle.

multiple transducer angulations at each site, using both the imaging and the nonimaging probes (83–85). These windows include the apical and left parasternal with the individual in the left lateral decubitus position; the right parasternal with the individual in right lateral decubitus; and the suprasternal, supraclavicular, or subcostal window with the individual in the supine position. Depending on which window is used, the direction of the jet in relation to the transducer will be depicted differently with respect to the baseline.

Having obtained an optimal maximal velocity signal of the stenotic jet, this can be converted into the systolic pressure gradient by applying the modified Bernoulli equation, $\Delta P = 4(V_2^2 - V_1^2)$, where ΔP is the pressure gradient (in mmHg), V_2 and V_1 are respective velocities (in m/s) of the aortic jet measured by CWD, and that of the left ventricular outflow tract (LVOT) measured by pulsed-wave Doppler. Because the LVOT velocity is usually less than 1 m/s, it is generally ignored in the above equation, which is further simplified to $\Delta P = 4V_2^2$. However, in cases of high output state, associated significant aortic regurgitation, or associated subvalvular obstructions, V_1 is usually more than 1 m/s and should be taken into consideration to avoid overestimation of the pressure gradient (84). The application of the simplified Bernoulli equation in measuring pressure gradient has been thoroughly validated for assessment of aortic stenosis severity, in animal experiments (86,87) as well as in humans, utilizing simultaneous Doppler and cardiac catheterization techniques for measuring transaortic gradient (88–90) and also by many nonsimultaneous studies (44,91–93). Excellent correlations between Doppler-derived and catheter-measured gradients have been reported.

It must be emphasized that the Doppler-derived pressure gradient represents a physiological and instantaneous gradient throughout the ejection period. On the other hand, the peak-to-peak gradient measured at catheterization is a nonphysiologic measurement because the peak left ventricular pressure and peak aortic pressure do not occur at the same time during ejection. Hence the Doppler maximum pressure gradient is conceptually different from the peak-to-peak gradient. More meaningful information about the transaortic gradient and the severity of AS is provided by the mean gradient measured by equipment software from the maximal velocity spectral signal. This was found to correlate well with the mean gradient obtained by catheterization (89,92–97).

In 1951, Gorlin and Gorlin (17) proposed an equation to measure stenotic valve area at cardiac catheterization that had two important variables: cardiac output and pressure gradient. When Doppler transaortic pressure gradient measurement became available and its accuracy was validated, various methods were described for determining cardiac output noninvasively (98,99). However, since 1985, when Skjaerpe (100) first proposed the application of Doppler echocardiography using the continuity principle for the calculation of AVA, several studies have validiated this method, which has become the method of choice for measuring AVA and assessing AS severity (92,96,101–106).

C. Continuity Principle for Measuring Aortic Valve Area

The continuity principle states that volume of flow per unit time is maintained constant at any two points in a given flow stream. Thus, in AS, volume of flow passing through the LVOT is equal to that passing through the stenotic orifice. Volume of flow is calculated by multiplying the cross-sectional area (CSA) by the flow velocity integral (FVI), which is the distance that the blood has traveled during the period of flow and which can be calculated by the equipment software from the velocity spectral signal across the respective area of flow. Thus:

$$FVI_{(LVOT)} \times CSA_{(LVOT)} = FVI_{(AV)} \times CSA_{(AV)}$$

and

$$CSA_{(AV)} = \frac{CSA_{(LVOT)} \times FVI_{(LVOT)}}{FVI_{(AV)}}$$

Assuming a circular geometry of LVOT, its area is calculated from its diameter as, area $= \pi r^2 = \pi D^2/4$.

Since the ejection times for the LVOT and aortic valve are identical, corresponding peak velocities can be substituted for the FVIs and the formula can be further modified as follows:

$$CSA_{(AV)} \ (cm^2) = \frac{\pi D^2 \times V_{(LVOT)}}{4 \times V_{(AV)}}$$

where $V_{(LVOT)}$ (in m/s) is the maximum left ventricular outflow tract velocity obtained by PWD from the apical window, with the sample volume about 1 cm proximal to the AV to avoid the velocity acceleration which occurs near the valve; $V_{(AV)}$ (in m/s) is the maximum transaortic velocity, obtained by CWD; and D (in cm) is the LVOT diameter measured by 2-DE at the points of attachment of the leaflets of the aortic valve in the parasternal long-axis or apical windows (102). Inter- and intraobserver variability in these measurement estimations have been assessed in several studies with good results (103,107).

In patients with AS, Doppler color flow imaging does not seem to play a major role in assessing severity. The turbulent flow resulting from the aliased high velocities will appear as a diffuse mosaic pattern in the ascending aorta. CFI is thus helpful in localizing the jet direction and in delineating an anteriorly directed mitral regurgitation jet from that of AS. It will also help to detect and quantify aortic regurgitation or associated mitral regurgitation. There have been few reports correlating the maximum height of the color signal of the stenotic jet, measured at the aortic valve level in the right parasternal long-axis view, to AVA estimated at catheterization with good correlation (108,109). However, the most useful role for CFI remains that of localizing the stenotic jet and determining its direction especially when eccentric, so that CWD can be aligned with it with accurate recording of the maximum velocities. Fan reported in his study that a satisfactory color signal was obtained in only 60% of their patients, although the number increased to 80% with improved expertise (110). He also reported a high correlation coefficient with respect to calculating

AVA when there was color-guided CWD examination, compared to non-color-guided examination ($r = 0.92$ compared to $r = 0.71$).

D. Limitations and Pitfalls

Because the Doppler-derived aortic valve pressure gradient depends, on flow in addition to valve area, the information it offers about aortic stenosis severity is incomplete. Quantitation of valvular stenosis, therefore, should include estimation of the valve area.

One must be aware of the limitations of the simplified Bernoulli equation. Obtaining maximum flow velocities by Doppler echocardiography is dependent on proper alignment between the ultrasound beam and direction of flow. Failure to achieve this results in lower velocities and, thus, predictable underestimation of the transaortic pressure gradient. A meticulous and systematic search utilizing all available acoustic windows is mandatory. Coexisting conditions that increase flow across the aortic valve, such as aortic regurgitation or high output states (e.g., anemia) will lead to increased flow, and thus increased velocity and gradient independent of severity of AS. In such patients, LVOT velocity, V_1, is proportionately accentuated and must not be ignored in the simplified Bernoulli equation (97,106,111), whereas conditions that decrease flow, such as impaired left ventricular function (95,103) or coexisting mitral regurgitation, will lead to decreased forward flow, velocity, and pressure gradient. The presence of atrial fibrillation will also affect gradients; velocities will vary with the wide variation in beat-to-beat stroke volumes secondary to changes in RR intervals (111). It is good practice to average 6–10 cycles.

An important limitation of the continuity equation technique remains that of the high level of expertise needed to obtain good recordings of the velocities by optimizing the angle of incidence between the Doppler beam and the stenotic jet, and in measuring LVOT diameter, where potential difficulties are expected to arise with a heavily calcific aortic valve. It is perhaps with this last calculation that the major limitation exists, because the value has to be squared and even small measurement errors can result in large errors in the calculation of aortic valve area. Oh et al. (101) suggested that a value of 25% or less for the ratio of LVOT velocity to peak transaortic jet is highly sensitive, though not specific for severe AS when LVOT diameter cannot be measured. Zoghbi et al. (112) also described a method for assessing AS severity that is independent of the measurement of aortic jet velocity, utilizing left ventricular ejection time and flow velocity integral. In spite of all this, the continuity equation for calculating AVA, being independent of left ventricular performance and of the presence of aortic regurgitation (106), remains a widely accepted, convenient, and accurate method for assessing the severity of AS.

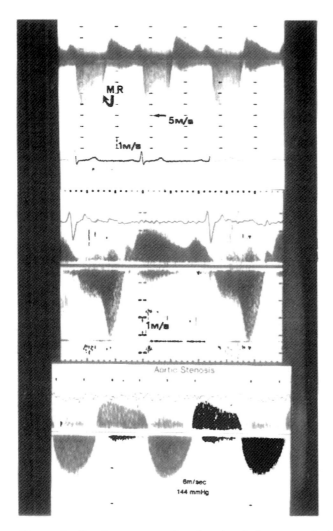

Figure 9 Continuous-wave Doppler signals from an apical window in a patient with mitral regurgitation (MR) (upper panel), a patient with dynamic left ventricular outflow tract obstruction (middle panel), and a patient with severe aortic stenosis (lower panel). Note that the MR Doppler signal (curved arrow) in the upper panel is holosystolic, with a maximum velocity of 5 m/s and the associated typical M-shaped diastolic mitral inflow signal, displayed above the zero line. The dynamic left ventricular outflow tract obstruction signal in the middle panel shows the characteristic late peaking of the velocity. Note the associated mitral stenosis, whose M-shaped inflow signal is displayed above the zero line in diastole with a maximum velocity of 2 m/s. The aortic stenosis Doppler signal in the lower panel has a maximum velocity of 6 m/s, corresponding to a gradient across the aortic valve of 144 mmHg, using the modified Bernoulli equation. Note the associated diastolic Doppler signal of aortic regurgitation above the zero line.

81

An important pitfall is to mistake mitral regurgitation high-velocity jet for AS, when the nonimaging probe is used. Careful attention to the timing and shape of the velocity spectral signal, and its relation to opening and closing valve sounds, and to diastolic signals, will help distinguish AS from MR signal (84,113) (Fig. 9). Mitral regurgitation signal will always be of higher velocity and of longer duration, covering both isovolumic contraction and relaxation periods.

E. Role of Transesophageal Echocardiography

More recently, Hoffman et al. (114) measured AVA by TEE, which allows better visualization of all leaflets, and accurate tracing of the valve orifice.

F. Summary

In summary, although a complete echocardiographic examination for assessing the severity of AS can be challenging and time-consuming, the information thus obtained is accurate, reliable, reproducible, and ideal for clinical decision making concerning the need for valve surgery in the symptomatic patient, and for longitudinal follow-up of those who are asymptomatic with less severity of the disease, thus virtually eliminating the need for catheterization. Coronary angiography is indicated if coexistent coronary artery disease is suspected, and invasive hemodynamics should be performed if Doppler echocardiographic data is incomplete or unsatisfactory.

IV. ECHOCARDIOGRAPHY IN MITRAL REGURGITATION

The mitral valve (MV) apparatus is a complex structure, consisting of the MV annulus, leaflets, chordae tendineae, papillary muscles, and the left ventricular myocardium adjacent to it (57). Competence of the MV depends on integrated normal function of this apparatus; any structural or functional abnormality in one or more of the components may result in mitral regurgitation (MR) (115).

A. Two-Dimensional Echocardiography

Two-dimensional echocardiography is particularly useful for imaging the valve apparatus in real time and identifying the structural abnormality underlying the etiology of MR, whether the transthoracic or transoesophageal approach is used (116,117). Mitral valve prolapse can be easily identified utilizing multiple views (118–120) (Fig. 10), although the parasternal long-axis view is particularly advised to avoid the overdiagnosis made by using other views, taking into consideration that the annulus is saddle shaped rather than planar (121,122). Associated leaflet thickening and redundancy, chordal thickening and elongation with or without rupture (123) and annular dilatation, can be demonstrated. 2-DE can demonstrate flail MV, with the loss of normal systolic leaflet coaptation and excessive systolic mitral leaflet motion, with or without prolapse into the left atrium (LA) (124,125), thickened rheumatic valve with or without associated stenosis (126), vegetations on the valve leaflets (127–129) (Fig. 11) with or without other complications such as chordal rupture, a flail leaflet (125,130,131), or a perivalvular abscess (132). A congenitally cleft mitral valve with (133) or without (134,145) associated ostium primum atrial septal defect, mitral annular calcification (136), and papillary muscle dysfunction with or without rupture (137,138) also can be identified. In addition, 2-DE can identify ischaemic heart disease as a possible underlying cause of MR by showing segmental wall motion abnormality (139,140), and papillary muscle dysfunction with incomplete mitral leaflet closure with or without rupture (141–144), or dilated cardiomyopathy as the underlying cause when global, severe ventricular dysfunction is demonstrated (145).

Transoesophageal echocardiography, due to the proximity of the high-frequency transducer to the LA and the MV, offers an excellent view of the MV and its apparatus and has become an excellent tool for assessing MV morphology (117), identifying vegetations on the valve with better yield compared to the transthoracic approach (129,146), and revealing complications such as abcesses, ruptured leaflets, or chordae. With color flow imaging capabilities, it has also become an excellent tool for assessing MR severity (147,148), which would be of particular use when evaluating the valve for repair and in assessing the repair intraoperatively (149).

B. Doppler Echocardiography

Doppler echocardiography allows for the unequivoval diagnosis of MR with high sensitivity and specificity, utilizing either pulsed-wave Doppler (Fig. 12, left), continuous-wave Doppler (Fig. 12, right), or color flow imaging (Fig. 13, see color plate), and permits noninvasive diagnosis of its severity. Minimal MR has been identified in normal subjects with no evidence of structural valve abnormality and has been referred to as physiological MR (150–153). It is usually detected only a short distance into the left atrium and does not last all through systole, which helps differentiate it from pathological MR.

Doppler interrogation for MR with PWD is best accomplished from an apical or a parasternal long-axis view. With the PWD range-dated sample volume positioned in the LA just proximal to the MV, the sample volume

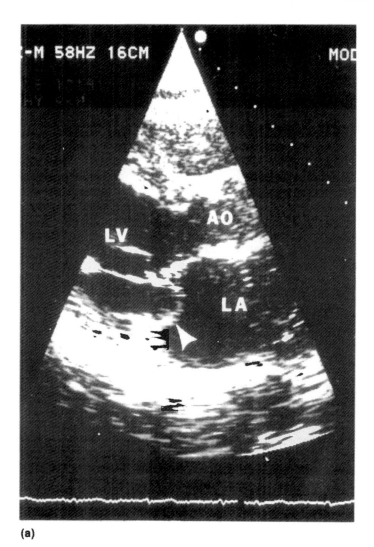

(a)

Figure 10 Two-dimensional echocardiogram, in the parasternal long-axis view from a patient with isolated prolapse of posterior leaflet of mitral valve (left panel) and a patient with prolapse of the anterior leaflet (right panel). Note the arching of the corresponding leaflet, in systole, beyond the plane of the mitral annulus into the left atrium (LA). AO = aorta, LV = left ventricle.

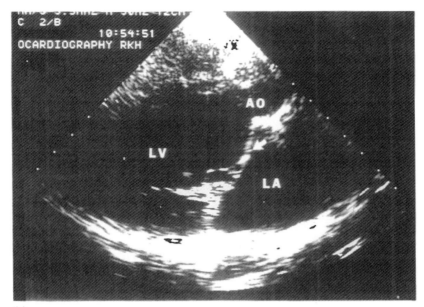

(b)

Figure 10 (*Continued*)

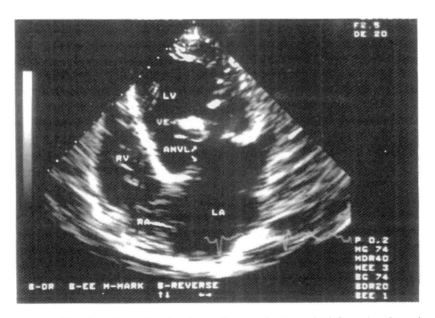

Figure 11 Two-dimensional echocardiogram in the apical four-chamber view showing a big vegetation (V) attached to the tip of the mitral valve anterior leaflet (AMVL), which itself shows a hole (two white oblique arrows). LA = left atrium, RA = right atrium, RV = right ventricle, LV = left ventricle.

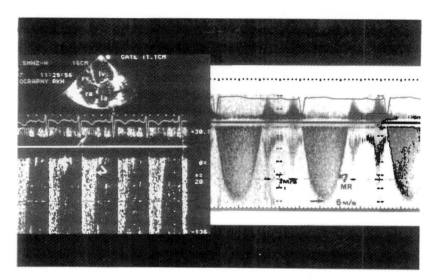

Figure 12 Pulsed-wave Doppler (left panel) and continuous-wave Doppler (right panel) velocity signals of mitral regurgitation (MR) obtained from the apical window. The pulsed-wave Doppler sample volume is placed in the left atrium (1a in the small inset picture). As the regurgitant jet velocity exceeds the Niquist limit, aliasing occurs and the velocity signal appears below (curved arrow) and above (oblique arrow) the zero reference line. The continuous-wave Doppler MR velocity signal in the right panel is of strong intensity, holosystolic, and of a maximum velocity of 6 m/s. Note the associated typical m-shaped mitral diastolic inflow velocity signal above the zero line. LV = left ventricle, RA = right atrium, RV = right ventricle.

is moved within the LA to detect the retrograde systolic blood flow (154–156). Small eccentric jets may be missed if interrogration with the PWD sample volume is not performed from different windows or transducer angulations, or if the mapping was incomplete. CFI, on the other hand, provides an excellent real-time visual display of the MR mosaic systolic jet originating at the MV and extending retrogradely into the LA (6,157–159). It is especially useful in detecting unusual eccentric jets. CWD is utilized to obtain the full MR velocity envelope, with a peak velocity that is usually high, exceeding 4.5 m/s, due to the high pressure difference between the left ventricle and LA. The peak velocity of the MR jet bears no relationship to MR severity. The best window for CWD interrogation is the apical, although multiple transducer angulations should be utilized to try and capture the complete regurgitant jet and to differentiate it from aortic stenosis or tricuspid regurgitation flow; careful attention to the timing and shape of the velocity spectral signal and its relation to opening and closing valve sounds, and to diastolic signals, will help in the differentiation (113).

C. Mitral Regurgitation Quantitation

Several methods have been devised to utilize Doppler in assessing MR noninvasively. Earlier techniques involved the use of PWD to map the spatial extension of the systolic regurgitant jet within the LA (155). The wider the jet and the further it was detected into the LA, the more severe the MR. Abbasi et al. (155) showed a good correlation between MR assessed in this manner and that assessed by angiography ($r = 0.88$). MR underestimation can be caused by eccentric jets which may be missed with incomplete mapping of the LA, by impaired left ventricular function which will make the regurgitant jet smaller, or in the presence of a huge LA.

CFI is now the most accepted and utilized methodology for semiquantitation of MR (Fig. 14, see color plate). Miyatake et al. (159) graded MR severity on the basis of both maximal jet length from valve orifice and the regurgitant jet area, with good correlation compared to angiographic grading of MR ($r = 0.87$ and $r = 0.83$, respectively). Maximum jet width, height, and area were utilized for grading MR severity with varying coefficient of correlation (158,160,161). However, the best correlation was obtained when the maximum regurgitant jet areas from three planes (parasternal long axis, parasternal short axis, and apical four-chamber) were expressed as a percentage of left atrial area. A value <20% indicated mild MR, while a value of 40% or above was in keeping with severe MR (158). The limitations inherent in CFI include its dependence on optimizing gain, filter, and transducer frequency (162), optimizing the angle of incidence between Doppler beam and the jet to as near zero as possible, and the dependence of the regurgitant jet area on left ventricular contractility and afterload (163). Color flow imaging may also underestimate the severity of MR if the jet is eccentric (wall jet).

Several features of the CWD signal provide clues as to the severity of the MR. Hatle and Angelsen (164) reported that there is a direct relationship between the intensity of signal judged by the gray scale on the full spectral display and that of severity of the MR, using the intensity of mitral forward diastolic flow as a reference. An early-occurring peak velocity to the MR signal with rapid deceleration is also indicative of a significant regurgitation causing rapid increase in LA pressure and equalization of pressure between it and the left ventricle. In the absence of mitral stenosis, an increased diastolic mitral forward flow velocity is indicative of a large regurgitant volume. Mitral regurgitation CWD signal is also utilized to measure the rate of left ventricular pressure rise (dP/dt) (Fig. 15), which can reflect left ventricular (LV) function; a faster rate reflects a better ejection fraction and thus better LV function (165,166).

The main quantitative method for assessing the severity of MR remains that of measuring the regurgitant volume and the regurgitant fraction, using combined 2-DE and PWD echocardiography (167–170). In the absence of shunts or other left-sided lesions, the difference between total forward MV inflow and that of net aortic valve outflow is the regurgitant volume (RV). The ratio of RV to the MV inflow is the regurgitant fraction. Flow at each respective valve is calculated by multiplying the corresponding area measured by 2-DE, by the flow valocity integral measured by PWD at the corresponding anulus (170). A major source of error for this method lies in the measurement of mitral and aortic anulus areas and in the accurate measurement of flow velocity, which necessitates meticulous care and experience in equipment gain setting and proper positioning of

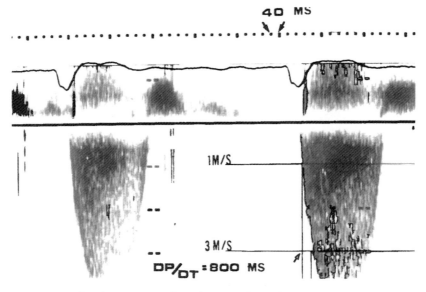

Figure 15 Continuous-wave Doppler recording of mitral regurgitation velocity signal in a patient with impaired left ventricular function, showing the calculation of the rate of pressure rise, dP/dT. The time for the velocity to increase from 1 m/s to 3 m/s is 0.04 s (two arrows), corresponding to a rate of pressure rise of 800 mmHg/s, which is below normal, reflecting an impaired left ventricular function. [$dP/dT = 4(3)^2 - 4(1)^2/0.04$ mmHg/s].

sample volume at the respective anulus to obtain a narrow angle of incidence between the Doppler beam and the jet. Recently, Jenni et al. (171)
described a method for quantitying MR that is independent of the need
to measure orifice areas. Even more recently, several studies have been
reported of measuring regurgitant flow utilizing the proximal isovelocity
surface area (PISA) technique by CFI, which takes advantage of the flow
convergence region proximal to the regurgitant orifice and its blue–red
interface to provide a method for measuring flow across it, applying the
continuity principle. The technique seems to be relatively insensitive to
changes in machine factors such as gain or wall filter, or to changes in
orifice size or shape. This method has been validated in both in-vitro
models (172–175) and in-vivo canine models (176), and its application has
been extended to patients with MR (177). Another method makes use of
the fluid dynamics principle of conservation of momentum of free turbulent jets and has been well validated in both in-vitro (178) and in-vivo
canine models (179); once it is validated in clinical situations, it holds
good promise of providing a quantitative measure of regurgitant flow from
information that is intrinsic to the jet alone.

D. Summary

Transthoracic echocardiography has emerged as the procedure of choice
for noninvasive assessment of MR, diagnosing it with high sensitivity and
specificity, determining its etiology, quantitating its severity, and assessing its impact on ventricular size and function. Its ability to provide close,
noninvasive, longitudinal follow-up of ventricular size and function, which
seems to play the major role in decision making concerning surgery, has
greatly improved our ability to manage patients with MR. Transesophageal
examination is ideal for delineation of valvular pathology and also for
semiquantitation of MR.

   The role of cardiac catheterization is primarily to detect associated
coronary disease and, rarely, for confirmation of severity of MR in patients with technically inadequate transthoracic 2-DE/Doppler examination.

V. ECHOCARDIOGRAPHY IN AORTIC REGURGITATION

Aortic regurgitation (AR) is usually the result of abnormalities of the aortic
valve, the aortic root, or both (180,181). Bedside diagnosis of AR can be
made easily by the peripheral signs and the characteristic decrescendo
diastolic blowing murmur at the base of the heart with radiation along the
sternal border (182,183). However, the ability to assess accurately the

severity of regurgitation remains a challenge. The duration of the diastolic murmur and the pulse pressure can provide a semiquantitative assessment of the severity of AR. ECG voltage changes (184), cardiothoracic ratio on chest roentgenograms (184,185), and radionuclide studies at rest and during exercise (186–188) can all help monitor progress of AR and identify clinical factors that detect early development of left ventricular dysfunction. Aortography can detect AR and semiquantitate its severity, but it is invasive and impractical as either a screening test or for repeated evaluations. Two-dimensional and Doppler echocardiography provide noninvasive means for accurate diagnosis and assessment of hemodynamic severity of AR and allow repeated evaluation over prolonged periods of followup for progression of disease and monitoring of LV function.

A. Two-Dimensional Echocardiography

Two-dimensional echocardiography, either transthoracic or transesophageal, can clearly define AV and aortic root anatomic abnormalities and thus characterize the etiology underlying the AR. The presence of a bicuspid (78,79) (Fig. 16) or a quadricuspid AV (189,190), or a rheumatic valve

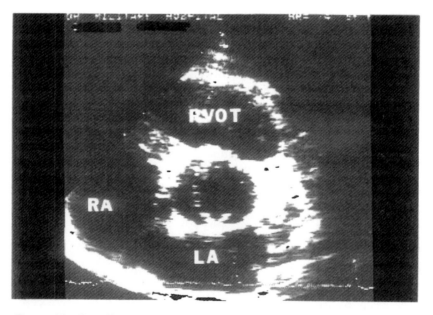

Figure 16 Two-dimensional echocardiogram in the parasternal short-axis view at the level of aortic valve, showing a bicuspid aortic valve in systole. LA = left atrium, RA = right atrium, RVOT = right ventricular outflow tract.

with leaftlet thickening and deformity, will be revealed by 2-DE utilizing the parasternal short-axis view. The parasternal long-axis view will demonstrate a flail or prolapsed aortic leaflet (191–195). Both parasternal and apical views will allow for direct visualization of vegetations (131,192,196) (Fig. 17) and other complications of endocarditis, such as aortic ring abscesses, with or without extension into surrounding structures (132,197–199), ruptured AV leaflets (191,192), or satellite lesions on surrounding structures (200). Transesophageal echocardiography aids in detection of small vegetations and perivalvular abscesses (146,201), and with the help of color flow imaging, Doppler localizes the regurgitant jet (202). Using right, left parasternal, and suprasternal views will help demonstrate aneurysmal dilatation of the aortic root (203–205) (Fig. 18) and demonstrate aortic dissection with the true and false lumens and the intimal flap (204–207) (Fig. 19). TEE has markedly increased the sensitivity of detection of aortic dissection and defining its extent (208–211).

2-D- and M-mode echocardiography can demonstrate the effect of AR on surrounding structures and the appearance of the valve itself. The high-frequency fluttering of anterior mitral leaflet and/or the interventricular septum have been the hallmark of aortic regurgitation (212–214) (Fig. 20). However, this feature lacks sensitivity and bears no relationship to sever-

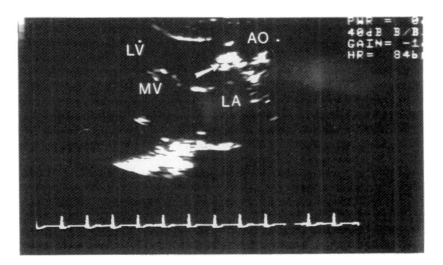

Figure 17 Two-dimensional echocardiogram in the parasternal long-axis view showing a large vegetation (arrow) attached to the noncoronary cusp of the aortic valve and prolapsing into left ventricular outflow tract in diastole (note the open position of the mitral valve, MV). AO = aorta, LA = left atrium, LV = left ventricle.

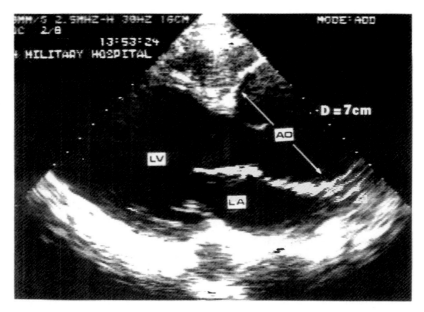

Figure 18 Two-dimensional echocardiogram in the parasternal long-axis view, in a patient with Marfan's syndrome and aortic regurgitation (note dilated left ventricle, LV). The ascending aorta (AO) is abnormally dilated with a diameter of 7 cm. LA = left atrium.

ity. M-mode is particularly useful in determining LV size and function by measuring LV end-diastolic and end-systolic dimensions, fraction shortening, and ejection fraction (215–217). In addition, wall thickness and systolic wall stress can be assessed (218–220). All these measurements reflect the effect of AR volume overload on the LV and can be periodically measured and serially followed for proper timing of surgery (216,217,219–224).

Acute AR, which usually results from endocarditis or aortic dissection, is an entity in itself, characterized by a fulminant course leading rapidly to death unless intensive medical therapy and surgery are undertaken urgently. 2-DE, by demonstrating the underlying cause, will establish the diagnosis, which can be supported by Doppler echocardiography. M-mode echocardiography will demonstrate premature diastolic closure of the mitral valve (225–228) (Fig. 21) with or without premature diastolic opening of the aortic valve (227,229,230). Both are the result of the hemodynamic effect of acute severe AR on markedly increasing left ventricular end-diastolic pressure, thus exceeding left atrial pressure—causing the prema-

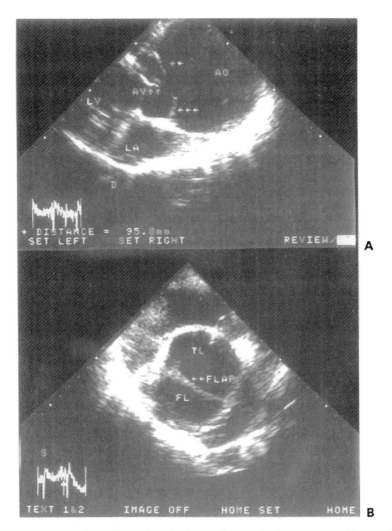

Figure 19 Two-dimensional echocardiogram in the parasternal long-axis (A) and the short-axis view at level of aortic root (B), in a patient with dissection of ascending aorta showing the true lumen of the aorta (AO), the false lumen of the dissection (FL), and the intimal flap in between. AV = aortic valve, LV = left ventricle, LA = left atrium.

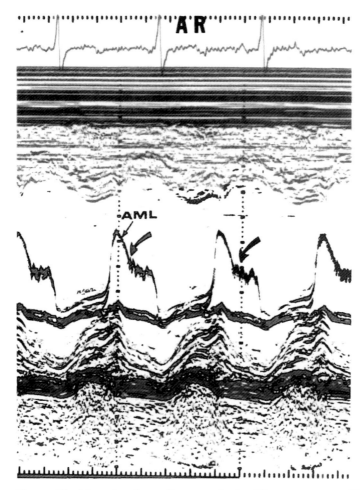

Figure 20 M-mode echocardiogram, obtained from a parasternal long-axis view, in a patient with aortic regurgitation, showing the high-frequency fluttering (curved arrow) of the anterior mitral leaflet (AML).

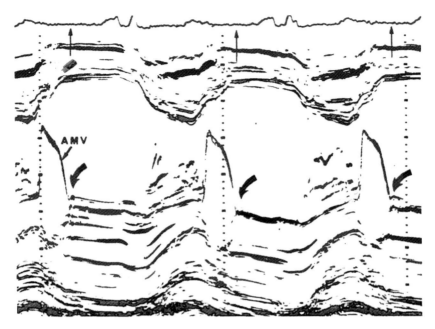

Figure 21   M-mode echocardiogram in a patient with aortic regurgitation showing low-frequency flutter of anterior mitral leaflet, AMV (short straight arrow), and premature closure of the mitral valve (curved arrow) before the beginning of systole and QRS complex (vertical thin arrow). The echogenecity in the left ventricular outflow tract to the left AML is related to the ruptured flail aortic leaflet, which is the underlying cause for this severe aortic regurgitation.

ture closure of MV, and the aortic diastolic pressure—causing the premature (diastolic) opening of the AV (231).

B. Doppler Echocardiography

The addition of Doppler echocardiography to the standard 2-D imaging markedly improved the sensitivity of diagnosing AR, allowed for direct demonstration of the diastolic regurgitant flow into the left ventricle, and provided a number of methods to evaluate the hemodynamic severity of the regurgitation.

Aortic regurgitation results in turbulent holodiastolic flow with a high velocity (in excess of 4 m/s), due to the high pressure difference between early diastolic aortic pressure and left ventricular diastolic pressure (Fig. 22). The flow direction and localization is variable, and different transducer positions are utilized to align the Doppler beam with that of the jet.

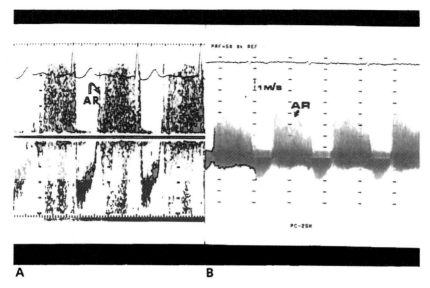

A   **B**

Figure 22   Pulsed-wave Doppler (A) and continuous-wave Doppler (B) velocity signals in two patients with aortic regurgitation, obtained from an apical window. The pulsed-wave Doppler sample volume is placed in the left ventricular outflow tract just below the aortic valve, and a holodiastolic velocity signal is picked with aliasing with the signal displayed both above the zero reference line (curved arrow) and below it. The continuous-wave Doppler signal is also holodiastolic, with a peak early diastolic velocity of 4.5 m/s, slow decay of velocity, and a high end-diastolic velocity, implying mild aortic regurgitation.

Scanning windows should include the apical, left and right parasternal., and suprasternal.

1. Pulsed-Wave Doppler

AR can be detected using pulsed-wave Doppler by positioning the sample volume in the left ventricular outflow tract to record the diastolic turbulent flow of AR (182,232–236). Many studies describe a sensitivity of 82–100% of PWD in detecting AR. Doppler is extremely sensitive and may detect AR even when no diastolic murmur is detected by auscultation (182,233,236).

   The original description for the quantitative assessment of AR by PWD described flow mapping of the spatial extent of the regurgitant jet in length, utilizing the parasternal long-axis view (234) with a good correlation (*n* = 0.88) when compared to angiographic assessment of AR. Veyrat et al. (232) also described a grading method for AR using PWD to map the regurgitant area in the parasternal short-axis view to calculate what was referred to as the "valvular regurgitant index," which is the ratio of the above to aortic valve orifice area in the same view. Both methods, however, are tedious and time-consuming and may lead to underestimation of the severity when the mapping is incomplete. When the right parasternal or suprasternal views are utilized to detect diastolic reversal in the aorta caused by AR, PWD alone or guided by CFI is useful for semiquantitative assessment of AR. A significant degree of AR causes substantial diastolic reversal of flow in both the ascending and descending aorta (237–240) (Fig. 23). The ratio of the reversed to the forward flow velocity integrals determines the AR fraction. Quinones et al. (238) proposed that a ratio of 30% or more reliably differentiates mild from moderate AR. One should note that a mild degree of flow reversal in the aorta occurs normally in early diastole immediately following AV closure, and that is why this method is less specific for diagnosis of mild AR. One should also exclude

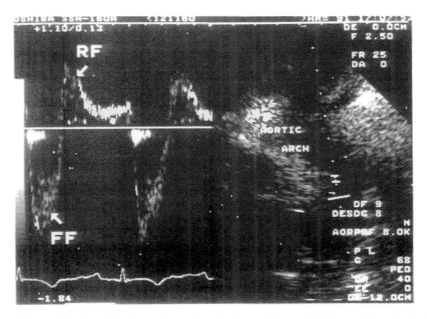

Figure 23 Combined two-dimensional echocardiogram (right panel) and pulsed-wave Doppler signal (left panel) obtained from the suprasternal window, with the pulsed-wave Doppler sampled volume placed in the descending aorta. Note the normal antegrade systolic forward flow signal (FF) displayed below the zero reference line and the holodiastolic retrograde flow signal (RF) of aortic regurgitation, displayed above the zero line.

the presence of a patent ductus arteriosus or surgical aortopulmonary shunts, which can cause diastolic reversal of aortic flow independent of the severity of AR. Reversal of flow in the subclavian artery and in the abdominal aorta has also been used to assess severity of AR (241).

2. Regurgitant Volume and Regurgitant Fraction

Combined 2-D and PWD echocardiography is utilized to determine regurgitant volume and regurgitant fraction as an absolute method for quantitation of severity of AR (170,242). This requires calculation of the total systolic flow volume across the AV and comparing it to the net forward flow volume at the mitral or pulmonary valve. Volumetric flow through these valves is calculated as the product of the cross-sectional area of the valve annulus, by the flow velocity integral (continuity equation: "What goes in, must come out"). The difference between these two flow volumes represents the regurgitant volume (RV), and the ratio of RV to the total flow volume through the aortic valve is the regurgitant fraction (RF). These measurements correspond closely to regurgitant fractions assessed at cardiac catheterization, whether the mitral ($n = 0.91$) (170) or the pulmonic ($n = 0.94$) (242) flows are used. This method, however, should not be used if there is coexistent (more than mild) mitral or pulmonary valvular regurgitation.

3. Color Flow Imaging

Color flow imaging has considerably facilitated the detection and semiquantitation of AR, with a reported sensitivity for detection ranging from 92% to 100% (157,243,244) (Fig. 24, see color plate). The regurgitant jet is composed of mosaic colors in the left ventricular outflow tract, and the length of the jet bears only a modest correlation to the angiographic grading of AR (243,245). Better correlation was found when the width/area of the jet was measured relative to width/area of LVOT in the parasternal long-axis and short-axis views, respectively (243,246). Perry et al. proposed that a ratio of the width of the AR jet to that of the LVOT less than 4% identifies grade I AR, 4–24% grade II, 25–59% grade III, and >60% grade IV (243).

Potential limitations exist for the use of CFI in assessing the degree of aortic regurgitation. The color flow signal varies with equipment gain setting, transducer frequency, and pulse repetition frequency (247). Hemodynamic factors such as blood pressure, peripheral resistance, size of LV and its compliance, left ventricular end diastolic pressure, and length of diastole all can affect the size of the jet. However, in spite of these limitations, CFI is widely applied and clinically useful for detection and semiquantitation of aortic regurgitation.

4. Continuous-Wave Doppler

Continuous-wave Doppler also offers quantitative assessment of AR. The intensity of this signal has been proposed to reflect the severity of AR semiquantitatively (248). Thus, patients with mild AR have a faint diastolic signal, while those with severe AR have a strong (dark) signal.

The diastolic flow velocity signal of AR by CWD is characterized by an increased early peak velocity with variable rate of deceleration (deceleration slope) depending on the severity of AR. This rate of deceleration is a measure of the rate with which aortic and left ventricular pressures equate during diastole and can be a reflection of the severity of AR (249–252). A rate higher than $3m/s^2$ is usually indicative of severe AR.

5. Doppler Pressure Half-Time

The deceleration slope is also used to calculate pressure half-time (249,252–254). It is the time taken for diastolic transaortic pressure gradient to decay by 50% (Fig. 25). The principle of the Doppler velocity $t^{1/2}$ is based on the fact that in severe AR the pressure gradient between the aorta and LV decreases rapidly through diastole with the rapid increase in left ventricular end-diastolic pressure (LVEDP). This $t^{1/2}$ has been shown to correlate well with AR assessed by aortography, with an inverse relationship. A $t^{1/2}$ of 400 ms has been proposed by Teague et al. (253) to divide moderate from moderately severe AR, with a specificity of 92% and a predictive positive value of 90%. A short pressure $t^{1/2}$ of less than 200 ms is associated with severe AR. Quantitation of AR using the pressure half-time method has its limitations. The decrease in gradient across the AV in diastole is influenced by other factors than the size of the regurgitant orifice: It is affected by aortic root and LV complicance, peripheral resistance, and by extreme elevation of LVEDP (53,253). However, it seems to be independent of heart rate and angle of incidence, which is why it is one of the widely applied parameters to assess AR.

Closely related to this mechanism of increasing left ventricular end-diastolic pressure by the aortic regurgitation is the effect of hemodynamically significant AR on reducing mitral valve deceleration time and increasing the early filling (E) wave velocity as shown by pulsed Doppler examination of mitral inflow (255). Also demonstrated is diastolic mitral regurgitation by both PWD (225) and CFI both in real time and M-mode (256) when LVEDP exceeds left atrial pressure in late diastole.

The flow velocity signal of AR can also be used to estimate left-ventricular end diastolic pressure by subtracting the end diastolic gradient [obtained by the modified Bernoulli equation: $4 \times$ (end diastolic velocity)^2] from the cuff diastolic blood pressure (251,254). It should be noted, however, that to obtain these measurements, high-quality spectral recording

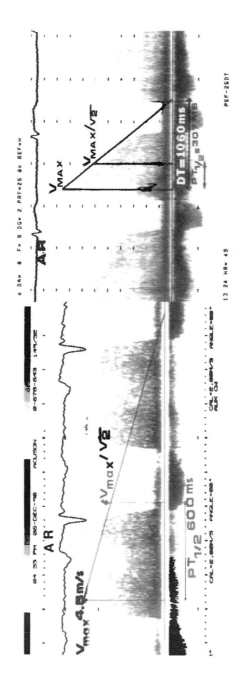

Figure 25 Continuous-wave Doppler signal, obtained from an apical window, in a patient with moderately severe (right panel) and mild (left panel) aortic regurgitation, showing the calculation of the pressure half-time. Note the faster slope of the line of velocity decay, with low end diastolic velocity of 2 m/s and the short pressure half-time ($PT^{1/2}$) of 307 ms in the right panel, compared to the slow slope of line of velocity decay, higher end-diastolic velocity of 4 m/s, and longer $PT_{1/2}$ of 600 in the left panel.

must be meticulously obtained, and a pitfall is the assumption that cuff diastolic blood pressure is essentially the same as aortic diastolic pressure.

C. Summary

In summary, for the diagnosis of AR and for assessment of its severity, all echocardiographic modalities should be employed and should be complementary to each other. Conventional 2-DE, supplemented more recently with the transesophageal approach, is still the diagnostic method of choice for determining the etiology of AR. Along with M-mode echocardiography, it is still an excellent noninvasive basis for evaluating LV size and function, lending support for a decision on timing of surgery. Pulsed-wave Doppler, continuous-wave Doppler, and color flow image echocardiography, in addition to identifying the regurgitation, also allow for quantitative assessment of the severity of AR. In expert hands, the above can supply all the information needed concerning the severity of the condition and timing of surgery, leaving preoperative cardiac catheterization to be considered only when there may be associated coronary artery disease or when suboptimal echocardiographic data are obtained.

VI. ECHOCARDIOGRAPHY IN PULMONARY VALVE DISEASE

Pulmonic valve stenosis (PS) is a common congenital cardiac malformation occurring in isolation or in association with other congenital abnormalities and accounting for 80% of cases of right ventricular outflow tract (RVOT) obstruction. Rarely it is acquired secondary to rheumatic or carcinoid heart disease, in which case it is usually associated with pulmonary regurgitation (PR) and other valve involvement. PR, on the other hand, is acquired secondary to pulmonary artery dilatation caused by pulmonary hypertension of any etiology, structural changes in the valve itself caused by rheumatic or carcinoid heart disease or endocarditis, or postsurgical treatment for PS.

A. Two-Dimensional Echocardiography

The pulmonic valve (PV) is best visualized utilizing the parasternal short-axis and the subcostal views. With lateral and superior angulation of the transducer in the parasternal position, optimal images can be obtained of the RVOT, of only two leaflets of the PV, and of the pulmonary artery (PA) and its bifurcations. Valve morphology and associated chamber changes can be evaluated. In PS, the leaflets are characteristically thickened, with restricted motion and systolic doming (257). Associated right ventricular (RV) hypertrophy and/or dilation will be demonstrated. The shortened, thickened, and fixed position of a carcinoid valve with associated tricuspid valve involvement (258,259), or a valve with vegetations, will also be demonstrated (260,261). Doppler echocardiogrphy is necessary, however, for direct demonstration of PS or PR.

B. Doppler Echocardiography

The sample volume of pulsed-wave Doppler moved from the RVOT across the valve and into the PA can help localize the level of obstruction. If PS is mild, a maximal velocity will be obtained by PWD without aliasing; however continuous-wave Doppler is utilized to record higher systolic velocities (V) (262) (Fig. 26). If there is associated subvalvular stenosis, velocities that originate proximal to the valve and the higher velocities across the valve itself can frequently be recorded superimposed on each other simultaneously (263) (Fig. 27). Utilizing V in the simplified Bernoulli equation (pressure gradient $= 4V^2$), a good estimate of the severity of the stenosis is obtained.

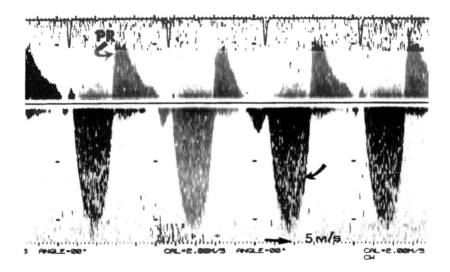

Figure 26 Continuous-wave Doppler signal obtained from a parasternal position in a patient with severe valvular pulmonary stenosis and combined pulmonary regurgitation (PR). The systolic signal peak velocity is 5 m/s, corresponding to a gradient across the pulmonary valve of 100 mmHg, using the modified Bernoulli equation.

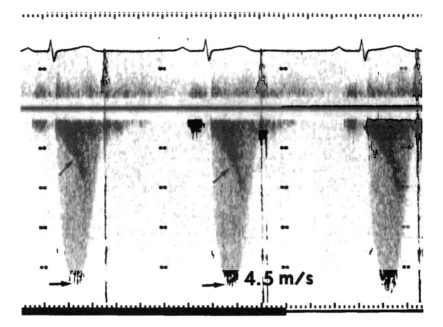

Figure 27 Continuous-wave Doppler signal, recorded from the parasternal position, showing two superimposed signals: one of severe valvular pulmonary stenosis with a peak velocity of 4.5 m/s corresponding to a valve gradient of 80 mmHg; and the superimposed one (oblique arrow), with late systolic peaking, in keeping with subvalvular dynamic obstruction.

Doppler-measured systolic gradients correlated highly with gradients measured at cardiac catheterization (262,264). Color flow imaging, which will demonstrate a mosaic pattern beginning at valve level and extending distally for variable distances into main PA, may be utilized to align the CWD beam with that of the stenotic jet to obtain the highest possible velocity. Pressure gradient is dependent on flow, in addition to valve area, and thus severity of obstruction may be underestimated in the presence of RV dysfunction, or overestimated in the presence of associated significant PR and other associated shunt lesions. Kosturakis et al. used ejection time and velocity across the stenosed PV to calculate PV areas, with good correlation with PV area obtained at cardiac catheterization (265). Theoretically also, estimation of PV area is possible by applying the continuity equation as applied for aortic valve area. The pressure gradient as measured by CWD, however, remains a good method for estimating severity of PS and is utilized to assess results post surgery or percutaneous balloon valvuloplasty (266–269) and to serially follow the patients (270,271).

Trivial PR, referred to as physiological PR, is seen in the majority of the normal population and is identified by the three Doppler modalities, although CFI is the most sensitive (152–153,272). It demonstrates an orange-red jet originating at the PV and extending retrogradely only for a short distance into the RVOT (usually for less than 1 cm). This limited extension of the PR jet will differentiate it from the pathological regurgitation in which the jet is mosaic and extends for longer distances into the RVOT (Fig. 28, see color plate). Nanda et al. (273) utilized CFI to assess the severity of PR, taking into consideration the maximum depth of the regurgitant jet into the RVOT, as well as the maximum width at its origin in the parasternal short-axis view at the level of the aortic valve. If a jet occupies at its origin more than 50% of RVOT diameter, or if it extends to within 1 cm of the tricuspid valve, it is considered to be associated with severe PR. However, this criterion lacks validation, as no angiographic "gold standard" exists.

Although PWD is utilized to localize and map PR jet (274–276), CWD is better for capturing the complete flow velocity signal of the regurgitant jet all through diastole (277). This flow velocity signal has a characteristic shape with maximal early diastolic peak velocity that gradually decreases, maintaining a stable velocity until end-diastole, with a characteristic decrease in the velocity with atrial contraction. The intensity of the velocity signal reflects the severity of the PR. The shape of the signal also reflects the severity: Significant PR will result in rapid deceleration with minimal velocity at end-diastole (Fig. 29), reflecting the rapid equalization of pressures between PA and right ventricle. Significant PR will also be associated with increased forward flow systolic velocities, and a late diastolic regurgitation across a partially closed tricuspid valve (278).

The CWD signal of PR can be utilized to calculate pulmonary artery pressure (PAP). Masuyama et al. (277) showed that end-diastolic pressure gradient calculated from end-diastolic PR velocity applying the Bernoulli equation, to which an estimate of RA pressure is added, correlated well with PA diastolic pressure ($r = 0.94$, SEE 4 mmHg) and that pressure gradient calculated similarly from early diastolic PR velocity correlated well with mean PAP obtained at cardiac catheterization ($r = 0.92$, SEE $= 7$ mmHg). The PWD velocity signal of the flow in the RVOT proximal to the PV also contains information about PAP utilizing acceleration time (which is the time from onset of ejection to peak velocity) (279,280), and/ or its ratio to RV ejection time (281–283), or the interval between PV closure to TV opening (284), with good correlation to PAP obtained at

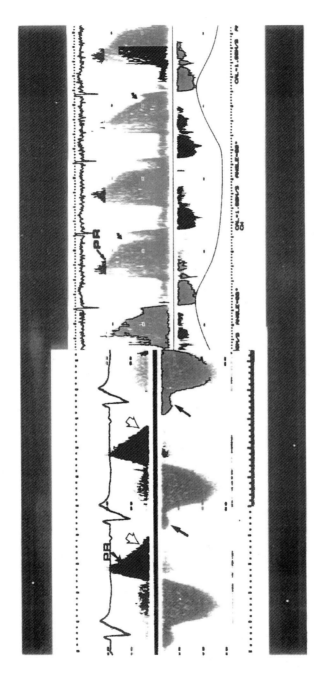

Figure 29 Continuous-wave Doppler signals, obtained from the parasternal position in a patient with mild pulmonary regurgitation (right panel) and a patient with severe pulmonary regurgitation (left panel). Note the rapid deceleration with minimal velocity at end-diastole in the latter (open arrows) compared to the slow deceleration and high velocity at end-diastole in the former (curved small arrows).

catheterization. In the absence of PS, the most commonly used method for measuring systolic PAP is to use the tricuspid regurgitation signal as described later under tricuspid valve disease.

Regurgitant volume and fraction calculated as for aortic regurgitation, comparing the total forward flow across the PV to the net forward flow across mitral, aortic, or tricuspid valves and assuming the excess flow at the PV to be due to the PR, can be utilized to assess the severity of PR quantitatively. Goldberg and Allen (274) also described a method for quantitating PR by comparing areas under forward and regurgitant velocity integrals utilizing PWD echocardiography.

C. Summary

Doppler echocardiography, in addition to identifying PS and PR and quantifying them, has opened new avenues for measuring PAP noninvasively, which is very important in clinical evaluation and decision making before therapeutic interventions are considered in many cardiac diseases.

VII. ECHOCARDIOGRAPHY IN TRICUSPID VALVE DISEASE

A. Tricuspid Stenosis

Tricuspid stenosis (TS) as an isolated lesion is rare and is almost always associated with tricuspid regurgitation (TR). It is rheumatic in origin in the majority of cases (285), and thus is invariably associated with mitral valve disease. Rarely, it could be associated with other conditions such as malignant carcinoid disease and use of ergot alkaloids (258,259,286).

1. Two-Dimensional Echocardiography

The tricuspid valve (TV) can be visualized easily from the parasternal RV inflow and short-axis views, apical, and subcostal four-chamber views. Two-dimensional echocardiographic findings of TS include valve thickening, restricted motion with diastolic doming (Fig. 30), increase in right atrial size, and associated other valvular involvement (287–291). TS severity is best determined by Doppler echocardiography.

2. Doppler Echocardiography

Tricuspid inflow Doppler signal is best obtained from the low-parasternal RV inflow or apical four-chamber views. With the pulsed-wave Doppler sample volume placed in the RV immediately distal to the TV, a velocity spectral signal is recorded that is qualitatively similar to that of mitral stenosis but with lesser magnitude and with respiratory variation (Fig. 31). As in MS, the early diastolic velocity is increased with decrease in

COLOR PLATES

Figure 6 Color-flow Doppler velocity signal in the apical four-chamber view in a patient with severe mitral stenosis, showing the characteristic flame-shaped, mosaic high-velocity signal, starting at the mitral valve (MV) and extending into the left ventricle. LA = left atrium, RA = right atrium.

Figure 13 Color-flow Doppler velocity map, in the parasternal long-axis view, demonstrating severe mitral regurgitation (MR). The mosaic color regurgitant signal (arrows) originates at the mitral valve (MV) and extends retrogradely to fill almost the whole of the left atrium (LA). LV = left ventricle, RV = right ventricle, AO = aorta.

Figure 14 Color-flow Doppler velocity map in a patient with severe mitral stenosis (A, parasternal long-axis view), showing the mosaic color regurgitant signal (arrow) occupying almost half of the left atrium (LA), and a patient with mild mitral regurgitation (B, apical four-chamber view) with a small mosaic color regurgitant signal (arrow) directed laterally. Note the prolapse of the anterior mitral leaflet in the lower panel, which is the cause underlying the mitral regurgitation in this patient. AO = aorta, LV = left ventricle.

Figure 24 Color-flow Doppler velocity map in a patient with aortic regurgitation (AR), in the apical four-chamber view (upper panel) and the parasternal long-axis view (right lower panel), showing the mosaic color regurgitant signal occupying the left ventricular outflow tract and extending into the body of the left ventricle. Note the m-mode color scan of AR in the left lower panel. LA = left atrium, LV = left ventricle, RA = right atrium, RV = right ventricle, AV = aortic valve.

Figure 28 Combined two-dimensional (right panel) and pulsed-Doppler (left panel) echocardiograms in the parasternal short-axis view at the level of the aortic root. The sample volume is placed in the right ventricular (RV) outflow tract, just proximal to the pulmonary valve (PV). The pulsed-wave Doppler signal shows the aliased diastolic high-velocity signal of pulmonary regurgitation (PR) (multiple arrows). LA = left atrium, RA = right atrium.

Figure 32 Color-flow Doppler velocity map, in the apical four-chamber view, in a patient with severe rheumatic tricuspid stenosis, showing the characteristic flame-shaped mosaic jet, starting at the tricuspid valve and extending into the right ventricle (RV). LA = left atrium, LV = left ventricle, RA = right atrium.

Figure 34 Color-flow Doppler velocity map in a patient with mild tricuspid regurgitation (TR), in the apical four-chamber view (arrow, upper panel), and a patient with severe TR, in the parasternal right ventricular inflow view, with the TR mosaic signal occupying more than half of the dilated right atrium (arrow, lower panel). LA = left atrium, RA = right atrium, RV = right ventricle, TV = tricuspid valve.

Figure 35 Color-flow Doppler velocity map of the inferior vena cava (IVC) and hepatic vein (HV), obtained from a subcostal view, showing retrograde systolic flow (note ECG gating) into them (red, toward transducer) in a patient with severe tricuspid regurgitation. RA = right atrium.

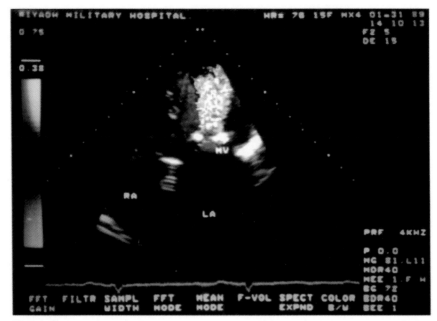

Figure 6

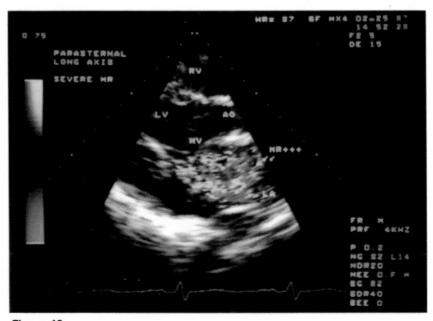

Figure 13

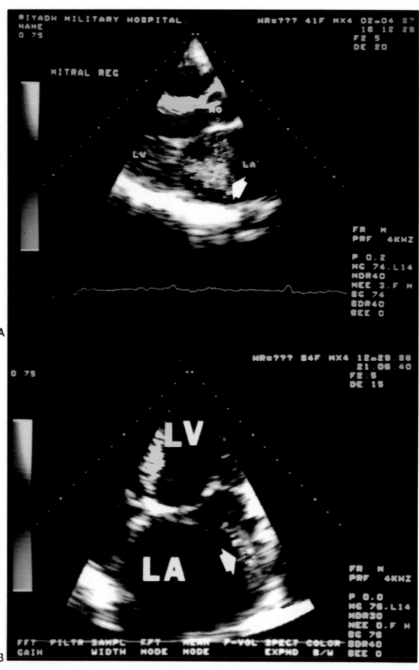

Figure 14

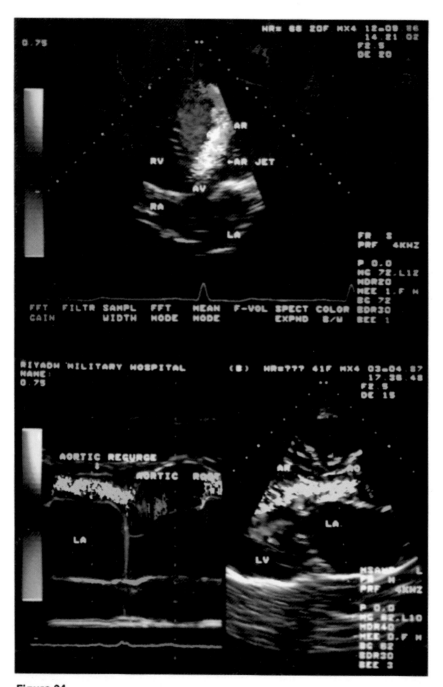

Figure 24

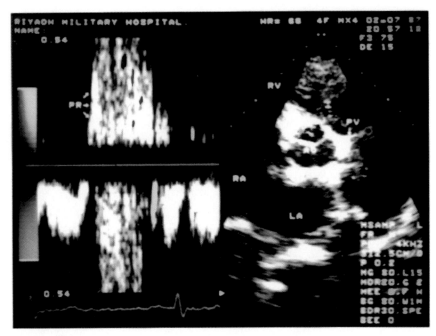

Figure 28

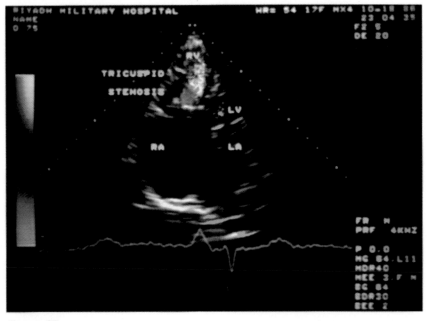

Figure 32

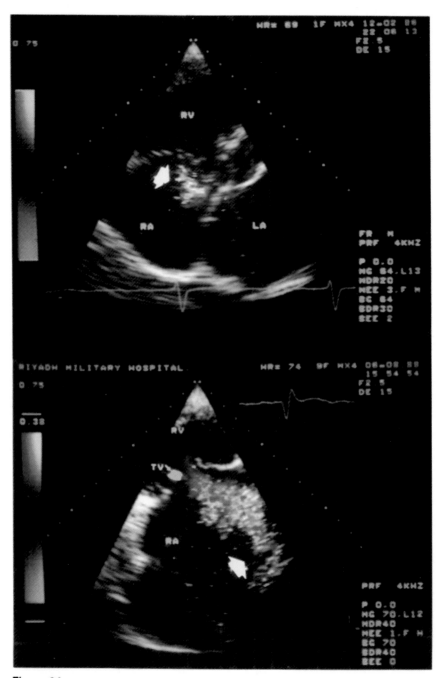

Figure 34

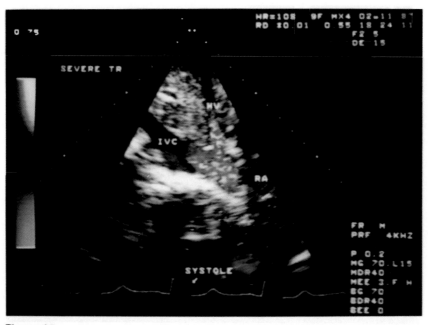

Figure 35

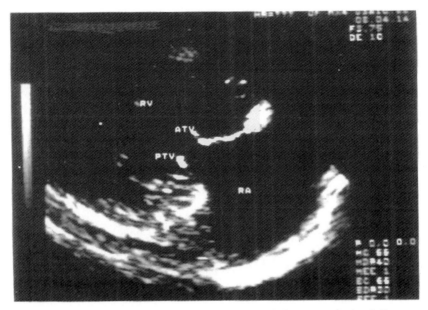

Figure 30 Two-dimensional echocardiogram of right ventricular inflow tract showing the anterior leaflet (ATV) and posterior leaflet (PTV) of a rheumatically stenosed tricuspid valve, with restriction, thickening of the leaflets, and a dilated right atrium (RA). RV = right ventricle.

its rate of decline (291–293). This velocity may still be within the velocity limits of the PWD system, even with severe TS, and thus is usually recorded without aliasing. Continuous-wave Doppler will provide the same information and is utilized when the velocity exceeds the velocity limits of the PWD system. Peak and mean gradients can be calculated from the flow velocity signal utilizing the simplified Bernoulli equation (291,293). Good correlation was found between mean pressure gradients measured by Doppler and those determined at cardiac catheterization (293). With color flow imaging, the characteristic flame-shaped jet described in mitral stenosis is seen (Fig. 32, see color plate). CFI can help identify the direction of the jet, especially when it is eccentric, and facilitate the optimum alignment of the CWD parallel to the stenotic jet (294). Pressure half-time of TV inflow signal can be measured, and TV area, utilizing the empirical constant of 220 in the equation proposed by Hatle and Angelsen, can be calculated and is found to correlate well with values obtained at catheterization (293).

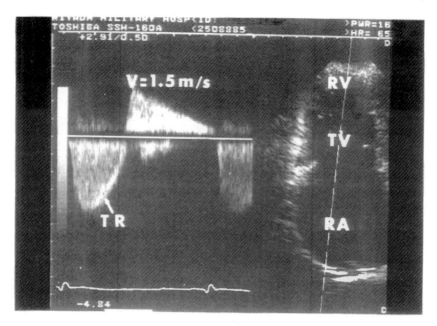

Figure 31 Simultaneous two-dimensional echocardiogram (right panel) and continuous-wave Doppler recording (left panel), obtained in the apical four-chamber view, in a patient with combined rheumatic tricuspid stenosis and regurgitation (TR) and atrial fibrillation. Note no a-wave in the antegrade tricuspid inflow signal, which shows an increased velocity of 1.5 m/s, corresponding to a gradient across the tricuspid valve of 9 mmHg, and slow deceleration. The tricuspid regurgitation signal below the zero line is holosystolic, with a peak velocity of 2.3 m/s. RV = right ventricle, TV = tricuspid valve, RA = right atrium.

B. Tricuspid Regurgitation

Tricuspid regurgitation can be functional, secondary to annular dilatation caused by RV pressure or volume overload, or organic, resulting from changes in leaflet morphology (rheumatic heart disease, Ebstein's anomaly, carcinoid heart disease, endocarditis, or prolapse) or in the supporting apparatus (endocarditis or myocardial infarction) (285,295).

1. Two-Dimensional Echocardiography

2-DE provides valuable information regarding the structural abnormality of the TV apparatus underlying the cause of TR (193,258,296–299), and can also identify changes secondary to TR, such as dilatation of tricuspid annulus, right-sided chambers, or inferior vena cava (IVC) and hepatic veins (HV) (300–302), and paradoxical septal motion characteristic of right-sided volume overload. Contrast 2-DE has been utilized to document regurgitation by showing the microbubble material moving back and forth across the TV or even into the IVC and HV in severe cases of TR (303–307). In current practice, detection and quantitation of TR are based on Doppler echocardiography.

2. Doppler Echocardiography

All three modalities of Doppler are very sensitive for the detection of TR (Figs. 33 and 34, [see color plate for Fig. 34]). Physiological TR is observed in the majority of normal subjects, even in the absence of auscultatory findings (151–153). With the PWD sample volume placed in the right atrium (RA) just proximal to the TV, utilizing any of the views previously

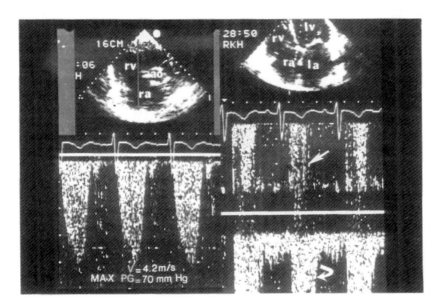

Figure 33 Pulsed-wave Doppler (right panel) and continuous-wave Doppler (left panel) signals of tricuspid regurgitation. The pulsed-wave Doppler signal is obtained in the apical four-chamber view, with the sample volume placed in the right atrium (ra). Because velocity is high, exceeding the Niquist limit, aliasing occurs and the signal appears both below (curved arrow) and above (oblique arrow) the zero reference line. The continuous-wave Doppler signal is obtained by a dual transducer with both two-dimensional and Doppler capabilities, from the parasternal position. The signal is holosystolic, below the reference line as flow is away from the transducer, and with a maximum velocity of 4.2 m/s. ao = aortica, la = left atrium, lv = left ventricle, rv = right ventricle.

mentioned, TR is diagnosed when turbulent retrograde systolic flow is recorded that usually shows aliasing due to the high velocity resulting from the pressure difference between the right ventricle (RV) and RA (308). This technique was utilized in several studies to quantitate TR, primarily by mapping the length and width of the TR jet into the RA or into systemic veins (302,307,309–312). As in mitral regurgitation, eccentric jets may be missed and lead to underestimation of TR severity. However, CFI is currently the method of choice for detection and semiquantitation of TR. A systolic mosaic jet is demonstrated starting at the TV and extending for variable distances into RA (313), or causing reversal of color into the IVC and HV in severe TR. The length of the jet (313), its area, and the ratio of regurgitant area to that of the RA measured from multiple views (301,314) are used to assess severity of TR semiquantitatively. Severe reversal of flow into the HV (Fig. 35, see color plate), appreciated with real-time CFI or color M-mode, is also indicative of severe TR. CFI also facilitates the optimal alignment of CWD parallel to the jet to obtain maximal velocity of TR flow velocity signal.

CWD displays the full envelope of the flow velocity signal with the characteristic rounded mid-systolic peak and a maximal velocity that can be measured accurately (315). Hatle and Angelsen (316) reported that the intensity of the TR signal is a reflection of its severity, when compared to the forward tricuspid inflow signal as a reference for comparison; the more intense the signal, the more severe is the TR. A sharp deceleration of the signal with low end-systolic velocities reflecting the fast equalization of pressure between RV and RA is also indicative of severe TR.

The CWD-derived maximal velocity can be translated into maximum pressure gradient utilizing the simplified Bernoulli equation. By adding an estimate of mean RA pressure obtained, either clinically, by examining the jugular venous pressure, or by using estimated values from regression equations (Currie suggested a value of 14 mmHg in the absence of severe TR), RV systolic pressure is calculated. It equals pulmonary artery systolic pressure (PAP) in the absence of right ventricular outflow tract obstruction. Several studies have shown good correlation between TR velocity Doppler-derived systolic PAP and that derived at cardiac catheterization (317–319).

C. Summary

Although catheterization has been a standard method for assessing TR severity, it is not without its drawbacks, and factitious TR can occur due to catheter placement. That is why Doppler echocardiography has emerged as the diagnostic method of choice for diagnosing TR, determining its etiology, assessing its severity, and measuring systolic PAP.

REFERENCES

1. Feigenbaum H. Echocardiography. Philadelphia: Lea & Febiger, 1986.
2. Weyman AE. Cross-Sectional Echocardiography. Philadelphia: Lea & Febiger, 1982.
3. Nanda NC. Textbook of Color Doppler Echocardiography. Philadelphia: Lea & Febiger, 1989.
4. DeMaria AN, Smith M, Branco M, et al. Normal and abnormal blood flow patterns by color Doppler flow imaging. Echocardiography 1986; 3:475–82.
5. Hatle L, Angelsen B. Doppler Ultrasound in Cardiology: Physical Principles and Clinical Application. 2d ed. Philadelphia: Lea & Febiger, 1985.
6. Miyatake K, Okamoto M, Kinoshita N, et al. Clinical application of a new type of real-time, two-dimensional Doppler flow imaging system. Am J Cardiol 1984; 54:857–68.
7. Omoto R, Kasai C. Physics and instrumentation of Doppler flow mapping. Echocardiography 1987; 4:467–83.
8. Stevenson JG. Appearance and recognition of basic Doppler concepts in color flow imaging. Echocardiography 1989; 6:451–66.
9. Doppler CJ: Cited by Hatle L, Angelsen B (5).
10. Olson LJ, Subramanian R, Ackerman DM, et al. Surgical pathology of the mitral valve: a study of 712 cases spanning 21 years. Mayo Clin Proc 1987; 62:22–34.
11. Hauk AJ, Edwards WD, Danielson GK, et al. Mitral and aortic valve disease associated with ergotamine therapy for migraine. Arch Pathol Lab Med 1990; 114:62–4.
12. Roberts WC, Perloff JK. Mitral valvular disease: a clinicopathologic survey of the conditions causing the mitral valve to function abnormally. Annals Int Med 1972; 77:939–75.
13. Al-Zaibag M, Ribeiro PA, Al Kassab S, et al. Percutaneous double balloon mitral mitral valvotomy for rheumatic mitral valve stensis. Lancet 1986; 1: 757–61.
14. McKay RG, Lock JE, Safian RD, et al. Balloon dilatation of mitral stenosis in adult patients: postmortem and percutaneous mitral valvuloplasty studies. J Am Coll Cardiol 1987; 9:723–31.
15. Palacios I, Block PC, Brandi S, et al. Percutaneous balloon valvotomy for patients with severe mitral stenosis. Circulation 1987; 75:778–84.
16. Inoue K, Owaki T, Nakamura T, et al. Clinical application of transvenous mitral commissurotomy by a new balloon catheter. J Thor Cardiovasc Surg 1984; 87:394–402.
17. Gorlin R, Gorlin SG. Hydraulic formula for calculation of the area of the

stenotic mitral valve, other cardiac valves, and central circulatory shunts. Am Heart J 1951; 41:1–29.

18. Duchack J, Chang S, Feigenbaum H. The posterior mitral echo and the echocardiographic diagnosis of mitral stenosis. Am J Cardiol 1972; 29: 628–32.

19. Levisman JA, Abbasi AS, Pearce ML. Posterior mitral leaflet motion in mitral stenosis. Circulation 1975; 51:511–4.

20. Cope GD, Kisslo JA, Johnson ML, et al. A reassessment of the echocardiogram in mitral stenosis. Circulation 1975; 52:664–70.

21. Henry L, Grifith JM, Michaelis LL, et al. Measurement of mitral orifice area in patients with mitral valve disease by real-time two-dimensional echocardiography. Circulation 1975; 51:827–31.

22. Nichol PM, Gilbert BW, Kisslo JA, et al. Two-dimensional echocardiographic assessment of mitral stenosis. Circulation 1977; 55:120–8.

23. Martin RP, Rakowski H, Kleiman JH, et al. Reliability and reproducibility of two-dimensional echocardiographic measurement of the stenotic mitral valve orifice area. Am J Cardiol 1979; 43:560–8.

24. Wann LS, Weyman AE, Feigenbaum H, et al. Determination of mitral valve area by cross-sectional echocardiography. Annals Int Med 1978; 88:337–41.

25. Feigenbaum H. Echocardiography. Philadelphia: Lea & Febiger, 1986: 249–62.

26. Smith MD, Handshoe R, Handshoe S, et al. Comparative accuracy of two-dimensional echocardiography and Doppler pressure half-time methods in assessing severity of mitral stenosis in patients with and without prior commissurotomy. Circulation 1986; 73:100–7.

27. Glover MU, Warren SE, Vieweg WVR, et al. M-mode and two-dimensional echocardiographic correlation with findings at catheterization and surgery in patients with mitral stenosis. Am Heart J 1983; 105:98–102.

28. Nanda NC, Gramiak R, Shah PM, et al. Mitral commissurotomy versus replacement: preoperative evaluation by echocardiography. Circulation 1975; 51:263–7.

29. Abascal VM, Wilkins GT, O'Shea JP, et al. Prediction of successful outcome in 130 patients undergoing percutaneous balloon mitral valvotomy. Circulation 1990; 82:448–57.

30. Palacios I, Block PC, Wilkins GT, et al. Follow-up of patients undergoing percutaneous mitral balloon valvotomy: analysis of factors determining restenosis. Circulation 1989; 79:573–9.

31. Wilkins GT, Weyman AE, Abasacal VM, et al. Percutaneous mitral valvotomy: an analysis of echocardiographic variables related to outcome and the mechanism of dilatation. Br Heart J 1988; 60:299–308.

32. Shrestha NK, Moreno FL, Narciso VF, et al. Two-dimensional echocardiographic diagnosis of left atrial thrombus in rheumatic heart disease: a clinicopathologic study. Circulation 1983; 67:341–7.

33. Herzog CA, Bass D, Kane M, et al. Two-dimensional echocardiographic imaging of left atrial appendage thrombi. J Am Coll Cardiol 1984; 3:1340–4.

34. Seward JB. Cardiac tumors and thrombus: transesophageal echocardio-

graphic experience. In: Erbel R, Khanderia BK, Brenneck R, et al., eds. Transesophageal Echocardiography: A New Window to the Heart. Springer-Verlag, Berlin. 1989:120–8.

35. Ascenberg W, Schluter M, Kremer P, et al. Transesophageal two-dimensional echocardiography for the detection of left atrial appendage thrombus. J Am Coll Cardiol 1986; 7:163–6.

36. Mugge A, Daniel WG, Hausmann D, et al. Diagnosis of left atrial appendage thrombi by transesophageal echocardiography: clinical implications and follow-up. Am J Cardiac Imaging 1990; 4:173–9.

37. Khanderia BK, Tajik AJ, Reeder GS, et al. Doppler color flowing imaging: a new technique for visualization and characterization of the blood flow jet in mitral stenosis. Mayo Clin Proc 1986; 61:623–30.

38. Kan M, Goyal RG, Helmcke F, et al. Color Doppler assessment of severity of mitral stenosis. Circulation 1986; 74(suppl III):145.

39. Holen J, Aaslid R, Landmark K, et al. Determination of pressure gradient in mitral stenosis with a noninvasive ultrasound Doppler technique. Acta Med Scand 1976; 199:455–60.

40. Hatle L, Brubakk A, Tromsdal A, et al. Noninvasive assessment of pressure drop in mitral stenosis by Doppler ultrasound. Br Heart J 1978; 40:131–40.

41. Holen J, Simonsen S. Determination of pressure gradient in mitral stenosis with Doppler echocardiography. Br Heart J 1979; 41:529–35.

42. Libanoff AJ, Rodband S. Atrioventricular pressure half-time measure of mitral valve orifice area. Circulation 1968; 38:144–50.

43. Hatle L, Angelsen B, Tromsdal A. Noninvasive assessment of atrioventricular pressure half-time by Doppler ultrasound. Circulation 1979; 60: 1096–104.

44. Stamm RB, Martin RP. Quantification of pressure gradients across stenotic valves by Doppler ultrasound. J Am Coll Cardiol 1983; 2:707–18.

45. Gonzalez MA, Child JS, Krovokapich J. Comparison of two-dimensional Doppler echocardiography and intracardiac hemodynamics for quantification of mitral stenosis. Am J Cardiol 1987; 60:327–32.

46. Bryg RJ, Williams GA, Labovitz AJ, et al. Effect of atrial fibrillation and mitral regurgitation on calculated mitral valve area in mitral stenosis. Am J Cardiol 1986; 57:634–8.

47. Sagar KB, Wann S, Paulson WJ, et al. Role of exercise Doppler echocardiography in isolated mitral stenosis. Chest 1987; 92:27–30.

48. Hatle L, Angelsen B. Doppler Ultrasound in Cardiology: Physical Principles and Clinical Application. 2d ed. Philadelphia: Lea & Febiger, 1985;110–24.

49. Nakatani S, Masuyama T, Kodama K, et al. Value and limitations of Doppler echocardiography in the quantification of stenotic mitral valve area: comparison of the pressure half-time and the continuity equation methods. Circulation 1988; 77:78–85.

50. Flachskampf FA, Weyman AE, Gillam L, et al. Aortic regurgitation shortens Doppler pressure half-time in mitral stenosis: clinical evidence, in vitro simulation, and theoretic analysis. J Am Coll Cardiol 1990; 16:396–404.

51. Moro E, Nicolosi GL, Zanuttini D, et al. Influence of aortic regurgitation

on the assessment of the pressure half-time and derived mitral valve area in patients with mitral stenosis. Eur Heart J 1988; 9:1010–17.

52. Grayburn PA, Smith MD, Gurley JC, et al. Effect of aortic reguritation on the assessment of mitral valve orifice area by Doppler pressure half-time in mitral stenosis. Am J Cardiol 1987; 60:322–6.

53. Thomas JD, Wilkins GT, Choong CYP, et al. Inaccuracy of mitral pressure half-time immediately after percutaneous mitral valvotomy: dependence on transmitral gradient and left atrial and ventricular compliance. Circulation 1988; 78:980–93.

54. Karp K, Teien D, Bjerle P, et al. Reassessment of valve area determinations in mitral stenosis by the pressure half-time method: impact of left ventricular stiffness and peak diastolic pressure difference. J Am Coll Cardiol 1989; 13:594–9.

55. Karp K, Teien D, Eriksson P. Doppler echocardiographic assessment of valve area in patients with atrioventricular valve stenosis by application of the continuity equation. J Intern Med 1989; 225:261–6.

56. Rodriguez L, Monterroso V, Mueller L, et al. Validation of a new method for valve area calculation using the proximal isovelocity surface area in patients with mitral stenosis. J Am Coll Cardiol 1990; 15:108A.

57. Roberts WC. The structure of the aortic valve in clinically isolated aortic stenosis: an autopsy study of 162 patients over 15 years of age. Circulation 1970; 42:91–7.

58. Pomerance A. Pathogenesis of aortic stenosis and its relation to age. Br Heart J 1972; 34:569–74.

59. Passik CS, Ackermann DM, Pluth JR, et al. Temporal changes in the causes of aortic stenosis: a surgical-pathologic study of 646 cases. Mayo Clin Proc 1987; 62:119–23.

60. Roberts WC, Perloff JK, Costantino T. Severe valvular aortic stenosis in patients over 65 years of age: a clinicopathologic study. Am J Cardiol 1971; 27:497–506.

61. Nylander E, Ekman I, Marklund T, et al. Severe aortic stenosis in elderly patients. Br Heart J 1986; 55:480–7.

62. Eddleman EE, Frommey WB, Lyle DP, et al. Critical analysis of clinical factors in estimating severity of aortic valve disease. Am J Cardiol 1973; 31:687–95.

63. Cheitlin MD, Gertz EW, Brundage BH, et al. Rate of progression of severity of valvular aortic stenosis in the adult. Am Heart J 1979; 98:689–700.

64. Nakamura T, Hultgren HN, Shettigar UR, et al. Noninvasive evaluation of the severity of aortic stenosis in adult patients. Am Heart J 1984; 107: 959–66.

65. Voelkel AG, Kendrick M, Pietro DA, et al. Noninvasive tests to evaluate the severity of aortic stenosis: limitations and reliability. Chest 1980; 77: 155–60.

66. Bonner AJ, Sacks HN, Tavel ME. Assessing the severity of aortic stenosis by phonocardiography and external carotid pulse recordings. Circulation 1973; 48:247–52.

67. Aronow WS, Harris CN. Treadmill exercise test in aortic stenosis and mitral stenosis. Chest 1975; 68:507–9.
68. Atwood JE, Kawanishi S, Myers J, et al. Exercise testing in patients with aortic stenosis. Chest 1988; 93:1083–7.
69. Ng ASH, Holmes DR, Smith HC, et al. Hemodynamic progression of adult valvular aortic stenosis. Cathet Cardiovas Diagnosis 1986; 12:145–50.
70. Wagner S, Selzer A. Patterns of progression of aortic stenosis: a longitudinal hemodynamic study. Circulation 1982; 65:709–12.
71. Nestico PF, DePace NL, Kimbris D, et al. Progression of isolated aortic stenosis: analysis of 29 patients having more than one cardiac catheterization. Am J Cardiol 1983; 52:1054–8.
72. Otto CM, Pearlman AS, Gardner CL. Hemodynamic progression of aortic stenosis in adults assessed by Doppler echocardiography. J Am Coll Cardiol 1989; 13:545–50.
73. Roger VL, Tajik AJ, Bailey KR, et al. Progression of aortic stenosis in adults: new application using Doppler echocardiography. Am Heart J 1990; 119:331–8.
74. Edwards JE. Pathology of acquired valvular disease of the heart. Semin Roentgenol 1979; 14:96–115.
75. Subramanian R, Olson LJ, Edwards WD. Surgical pathology of pure aortic stenosis: a study of 374 cases. Mayo Clin Proc 1984; 59:683–90.
76. DeMaria AN, Bommer W, Joye J, et al. Value and limitations of cross-sectional echocardiography of aortic valve in the diagnosis and quantification of valvular aortic stenosis. Circulation 1980; 62:304–12.
77. Weyman AE, Feigenbaum H, Dillon JC, et al. Cross-sectional echocardiography in assessing the severity of valvular aortic stenosis. Circulation 1975; 52:828–34.
78. Fowles RE, Martin RP, Abrams JM, et al. Two-dimensional echocardiographic features of bicuspid aortic valve. Chest 1979; 75:434–40.
79. Brandenburg RO, Tajik AJ, Edwards WD, et al. Accuracy of two-dimensional echocardiographic diagnosis of congenitally bicuspid aortic valve: echocardiographic-anatomic correlation in 115 patients. Am J Cardiol 1983; 51:1469–73.
80. Chang S, Clements S, Chang J. Aortic stenosis: echocardiographic cusp separation and surgical description of aortic valve in 22 patients. Am J Cardiol 1977; 39:499–504.
81. Leo LR, Barrett MJ, Leddy CL, et al. Determination of aortic valve area by cross-sectional echocardiography. Circulation 1979; 609(suppl II):203.
82. Godley RW, Green D, Dillon JC, et al. Reliability of two-dimensional echocardiography in assessing the severity of valvular aortic stenosis. Chest 1981; 79:657–62.
83. Williams GA, Labovitz AJ, Nelson JG, et al. Value of multiple echocardiographic views in the evaluation of aortic stenosis in adults by continuous-wave Doppler. Am J Cardiol 1985; 55:445–9.
84. Hatle L, Angelsen B. Doppler Ultrasound in Cardiology: Physical Principles and Clinical Application. 2d ed. Philadelphia: Lea & Febiger, 1985:124–43.

85. Hatle L, Angelsen B, Tromsdale A. Noninvasive assessment of aortic steno-sis by Doppler ultrasound. Br Heart J 1980; 43:284–92.
86. Callahan MJ, Tajik AJ, Su-Fan Q, et al. Validation of instantaneous pres-sure gradients measured by continuous-wave Doppler in experimentally induced aortic stenosis. Am J Cardiol 1985; 56:989–93.
87. Smith MD, Dawson PL, Elion JL, et al. Correlation of continuous-wave Doppler velocities with cardiac catheterization gradient: an experimental model of aortic stenosis. J Am Coll Cardiol 1985; 6:1306–14.
88. Smith MD, Dawson PL, Elion JL, et al. Systematic correlation of continu-ous-wave Doppler and hemodynamic measurements in patients with aortic stenosis. Am Heart J 1986; 111:245–52.
89. Currie PJ, Hagler DJ, Seward JB, et al. Instantaneous pressure gradient: a simultaneous Doppler and dual catheter correlative study. J Am Coll Cardiol 1986; 7:800–6.
90. Teien D, Karp K, Eriksson P. Noninvasive estimation of the mean pressure difference in aortic stenosis by Doppler ultrasound. Br Heart J 1986; 56: 450–4.
91. Berger M, Berdoff RL, Gallerstein PE, et al. Evaluation of aortic stensosis by continuous-wave Doppler ultrasound. J Am Coll Cardiol 1984; 3:150–6.
92. Danielsen R, Nordrehaug JE, Vik-Mo H, et al. Factors affecting Doppler echocardiographic valve area assessment in aortic stenosis. Am J Cardiol 1989; 63:1107–11.
93. Hegrenaes L, Hatle L. Aortic stenosis in adults: noninvasive estimation of pressure differences by continuous-wave Doppler echocardiography. Br Heart J 1985; 54:396–404.
94. Currie PJ, Seward JB, Reeder GS, et al. Continuous-wave Doppler echocar-diographic assessment of severity of calcific aortic stenosis: a simultaneous Doppler-catheter study in 100 adult patients. Circulation 1985; 71:1162–9.
95. Yaeger M, Yock PG, Popp RL. Comparison of Doppler derived pressure gradient to that determined at cardiac catheterization in adults with aortic valve stenosis: implications for management. Am J Cardiol 1986; 57:644–8.
96. Teirstein P, Yaeger M, Yock PG, et al. Doppler echocardiographic measure-ment of aortic valve area in aortic stenosis: a noninvasive application of the Gorlin formula. J Am Coll Cardiol 1986; 8:1059–65.
97. Krafcheck J, Robertson JH, Radford M, et al. A reconsideration of Doppler assessed gradients in suspected aortic stenosis. Am Heart J 1985; 110: 765–73.
98. Ohlsson J, Wranne B. Noninvasive assessment of valve area in patients with aortic stenosis. J Am Coll Cardiol 1986; 7:501–8.
99. Goli VD, Teague SM, Prasad R, et al. Noninvasive evaluation of aortic stenosis severity utilizing Doppler ultrasound and electrical bioimpedance. J Am Coll Cardiol 1988; 11:66–71.
100. Skjaerpe T, Hegrenaes L, Hatle L. Noninvasive estimation of valve area in patients with aortic stenosis by Doppler ultrasound and two-dimensional echocardiography. Circulation 1985; 72:810–8.
101. Oh JK, Taliercio CP, Holmes DR, et al. Prediction of the severity of aortic

stenosis by Doppler Aortic area determination: prospective Doppler-catheterization correlation in 100 patients. J Am Coll Cardiol 1988; 11:1227–34.

102. Zoghbi WA, Farmer KL, Soto JG, et al. Accurate noninvasive quantification of stenotic aortic valve area by Doppler echocardiogrphy. Circulation 1986; 73:452–9.

103. Otto CM, Pearlman AS, Comess KA, et al. Determination of the stenotic aortic valve area in adults using Doppler echocardiography. J Am Coll Cardiol 1986; 7:509–17.

104. Harrison MR, Gurley JC, Smith MD, et al. A practical application of Doppler echocardiography for the assessment of severity of aortic stenosis. Am Heart J 1988; 115:622–8.

105. Come PC, Riley MF, McKay RG, et al. Echocardiographic assessment of aortic valve area in elderly patients with aortic stenosis and changes in valve area after percutaneous balloon valvuloplasty. J Am Coll Cardiol 1987; 10:115–24.

106. Grayburn PA, Smith MD, Harrison MR, et al. Pivotal role of aortic valve area calculation by the continuity equation for Doppler assessment of aortic stenosis in patients with combined aortic stenosis and regurgitation. Am J Cardiol 1988; 61:376–81.

107. Myreng Y, Molstad P, Endresen K, et al. Reproducibility of echocardiographic estimates of the area of stenosed aortic valves using the continuity equation. Int J Cardiol 1990; 26:349–54.

108. Fan PH, Kapur KK, Nanda NC. Color-guided Doppler echocardiographic assessment of aortic valve stenosis. J Am Coll Cardiol 1988; 12:441–9.

109. Morris AM, Roitman DI, Nanda NC, et al. Color Doppler assessment of stenotic aortic valve area. Circulation 1985; 72(suppl III):100.

110. Nanda NC. Textbook of Color Doppler Echocardiography. Philadelphia: Lea & Febiger, 1989:178–89.

111. Panidis IP, Mintz GS, Ross J. Value and limitations of Doppler ultrasound in the evaluation of aortic stenosis: a statistical analysis of 70 consecutive patients. Am Heart J 1986; 112:150–8.

112. Zoghbi WA, Galan A, Quinones MA. Accurate assessment of aortic stenosis severity by Doppler echocardiography independent of aortic jet velocity. Am Heart J 1988; 116:855–63.

113. Oh JK, Nishimura RA, Seward JB, et al. Differentiation of aortic stenosis jet from mitral regurgitation by analysis of continuous-wave Doppler spectrum: illustrative cases. Echocardiography 1986; 3:55–60.

114. Hoffman T, Kasper W, Meinertz T, et al. Determination of aortic valve orifice area in aortic valve stenosis by two-dimensional transesophageal echocardiography. Am J Cardiol 1987; 59:330–5.

115. Waller BF, Morrow AG, Maron BJ, et al. Etiology of clinically isolated severe chronic pure mitral regurgitation: analysis of 97 patients over 30 years of age having mitral valve replacement. Am Heart J 1982; 104:276–88.

116. Mintz GS, Kotler MN, Segal BL, et al. Two-dimensional echocardiographic evaluation of patients with mitral insufficiency. Am J Cardiol 1979; 44:670–7.

117. Himelmann RB, Kusumoto F, Oken K, et al. The flail mitral valve: echocardiographic findings by precordial and transesophageal imaging and Doppler color flow mapping. J Am Coll Cardiol 1991; 17:272–9.

118. Gilbert BW, Scatz RA, Von Ramm OT, et al. Mitral valve prolapse: two-dimensional echocardiographic and angigraphic correlation. Circulation 1976; 54:716–23.

119. Alpert MA, Carney RJ, Flaker GC, et al. Sensitivity and specificity of two-dimensional echocardiographic signs of mitral valve prolapse. Am J Cardiol 1984; 54:792–6.

120. Krivokapich J, Child JS, Dadourian BJ, et al. Reassessment of echocardiographic criteria for diagnosis of mitral valve prolapse. Am J Cardiol 1988; 61:131–5.

121. Levine RA, Stathogiannis E, Newell JB, et al. Reconsideration of echocardiographic standards for mitral valve prolapse: lack of association between leaflet displacement isolated to the apical four-chamber view and independent echocardiographic evidence of abnormality. J Am Coll Cardiol 1988; 11:1010–9.

122. Levine RA, Triulzi MO, Harrigan P, et al. The relationship of mitral annular shape to the diagnosis of mitral valve prolapse. Circulation 1987; 75:756–67.

123. Ballester M, Foale R, Presbitero P, et al. Cross-sectional echocardiographic features of ruptured chordae tendineae. Eur Heart J 1983; 4:795–802.

124. Child JS, Skorton J, Taylor RD, et al. M-mode and cross-sectional echocardiographic features of flail posterior mitral leaflets. Am J Cardiol 1979; 44: 1383–9.

125. Mintz GS, Kotler MN, Segal, et al. Two-dimensional echocardiographic recognition of ruptured chordae tendineae. Circulation 1978; 57:244–50.

126. Wann LS, Feigenbaum H, Weyman AE, et al. Cross-sectional echocardiographic detection of rheumatic mitral regurgitation. Am J Cardiol 1978; 41: 1258–63.

127. Martin RP, Meltzer RS, Chia BL, et al. Clinical utility of two-dimensional echocardiography in infective endocarditis. Am J Cardiol 1980; 46:379–85.

128. O'Brien JT, Geiser EA. Infective endocarditis and echocardiography. Am Heart J 1984; 108:386–94.

129. Mugge A, Daniel WG, Frank G, et al. Echocardiography in infective endocarditis: reassessment of prognostic implications of vegetation size determined by the transthoracic and the transesophageal approach. J Am Coll Cardiol 1989; 14:631–8.

130. Mintz GS, Kotler MV, Segal BL, et al. Comparison of two-dimensional and M-mode echocardiography in the evaluation of patients with infective endocarditis. Am J Cardiol 1979; 43:738–44.

131. Jaffe WM, Morgan DE, Pearlman AS, et al. Infective endocarditis, 1983–1988: echocardiographic findings and factors influencing morbidity and mortality. J Am Coll Cardiol 1990; 15:1227–33.

132. Ellis SG, Goldstein J, Poppe RL, et al. Detection of endocarditis-associated paravalvular abcesses by two-dimensional echocardiography. J Am Coll Cardiol 1985; 5:647–53.

133. Beppu S, Nimura Y, Sakakibara H, et al. Mitral cleft in ostium primum atrial septal defect assessed by cross-sectional echocardiography. Circulation 1980; 62:1099–107.
134. DiSegni E, Bass JL, Lucas RY, et al. Isolated cleft mitral valve: a variety of congenital mitral regurgitation identified by two-dimensional echocardiography. Am J Cardiol 1983; 51:927–31.
135. Smallhorn JF, DeLeval M, Stark J, et al. Isolated anterior mitral cleft: two-dimensional echocardiographic assessment and differentiation from "clefts" associated with atrioventricular septal defect. Br Heart J 1982; 48: 109–16.
136. Nestico PF, DePace NL, Morganroth J, et al. Mitral annular calcification: clinical, pathophysiology, and echocardiographic review. Am Heart J 1984; 107:988–96.
137. Erbel R, Schweizer P, Bardos P, et al. Two-dimensional echocardiographic diagnosis of papillary muscle rupture. Chest 1981; 79:595–9.
138. Nishimura RA, Tajik AJ. Determination of left-sided pressure gradients utilizing Doppler aortic and mitral regurgitant signals: validation by simultaneous dual catheter and Doppler studies. J Am Coll Cardiol 1988; 11: 317–21.
139. Weiss JL, Bulkley BH, Hutchins GM, et al. Two-dimensional echocardiographic recognition of myocardial injury in man: comparison with postmortem studies. Circulation 1981; 63:401–8.
140. Horowitz RS, Morganroth J. Immediate detection of early high-risk patients with acute myocardial infarction using two-dimensional echocardiographic evaluation of left ventricular regional wall motion abnormalities. Am Heart J 1982; 103:814–21.
141. Godley RW, Wann LS, Rogers EW, et al. Incomplete mitral leaflet closure in patients with papillary muscle dysfunction. Circulation 1981; 63:565–71.
142. Izumi S, Miyatake K, Beppu S, et al. Mechanism of mitral regurgitation in patients with myocardial infarction: a study using real-time two-dimensional Doppler flow imaging and echocardiography. Circulation 1987; 76:777–85.
143. Donaldson RM, Rubens MB, Ballester M, et al. Echocardiographic visualization of the anatomic causes of mitral regurgitation resulting from myocardial infarction. Post Grad Med 1982; 58:257–63.
144. Mintz GS, Victor MF, Kotler MN, et al. Two-dimensional echocardiographic identification of surgically correctable complications of myocardial infarction. Circulation 1981; 64:91–6.
145. Shah PM. Echocardiography in congestive or dilated cardiomyopathy. J Am Soc Echocardiogr 1988; 1:20–30.
146. Erbel R, Rohmann S, Drexler M, et al. Improved diagnostic value of echocardiography in patients with infective endocarditis by transesophageal approach. Eur Heart J 1988; 9:43–53.
147. Yoshida K, Yoshikawa J, Yamaura Y, et al. Assessment of mitral regurgitation by biplane transesophageal color Doppler flow mapping. Circulation 1990; 82:1121–6.
148. Kleinman JP, Czer LSC, DeRobertis M, et al. A quantitative comparison

of transesophageal and epicardial color Doppler echocardiography in the intraoperative assessment of mitral regurgitation. Am J Cardiol 1986; 64: 1168–72.

149. Currie PJ, Stewart WJ. Intraoperative echocardiography in mitral repair for mitral regurgitation. Am J Cardiac Imaging 1990; 4:192–206.

150. Nimura Y, Miyatake K, Izumi S. Physiological regurgitation identified by Doppler techniques. Echocardiography 1989; 6:385–92.

151. Yoshida K, Yoshikawa J, Shakudo M, et al. Color Doppler evaluation of valvular regurgitation in normal subjects. Circulation 1988; 78:840–7.

152. Kostuchi W, Vandenbossche J, Friart A, et al. Pulsed Doppler regurgitant flow patterns of normal valves. Am J Cardiol 1986; 58:309–13.

153. Berger M, Hecht SR, van Tosh A, et al. Pulsed- and continuous-wave Doppler echocardiographic assessment of valvular regurgitation in normal subjects. J Am Coll Cardiol 1989; 13:1540–5.

154. Blanchard D, Diebold B, Peronneau P, et al. Noninvasive diagnosis of mitral regurgitation by Doppler echocardiography. Br Heart J 1981; 45:589–93.

155. Abbasi AS, Allen MW, DeCristofaro D, et al. Detection and estimation of the degree of mitral regurgitation by range-gated pulsed Doppler echocardiography. Circulation 1980; 61:143–7.

156. Miyatake K, Kinoshita N, Nagala S, et al. Intracardiac flow pattern in mitral regurgitation studied with combined use of the ultrasonic pulsed Doppler technique and cross-sectional echocardiography. Am J Cardiol 1980; 45: 155–62.

157. Omoto R, Yokote Y, Takamoto S, et al. The development of real-time, two-dimensional Doppler echocardiography and its clinical significance in acquired valvular disease. Jpn Heart J 1984; 25:325–40.

158. Helmcke F, Nanda NC, Hsuing MC, et al. Color Doppler assessment of mitral regurgitation with orthogonal planes. Circulation 1987; 75:175–83.

159. Miyatake K, Izumi S, Okamoto M, et al. Semiquantitative grading of severity of mitral regurgitation by real-time, two-dimensional Doppler flow imaging technique. J Am Coll Cardiol 1986; 7:82–8.

160. Spain MG, Smith MD, Grayburn PA, et al. Quantitative assessment of mitral regurgitation by Doppler color flow imaging: angiographic and hemodynamic correlations. J Am Coll Cardiol 1989; 13:585–90.

161. Mohr-Kahaly S, Erbel R, Zenker G, et al. Semiquantitative grading of mitral regurgitation by color-coded Doppler echocardiography. Int J Cardiol 1989; 23:223–30.

162. Stevenson JG. Two-dimensional color Doppler estimation of the severity of atrioventricular valve regurgitation: important effects of instrument gain setting, pulse repetition frequency, and carrier frequency. J Am Soc Echocardiogr 1989; 2:1–10.

163. Saenz CB, Deumite J, Roitman DI, et al. Limitation of color Doppler in quantitative assessment of mitral regurgitation. Circulation 1985; 72(supl III):99.

164. Hatle L, Angelsen B. Doppler Ultrasound in Cardiology: Physical Principles and Clinical Application. 2d ed. Philadelphia: Lea & Febiger, 1985:176–88.

165. Pai RG, Bansal RC, Shah PM. Doppler-derived rate of left ventricular pressure rise: its correlation with the postoperative left ventricular function in mitral regurgitation. Circulation 1990; 82:514–20.

166. Bargiggia GS, Bertucci C, Recusani F, et al. A new method for estimating left ventricular dP/dt by continuous-wave Doppler echocardiography: validation studies at cardiac catheterization. Circulation 1989; 80:1287–92.

167. Stewart WJ, Palacios I, Jiang L, et al. Doppler measurement of regurgitant fraction in patients with mitral regurgitation: a new quantitative technique. Circulation 3; 1983; 68(suppl III):111.

168. Zhang Y, Ihlen H, Myhre E, et al. Measurement of mitral regurgitation by Doppler echocardiography. Br Heart J 1985; 54:384–91.

169. Blumlein S, Bouchard A, Schiller N, et al. Quantitation of mitral regurgitation by Doppler echocardiography. Circulation 1986; 74:306–14.

170. Rokey R, Sterling LL, Zoghbi WA, et al. Determination of regurgitant fraction in isolated mitral or aortic regurgitation by pulsed Doppler two-dimensional echocardiography. J Am Coll Cardiol 1986; 7:1273–8.

171. Jenni R, Ritter M, Eberli F, et al. Quantification of mitral regurgitation with amplitude-weighted mean velocity from continuous-wave Doppler spectra. Circulation 1989; 79:1294–9.

172. Rodriguez L, Flachskampf FA, Abascal VM, et al. Regurgitant flow rate calculated by proximal isovelocity surface area is independent of orifice area. Circulation 1989; 80(suppl II):570.

173. Cape EG, Yoganathan AP, Rodriguez L, et al. The proximal flow convergence method can be extended to calculate regurgitant stroke volume: in vitro application of the color Doppler M-mode. J Am Coll Cardiol 1990; 15: 109A.

174. Utsunomiya T, Ogawa T, Patel D, et al. Color flow Doppler "proximal isovelocity surface area" method for estimating volume flow: independence from machine factors. Circulation 1989; 80[4(suppl II)]:571.

175. Utsunomiya T, Doshi R, Patel D, et al. Effect of orifice shape on Doppler color flow "proximal isovelocity surface area" method for estimating volume flow rate. Circulation 1989; 80[4(suppl II)]:570.

176. Rodriguez L, Vlahakes GJ, Yoganathan AP, et al. Quantification of regurgitant flow rate using the proximal flow convergence method: in vivo validation. Circulation 1989; 80(suppl II):571.

177. Utsonomiya T, Nguyen D, Doshi R, et al. Regurgitant volume estimation in mitral regurgitation by color Doppler using the "proximal isovelocity surface method." Circulation 1989; 80[4(suppl II)]:577.

178. Cape EG, Skoufis EG, Weyman AE, et al. A new method for noninvasive quantification of valvular regurgitation based on conservation of momentum: in vitro validation. Circulation 1989; 79:1343–53.

179. Rodriguez L, Vlahakes GJ, Cape EG, et al. In vitro validation of a new method for noninvasive quantification of mitral regurgitation. Circulation 1989; 80(suppl II):577.

180. Edwards JE. Pathology of acquired valvular disease of the heart. Semin Roentgenol 1979; 14:96–115.

181. Olson LJ, Subramanian R, Edwards WD. Surgical pathology of pure aortic insufficiency: a study of 225 cases. Mayo Clin Proc 1984; 59:835–41.
182. Grayburn PA, Smith MD, Handshoe R, et al. Detection of aortic insufficiency by standard echocardiography, pulsed Doppler echocardiography, and auscultation: a comparison of accuracies. Annals Intern Med 1986; 104: 599–605.
183. Meyers DG, Olson TS, Hansen DA. Auscultation, M-mode, and pulsed Doppler echocardiography compared with angiography for diagnosis of chronic aortic regurgitation. Am J Cardiol 1985; 56:811–2.
184. Spagnuolo M, Kloth H, Taranta A, et al. Natural history of rheumatic aortic regurgitation: criteria predictive of death, congestive heart failure, and angina in young patients. Circulation 1971; 44:368–80.
185. Braun LO, Kincaid OW, McGoon D, et al. Prognosis of aortic valve replacement in relation to the preoperative heart size. J Thor Cardiovasc Surg 1973; 65:381–5.
186. Borer JS, Bacharach SL, Green MV, et al. Exercise-induced left ventricular dysfunction in symptomatic and asymptomatic patients with aortic regurgitation: assessment with radionuclide cineangiography. Am J Cardiol 1978; 42:351–57.
187. Lumia FJ, MacMillan RM, Germon PA, et al. Rest-exercise radionuclide angiographic assessment of left ventricular function in chronic aortic regurgitation: significance of serial studies in medically versus surgically treated groups. Clin Cardiol 1985; 8:465–76.
188. Bonow RO, Rosing DR, McIntosh CL, et al. The natural history of asymptomatic patients with aortic regurgitation and normal left ventricular function. Circulation 1983; 68:509–17.
189. Feldman BJ, Khandheria BK, Warnes CA, et al. Incidence, description, and functional assessment of isolated quadricuspid aortic valve. Am J Cardiol 1990; 65:937–8.
190. Barbosa MM, Motta MS. Quadricuspid aortic valve and aortic regurgitation diagnosed by Doppler echocardiography: report of two cases and review of the literature. J Am Soc Echocardiogr 1991; 4:69–74.
191. Krivokapich J, Child JS, Skorton DJ, et al. Flail aortic valve leaflets: M-mode and two-dimensional echocardiographic manifestations. Am Heart J 1980; 99:425–37.
192. Berger M, Gallerstein PE, Benhuri P, et al. Evaluation of aortic valve endocarditis by two-dimensional echocadiographyphy. Chest 1981; 80:61–7.
193. Ogawa S, Hayashi J, Sasaki H, et al. Evaluation of combined valvular prolapse syndrome by two-dimensional echocardiography. Circulation 1982; 65:174–80.
194. Woldow AB, Parameswaren R, Hartman J, et al. Aortic regurgitation due to aortic valve prolapse. Am J Cardiol 1985; 55:1435–7.
195. Mardelli TJ, Morganroth J, Naito M, et al. Cross-sectional echocardiographic detection of aortic valve prolapse. Am Heart J 1980; 100:295–301.
196. Gilbert BW, Haney RS, Crawford F, et al. Two-dimensional echocardiographic assessment of vegetative endocarditis. Circulation 1977; 55:346–53.

197. Saner HE, Asinger RW, Homans DC, et al. Two-dimensional echocardiographic identification of complicated aortic root endocarditis: implication
for surgery. J Am Coll Cardiol 1987; 10:859–68.
198. Scanlan JG, Seward JB, Tajik AJ. Valve ring abcess in infective endocarditis: visualization with wide-angle two-dimensional echocardiography. Am
J Cardiol 1982; 49:1794–800.
199. Pollak SJ, Felner JM. Echocardiographic identification of aortic valve ring
abcess. J Am Coll Cardiol 1986; 7:1167–73.
200. Nguyen NX, Kessler KM, Bilsker MS, et al. Echocardiographic demonstration of satellite lesions in aortic valvular endocarditis. Am J Cardiol 1985;
55:1433–5.
201. Daniel WG, Mugge A, Martin RP, et al. Improvement in the diagnosis of
abcesses associated with endocarditis by transesophageal echocardiography. N Engl J Med 1991; 324:795–800.
202. Stewart WJ, Agler DA, Michael J, et al. Color flow mapping diagnosis and
localization of paravalvular aortic regurgitation. Circulation 1987; 76(suppl
IV):448.
203. DeMaria AN, Bommer W, Neumann A, et al. Identification and localization
of aneurysms of ascending aorta by cross-sectional echocardiography. Circulation 1979; 59:755–61.
204. Victor MF, Mintz GS, Kotler MN, et al. Two-dimensional echocardiographic diagnosis of aortic dissection. Am J Cardiol 1981; 48:1155–9.
205. Mathew T, Nanda NC. Two-dimensional and Doppler echocardiographic
evaluation of aortic aneurysm and dissection. Am J Cardiol 1984; 54:379–85.
206. Khandheria BK, Tajik AJ, Taylor CL, et al. Aortic dissection: review of
value and limitation of two-dimensional echocardiography in a six-year experience. J Am Soc Echocardiogr 1989; 2:17–24.
207. Smuckler AL, Nomeir AM, Watts LE, et al. Echocardiographic diagnosis
of aortic root dissection by M-mode and two-dimensional techniques. Am
Heart J 1982; 103:897–904.
208. Erbel R, Borner N, Steller D, et al. Detection of aortic dissection by transesophageal echocardiography. Br Heart J 1987; 58:45–51.
209. Erbel R, Engberding R, Daniel W, et al. Echocardiography in diagnosis of
aortic dissection. Lancet 1989; 1:457–61.
210. Hashimoto S, Kumada T, Osaka G, et al. Assessment of transesophageal
echocardiography in dissecting aortic aneurysm. J Am Coll Cardiol 1989;
14:1253–62.
211. Iliceto S, Nanda NC, Rizzon P, et al. Color Doppler evaluation of aortic
dissection. Circulation 1987; 75:748–55.
212. D'Cruz I, Cohen HC, Prabhu R, et al. Flutter of left ventricular structures
in patients with aortic regurgitation with special reference to patients with
associated mitral stenosis. Am Heart J 1976; 92:684–91.
213. Pridie RB, Benham R, Oakley CM. Echocardiography of the mitral valve
in aortic disease. Br Heart J 1971; 33:296–304.
214. Johnson AD, Gosnik BB. Oscillation of left ventricular structures in aortic
regurgitation. J Clin Ultrasound 1977; 5:21–4.

215. McDonald IG. Echocardiographic assessment of left ventricular function in aortic valve disease. Circulation 1976; 53:860–4.

216. Henry WL, Bonow RO, Borer JS, et al. Observations on the optimum time for operative intervention for aortic regurgitation: I. Evaluation of the results of aortic valve replacement in symptomatic patients. Circulation 1980; 61:471–83.

217. Henry WL, Bonow RO, Rosing DR, et al. Observations on the optimum time for operative intervention for aortic regurgitation: II. Serial echocardiographic evaluation of asymptomatic patients. Circulation 1980; 61: 484–92.

218. Reichek N, Wilson J, St-John Sutton M, et al. Noninvasive determination of left ventricular end-systolic stress: validation of the method and initial application. Circulation 1982; 65:99–108.

219. Bonow RO, Todd JT, Maron J, et al. Long-term serial changes in left ventricular function and reversal of ventricular dilation after valve replacement for chronic aortic regurgitation. Circulation 1988; 78:1108–20.

220. Kumpuris AG, Quinones MA, Waggoner AD, et al. Importance of preoperative hypertrophy, wall stress, and end-systolic dimensions as predictors of normalization of left ventricular dilation after valve replacement in chronic aortic insufficiency. Am J Cardiol 1982; 49:1091–100.

221. Fioretti P, Roelandt J, Bos RJ, et al. Echocardiography in chronic aortic insufficiency: is valve replacement too late when left ventricular end-systolic dimension reaches 55 mm? Circulation 1983; 67:216–21.

222. Cunha CLP, Giuliani ER, Fuster V, et al. Preoperative M-mode echocardiography as a predictor of surgical results in chronic aortic insufficiency. J Thorac Cardiovasc Surg 1980; 79:256–65.

223. Gaasch WH, Caroll JP, Levine HJ, et al. Chronic aortic regurgitation: prognostic value of left ventricular end-systolic radius/thickness ratio. J Am Coll Cardiol 1983; 1:775–82.

224. McDonald IG, Jelinek VM. Serial M-mode echocardiography in severe chronic aortic regurgitation. Circulation 1980; 62:1291–6.

225. Downes TR, Nomeir AM, Hackshaw BT, et al. Diastolic mitral regurgitation in acute but not chronic aortic regurgitation: implication regarding the mechanism of mitral closure. Am Heart J 1989; 117:1106–12.

226. Botvinick EH, Schiller NB, Wickramasekaran R, et al. Echocardiographic demonstration of early mitral valve closure in severe aortic insufficiency: its clinical implications. Circulation 1975; 51:836–47.

227. Meyer T, Sareli P, Pocock WA, et al. Echocardiographic and hemodynamic correlates of diastolic closure of mitral valve and diastolic opening of aortic valve in severe aortic regurgitation. Am J Cardiol 1987; 59: 1144–8.

228. Mann T, McLaurin L, Grossman W, et al. Assessing the hemodynamic severity of acute aortic regurgitation due to infective endocarditis. N Engl J Med 1975; 293:108–13.

229. Weaver WF, Wilson CS, Bourke T, et al. Mid-diastolic aortic valve opening in severe aortic regurgitation. Circulation 1977; 55:145–8.

230. Pietro DA, Parisi AF, Harrington JJ, et al. Premature opening of the aortic

valve: an index of highly advanced aortic regurgitation. J Clin Ultrasound 1978; 6:170–2.

231. Tajik AJ, Giuliani ER. Diastolic opening of aortic valve: an echocardiographic observation. Mayo Clin Proc 1977; 52:112–6.

232. Veyrat C, Lessana A, Abitol G, et al. New indexes for assessing aortic regurgitation with two-dimensional Doppler echocardiographic measurements of regurgitant aortic valvular area. Circulation 1983; 68:998–1005.

233. Ward JM, Baker DW, Rubenstein SA, et al. Detection of aortic insufficiency by pulsed Doppler echocardiography. J Clin Ultrasound 1977; 5:5–10.

234. Ciobanu M, Abbasi AS, Allen M, et al. Pulsed Doppler echocardiography in the diagnosis and estimation of severity of aortic insufficiency. Am J Cardiol 1982; 49:339–43.

235. Boughner DR. Assessment of aortic insufficiency by transcutaneous Doppler ultrasound. Circulation 1975; 52:874–9.

236. Esper RJ. Detection of mild aortic regurgitation by range-gated pulsed Doppler echocardiography. Am J Cardiol 1982; 50:1037–43.

237. Favvuzi A, Pennestri F, Biasucci LM, et al. Pulsed-wave Doppler quantitation of aortic regurgitation associated with mitral stenosis. Cardiologia 1988; 33:485–91.

238. Quinones MA, Young JB, Waggoner AD, et al. Assessment of pulsed Doppler echocardiography in detection and quantification of aortic and mitral regurgitation. Br Heart J 1980; 44:612–20.

239. Diebold B, Peronneau P, Blanchard D, et al. Noninvasive quantification of aortic regurgitation by Doppler echocardiography. Br Heart J 1983; 49: 167–73.

240. Touche T, Prasquir R, Nitenberg A, et al. Assessment and follow-up of patients with aortic regurgitation by an updated echocardiographic measurement of the regurgitant fraction in the aortic arch. Circulation 1985; 72: 819–24.

241. Takenaka K, Dabestani A, Gardin JM, et al. A simple Doppler echocardiographic method for estimating severity of aortic regurgitation. Am J Cardiol 1986; 57:1340–3.

242. Kitabatake A, Ito H, Inoue M, et al. A new approach to noninvasive evaluation of aortic regurgitant fraction by two-dimensional Doppler echocardiography. Circulation 1985; 72:523–9.

243. Perry GH, Helmcke F, Nanda NC, et al. Evaluation of aortic insufficiency by Doppler color flow mapping. J Am Coll Cardiol 1987; 9:952–9.

244. Pearlman AS, Otto CM, Janko CL, et al. Direction and width of aortic regurgitant jets: assessment by Doppler color flow mapping. J Am Coll Cardiol 1986; 7:100A.

245. Switzer DF, Yoganathan AP, Nanda NC, et al. Calibration of color Doppler flow mapping during extreme hemodynamic conditions in vitro: a foundation for a reliable quantitative grading system for aortic incompetence. Circulation 1987; 75:837–46.

246. Baumgartner H, Kratzer H, Helmreich G, et al. Quantitation of aortic regurgitation by color-coded cross-sectional Doppler echocardiography. Eur Heart J 1988; 9:380–7.

247. Bolger AF, Eiger NL, Pfaff JM, et al. Relationship of color Doppler jet area to flow volume: reliability and limitations. Circulation 1986; 74(suppl II):216.

248. Hatle L, Angelsen B. Doppler Ultrasound in Cardiology: Physical Principles and Clinical Application. 2d ed. Philadelphia: Lea & Febiger, 1985:154–62.

249. Masuyama T, Kodama K, Kitabatake A, et al. Noninvasive evaluation of aortic regurgitation by continuous-wave Doppler echocardiography. Circulation 1986; 73:460–6.

250. Beyer RW, Ramirez M, Josephson MA, et al. Correlation of continuous-wave Doppler assessment of chronic aortic regurgitation with hemodynamics and angiography. Am J Cardiol 1987; 60:852–6.

251. Grayburn PA, Handshoe R, Smith MD, et al. Quantitative assessment of the hemodynamic consequences of aortic reguritation by means of continuous-wave Doppler readings. J Am Coll Cardiol 1987; 10:135–41.

252. Labovitz AJ, Ferrara RP, Kern MJ, et al. Quantitative evaluation of aortic insufficiency by continuous-wave Doppler echocardiography. J Am Coll Cardiol 1986; 8:1341–7.

253. Teague SM, Heinsimer JA, Anderson JL, et al. Quantification of aortic regurgitation utilizing continuous-wave Doppler ultrasound. J Am Coll Cardiol 1986; 8:592–9.

254. Nishimura RA, Tajik AJ. Determination of left-sided pressure gradients by utilizing Doppler aortic and mitral regurgitant signals; validation by simultaneous dual catheter and Doppler studies. J Am Coll Cardiol 1988; 11:317–21.

255. Oh JK, Hatle LK, Sinak LJ, et al. Characteristic Doppler echocardiographic pattern of mitral inflow velocity in severe aortic regurgitation. J Am Coll Cardiol 1989; 14:1712–7.

256. Vandenbossche JL, Englert M. Doppler color flow mapping demonstration of diastolic mitral regurgitation in severe acute aortic regurgitation. Am Heart J 1987; 114:889–90.

257. Weyman AE, Hurwitz RA, Girod DA, et al. Cross-sectional echocardiographic visualization of the stenotic pulmonary valve. Circulation 1977; 56:769–74.

258. Callahan JA, Wroblewski EM, Reeder GS, et al. Echocardiographic features of carcinoid heart disease. Am J Cardiol 1982; 50:762–8.

259. Come PC, Come SE, Hawley CR, et al. Echocardiographic manifestation of carcinoid heart disease. J Clin Ultrasound 1982; 10:233–7.

260. Cremieux A, Witchitz S, Malergue M, et al. Clinical and echocardiographic observations in pulmonary valve endocarditis. Am J Cardiol 1985; 56:610–3.

261. Nakamura K, Satomi G, Sakai T, et al. Clinical and echocardiographic features of pulmonary valve endocarditis. Circulation 1983; 67:198–204.

262. Johnson GL, Kwan OL, Handshoe S, et al. Accuracy of combined two-dimensional echocardiography and continuous-wave Doppler recordings in the estimation of pressure gradient in right ventricular outlet obstruction. J Am Coll Cardiol 1984; 3:1013–8.

263. Hatle L, Angelsen B. Doppler Ultrasound in Cardiology: Physical Principles and Clinical Application. 2d ed. Philadelphia: Lea & Febiger, 1985:143–51.
264. Lima CO, Sahn DJ, Valdes-Cruz LM, et al. Noninvasive prediction of transvalvular pressure gradient in patients with pulmonary stenosis by quantitative two-dimensional echocardiographic Doppler studies. Circulation 1983; 67:866–71.
265. Kosturakis D, Allen HD, Goldberg SJ, et al. Noninvasive quantification of stenotic semilunar valve areas by Doppler echocardiography. J Am Coll Cardiol 1984; 3:1256–62.
266. Kan JS, White RI, Mitchell SE, et al. Percutaneous transluminal balloon valvuloplasty for pulmonary valve stenosis. Circulation 1984; 69:554–60.
267. Lababidi Z, Wu J. Percutaneous balloon pulmonary valvuloplasty. Am J Cardiol 1983; 52:560–2.
268. Mullins CE, Ludomirsky A, O'Laughlin MP, et al. Balloon valvuloplasty for pulmonic valve stenosis: two-year follow-up: hemodynamic and Doppler evaluation. Cathet Cardiovasc Diagnosis 1988; 14:76–81.
269. Robertson M, Benson LN, Smallhorn JS, et al. The morphology of the right ventricular outflow tract after percutaneous pulmonary valvotomy: long-term follow-up. Br Heart J 1987; 58:239–44.
270. Rao PS, Fawzy ME, Solymar L, et al. Long-term results of balloon pulmonary valvuloplasty of valvar pulmonic stenosis. Am Heart J 1988; 115: 1291–6.
271. Kveselis DA, Rocchini AP, Snider AT, et al. Results of balloon valvuloplasty in treatment of congenital valvar pulmonary stenosis in children. Am J Cardiol 1985; 56:527–32.
272. Takao S, Miyatake K, Izumi S, et al. Physiological pulmonary regurgitation detected by the Doppler technique and its differential diagnosis. J Am Coll Cardiol 1985; 5:499.
273. Nanda NC. Textbook of Color Doppler Echocardiography. Philadelphia: Lea & Febiger, 1989:164–89.
274. Goldberg SJ, Allen HD. Quantitative assessment by Doppler echocardiography of pulmonary or aortic regurgitation. Am J Cardiol 1985; 56:131–5.
275. Patel AK, Rowe GG, Dhanni SP, et al. Pulsed Doppler echocardiography in diagnosis of pulmonary regurgitation: its value and limitations. Am J Cardiol 1982; 49:1801–5.
276. Miyatake K, Okamoto M, Konoshita N, et al. Pulmonary regurgitation studied with the ultrasonic pulsed Doppler technique. Circulation 1982; 65: 969–76.
277. Masuyama T, Kodama K, Kitabatake A, et al. Continuous-wave Doppler echocardiographic detection of pulmonary regurgitation and its application to noninvasive estimation of pulmonary artery pressure. Circulation 1986; 74:484–92.
278. Hatle L, Angelsen B. Doppler Ultrasound in Cardiology: Physical Principles and Clinical Application. 2d ed. Philadelphia: Lea & Febiger, 1985:162–76.
279. Matsuda M, Sekiguchi T, Sugishita Y, et al. Reliability of noninvasive esti-

mates of pulmonary hypertension by pulsed Doppler echocardiography. Br Heart J 1986; 56:158–64.

280. Isobe M, Yazaki Y, Takaku F, et al. Prediction of pulmonary arterial pressure in adults by pulsed Doppler echocardiography. Am J Cardiol 1986; 57: 316–21.

281. Graettinger WF, Greene ER, Voyles WF. Doppler predictions of pulmonary artery pressure and resistance in adults. Am Heart J 1987; 113:1426–37.

282. Martin-Duran R, Larman M, Trugeda A, et al. Comparison of Doppler-determined elevated pulmonary arterial pressure with pressure measured at cardiac catheterization. Am J Cardiol 1986; 57:859–63.

283. Kitabatake A, Inoue M, Asao M, et al. Noninvasive evaluation of pulmonary hypertension by pulsed Doppler technique. Circulation 1983; 68:302–9.

284. Hatle L, Angelsen BAJ, Tromsdal A. Noninvasive estimation of pulmonary artery systolic pressure with Doppler ultrasound. Br Heart J 1981; 45: 157–65.

285. Hauk AJ, Freeman DP, Ackermann DM, et al. Surgical pathology of the tricuspid valve: a study of 363 cases spanning 25 years. Mayo Clin Proc 1988; 63:851–63.

286. Redfield MM, Holmes DR, Edwards WD, Tajik AJ. Valve disease associated with ergot alkaloid use: echocardiographic and pathologic correlations. Annals Intern Med 1992; 117:50–2.

287. Daniels SJ, Mintz GS, Kotler MN. Rheumatic tricuspid valve disease: two-dimensional echocardiographic, hemodynamic, and angiographic correlations. Am J Cardiol 1983; 51:492–6.

288. Nanna M, Chandraranta A, Reid C, et al. Value of two-dimensional echocardiography in detecting tricuspid stenosis. Circulation 1983; 67:221–4.

289. Shimada R, Takeshita A, Nakamura M, et al. Diagnosis of tricuspid stenosis by M-mode and two-dimensional echocardiography. Am J Cardiol 1984; 53: 164–8.

290. Guyer DE, Gillam LD, Foale RA, et al. Comparison of the echocardiographic and hemodynamic diagnosis of rheumatic tricuspid stenosis. J Am Coll Cardiol 1984; 3:1135–44.

291. Parris TM, Panidis IP, Ross J, et al. Doppler echocardiographic findings in rheumatic tricuspid stenosis. Am J Cardiol 1987; 60:1414–6.

292. Perez JE, Ludbrook PA, Ahumada GG. Usefulness of Doppler echocardiography in detecting tricuspid stenosis. Am J Cardiol 1985; 55:601–3.

293. Denning K, Henneke K, Rudolph W. Assessment of tricuspid stenosis by Doppler echocardiography. J Am Coll Cardiol 1987; 9(suppl A):237.

294. Nanda NC. Textbook of Color Doppler Echocardiography. Philadelphia: Lea & Febiger, 1989:175–6.

295. Waller BF, Morarty AT, Eble JN, et al. Etiology of pure tricuspid regurgitation based on anular circumference and leaflet area: analysis of 45 necropsy patients with clinical and morphological evidence of pure tricuspid regurgitation. J Am Coll Cardiol 1986; 7:1063–74.

296. Mardelli TJ, Morganroth J, Chen CC, et al. Tricuspid valve prolapse diagnosed by cross-sectional echocardiography. Chest 1981; 79:201–5.

297. Oliver J, Benito F, Garcia-Gallepo F, et al. Echocardiographic findings in ruptured chordae tendineae of the tricuspid valve. Am Heart J 1983; 105: 1033–5.
298. Panidis IP, Kotler MN, Mintz GS, et al. Right heart endocarditis: clinical and echocardiographic features. Am Heart J 1984; 107:759–64.
299. Shiina A, Seward JB, Edwards WD, et al. Two-dimensional echocardiographic spectrum of Ebestein's anomaly: detailed anatomic assessment. J Am Coll Cardiol 1984; 3:356–70.
300. Moreno FL, Hagan AD, Holmen JR, et al. Evaluation of size and dynamics of the inferior vena cava as an index of right-sided cardiac function. Am J Cardiol 1984; 53:579–85.
301. Fisher EA, Goldman ME. Simple, rapid method for quantification of tricuspid regurgitation by two-dimensional echocardiography. Am J Cardiol 1989; 63:1375–8.
302. Sakai K, Nakamura K, Satomi G, et al. Evaluation of tricuspid regurgitation by blood flow pattern in the hepatic vein using pulsed Doppler technique. Am Heart J 1984; 108:516–23.
303. Curtius JM, Thyssen M, Breuer HM, et al. Doppler versus contrast echocardiography for diagnosis of tricuspid regurgitation. Am J Cardiol 1985; 56: 333–6.
304. Lieppe W, Behar VS, Scallion R, et al. Detection of tricuspid regurgitation with two-dimensional echocardiography and peripheral vein injections. Circulation 1978; 57:128–32.
305. Meltzer RS, van Hoogenhuyze F, Serruys PW, et al. Diagnosis of tricuspid regurgitation by contrast echocardiography. Circulation 1981; 63:1093–9.
306. Chen CC, Morganroth J, Mardelli TJ, et al. Tricuspid regurgitation in tricuspid valve prolapse demonstrated with contrast cross-sectional echocardiography. Am J Cardiol 1980; 46:938–87.
307. Nimura Y, Miyatake K, Okamoto M, et al. Pulsed Doppler echocardiography in the assessment of tricuspid regurgitation. Ultrasound Med Biol 1984; 10:239–47.
308. Waggoner AD, Quinones MA, Young JB, et al. Pulsed Doppler echocardiographic detection of right-sided valve regurgitation. Am J Cardiol 1981; 47: 279–86.
309. Miyatake K, Okamoto M, Konishata N, et al. Evaluation of tricuspid regurgitation by pulsed Doppler and two-dimensional echocardiography. Circulation 1982; 66:777–84.
310. Pennestri F, Loperfido F, Salvatori MP, et al. Assessment of tricuspid regurgitation by pulsed Doppler ultrasonography of the hepatic veins. Am J Cardiol 1984; 54:363–8.
311. Dabestani A, French J, Gardin J, et al. Doppler hepatic vein blood flow in patients with tricuspid regurgitation. J Am Coll Cardiol 1983; 1(2):658.
312. Diebold B, Touati R, Blanchard D, et al. Quantitative assessment of tricuspid regurgitation using pulsed Doppler echocardiography. Br Heart J 1983; 50:443–9.
313. Suzuki Y, Kambara H, Kadota K, et al. Detection and evaluation of tricus-

pid regurgitation using real-time, two-dimensional, color-coded Doppler flow imaging system: comparison with contrast two-dimensional echocardiography and right ventriculography. Am J Cardiol 1986; 57:811–5.

314. Chopra HK, Nanda NC, Fan P, et al. Can two-dimensional echocardiography and Doppler color flow mapping identify the need for tricuspid valve repair? J Am Coll Cardiol 1989; 14:1266–74.

315. Minagoe S, Rahimtoola SH, Chandraratna PA. Significance of laminar systolic regurgitant flow in patients with tricuspid regurgitation: a combined pulsed-wave, continuous-wave Doppler, and two-dimensional echocardiographic study. Am Heart J 1990; 119:627–35.

316. Hatle L, Angelsen B. Doppler Ultrasound in Cardiology: Physical Principles and Clinical Application. 2d ed. Philadelphia: Lea & Febiger, 1985:170–6.

317. Currie PJ, Seward JB, Chan KL, et al. Continuous-wave Doppler determination of right ventricular pressure: a simultaneous Doppler-catheterization study in 127 patients. J Am Coll Cardiol 1985; 6:750–6.

318. Yock PG, Popp RL. Noninvasive estimation of right ventricular systolic pressure by Doppler ultrasound in patients with tricuspid regurgitation. Circulation 1984; 70:657–62.

4

Radiological Examination in Valvular Heart Disease

Richard Coulden and Martin J. Lipton
University of Chicago
Chicago, Illinois

The imaging of valvular heart disease, like all other areas of cardiac investigation, has changed dramatically over recent years. The old standbys of chest radiography and cardiac catheterization have been supplemented and at times replaced by newer techniques. A prime example of this is ultrasound. Over the space of 15 years, echocardiography has been transformed from Kisslo's first report to being an invaluable part of everyday diagnosis and management (1). Ultrafast computed tomography (UFCT) and magnetic resonance imaging (MRI) are still in their infancy, but continuing development will undoubtedly make them more important (2–4).

Before the clinician can establish a rational approach to imaging, it is important to have a clear understanding of the capabilities and limitations of the modalities available. This chapter describes the basics of technique, anatomy, and pathology with regard to the chest radiograph, UFCT, and MRI. As echocardiography and cardiac catheterization have been dealt with elsewhere, they will not be considered.

I. THE CHEST RADIOGRAPH

The chest radiograph is inexpensive, noninvasive, and universally available. Although it has been overshadowed by newer techniques, it remains the most frequently requested cardiac examination. It provides important information concerning cardiac size, chamber enlargement, pulmonary circulation, and cardiac calcification. Understanding the chest radiograph is a vital precursor to understanding much of cardiac radiology.

A. Technique

The cardiac patient's first series of radiographs should include frontal and lateral views. Both are necessary for a complete assessment of chamber size and cardiac calcification. With this as a baseline, follow-up examinations may require only a frontal view. Oblique views are rarely indicated.

The frontal view should be performed postero-anteriorly (PA), with the subject erect and in full inspiration. The distance from X-ray source (focus) to film is standardized at 6 ft, allowing easy comparison between interval studies. If the patient is unable to come to the radiology department, mobile X-ray equipment can be used. In this situation, an antero-posterior (AP) view is usually obtained; this may be erect or supine. Differences in position and projection have important effects on heart size and appearance. Both AP and PA views cause cardiac magnification, but this is greater for the AP, where the heart is farther from the film. In the supine position, the combination of a short focus–film distance and AP projection cause the greatest magnification.

X-ray exposure factors and the type of equipment used will also have important effects on the image. The X-ray tube kilovoltage (kV) determines the level of tissue contrast. Conventionally, a low-kV technique is used (60–80 kV). This gives high contrast, demonstrating lung and bone well, but penetrating the mediastinum poorly. Using a higher kV (120–150 kV) lowers contrast but improves visualization of the mediastinum and hidden areas of lung, i.e., behind the heart and diaphragm. There is always a compromise between contrast and penetration, parameters being altered to meet the needs of the viewer. New developments in digital and computed radiography (CR) may help solve this conflict. CR is particularly appealing, as it represents a "halfway house" between conventional and digital radiography (5). Images are obtained with standard X-ray equipment, making it ideal for use on wards and intensive-care units (6), but it still has the advantages of digital imaging, wide exposure latitude, reduced radiation dose, and the capacity for image manipulation. In its simplest form, image manipulation means that "window level and width" can be adjusted, just as for CT or MRI; a range of contrasts and depths of penetration can then be created from a single exposure.

B. Anatomy

The X-ray attenuating characteristics of different tissues determine their appearance on the chest radiograph. Four levels of attenuation are recognized: air, fat, soft tissue, and bone. Adjacent structures can be separated only by differences in their radiographic density. If they both have the same density, they appear as one. For the mediastinum, this means that most diagnostic information is contained in the borders which abut air-filled lung, i.e., the cardiac silhouette. Internal borders are lost, as the soft tissue structures in the mediastinum have the same radiographic density. Interpreting the chest radiograph, therefore, requires an understanding of both mediastinal anatomy and the way this relates to the visualized boundaries.

Figures 1A–1D show the relationship of the cardiac chambers, great vessels, and valves to the mediastinal boundaries on frontal and lateral views. Although the AV and semilunar valves cannot normally be identified, they may calcify when diseased. The appearance and position of this calcification indicates the valve involved and may predict the nature of the underlying process.

C. Heart Size

Heart size is best assessed by measurement of transverse diameter (7,8). This can be expressed as an absolute value or as a cardio-thoracic ratio (CTR). Considering a routine PA projection, the transverse diameter should be no more than 15.5 cm in men and 15 cm in women. A change of more than 1.5 cm between examinations is significant. The CTR is the ratio between cardiac transverse diameter and maximum width of the thorax above the costophrenic angles (Fig. 2). The upper limit of normal is quoted as 0.50, but if it is adhered to too rigidly this will lead to false positive and negative diagnoses. In ischemic heart disease, the left ventricle may enlarge inferiorly and posteriorly, with the CTR remaining within normal limits. Conversely, chest deformities such as scoliosis or pectus excavatum may lead to an increase in CTR without genuine cardiomegaly. In situations where the heart size is in doubt, a review of old radiographs is more helpful than a solitary CTR measurement. The normal CTR in children is over 0.5 (up to 0.6 in neonates). This varies inversely with age and must be taken into account when making serial measurements in children with congenital heart disease. CTR may also be used for supine AP films, although the short film–focus distance will increase magnification. In this setting, the upper limit of normal is 0.57 (9).

Previously accepted radiographic methods for calculating heart volume have become outdated with the introduction of cross-sectional imaging techniques, namely, echocardiography, CT, and MRI.

D. Specific Patterns of Cardiac Chamber Enlargement

In valvular heart disease, the changes observed are generally the result of pressure overload, volume overload, or both. In this context, pressure

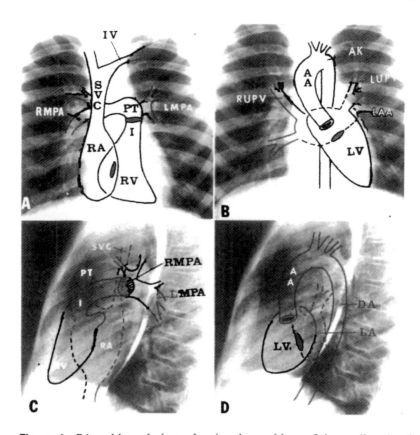

Figure 1 PA and lateral views showing the positions of the cardiac chambers, valves, and major pulmonary and systemic vessels. A and C demonstrate the right heart, B and D demonstrate the left. AA, ascending aorta; AK, aortic knob; DA, descending aorta; I, infundibulum; IV, innominate vein; LA, left atrium; LAA left atrial appendage; LMPA, left main pulmonary vein; LUPV, left upper pulmonary vein; LV, left ventricle; PT, pulmonary trunk; RA, right atrium; RMPA, right main pulmonary artery; RUPV, right upper pulmonary vein; RV, right ventricle; SVC, superior vena cava. (From Elliott and Scheibler. The X-Ray Diagnosis of Congenital Heart Disease in Infants, Children and Adults. 2d ed. Springfield, Ill.: Charles C Thomas, 1979. Reproduced with permission.)

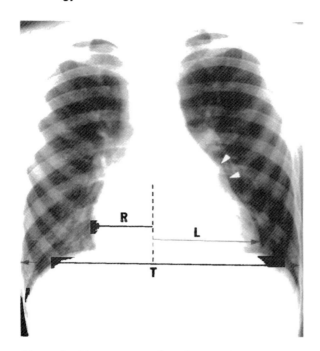

Figure 2 Measurement of cardiothoracic ratio (CTR). CTR = R + L/T = 0.59. Moderate cardiomegaly due to mixed mitral valve disease. Large left atrial appendage (white arrow heads) and increased convexity right heart border, the latter indicates right atrial enlargement.

overload is caused by valvular stenosis or outlet obstruction; volume overload is caused by regurgitation. The result, in terms of dilatation and/or hypertrophy, depends on the chamber involved, the severity and duration of the insult, and the presence or absence of myopathy. For example, pressure overload due to aortic stenosis produces left ventricular hypertrophy without dilatation. Even marked hypertrophy may not cause radiographic evidence of chamber enlargement. The presence of dilatation indicates the presence of ventricular failure or associated regurgitation. In mitral stenosis, by contrast, the thin-walled left atrium responds by hypertrophy and dilatation. The atrial myopathy, which often underlies rheumatic mitral disease, may make this dilatation severe.

Volume overload produces dilatation. Although there may be an increase in myocardial mass, chamber dilatation often masks the increase in wall thickness. This is true for atria, ventricles, and mediastinal vessels alike.

The severity of the lesion is also an important. While the degree of stenosis may not be mirrored by chamber enlargement, dilatation secondary to regurgitation does show a broad correlation. The duration of the process should also be taken into account. For example, a patient with longstanding aortic regurgitation may have marked left ventricular enlargement but no evidence of failure; whereas another patient with acute regurgitation due to a disrupted aortic prosthesis has little dilatation but severe failure.

The recognition of specific chamber enlargement is fraught with difficulties. As blood and soft tissue both have the same radiographic density, one cannot clearly distinguish one chamber from another. Diagnosis is based largely on a subjective assessment of the cardiac contour and the way this fits in with accepted patterns. These are outlined below. Although they may be helpful, one must remember that these patterns may be lost in complex valve disease and multichamber enlargement.

1. Right Atrium

The superior vena cava, right atrium and inferior vena cava form the right heart border. As the right atrium enlarges, the right heart border bulges to the right (Fig. 3). When dilatation is severe, the atrial appendage is involved and projects anteriorly and superiorly on the lateral view. Assessment of right atrial enlargement is particularly difficult, as abnormal convexity of the right heart border may be a feature of left atrial or right ventricular enlargement. When right atrial enlargement is associated with elevated pressures, the cavae and azygos vein also become distended, the degree of azygos distension being broadly correlated with mean right atrial pressure (Fig. 4) (10). The lateral border of the superior vena cava normally lies within 1 cm of the spine, and the azygos vein, as it crosses above the right main bronchus, is less than 1 cm in diameter. These values are only a guide and vary with intrathoracic pressure and position.

2. Right Ventricle

The normal right ventricle lies anteriorly and is border-forming only on the lateral view. As the triangular ventricle enlarges, it displaces the left ventricle and heart border laterally. The cardiac apex moves superiorly (Fig. 5). With further enlargement, the left ventricle is rotated posteriorly and the right ventricle may form the left heart border. On the lateral view, enlargement produces an increase in the anterior bulk of the heart and displacement of the anterior border anteriorly and superiorly. Contact of more than half the body of the sternum with the cardiac silhouette is a late sign of dilatation. This sign should be treated with caution; it may be misleading in patients with a hyperinflated chest or pectus excavatum.

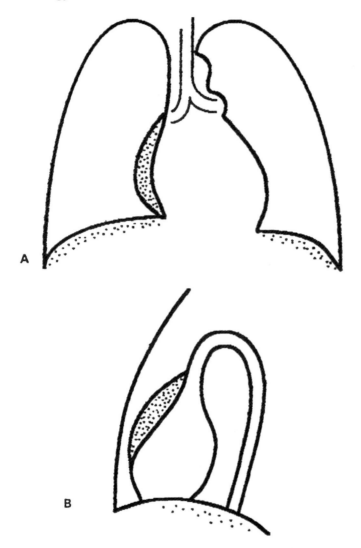

Figure 3   PA (A) and lateral (B) cardiac silhouettes indicating pattern of right atrial enlargement. On the lateral, the right atrial appendage enlarges antero-superiorly.

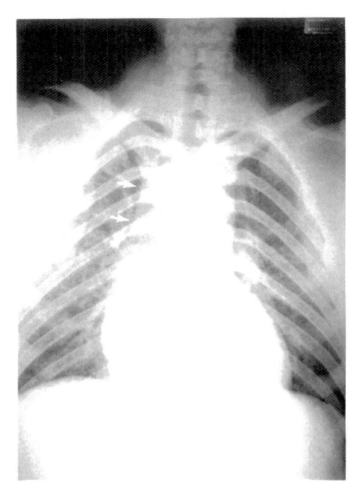

Figure 4 Widened superior mediastinum to the right of the midline (white arrows) due to fluid overload and dilatation of the SVC and innominate vein.

3. Left Atrium

The left atrium lies in the midline posteriorly, the atrial appendage forming
a small part of the left heart border below the left main bronchus. On the
lateral view it forms the superior aspect of the posterior heart border.
This border is often obscured by converging pulmonary veins. The right
pulmonary venous confluence is sometimes visible on the PA view and
may be mistaken for a mass. Left atrial enlargement may be to the left,
the right, superiorly or posteriorly (Fig. 6).

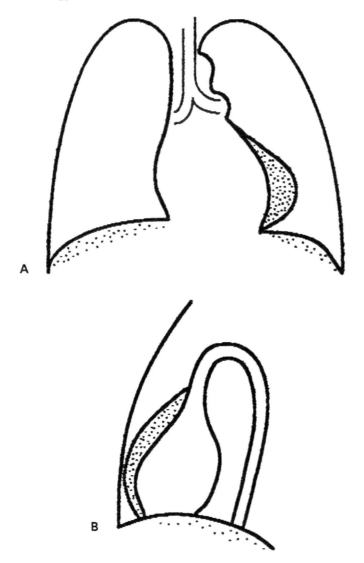

Figure 5 PA (A) and lateral (B) cardiac silhouettes indicating pattern of right ventricular enlargement. Cardiac apex moves supero-laterally. On the lateral, the anterior mediastinal window is lost and there is increased contact between the right ventricle and sternum (>50%).

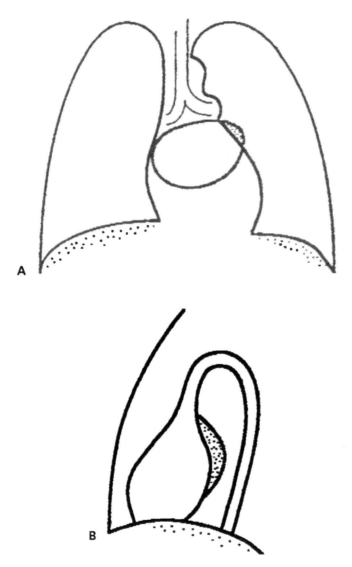

Figure 6   PA (A) and lateral (B) cardiac silhouettes indicating pattern of left atrial enlargement. Atrial appendage produces convexity below pulmonary trunk and carina is splayed. On the lateral, posterior enlargement does not involve the inferior aspect of the cardiac outline.

Enlargement to the left is seen as convexity of the atrial appendage. Occasionally, however, a normal appendage may produce a slight bulge, and a large appendage, no bulge. If coexisting right ventricular enlargement extends to the left heart border, this may mask a large appendage. A prominent appendage is typical of rheumatic mitral valve disease but is rare in other causes of left atrial enlargement. Moderate dilatation to the right produces a convex shadow within the right heart border (double right heart border). Any further increase may make the left atrium border-forming, rotating the right atrium anteriorly. If both atrial borders are superimposed, the diagnosis of left atrial enlargement can easily be missed on the PA radiograph alone. Enlargement superiorly bows the left main and lower lobe bronchi superiorly and laterally. Eventually the carina becomes splayed. Although the carinal angle is increased in short, stout normal subjects, it is not less than 90°.

Posterior enlargement is best seen on the lateral view, but this is sometimes masked by overlying pulmonary veins. On the PA, there may be increased density within the cardiac silhouette and displacement of the mid descending thoracic aorta laterally. This latter sign is of value only in young patients, before the aorta becomes elongated. Compression of the esophagus may cause dysphagia, although both dysphagia and aortic displacement are more likely in subjects with narrow AP chest diameters.

4. Left Ventricle

The left ventricle forms the left heart border below the left atrial appendage and the posterior border below the left atrium. Inferiorly, the posterior outline is made by the inferior vena cava as it passes through the diaphragm. When the left ventricle enlarges, the left heart border is displaced laterally and the apex inferiorly. Posteriorly, the free wall of the ventricle migrates behind the inferior vena cava (Fig. 7). In valve disease, these changes are usually symmetrical; a focal abnormality suggests concomitant ischemia or infarction.

Biventricular enlargement is more complex. When the right ventricle is very large, the left ventricle is displaced posteriorly. The right ventricle can then form the left heart border, giving a false impression of left ventricular enlargement. The correct diagnosis is suggested by increased bulk anterior to the right ventricle on a lateral view. Left ventricular enlargement alone will not produce this appearance.

5. Aorta

The ascending aorta normally lies within the cardiac silhouette. After the age of 40, elongation may make it bulge laterally beyond the superior vena cava. Before this, prominence is a good sign of aortic aneurysm or

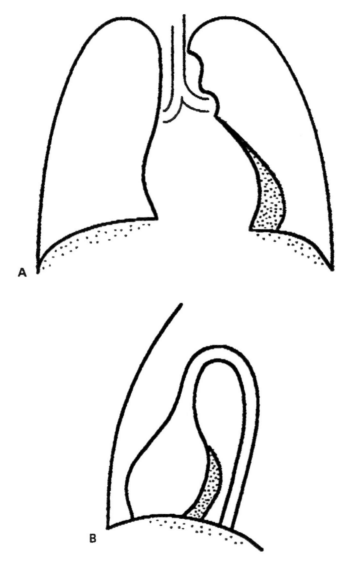

Figure 7 PA (A) and lateral (B) cardiac silhouettes indicating pattern of left ventricular enlargement. Apex is displaced infero-laterally. On the lateral, inferior aspect of the cardiac outline is displaced posteriorly.

poststenotic dilatation. In aortic regurgitation, diffuse enlargement of the ascending aorta may occur, sometimes extending to the arch and beyond. When the aorta is compliant, as in young patients, dilatation may be seen only in systole.

The normal descending aorta lies within the mediastinum. With age and elongation it extends to the left, forming a boundary with lung and making it visible on the PA film.

6. Pulmonary Artery

The pulmonary trunk and left pulmonary artery form part of the left heart border between the aortic knuckle and the left atrial appendage. In infants it may be obscured by the thymus, and in children and young women it is often distinctly convex. By the age of 20, the adult pattern is attained, giving a straight or only slightly convex outline. Enlargement occurs in pulmonary hypertension and pulmonary regurgitation. In poststenotic dilatation, only the pulmonary trunk and left pulmonary artery are affected; the right pulmonary artery is usually normal. This situation is reversed in corrected transposition, where altered flow leads to poststenotic dilatation of the right pulmonary artery.

E. Cardiac Calcification

Calcification may be dystrophic or metastatic. For most purposes cardiac calcification is dystrophic, i.e., it occurs in dead or degenerate tissue, and the serum calcium level is normal. The location and morphology of the calcification can often provide valuable diagnostic clues to the underlying pathological process.

1. Cardiac Chambers

Endocardial and myocardial calcification lie within the cardiac silhouette. The former occurs in organized thrombus; the latter tends to be linear and is deposited in infarcted muscle, most frequently in left ventricular aneurysms. Left atrial calcification is also thin and linear, but this develops as a result of rheumatic involvement of the atrial wall (Fig. 8). The septum is rarely involved. Occasionally, thrombus in the left atrial appendage will also calcify.

2. Pericardial Calcification

Pericardial calcification arises initially in the AV grooves and spreads irregularly over the epicardial surface. It may appear as amorphous mass-like deposits or as multiple layers resembling onion rings. There need not be pericardial constriction. Calcification is secondary to organized blood or exudate in the pericardium and commonly follows tuberculous or rheu-

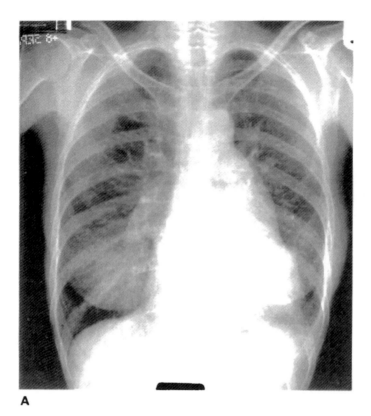

A

Figure 8 PA (A) and lateral (B) showing curvilinear calcification in an enlarged left atrium. This is secondary to rheumatic mitral valve disease. On the lateral, left atrial enlargement displaces the cardiac outline posteriorly (white arrows). Left ventricular enlargement is indicated by displacement of the posterior wall of the left ventricle behind the IVC (curved black arrow).

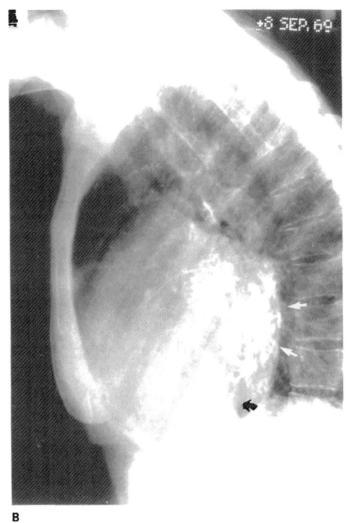

B

matic pericarditis. It is characteristically seen at the edge of the cardiac silhouette, and often appears more impressive and severe in a lateral projection, where it commonly lies adjacent to the diaphragm.

3. Valve Calcification

Aortic valve calcification lies above the line extending from the carina to the anterior costophrenic angle on the lateral film (Fig. 9). Mitral calcification usually lies below this line. Mitral calcification may be rheumatic or senile. In rheumatic valve disease it is more common in stenosis than in regurgitation and is usually present after the age of 50. Calcification involves the posterior valve leaflet and extends onto the adjacent posterior ventricular wall. This extension may be associated with heart block. Senile calcification is subvalvular and gives rise to a reversed C shape, which is incomplete medially (Fig. 10). It very rarely causes any hemodynamic

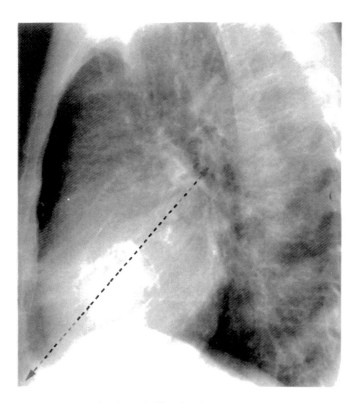

Figure 9 Aortic ring calcification in congenital aortic stenosis. Calcification lies predominantly above the line joining the anterior costophrenic angle and the hilum; mitral calcification usually lies below.

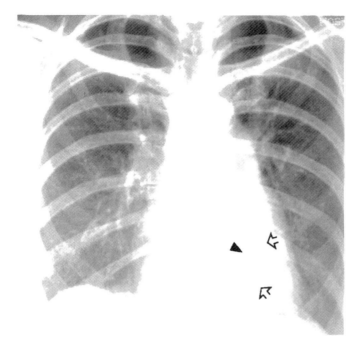

Figure 10 Mitral ring and leaflet calcification. Subvalvar ring calcification (open arrows) is typical of senile calcification and is of little significance. However, calcification of the posterior mitral leaflet (arrow head) suggests additional rheumatic involvement. This is supported by the cardiomegaly and prominent left atrial appendage.

disturbance, unlike aortic sclerosis. Calcification of both mitral and aortic valves indicates rheumatic valve disease, unless the patient is over 60, when it may be senile.

Aortic calcification occurs in bicuspid valves, rheumatic endocarditis, senile degeneration, syphilis, ankylosing spondylitis, and following bacterial endocarditis—in descending order of frequency. Only the first three will cause stenosis. Bicuspid valves may demonstrate commissural or ring calcification; the others usually show plaquelike calcification. The incidence of bacterial endocarditis is higher on calcified than noncalcified valves.

Calcification of right-sided valves is uncommon. In the tricuspid position it is rheumatic, and in the pulmonary it is most frequently due to congenital stenosis. Following surgery, conduits in the pulmonary outflow tract frequently calcify, often within the first 12 months, but this is rarely of clinical significance. Vascular calcification in the aorta and coronary arteries is common. It is always associated with atherosclerosis, although the extent does not correlate with severity. When calcification occurs in the proximal pulmonary arteries, it is a good indication of severe, long-standing pulmonary hypertension, regardless of cause.

F. Pulmonary Vasculature

1. Anatomy

The pulmonary trunk gives rise to right and left pulmonary arteries. The right passes horizontally in front of the right main bronchus, the left arches superiorly over the left main bronchus. The intrapulmonary arterial branches are closely related to the bronchi. Branching is either by bifurcation or collateral branching. In the latter, the main vessel follows a straight path with small side branches arising at right angles. Collateral branching is responsible for the even, reticular pattern of vessels seen in the periphery of the lung. The arrangement of veins differs from that of the arteries. The veins are not related to the broncho-arterial unit, tending to lie in the interlobular septa. Centrally they become intersegmental, whereas the arteries are intrasegmental. The upper-lobe veins descend lateral to the arteries and cross in front of the lower-lobe arteries to reach the left atrium. These crossing points are used as landmarks for measuring the diameters of the lower-lobe arteries and assessing the relative positions of the hila (hilar points). For the right lower-lobe artery, the upper limit of normal is 16 mm for men and 15 mm for women (11). Four veins enter the left atrium. The right middle lobe usually drains to the upper-lobe vein, but may enter the left atrium separately. The confluence of right upper- and lower-lobe veins as they enter the left atrium may occasionally mimic a mass on the frontal film.

2. Physiology

The pulmonary vascular bed is a low-pressure, low-resistance system which receives the entire cardiac output. With changes in output between rest and exercise, there may be a sixfold increase in flow. To accommodate this without a rise in pressure, there must be considerable vascular reserve. In an erect subject, the chest radiograph shows a gradation in vessel size from lung apex to base (larger vessels at the base). The relative hyperperfusion of the base is matched by relative hyperventilation. In the supine position, the gradation is from front to back, with equal perfusion of apex and base. As cardiac output increases, there is gradual recruitment of vessels in the hypoperfused upper zones. This is seen as an increase in upper-zone vessel size, until they are equal to or larger than those in the lower zones. While the radiographic assessment of vessel size is largely subjective, there are objective criteria which can be helpful. In the perihilar region an artery and its accompanying bronchus are often seen end on. The normal artery is smaller or equal in diameter to the bronchus. If there is recruitment, it will appear larger. Under normal circumstances, vessels in the interspace below the first rib anteriorly should be less than 3 mm in diameter, if they are larger, there is recruitment. Once recruitment has been recognized, other radiological features may be used to place it in one of four main categories: (1) pulmonary venous hypertension, (2) pulmonary arterial hypertension, (3) increased right ventricular output, or (4) secondary to parenchymal lung disease. Although these conditions may occur independently, they often coexist.

3. Pulmonary Venous Hypertension

Pulmonary venous hypertension is most commonly caused by mitral stenosis or left ventricular failure. In both conditions the increase in upper-zone vessel size may be marked and not simply a process of recruitment. When pulmonary venous hypertension is longstanding or severe, there is vasoconstriction in the lower zones, leading to upper zone redistribution. The exact mechanism for this is unclear, but it is likely to be due to perivascular edema or hypoxic vasoconstriction. In untreated pulmonary venous hypertension, there is a broad correlation between left atrial pressure and the radiographic appearance (12). When left atrial pressure is <12 mmHg, appearances are normal; at 12–18 mmHg, there is upper-lobe vascular redistribution; between 18 and 22 mmHg there is interstitial edema; and above 22 mmHg alveolar edema develops. These figures are a general guide. They take no account of individual variations in plasma osmotic pressure, the efficiency of lymphatic clearance, or the chronicity of venous hypertension.

Pulmonary venous hypertension may produce passive pulmonary arterial hypertension. When this is longstanding, changes in the arteriolar walls lead to increased pulmonary vascular resistance and the development of active hypertension. In this situation, pulmonary hemosiderosis or ossification can develop. Hemosiderosis gives rise to a diffuse reticular pattern, resembling interstitial edema, but with no response to treatment (Fig. 11). Pulmonary ossification occurs with or without hemosiderosis. The nodules arise in areas of organized intraalveolar edema and are found predominantly in the lower zones (Fig. 12).

4. Pulmonary Arterial Hypertension

Pulmonary arterial hypertension is defined as a pulmonary systolic pressure >30 mmHg. This is usually secondary to lung disease, pulmonary

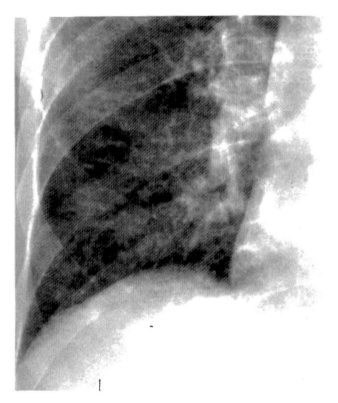

Figure 11 Pulmonary hemosiderosis in chronic pulmonary venous hypertension. Coarse linear streaks extending to the pleural surface represent septal lines. Although these may be a feature of interstitial edema, their failure to clear with appropriate therapy suggests hemosiderin deposition.

emboli, pulmonary venous hypertension, or shunts; rarely it is ideopathic. Although upper-lobe recruitment is a feature of these conditions, the major abnormality is enlargement of the proximal pulmonary arteries with relative peripheral pruning. The peripheral vessel may be normal or slightly diminished, only appearing "pruned" when compared with the large central arteries.

It is sometimes difficult to distinguish between pulmonary arterial and venous hypertension. One discriminator that can be helpful is the obtuse angle formed by the right upper-lobe vein and the lower-lobe artery (13). With venous hypertension, the enlarged upper-lobe vein obliterates the angle, while in arterial hypertension the enlarged lower-lobe artery main-

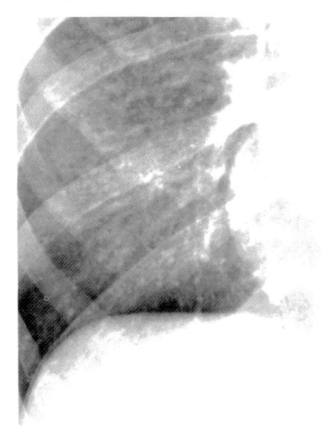

Figure 12 Pulmonary ossification. Discrete dense pulmonary nodules occurring in chronic mitral valve disease. They may, or may not, be associated with pulmonary hemosiderosis.

tains or increases the angle. Additional information can usually be gained by examining the cardiac configuration for evidence of right or left ventricular enlargement, valvular calcification, etc.

5. Increased Right Ventricular Output

Classically, increased right ventricular output is seen in left-to-right shunts, but similar appearances are seen in fluid overload from transfusion or renal failure.

Increased flow produces upper-zone recruitment, but the vessels in both upper and lower zones become enlarged. Vessels are then seen extending to the outer third of the lung, where they are not normally visible. Pulmonary to systemic shunts of less than 2:1 rarely cause these appearances. Plethora in a cyanosed subject indicates bidirectional shunting.

6. Parenchymal Lung Disease

Emphysema is the most frequent lung disease to cause pulmonary vascular disturbance. Like recurrent pulmonary emboli, parenchymal lung disease produces redistribution by destruction of the vascular bed. Vessel recruitment is of previously hypoperfused areas and may be necessary to accommodate the resting cardiac output. Theoretically, redistribution could occur without pulmonary arterial hypertension, but in practice this is unusual. The radiographic diagnosis of lung disease is suggested by the patchy nature of redistribution and the distortion of normal vascular branching. Additional features include hyperinflation, "barrel" chest, and flattened diaphragm. Abnormal branching, together with areas of lung destruction, may produce atypical patterns of pulmonary edema in these patients.

G. Pulmonary Edema

Radiologically, pulmonary edema falls into three main categories: left ventricular failure edema (which includes mitral stenosis), fluid overload edema, and membrane permeability edema.

Left ventricular failure and fluid overload edema occur when there is an imbalance between the hydrostatic and osmotic forces acting on the pulmonary capillary bed. This results in a net loss of fluid into the extracellular space, the protein content of that fluid being dependent on the level of imbalance (14). In both varieties, the initial radiographic findings are of interstitial edema with septal lines and peribronchial cuffing. Peribronchial "cuffing" is indicated by thickening of the bronchial wall, which is usually pencil thin (less than one-seventh of the bronchial diameter). This is best demonstrated around end-on bronchi near the hilum and reflects the accumulation of extracellular fluid and distended lymphatics in the bronchovascular sheath. Further elevation of left atrial pressure precipitates frank pulmonary edema and the development of subpleural or pulmonary effusions. Although there are similarities between left ventricular failure and fluid overload, there are also important differences which may be of diagnostic value. In left ventricular failure, a small increase in circulating volume leads to a rise in atrial filling pressure which is not matched by increased cardiac output. Interstitial edema develops at the lung bases, and local hypoxia causes vasoconstriction and redistribution of blood flow to the apices. The vessels at the lung apices appear significantly larger than those at the base. In fluid overload/renal failure, circulating volume is considerably increased and there is an attendant increase in cardiac output. The capacitance vessels at the lung apices are already full, and redistribution cannot occur. Vessels at apex and base therefore remain of similar size (15). These changes are all well represented on the chest radiograph.

Differences also exist in the distribution of pulmonary edema. In left heart failure, the shadowing is homogeneous, perihilar, and basal, with extension to the costophrenic angles; whereas in fluid overload edema, it tends to be perihilar and central, sparing the costophrenic angles (16). While these signs are not infallible, i.e., they may not be valid in acute failure or in lung disease, they are a useful guide to the underlying process.

Membrane permeability edema is of a different etiology. It is not related to atrial pressure and results instead from an injury to the pulmonary capillary basement membrane. This becomes "leaky," and fluid with the same protein content as plasma escapes into the extracellular space. While there are many possible precipitants, the most common are trauma and severe sepsis (ARDS). Radiographically, membrane permeability edema is characterized by widespread patchy opacities which tend to be peripheral. Air bronchograms are common. Heart size and pulmonary vascular pattern are normal, and there is no evidence of peribronchial cuffing/septal lines. Pleural effusions are rare unless there is a separate underlying cause, i.e., pulmonary sepsis or superadded fluid overload. Figure 13 illustrates some of the important features of each of these patterns of edema.

H. Specific Patterns in Valve Disease

1. Mitral Stenosis

Mitral stenosis is most commonly caused by rheumatic endocarditis. This results in progressive scarring and narrowing of the valve orifice over the next 10–30 years. In the Orient the process may be more rapid, with the disease presenting in childhood or adolescence. Although mitral stenosis may occur in isolation, tethering and fibrosis of the chordae often result in varying degrees of regurgitation. Calcification is a common late finding and arises in the valve itself, where it is irregular and localized, unlike senile or annular calcification. Occasionally, calcification may also be seen in the walls of the left atrium, where it is an important sign, confirming the rheumatic nature of the mitral valve disease. When it is present it indicates a fragile, brittle atrial wall which can bleed profusely and is difficult to suture at the time of surgery. Atrial calcification is more common in combined mitral stenosis and regurgitation.

Other features classically seen in mitral stenosis are enlargement of the left atrium and its appendage, enlargement of the right ventricle, and blood

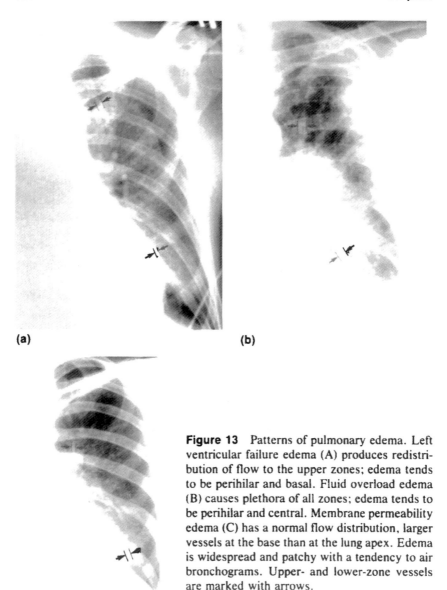

(a)   (b)

Figure 13 Patterns of pulmonary edema. Left ventricular failure edema (A) produces redistribution of flow to the upper zones; edema tends to be perihilar and basal. Fluid overload edema (B) causes plethora of all zones; edema tends to be perihilar and central. Membrane permeability edema (C) has a normal flow distribution, larger vessels at the base than at the lung apex. Edema is widespread and patchy with a tendency to air bronchograms. Upper- and lower-zone vessels are marked with arrows.

(c)

diversion to the upper lobes. These changes are due to pressure overload on the left atrium which is transmitted through the pulmonary vasculature to the right ventricle. Neither left atrial size nor pressure correlates with the severity or the duration of the disease. In the absence of mitral regurgitation, the left ventricle is normal. Pure or predominant mitral stenosis produces modest left atrial enlargement, although enlargement of the appendage is more common than in other causes of left atrial hypertension. The development of chronic pulmonary arterial hypertension leads to dilatation of both main and proximal pulmonary arteries. This may vary in degree but in some patients can dominate the appearance of the chest radiograph (Fig. 14).

Changes in the lungs are typically those of elevated venous pressure with diversion of blood to the upper lobes and the appearance of Kerley B or septal lines. Occasionally, patients with chronic mitral stenosis and pulmonary venous hypertension develop ossific nodules or hemosiderin deposits in the lungs. Pulmonary ossicles are found in 1–2% of patients and are of no clinical or prognostic significance. In keeping with other causes of pulmonary venous hypertension, patients with mitral disease are prone to develop pulmonary emboli (Fig. 15).

The diagnosis of mitral stenosis is normally a clinical one; the role of radiology is to assess severity and to identify any associated problems. One exception to this rule is in the presence of severe pulmonary arterial hypertension, when the typical mitral murmur may be lost due to low cardiac output.

Apart from congenital causes, described elsewhere, mitral stenosis may also be caused by left atrial myxoma or carcinoid syndrome (17). Left atrial myxomas commonly arise from the intraatrial septum and are usually pedunculated. As the tumor prolapses into the mitral valve orifice, it causes functional mitral stenosis. It can disturb mitral valve function even during systole, and it is often associated with mitral regurgitation. Myxomas rarely cause detectable calcification and have no other specific radiographic features. Carcinoid valve disease is predominantly right sided and related to hepatic metastases, mitral and aortic valve lesions being caused by primary bronchial tumors.

Tricuspid regurgitation may occur in conjunction with mitral stenosis. Regurgitation alone is usually functional; right-sided pressures are high, and the right ventricular enlargement dilates the tricuspid annulus. The heart is considerably enlarged. Once tricuspid regurgitation occurs, the appearance of the lungs alters from that of typical, pure mitral stenosis. There may be little or no upper-lobe redistribution and no interstitial edema, the near-normal lungs sometimes masking the underlying mitral lesion. Tricuspid incompetence appears to decompress the pulmonary

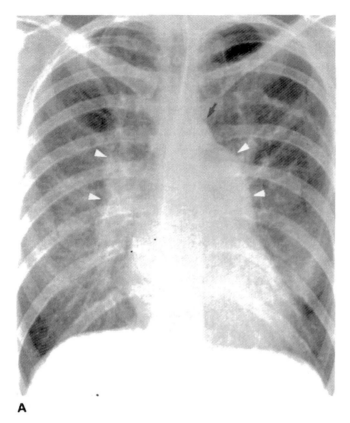

A

Figure 14 Pure mitral stenosis with pulmonary hypertension. A. pulmonary trunk and both proximal pulmonary arteries are enlarged (white arrow heads). Small aortic knob (arrow). Left fifth rib has remodeled following a closed mitral valvotomy. As part of this procedure, left atrial appendage was excised.

vascular changes, but this is at the expense of reduced cardiac output. The patient often has poor exercise tolerance despite the relative improvement in pulmonary vasculature.

2. Mitral Regurgitation

Mitral regurgitation is either functional or anatomical. Functional lesions are usually related to left ventricular dilatation and disturbance of papillary muscle function. The latter may be due to altered geometry as the ventricle enlarges or the consequence of ischemic heart disease and dyskinesia.

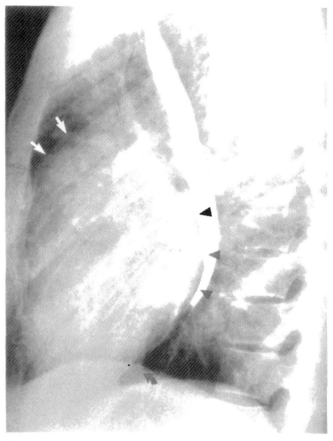

B

B. large left atrium outlined by barium (black arrow heads). Left ventricle is not enlarged, IVC lies behind left ventricle (curved arrow). Large right ventricle "fills in" anterior mediastinal window (white arrows).

Anatomical causes are numerous. Congenital mitral regurgitation may be due to a cleft in one of the leaflets, accessory leaflet tissue, or deficient leaflet tissue. This is discussed in greater detail in Chapter 1. Ideopathic mitral prolapse affects 6% of women and 2% of men, making it the most common cause of regurgitation in the Western world. Myxomatous degeneration of the valve apparatus and chordae leads to elongation of the chordae and enlargement of the leaflets. The process is usually asymmet-

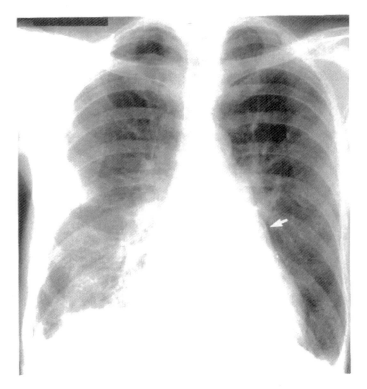

Figure 15 Mitral stenosis and right mid-zone pulmonary infarct. Large left atrial appendage (white arrow).

ric and gives rise to eccentric regurgitation which is rarely severe. As expected, the chest radiograph is normal unless the hemodynamic abnormality is significant. Inherited collagen disorders such as Marfan's syndrome, Ehlers-Danlos, and osteogenesis imperfecta may also cause mitral valve prolapse, but in these cases important regurgitation is more frequent. Other etiologies include rheumatic endocarditis, bacterial endocarditis, and ruptured chordae. A ruptured chorda occurs most frequently in association with myocardial infarction but has also been described in rheumatic mitral valve disease, bacterial endocarditis, and rarely following steering wheel injuries and cardiac trauma.

Radiographic features depend on severity and chronicity. If the lesion is chronic and there is no other significant disease, heart size broadly reflects severity. This is not true for pulmonary venous pressure, unlike mitral stenosis. The left atrium is large, and this may be marked if there is added mitral stenosis. The large, compliant left atrium seems to moderate the effects of mitral regurgitation on the pulmonary circulation. As such, most patients with compensated mitral regurgitation have little or no evidence of pulmonary venous hypertension. Increased pulmonary vascular resistance is rare unless regurgitation is severe or longstanding. A "giant" left atrium may occur in both mitral stenosis and regurgitation but is more common in the latter. Acute regurgitation, as seen in a ruptured chordae, is characterized by severe pulmonary venous hypertension, pulmonary edema, and little or no cardiomegaly. The left atrium is not usually enlarged.

Combined stenosis and regurgitation is virtually always rheumatic, the notable exceptions being atrial myxoma and carcinoid syndrome. The chest radiograph is often unhelpful. The heart is enlarged, and left atrial dilatation is obvious. Distinguishing the dominant lesion may be impossible, but in general, elevated pulmonary venous pressure out of keeping with left atrial enlargement suggests mitral stenosis, whereas marked atrial enlargement out of keeping with the pulmonary venous pressure suggests mitral regurgitation.

3. Aortic Stenosis

Isolated aortic valve stenosis is usually congenital. In the severe forms, i.e., those with monocuspid or fused bicuspid valves, presentation is in infancy; the less severe, with nonobstructive bicuspid valves at birth, present later, typically in adolescence or adulthood. The specific types of congenital aortic valve stenosis and their associations is discussed elsewhere in Chapters 1 and 8. Isolated rheumatic aortic valve stenosis is rare (<1%), and when it does occur, aortic regurgitation usually coexists. In the majority of patients, therefore, both mitral and aortic disease is present. Aortic stenosis can occasionally be related to senile aortic sclerosis or familial hypercholesterolemia. Both pathologies have a similar mechanism. In one, heavy calcification of the valve ring and cusp bases results in restricted valve motion; in the other, the valve is splinted by large, calcified cholesterol deposits in the valve sinuses.

Pure aortic valve obstruction does not produce a large heart unless complications occur. The left ventricle is hypertrophied, and the cavity is small and heavily trabeculated. The aortic knob is small, and there may be dilatation of the ascending aorta on the PA chest film (Fig. 16). Poststenotic dilatation seems to be related primarily to the duration of the disease. Changes in the ascending aorta are useful only in patients below the age of 40; above this, unfolded and dilated aortas are commonplace. In the older patient, it is important to look for aortic valve calcification to make the diagnosis. This is often best seen on the lateral film, which

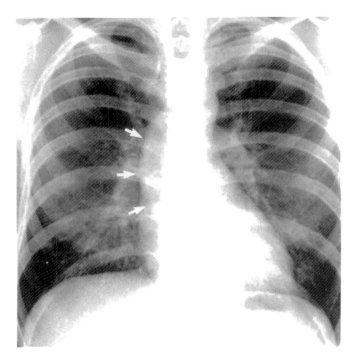

Figure 16 Aortic stenosis with posstenotic aortic dilatation of the ascending aorta (white arrows). Absence of left ventricular enlargement and normal aortic knob exclude significant aortic regurgitation.

should always be obtained in suspected valve disease. Calcification is more common in males than females and is almost invariable in men over 40. The degree and extent of the calcification correlates with the severity of stenosis (18). Once left ventricular failure occurs, cardiac enlargement ensues. In these patients, physical signs are less obvious and the radiographic findings may be particularly important in making or suggesting the diagnosis.

Subvalvar aortic stenosis occurs when there is a congenital diaphragm or ring below the aortic valve. Septal thickening, as in hypertrophic cardiomyopathy, can have the same effect, but the obstruction to outflow is typically mid-systolic. In both situations, left ventricular hypertrophy is severe. Even mild degrees of regurgitation lead to cardiomegaly, which is rare in uncomplicated aortic stenosis. The chest radiograph is generally unhelpful in distinguishing aortic stenosis from subvalvar stenosis. Both have a small aortic knob and dilated ascending aorta. Further studies (echocardiography/MRI) are always needed to make this diagnosis. Left atrial enlargement occurs in the presence of failure, and the plain films may then resemble mitral or aortic disease.

4. Aortic Regurgitation

The causes of aortic regurgitation fall into two main groups: diseases of the valve cusps and diseases of the aortic wall. Conditions involving the aortic cusps include rheumatic endocarditis, subacute bacterial endocarditis, syphilis, and a number of connective tissue disorders. Diseases of the aortic wall cause dilatation or dissection and can therefore lead to regurgitation; these include hypertension, syphilis, cystic medionecrosis, Marfan's syndrome, Ehlers Danlos syndrome, and osteogenesis imperfecta. Aneurysms of the aortic sinus are rare but cause regurgitation by disturbing valve closure.

In most instances, aortic regurgitation is chronic. Volume overload leads to dilatation of the left ventricle and a compensatory increase in stroke volume. The left ventricle hypertrophies and eventually fails. Further dilatation will often precipitate functional mitral regurgitation; the left atrium then dilates and pulmonary venous pressure rises. Dilatation of the left atrium is slight in the absence of a mitral abnormality. Eventually, increased pulmonary vascular resistance and pulmonary hypertension lead to enlargement of the right-sided chambers and marked cardiomegaly. Dilatation of the ascending aorta and arch is typical. Systolic hypertension elongates the descending aorta but does not dilate it. In acute aortic regurgitation there is not time for these changes to develop, and the left ventricle and atrium remain small or are minimally enlarged. The increase in end-diastolic pressure is transmitted straight to the pulmonary vasculature, upper-lobe vessels become engorged, and there is often severe pulmonary edema.

Aortic disease is often mixed, with evidence of both stenosis and regurgitation. The combination imposes pressure and volume loads on the ventricle, leading to dilatation and hypertrophy. In the absence of failure, the degree of cardiomegaly can be used as a guide to the dominance of stenosis or regurgitation. In dominant stenosis there is less enlargement and vice versa. Valve calcification is more frequent in dominant stenosis.

5. Mitral and Aortic Disease

Rheumatic valve disease often involves both aortic and mitral valves. Although carcinoids can also affect both valves, this is rare. In rheumatic disease, mitral stenosis and aortic regurgitation are usually dominant. Mitral stenosis lowers cardiac output, and some of the clinical features of aortic valve disease may be lost. It is therefore important to recognize

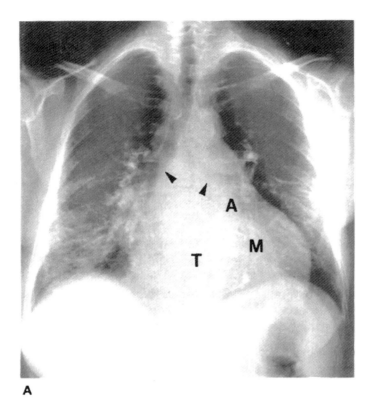

A

Figure 17 Triple valve replacement and generalized cardiomegaly. A. Braunwald-Cutter prostheses in the aortic (A), mitral (M) and tricuspid (T) positions. All four chambers are enlarged. Left atrial enlargement is suggested by splaying of the carina (arrow heads).

signs which suggest the presence of both kinds of lesions. In isolated mitral stenosis, the aorta is small; any prominence of the ascending aorta suggests added aortic valve disease. In simple aortic regurgitation, the left atrium and pulmonary venous pressure are unremarkable; if moderate or marked pulmonary venous hypertension is present, one must also suspect mitral stenosis.

When three valves are involved—mitral, aortic, and tricuspid—there will be features of all. Not surprisingly, one of the lesions is often missed. If all four chambers are dilated and there are severe pulmonary vascular changes, this diagnosis should be considered (Fig. 17).

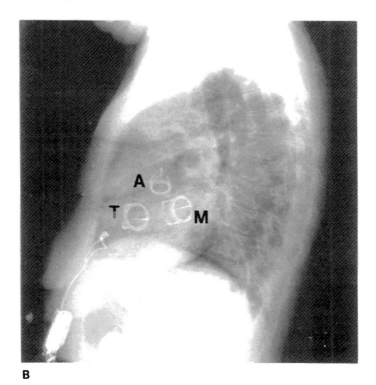

B

B. Aortic prosthesis lies antero-superior to mitral. Enlargement of right sided chambers is indicated by "filling in" of the anterior mediastinal window.

6. Tricuspid Valve Disease

The causes of tricuspid stenosis are the same as those for the mitral valve. Congenital lesions are rare. They occur in isolation or in combination with right ventricular hypoplasia. Acquired tricuspid stenosis is nearly always rheumatic and associated with mitral disease. Its importance lies in the fact that it may reduce the pulmonary vascular effects of mitral stenosis. The right atrium enlarges, but it is often impossible to distinguish enlargement due to tricuspid stenosis from the consequences of pulmonary hypertension.

Tricuspid regurgitation, like mitral regurgitation, may be functional or anatomical. The most common congenital lesion of the tricuspid valve is

Ebstein's anomaly. In this condition, the inferior and septal leaflets are displaced into the body of the ventricle; only the anterior leaflet remains attached to the valve ring. The degree of right atrial dilatation depends on the severity of regurgitation, but this is usually severe. The pulmonary trunk and aorta are usually small.

Acquired tricuspid regurgitation is usually functional, but this does not occur in the absence of pulmonary hypertension. Anatomical causes of tricuspid regurgitation are the same as for the mitral valve, but carcinoids and infective endocarditis are more common. The latter relates to the risk of infection in intravenous drug abusers. Radiographic signs of regurgitation include right atrial enlargement and dilatation of the superior and inferior vena cava. Cardiomegaly is usually marked.

7. Pulmonary Valve Disease

Pulmonary valve stenosis is one of the commonest congenital lesions. It may be associated with Noonan's syndrome and congenital rubella. In the rubella syndrome it is part of a complex picture involving branch pulmonary artery stenoses, cardiomyopathy, and septal defects. As with aortic stenosis, there is postvalvar dilatation. This affects the main pulmonary artery and extends down the left pulmonary artery (Fig. 18). The heart is usually normal in size, but if the case is severe there may be evidence of right ventricular enlargement. This produces straightening of the left heart border and may tilt the cardiac apex upward. The right atrium remains normal unless the heart enlarges. The aorta is usually normal; it may be small when the stenosis is severe enough to reduce cardiac output. In this situation, the lungs would also appear oligemic. Infundibular stenosis is usually associated with other congenital heart defects. It is indistinguishable from pulmonary valve stenosis on radiological grounds. Acquired causes of pulmonary stenosis include aneurysms of the ascending aorta and masses/tumors of the mediastinum.

Significant congenital pulmonary regurgitation is rare. However, recent Doppler studies have shown that minor degrees of pulmonary regurgitation are common (19). Acquired pulmonary regurgitation is usually due to dilatation of the valve ring following valvotomy for stenosis. Functional regurgitation occurs in association with processes which stretch the valve ring and is therefore common in pulmonary hypertension. Ideopathic enlargement of the pulmonary trunk, considered to be a "forme fruste" of Marfan's syndrome (20), may also lead to regurgitation. Rarer causes include bacterial endocarditis, as a result of intravenous drug abuse or pulmonary sepsis, and rheumatic endocarditis. Clinically significant pulmonary regurgitation is rare. There is little radiographic evidence of regurgitation unless tricuspid regurgitation intervenes. When this hap-

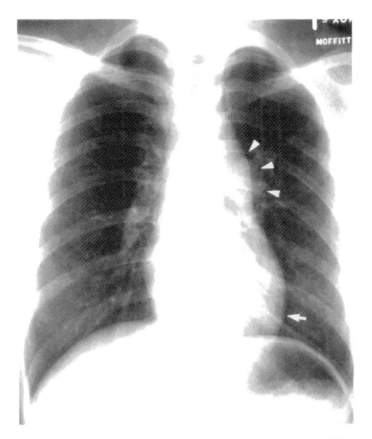

Figure 18 Pulmonary stenosis. Large pulmonary trunk and left pulmonary artery (white arrow heads). Right pulmonary artery is normal. Right ventricular enlargement is suggested by the upturned apex (white arrow).

pens, the features are of cardiomegaly and right-sided chamber enlargement.

8. Prosthetic Valves

There are over 40 cardiac prostheses available in the United States. They are designed for specific valve locations and are also used in conduits. The major varieties are of the caged-ball type, the low-profile caged-disk valve, the hinged-leaflet valve, the cageless tilting valve, and the tissue valves. Figure 19 illustrates the valve types, their X-ray appearance, and their main feature allowing identification.

Imaging of valve protheses is directed at demonstrating complications.

Ball Valves

Valve	Shape	X-Ray Film	X-Ray Outline	Mitral/Tricuspid	Aortic	Identifying Features	Complications
Starr-Edwards 6000	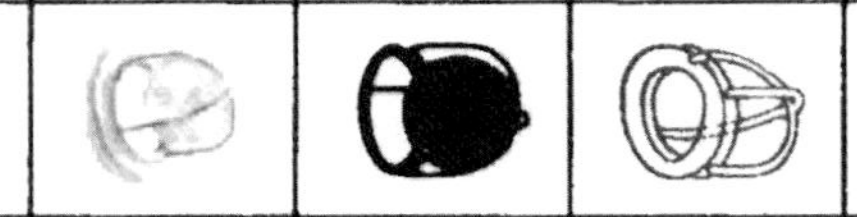			●		1. Double Doughnut 2. Four Struts Joined at Apex 3. Radiolucent Poppet (Some With Barium)	1. Thromboemboli 2. Ball Variance 3. Left Ventricular Incorporation of Cage
6300	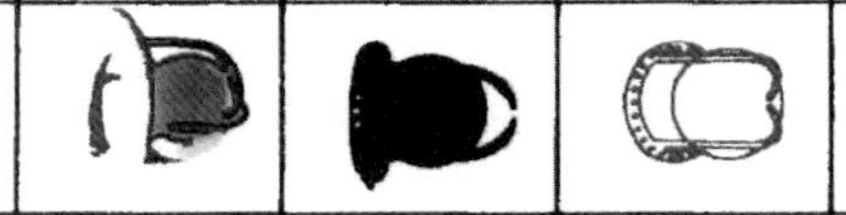			●		1. Concave Perforations 2. Four Thin Struts Not Joined at Apex 3. Radiopaque Poppet (In Systole Sits Far From Equator)	1. Thromboemboli 2. Bacterial Endocarditis
1000	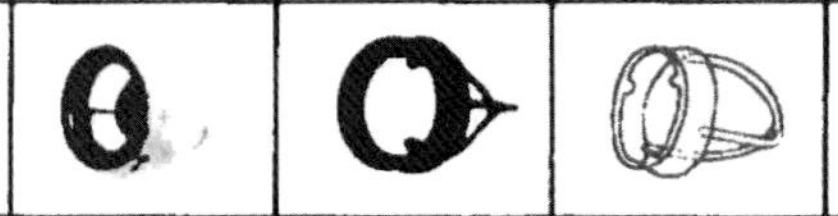				●	1. Conical Valve With Three Feet in Orifice 2. Three Thin Struts Joined at Apex 3. Radiolucent Poppet	1. Thromboemboli 2. Ball Variance
1200	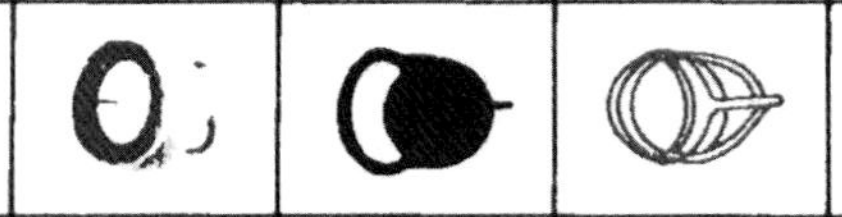				●	1. Tapered Support at Each Strut Junction 2. Three Thin Struts Fused at Apex 3. Some Barium Poppets	1. Thromboemboli 2. Ball Variance
2310	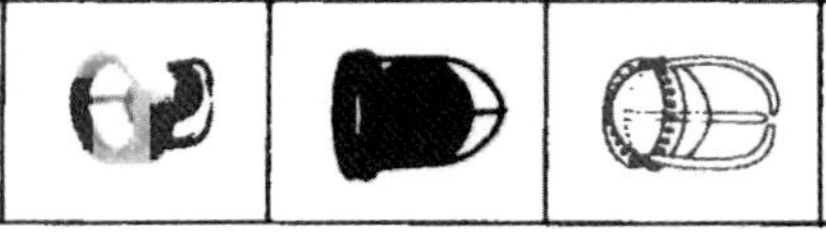				●	1. Perforated Concave Valve Base 2. Three Thin Struts Joined at Apex After 12/68 3. Radiopaque Poppet (Diastole Sits Close to Equator)	1. Close-Clearance Model With Poppet Impacted in Open Position

A

Figure 19 Valve prostheses available in the United States (A to E). Description of type, identifying features, and major complications. (From Chun P, Nelson W. JAMA 1977; 238:401–3. Reproduced with permission.)

Ball Valves

Valve	Shape	X-Ray Film	X-Ray Outline	Mitral/Tricuspid	Aortic	Identifying Features	Complications
Braunwald-Cutter				●	●	1. Open-Ended Cage 2. Radiolucent Poppet	1. Thromboemboli 2. Ball Variance 3. Hemolysis 4. Cloth Wear at Apex 5. Perivalvular Leaks
Smeloff-Cutter				●	●	1. Open-Ended Cage 2. Three Struts 3. Full-Flow Orifice Ball Valve 4. Radiolucent Poppet	1. Thromboemboli 2. Hemolysis 3. Ball Variance 4. Open Top Buried in Ventricular Septum*
McGovern-Cromie				●	●	1. Sutureless Mechanical Fixation Prosthesis 2. Open-Ended Cage 3. Three Struts 4. Vertical Fixation Pins 5. Radiopaque Poppet	1. Thromboemboli 2. Hemolysis 3. Ball Variance
DeBakey-Surgitool					●	1. Closed-Ended Cage 2. Three Struts 3. Serrated Ring 4. Radiolucent Poppet	

B

Low-Profile Valves—A Disk Valves

Valve	Shape	X-Ray Film	X-Ray Outline	Metal/Tricuspid	Aortic	Identifying Features	Complications
Starr-Edwards 6500	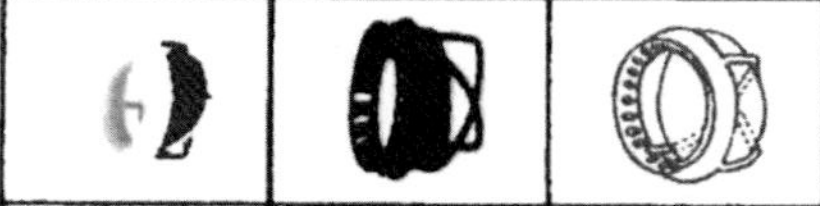			•		1 Low-Profile Cage 2 Cross Struts 3 Radiopaque Poppet 4 Concave Perforations	1 Thromboemboli 2 Cocking of Disk
6520	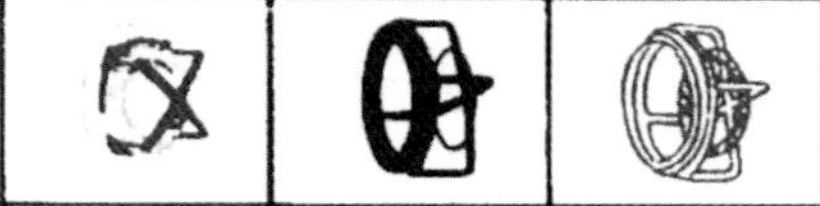			•		1 Low-Profile Cage 2 Cross Struts 3 Radiolucent Poppet With Radiopaque Ring In Poppet	
Kay-Shiley	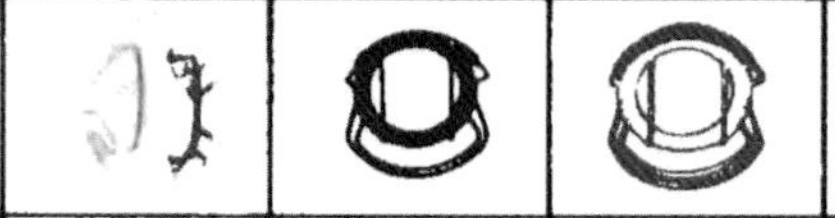			•	•	1 Single or Double Muscle Guard 2 Two Parallel Struts 3 Radiolucent Poppet	1 Thromboemboli 2 Sudden, Unexpected, Unexplained Death 3 Grooving and Disk Wear 4 Restenosis With Ingrowth 5 Perivalvular Leaks 6 Disk Cocking, Variance
Kay-Suzuki	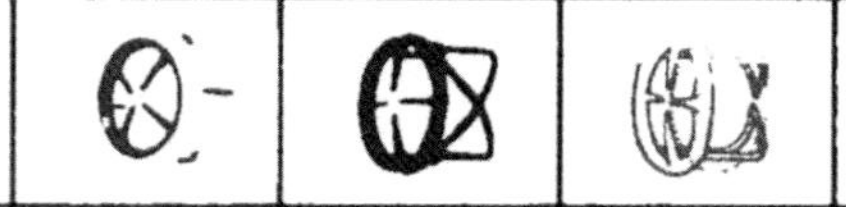			•		1 Cross-Ended Cage 2 Four Struts 3 Four Short, Open-Base Struts 4 Double-Ring Valve Base 5 Radiolucent Poppet	1 Thromboemboli 2 Disk Variance
Cross-Jones	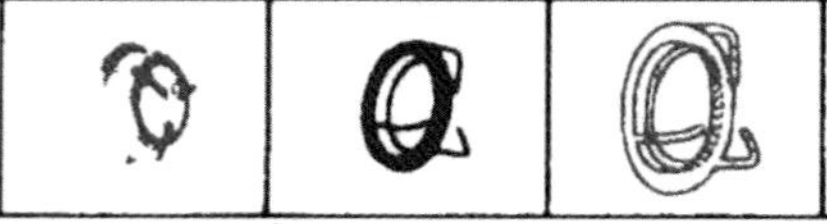			•		1 Open-Ended Cage 2 Radiolucent Poppet With Radiopaque Ring In Poppet	1. Thromboemboli 2. Cocking of Disk 3. Disk Variance

Figure 19C

Low-Profile Valves—A. Disk Valves

Valve	Shape	X-Ray Film	X-Ray Outline	Mitral/Tricuspid	Aortic	Identifying Features	Complications
Beall	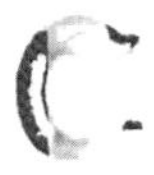	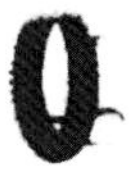	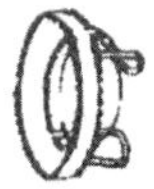	•		1. Two Parallel Indented Struts 2. Radiopaque Poppet	1. Obstruction of Prosthesis Orifice by Thrombus 2. Cocking of Disk 3. Hemolysis 4. Disk Variance 5. Gallstones*
Harken	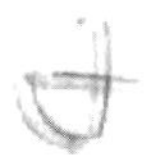	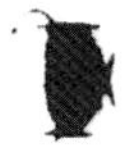			•	1. Thin Cross Struts 2. Radiopaque Poppet	1. Thromboemboli 2. Disk Variance
Cooley-Bloodwell-Cutter	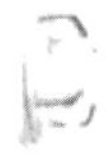	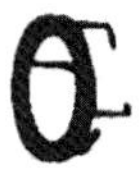	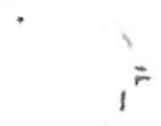	•	•	1. Discoid Valve 2. Open-Ended Cage 3. Four Struts 4. Radiolucent Poppet	1. Thromboemboli 2. Prosthetic Leaks 3. Thrombotic Valve Occlusion

Figure 19D

Low-Profile Valves—B. Hinged-Leaflet Valve

Valve	Shape	X-Ray Film	X-Ray Outline	Mitral/Tricuspid	Aortic	Identifying Features	Complications
Gott-Daggett	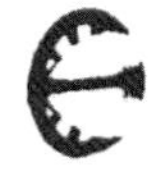	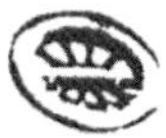			•	1. Central Cross Strut 2. Multiple Projecting Prongs From Ring 3. Radiolucent Leaflets	1. Thromboemboli 2. Hemolysis 3. Gallstones*

Low-Profile Valves—C. Central-Flow, Eccentric Monocusp Valves

Valve	Shape	X-Ray Film	X-Ray Outline	Mitral/Tricuspid	Aortic	Identifying Features	Complications
Lillehei-Kaster	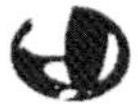	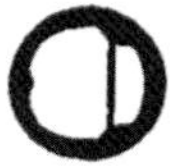	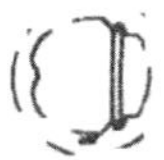	•		1. Two Teardrop-Shaped Pivots 2. Two Lateral Disk Guide-Shields 3. Radiolucent Poppet	1 Thromboemboli
Wada-Cutter	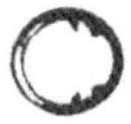	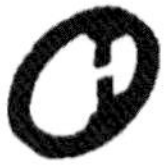		•	•	1. Base Ring With Two Notches 2. Disk With Two Notches 3. Radiolucent Poppet	1. Early Disk Wear 2. Total Valve Thrombosis 3. Thromboemboli 4. Perivalvular Leaks With Notable Regurgitation
Bjork-Shiley	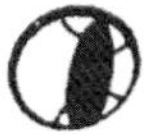	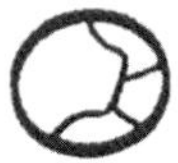	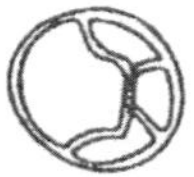	•	•	1 Two Eccentrically Located Support Struts 2. Radiolucent Poppet	1 Thromboemboli

E

Figure 19 (Continued)

These include valvar insufficiency and stenosis, thrombosis/embolism, fatigue and disruption of the valve, degeneration of bioprostheses, and bacterial endocarditis. The role of plain-film radiography is limited. It may show the type of valve that has been used and will occasionally show hingeing or valve disruption. Formal examination of mechanical valves requires fluoroscopy and/or cine. This reliably detects hingeing and will allow assessment of valve excursion. A normal prosthetic valve should not hinge from its resting plane by more than 11°. Angles greater than this always indicate a major dehiscence of the suture line; lesser degrees are more accurately assessed by Doppler echocardiography. Valve excursion can also be evaluated by echocardiography, but its success depends on the type of valve in question and the amount of reverberation artifact it causes. Bioprostheses and suspected bacterial endocarditis need to be investigated by echocardiography and Doppler. In difficult cases, where fluoroscopy and echocardiography have been unhelpful, UFCT should be considered. MRI is of little value in assessing the valve itself, but it may be useful when examining the aorta for postoperative complications.

II. ULTRAFAST COMPUTED TOMOGRAPHY

CT scanning provides the same cross-sectional format as echocardiography, tomographic radionuclide scintigraphy, and MRI. With UFCT, the images are acquired in milliseconds rather than seconds, eliminating blurring due to cardiac motion. The technique has two main advantages over MRI and nuclear cardiology. One is the freedom from respiratory artifacts; the other is that ECG gating is not required. In the cine mode, all CT images at one level are derived from a single cardiac cycle. There are none of the difficulties associated with averaging multiple cycles, and the problems of examining patients with irregular rhythms are reduced. The imaging plane is flexible due to the wide patient gantry and the table swivel and tilt capability. This allows the heart to be imaged in short- or long-axis planes depending on the clinical problem (2). Unlike echocardiography, image quality is independent of patient size and shape, and there are no restrictions from limited acoustic windows. Multiplane image reconstruction is also possible, provided contiguous multilevel scans are acquired.

UFCT demonstrates calcification with far greater sensitivity and precision than is possible with either angiography or MRI. Not only is valve and pericardial calcification well seen, but so is the fine calcification often present with coronary atherosclerosis. When used to quantify coronary calcification, UFCT has been shown to be a reliable predictor of coronary artery disease. More important, a negative test for coronary calcification has a strong negative predictive value of 98% (21). Young middle-age patients with valve disease often go to surgery without cardiac catheterization; in this setting there is potential for UFCT to be used as a noninvasive screening test for ischemic heart disease.

Contrast medium is needed to visualize the cardiac chambers, but this may be injected intravenously from a peripheral vein and only relatively small boluses (20–60 ml) are required. On contrast-enhanced images, the semilunar and AV valves are well demonstrated. Thickening/distortion or abnormal motion can be detected, but the current relatively low frame rate (17 frames/s) means that for most patients echocardiography is superior (Fig. 20).

Cardiac chamber size (22), shape, ventricular thickening (23), and mass (24) can all be quantitated with great accuracy from UFCT images. These measurements are more reliable than those from echocardiographic stud-

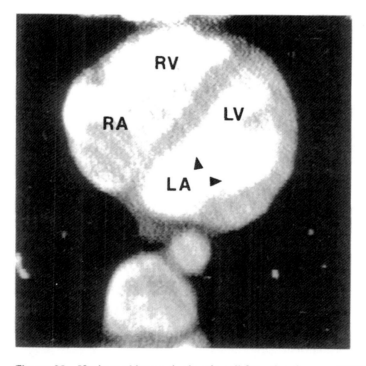

Figure 20 Horizontal long axis showing all four chambers on UFCT. Thickened mitral valve leaflets are well demonstrated during diastole (arrow heads). Lack of "doming" and wide orifice exclude stenosis. LA, left atrium; LV, left ventricle; RA, right atrium; RV, right ventricle.

ies because no geometric assumptions are made; all calculations are based on Simpson's rule. In this respect, UFCT and MRI, which shares the same advantages, are the ideal modalities for longitudinal studies of ventricular mass or volume. If only one valve is regurgitant, the regurgitant volume may be calculated by comparison of right and left ventricular stroke volumes (25). At present, there is no way of quantitating flow velocity and hence no established method of determining gradients across stenotic lesions.

Pacing wires, intravascular catheters, pericardial effusions, and/or constriction can all be identified, as well as intracardiac masses. Figure 21 shows a left atrial myxoma simulating mitral stenosis. UFCT provides a dynamic evaluation of tumor size, location, and wall attachment. Thrombus can frequently be distinguished from tumor by CT density measurement and the absence of enhancement following intravenous contrast medium. In certain areas, the left atrial appendage and the ventricular

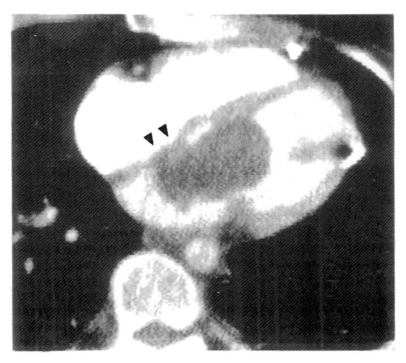

Figure 21 UFCT showing large left atrial myxoma prolapsing through the mitral valve during diastole. Broad attachment to the interatrial septum is well demonstrated (arrow heads).

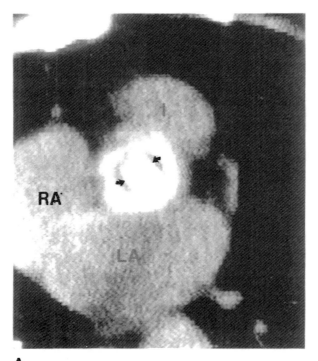

A

Figure 22 UFCT of a St. Jude prosthesis in the aortic area. A. Systole with leaflets open (arrows). B. Diastole with leaflets closed. Note that the infundibulum contracts in systole. LA, left atrium; I, infundibulum; RA, right atrium.

apex, thrombus is not well seen by transthoracic echocardiography. In this situation, UFCT is the noninvasive technique of choice. Unfortunately, it is underutilized even in those centers that are suitably equipped. Further understanding and experience may change this situation.

Figure 22 illustrates the appearance of a prosthetic valve in the aortic area. This is a St. Jude prosthesis, which is often difficult to evaluate by either echocardiography or X-ray fluoroscopy, its hinged flaps being virtually nonradioopaque. Rapid image acquisition reduces motion artifact and lessens the streaking usually seen with metal implants. In cases where fluoroscopy has been unhelpful, UFCT is a reliable alternative for assessing valve prostheses. It has distinct advantages over both echocardiography and MRI. In the former, reverberation artifacts from the prosthesis degrade image quality, and in the latter, susceptibility artifacts from the metal components of the valve cause marked signal loss.

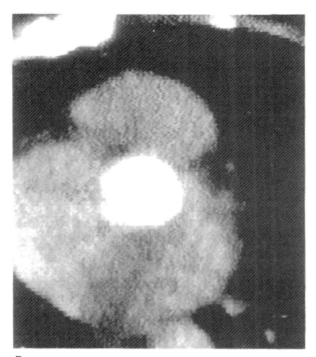

B

III. MAGNETIC RESONANCE IMAGING

Cardiac MRI provides the opportunity to image structure and function with one modality. It does not have the constraints of CT or echocardiography, with regard to image plane or acoustic window, and as such has distinct advantages over these techniques.

The most useful pulse sequences in cardiac imaging are the spin echo (SE) and gradient refocused echo (GRE) sequences. While a full understanding of the principles of MRI is not necessary, it is important to know something of the factors affecting image quality and production. All imaging sequences require multiple radiofrequency excitations (pulses) and echo acquisitions. The number of excitations/acquisitions needed to create an image depends on the spatial and contrast resolution required; for most cardiac purposes this is 256 or 512. Conventional SE imaging uses a 90° excitation pulse followed by a 180° pulse to generate the echo. The echo is collected at a time TE. Before another excitation pulse can be given, the tissues have to recover their original magnetization, introducing a delay between excitations (TR). The values of TE and TR are adjusted to alter the T1 or T2 properties of the final image. T1 is a measure of the spin-lattice relaxation time and T2 the spin-spin relaxation time. As a general guide, T1 images are best for demonstrating anatomy and T2 images for detecting pathology. For T1 weighted, cardiac SE images, a TE in the region of 26 ms and TR of 700–1000 ms is used. To eliminate cardiac motion, ECG gating is needed (Fig. 23). This triggers a new excitation pulse on the R wave of ECG. If this occurs on every R wave, the TR is equal to the R-R interval of the ECG; if it occurs on every other R wave

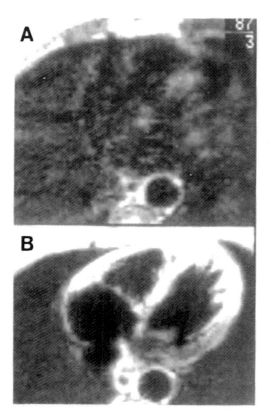

Figure 23 Ungated (A) and gated (B) images of the horizontal long axis on a SE sequence. Cardiac gating is a prerequisite for adequate visualization of the cardiac chambers.

the TR is 2× the R-R interval. Although several levels can be acquired simultaneously, it takes 256 or 512 heart beats to generate a set of T1 weighted images (3–7 min, depending on heart rate). To examine the whole heart, at various phases of systole and diastole, this means an hour or more in the magnet. As each image is a composite of numerous similar cardiac cycles, patients with arrhythmias and fluctuating R-R intervals give poor images.

Respiratory motion may also degrade image quality, but the effect is minor and does not prevent the technique from being a useful tool in cardiac patients.

GRE images employ a smaller excitation pulse (<90°) and can have very much shorter TR times (i.e., TE 12 ms and TR 21 ms for magnets operating at 1.5T). In this setting multiple repetitions can be performed in a single R-R interval. Fast MRI still requires ECG gating, but it does mean that multiple images at the same level can be obtained during the cardiac cycle. Combining these images into a cine loop gives an accurate demonstration of cardiac motion at that level. The problems of imaging patients with irregular rhythms still apply, but retrospective gating can sometimes be used to good effect.

These two types of sequence give very different images (Fig. 24). SE images have a high level of contrast between fast-flowing blood, which appears black, and the surrounding soft tissues. Slow-flowing blood or flow within the imaging plane gives a variable signal, which may make it difficult to distinguish slow flow from adjacent endocardium or thrombus. In most situations this is not a problem, and the SE sequence remains the sequence of choice for demonstrating anatomy. On GRE images, flowing blood is of high signal, providing contrast between the vascular spaces and surrounding myocardium. GRE images are generally noisier than SE images and are reserved for functional studies, i.e., cine imaging and examining flow.

Like UFCT, MRI is well established as an accurate technique for quantifying a range of cardiac parameters; LV and RV mass (26), LV and RV volumes (27), ejection fraction, cardiac output, and wall motion abnormalities (28). The accuracy of these values, just as for UFCT, has allowed reliable quantitation of univalvular regurgitation (29). Although valve anatomy may be demonstrated by MRI, relatively poor contrast and spatial resolution make echocardiography superior (Fig. 25). Multiplaner imaging makes MRI the ideal modality for imaging the thoracic aorta; it is therefore particularly useful in patients with aortic regurgitation due to a stretched valve ring. Some authorities now believe that it is the technique of choice when investigating subacute or chronic aortic aneurysm or dissection (30,31).

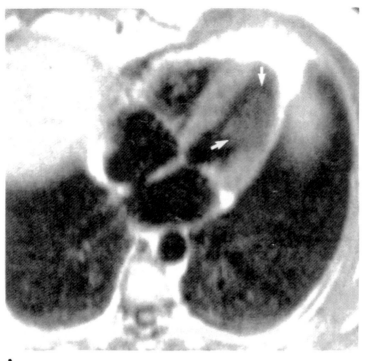

A

Figure 24 SE (A) and GRE (B) images of the horizontal long axis in the same subject. Flowing blood is low signal (black) on SE images. Slow flow or in-plane flow may give some signal-making delineation of the endocardium difficult (white arrows). Laminar flow on GRE images is high signal and appears white. When flow is fast or turbulent, however, there may be signal loss as seen in the descending aorta (curved white arrow).

The major advantage of MRI over UFCT is the ability to image and quantitate flow velocity. GRE images are sensitive to flow; as flow velocity increases, the development of turbulence leads to loss of signal. This signal loss correlates with the extent of turbulence and can be used to estimate velocity gradients across stenotic valves (Fig. 26) (32). Areas of signal loss are also seen in regurgitant jets, but they have proved less valuable in determining the severity of regurgitation (Fig. 27). Modifications of the GRE technique have been developed to quantitate flow velocity in absolute terms (33). This makes MRI equivalent or superior to Dopp-

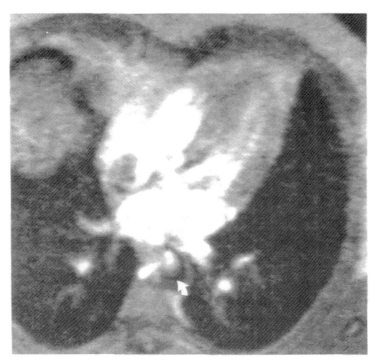

B

ler echocardiography. In some respects MRI velocity measurements are superior, as there are no restrictions as to imaging plane and no assumptions are made about the angle of flow relative to the imaging plane. MRI also has the advantage of being able to evaluate flow in regions that are inaccessible to the Doppler beam.

When prosthetic valves are studied by MRI, they usually cause local signal loss and therefore are not seen adequately. Early concerns regarding radiofrequency energy deposition and heating have largely been put to rest. There are no reports of MRI complications due to a valve prosthesis. Nevertheless, it is advised that those few patients with valves that are strongly ferromagnetic, i.e., Starr-Edwards valves pre-6000, should not be scanned (34).

When so many noninvasive modalities are available, the clinician must

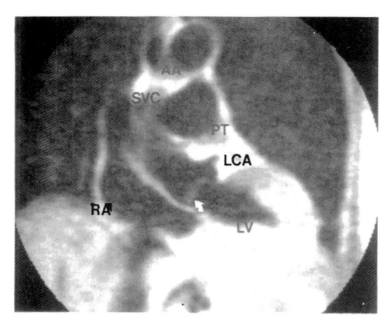

Figure 25 Oblique coronal SE image showing a thickened aortic valve (white arrow) and left ventricular hypertrophy in aortic stenosis. AA, aortic arch; LCA, left coronary artery; LV left ventricle; PT, pulmonary trunk; RA, right atrium; SVC, superior vena cava.

Table 1 Relative Value of Echocardiography, UFCT, and MRI in Valvular Heart Disease

	Echo	UFCT	MRI
Evaluation of atrio-ventricular valves	***	*	*
Evaluation of semilunar valves	***	*	*
Evaluation of aorta	**	***	***
Evaluation of valve prostheses	**	***	—
Quantitation of LV and RV mass	*	***	***
Quantitation of LV and RV volumes	*	***	***
Quantitation of ejection fraction	*	***	***
Quantitation of regurgitant volumes	*	***	***
Quantitation of valve gradients	***	*	***
Evaluation of intracardiac thrombus	*	***	**
Evaluation of segmental wall motion abnormalities	***	***	***
Evaluation of cardiac calcification	—	***	—

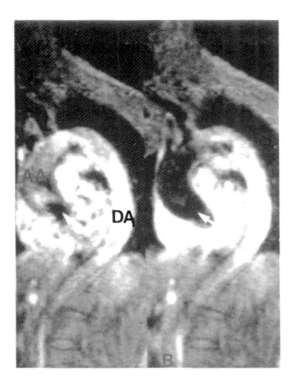

Figure 26 Sagittal oblique GRE images of the aorta at early (A) and mid-systole (B). The length of signal loss (white arrows) due to turbulence from a stenotic aortic valve increases during systole. The maximum length of signal loss correlates broadly with the severity of stenosis. AA, ascending aorta; DA, descending aorta.

be familiar with the strengths and weaknesses of each. Table 1 compares the relative values of echocardiography, UFCT, and MRI in the evaluation of valvular heart disease.

Despite its promise, cardiac MRI has not been widely disseminated. It continues to be held back by problems of motion artifact and long imaging times. The development of new, faster sequences promises to be a major step forward. Echo planar imaging (EPI) is the fastest of these new techniques (35). EPI using a single excitation pulse and its echo train to create an image. With total acquisition times between 30 and 100 ms, real-time MRI is a genuine hope. Progress is rapid; perhaps the next 15 years will see the same growth in cardiac MRI as we have seen in echocardiography over the last 15.

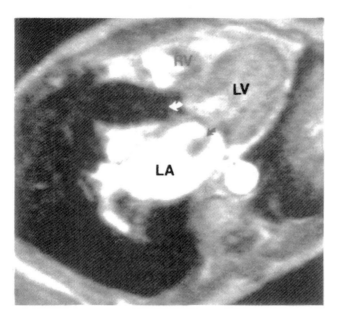

Figure 27   GRE vertical long axis in a patient with mitral and aortic valve disease. This systolic image shows signal loss in the aorta from aortic stenosis (white arrow) and in the left atrium from mitral regurgitation (black arrow). LA, left atrium; LV, left ventricle; RA, right atrium.

REFERENCES

1.   Kisslo J, von Ramm OT, Thurstone FL. Cardiac imaging using a phased array ultrasound system. II. Clinical technique and application. Circulation 1976; 53:262–8.
2.   Rumberger JA, Lipton MJ. Ultrafast cardiac CT scanning. In: Wolfe C, ed. Cardiology Clinics. Vol. 7(3). Philadelphia: Saunders, 1989: 713–34.
3.   Lipton JM. Computed tomography, positron emission tomography and nuclear magnetic resonance in cardiology. Fast CT of the heart. In: Rudolf W, ed. Herz Kardiovaskuläre Erkrankungen. Vol 12(1): 1987: 1–12.
4.   Sechtem V, Pflugfelder PW, White RD, et al. Cine MR imaging: potential for the evaluation of cardiovascular fucntion. Am J Radiol 1987; 148:239–46.
5.   Schaefer CM, Greene R, Oestmann JW, et al. Digital phosphor storage imaging versus conventional film radiography in CT-documented chest disease. Radiology 1900; 174:207–10.
6.   Merlo I, Bighi P, Cervi PM, Lupi L. Computed radiography in neonatal intensive care. Pediatr Radiol 1991; 21:94–6.
7.   Ungerleider HE, Gubner R. Evaluation of heart size measurements. Am Heart J 1942; 24:494–8.

8.   Jefferson K, Rees S. Clinical Cardiac Radiology. (2d ed.) London: Butterworths, 1980.
9.   Milne ENC, Burnett K, Aufrichtig D, et al. Assessment of cardiac size on portable chest films. J Thorac Imag 1988; 3(2):64–9.
10. Pistolesi M, Milne ENC, Miniati M, Giuntini C. The vascular pedicle of the heart and the azygos vein. Part II. In acquired heart disease. Radiology 1984; 152:9–17.
11. Higgins CB, Lipton MJ. Pulmonary circulation. In: Grainger RG, Allison D, eds. Diagnostic Radiology: An Anglo-American Textbook of Imaging. London: Churchill Livingston, 1986.
12. Lavender JP, Doppman J, Shawdon H, Steiner RE. The pulmonary veins in left ventricular failuire and mitral stenosis. Br J Radiol 1962; 35:293–7.
13. Doppman JL, Lavender JP. The hilum and large left ventricle. Radiology 1963; 80:931–6.
14. Bradley RD. Acute heart failiure. In: Julian DG, et al. eds. Diseases of the Heart. London: Balliere Tindall, 1989.
15. Hughes JM, Glazier JB, Maloney JE, et al. Effect of interstitial pressure on pulmonary blood flow. Lancet 1967; i:192–4.
16. Miniati M, Pistolesi M, Paoletti, et al. Objective radiographic criteria to differentiate cardiac, renal and injury lung edema. Invest Radiol 1988; 23: 433–40.
17. Roberts WC, Msjaerdisma A. The cardiac disease associated with carcinoid syndrome (carcinoid heart disease). Am J Med 1964; 36:5–34.
18. Spindola-Franco H, Fish BG, Dachman A. Recognition of bicuspid aortic valve by plain film calcification pattern. Am J Radiol 1982; 139:867–71.
19. Hall R. Other valve disorders: tricuspid pulmonary and mixed lesions. In: Julian DG, et al. eds. Diseases of the Heart. London: Balliere Tindall, 1989.
20. Edwards JE. Congenital pulmonary vascular disorders. In: Pulmonary vascular diseases. Moser KM, et al., eds. New York: Marcel Dekker, 1979.
21. Agaston AS, Janowitz WR, Hildner FJ, et al. Quantification of coronary calcification using ultrafsta computed tomography. J Am Coll Cardiol 1990; 15:827–32.
22. Reiter SJ, Rumberger JA, Stanford W. Precision of right and left ventricular stroke volume measurements by rapid acquisition cine computed tomography. Circulation 1986; 74:890–900.
23. Lipton MJ, Rumberger JA. Exercise ultrafast computed tomography for the detection of coronary artery disease (Riog et al.): editorial comment. J Am Coll Cardiol 1989; 13:1082–4.
24. Diethelm L, Simonsen JS, Dery R, et al. Measurement of LV mass by ultrafast CT and 2-D echocardiography. Radiology 1989; 171:213–7.
25. Stark CA, Rumberger JA, Reiter SJ, Marcus ML. Use of cine CT in assessing the severity of aortic regurgitation in patients. Circulation 1986; 74:II-4.
26. Katz J, Milken MC, Stray-Gunderson J, et al. Estimation of human myocardial mass with MR imaging. Radiology 1988; 169:495–8.
27. Longmore DB, Klipstein RH, Underwood SR, et al. Dimensional accuracy of magnetic resonance in studies of the heart. Lancet 1985; i:1360–2.

28. White RD, Holt WW, Cheitlin MD, et al. Estimation of the functional and anatomical extent of myocardial infarction using magnetic resonance imaging. Am Heart J 1988; 115:740–8.

29. Underwood SR, Klipstein RH, Firmin DN, et al. Magnetic resonance assessment of aortic and mitral regurgitation. Br Heart J 1986; 56:455–62.

30. Kersting-Sommerhoff BA, Sechtem VP, Schiller NB, et al. MRI of the thoracic aorta in Marfan patients. Radiology 1987; 162:181–6.

31. Kersting-Sommerhoff BA, Higgins CB, White RD, et al. Aortic dissection sensitivity and specificity of MR imaging. Radiology 1988; 166:651–5.

32. Mitchell L, Jenkins JPR, Watson Y, et al. Diagnosis and assessment of mitral and aortic valve disease by cine flow magnetic resonance imaging. Magn Reson Med 1989; 12:181–97.

33. Naylor GL, Firmin DN, Longmore DB. Blood flow imaging by cine magnetic resonance. JCAT 1986; 10:715–22.

34. Soulen RL, Buddinger TE, Higgins CB. Magnetic resonance imaging of prosthetic heart valves. Radiology 1985; 154:705–7.

35. Stehling MK Turner R, Mansfield P. Echo-planar imaging: magnetic resonance imaging in a fraction of a second. Science 1991; 254:43–50.

Part II

5

Mitral Valve Regurgitation

Muayed Al Zaibag
Armed Forces Hospital, Riyadh, Saudi Arabia, and Loma Linda University Medical Center, Loma Linda, California

Murtada A. Halim
Armed Forces Hospital, Riyadh, Saudi Arabia

The mitral valve apparatus is complex in both structure and function. The accurate evaluation of the pathophysiological mechanism responsible for valve dysfunction is of paramount importance and has major clinical and therapeutic implications.

I. ANATOMY OF THE MITRAL VALVE

The mitral valve consists of an annulus, two leaflets, approximately 120 chordae tendinaea, and two papillary muscles. The papillary muscles and the adjacent part of the left ventricular wall act as one unit. Both the left ventricle and the atrium play an important role in the pathophysiology of the diseased mitral valve (1).

The annulus fibrosis is an ill-defined fibro-muscular ring. Two fibrous trigones form part of the mitral ring (2), of which the right—the central fibrous body—is the most important. These fibrous structures act as an anchor for myocardial contraction. The anterior portion of the annulus is rich in fibrous tissue and, therefore, has minimal mobility during cardiac contraction. In contrast, the posterior part of the annulus is devoid of fibrous tissue and is encircled by the myocardium of the left ventricle and atrium (3). Contraction of the annulus results in a 20% to 40% reduction of the annular area, and its nonhomogenous structure produces an eccentric narrowing.

187

The anterior leaflet is large and attached to only one-third of the annulus, but it is responsible for about two-thirds of the mitral valve closing area. In contrast, the small posterior mitral leaflet, which is attached to two-thirds of the annulus, contributes to only one-third of the mitral valve closing area. The anterior mitral leaflet is the more mobile leaflet and has the dominant role in the closure of the mitral valve. The combined surface of both leaflets is 1.5 to 2 times that of the relaxed mitral orifice. The area of coaptation will be even more increased during annular contraction; the area of the anterior leaflet alone becomes larger than the mitral orifice.

The chordae have their own complex features (4). Each chorda subdivides in a gradual fashion toward its insertion on the leaflet. This subdivision occurs in three steps, resulting in primary, secondary, and tertiary chordae. There are 12 primary chordae tendinaea attached to the six heads of each of the two papillary muscles, and 60 tertiary chordae are inserted into each leaflet. Each head of the papillary muscle is attached to two primary chordae, ultimately supporting 10 tertiary chordae. Chordae from either papillary muscle are inserted into both leaflets (4).

The anterolateral papillary muscle has extensive blood supply from both the diagonal branches of the left anterior descending and the obtuse marginal branches of the left circumflex coronary arteries. In contrast, the posteromedial papillary muscle has a single source of blood supply from the posterior descending artery. The latter originates from the dominant (85%) or codominant (7%) right coronary artery in 92% of the patients, or from the dominant left circumflex artery in about 7% of patients (5).

II. PATHOLOGY

The most common underlying pathological processes causing mitral regurgitation (MR) are rheumatic heart disease, mitral valve prolapse—myxomatous degeneration with or without ruptured chordae—infective endocarditis, and papillary muscle dysfunction.

Pure MR was detected in 10% of 1414 patients who underwent cardiac valve replacement (6), and in 16% of 1010 patients studied at necropsy. Forty-eight percent of the latter patients had rheumatic heart disease (7). In patients above 50 years of age, without mitral stenosis (MS) or aortic valve involvement, 78–98% of pure MR was of nonrheumatic etiology (8,9): The causes included floppy valve, infection, and papillary muscle dysfunction. A major changing trend has been observed in the prevalence of mitral valve prolapse (MVP). In a necropsy study published in 1973, MVP accounted for only 4% of the cases of pure MR (9). In contrast, a more recent study showed MVP to be the most common cause of MR in patients requiring mitral surgery, i.e., 62% of cases (8).

In elderly patients, myxomatous degeneration of the mitral leaflets, papillary muscle dysfunction following myocardial infarction and mitral annulus calcification, are the most common underlying pathologies of MR (10–12). Spontaneous chordae rupture, acute ischemic coronary syndromes, and infective endocarditis are the most common causes of acute severe MR (see Chapter 11).

Mitral regurgitation results from a variety of different pathological processes, frequently affecting more than one component of the mitral valve apparatus. For instance, MR secondary to mitral valve prolapse may be due to elongation of chordae with or without rupture, prolapse of the leaflet, and/or mitral annular dilatation. The involvement of more than one component of the mitral valve by a single disease process, and the complex structure and performance of the mitral valve, preclude classification of the causes of MR solely on the basis of an anatomical or pathological involvement, or clinical presentation (acute versus chronic). For didactic purposes, we will classify the causes of MR according to the anatomical involvement of the mitral valve apparatus according to the various underlying pathological processes (Table 1).

A. Disorders of the Mitral Annulus

Morphologically, the mitral annulus has a circumference of 8.5–10 cm. The muscular component contracts in systole, causing constriction of the annulus, which contributes to the mechanism of mitral valve closure. Significant MR may result from dilatation of the annulus, which occurs when the left ventricle dilates, such as in dilated cardiomyopathy. Some authors have suggested that MR caused by severe left ventricular (LV) dilatation is more likely to be due to malalignment of the papillary muscles rather than due to mitral annular dilatation (1). A recent elegant animal experiment has demonstrated that MR in a dilated left ventricle is caused by incomplete mitral leaflet closure (IMLC) (13).

As the degree of MR increases, this will result in further LV dilatation, which in turn will exacerbate the mitral annular dilatation, worsening the degree of MR (11). In view of this phenomenon, it may be difficult to pinpoint the primary etiological factor in patients who present for the first time with both severe LV dilatation and MR.

In the elderly, mitral annular calcification is a natural degenerative aging process and is a common cause of MR (10). It is three times more prevalent in women than men. Calcification may interfere with the normal

Table 1   Causes of Mitral Regurgitation

A. Disorders of the mitral annulus
    1. Annular dilatation: conditions that lead to left ventricular dilatation, i.e., dilated cardiomyopathy
    2. Annular calcifications:
        (a) Idiopathic or degenerative
        (b) Conditions that raise left ventricular pressure; hypertension, aortic stenosis, and hypertrophic cardiomyopathy
        (c) Diabetes mellitus
        (d) Marfan's syndrome
        (e) Chronic renal failure and hypercalcemia
B. Disorders of mitral valve leaflets
    1. Rheumatic heart disease
    2. Mitral valve prolapse (myxomatous degeneration)
    3. Infective endocarditis
    4. Systemic lupus erythematosus (Libman-Sacks lesion)
    5. Trauma, blunt and penetrating, including percutaneous mitral balloon valvotomy
    6. Acute rheumatic fever
    7. Interference with its closure, i.e., atrial myxoma
C. Disorders of chordae tendinaea
    1. Chordae rupture, i.e., idiopathic
    2. Myxomatous degeneration: mitral valve prolapse, Marfan's syndrome
    3. Infective endocarditis
    4. Acute myocardial infarction
    5. Acute rheumatic fever
    6. Trauma, blunt and penetrating, including percutaneous mitral balloon valvotomy
    7. Acute left ventricular dilatation
D. Disorders of papillary muscles
    1. Coronary artery disease: acute reversible ischemia, acute myocardial infarction
    2. Other rare causes
        (a) Infiltrative diseases: sarcoidosis, amyloidosis, and tumors
        (b) Congenital: parachute mitral valve
        (c) Conditions that cause localized fibrosis: hypertension, myocarditis, and cardiomyopathy
        (d) Trauma

systolic annular contraction, thus preventing normal leaflet coaptation
(1). Calcification of the mitral annulus is usually accelerated by systemic
hypertension, aortic stenosis, and hypertrophic cardiomyopathy (7,14). It
may also occur in young patients with chronic renal failure (15), diabetes
mellitus (7), mitral valve prolapse (7), and Marfan's syndrome (16). The
calcification may extend toward adjacent structures and invade the conduction system, leading to various degrees of atrio-ventricular conduction
blocks. In rare instances, extensive annular calcification may cause functional MS (17,18).

B. Disorders of the Mitral Leaflets

Mitral regurgitation due to rheumatic heart disease is prevalent in the
developing countries. The pathological abnormalities include scarring and
contraction of the leaflets as sequelae of rheumatic inflammation, leading
to a lack of coaptation of the leaflets and resulting in MR. The rheumatic
process may also involve the chordae, producing shortening and fusion,
and may interfere with the mechanism of normal valve closure.

The leaflets may also be affected by infective endocarditis, which was
found to be the cause of MR in 5% of the cases studied (7,19). Acute or
subacute endocarditis may cause leaflet perforation with moderate or severe acute MR and pulmonary edema. Scarring and deformity of the mitral
leaflets causing MR may occur after the healing phase of endocarditis.
Other mechanisms by which infective endocarditis may induce MR include chordae rupture and the presence of vegetations that may interfere
mechanically with valve closure.

Percutaneous mitral balloon valvotomy, a recently established technique for the treatment of severe MS, is a rare cause of iatrogenic MR
(20,21). The mechanism of this iatrogenic type of MR appears to be mitral
leaflet tear or excessive splitting of the fused commissures by the inflated
balloon catheters. Mild to moderate MR develops after this therapeutic
procedure in 36% of cases, but the incidence of severe MR requiring
emergency surgery is only 1.5% (22).

C. Disorders of the Chordae Tendineae

Twenty percent of all cases of MR are caused by chordae rupture (19),
invariably occurring spontaneously. The most common etiology of spontaneous chordal rupture is idiopathic. Other causes include infective endocarditis and myxomatous degeneration—as in mitral valve prolapse and
Marfan's syndrome. The spectrum of severity of MR is variable, depending on the number and type of ruptured chordae.

In the degenerative variety, the thinner chordae of the posterior leaflet rupture more frequently than those of the anterior leaflet. It would be expected that the normal chordae tendinaea are more vulnerable to rupture than the thickened chordae produced by a previous pathological process. Pathologically, the myxomatous process in MVP syndrome can affect the mitral annulus, leaflets, and chordae tendinaea. (Refer to the detailed description of the pathological changes in MVP and Marfan's syndrome in Chapter 1.)

Mitral regurgitation may develop when the chordae to the anterior mitral leaflet are damaged by "jet lesions" secondary to aortic valve endocarditis with aortic regurgitation (AR). Other rare causes of MR are mentioned in Table 1.

D. Disorders of the Papillary Muscle

Ten percent of cases of MR are due to papillary muscle dysfunction (19), and the most common cause of the latter is coronary ischemia (7). The posteromedial papillary muscle is more often involved than the anterolateral, because of the pattern of its blood supply. During acute ischemia, the papillary muscle dysfunction may be transient and variable in severity, causing a wide spectrum of degree of MR. *Flashing episodes* of acute pulmonary edema have been more recently recognized during episodes of acute reversible myocardial ischemia (q.v., see Chapter 11).

If ischemia of the papillary muscle territory persists, necrosis may develop and cause permanent MR without chordal rupture. Less commonly, a rupture of a portion of the papillary muscle may occur. Ischemic necrosis rarely causes complete rupture of the entire papillary muscle. Mitral regurgitation has been detected in 15% of the anterior and 40% of the posteroinferior wall infarcts (23). Despite the fact that most of these MR episodes may be transient, some degree of ischemic necrosis of the papillary muscles has been confirmed in 20–50% of those patients who die after acute myocardial infarction (23,24). Thirty percent of patients undergoing coronary bypass surgery have some degree of MR (25,26).

Partial rupture of a papillary muscle, which usually occurs toward the end of the first week after myocardial infarction, may cause severe MR with hemodynamic instability and warrant emergency surgical intervention. Complete rupture of a papillary muscle secondary to acute myocardial infarction is rare and invariably fatal (4,7). Such complete transsection of the papillary muscle will result in rupture of about 60 tertiary chordae tendinaea (q.v. Section I).

III. PATHOPHYSIOLOGY

The onset of symptoms and/or early detection of signs of LV dysfunction are of paramount importance. Appreciation of the precise pathophysiological changes following the development of chronic MR is essential to begin to recognize the difficulty in detecting the onset of LV dysfunction in such a volume overload-dependent disorder. The onset of symptoms in conditions characterized by volume overload (i.e., chronic MR and AR) affects their natural history and prognosis adversely. (Refer to Chapters 16 and 17 for further details.)

The hemodynamic consequence of MR depend on: (1) the size of the regurgitant orifice, and (2) the pressure gradient across the incompetent mitral valve in systole (27,28). This pressure gradient depends on the LV function, left atrial compliance, and the state of the afterload (peripheral vascular resistance). The regurgitant orifice is affected by the extent of the pathological involvement of the mitral valve apparatus and by the dynamic changes in the mitral valve annulus in the absence of annular calcification. Consequently, conditions that are associated with increased LV systolic pressure and dilatation will lead to an increase in the degree of MR. On the other hand, medications that reduce the peripheral vascular resistance, decrease the LV size, and/or improve the LV contractility (e.g., vasodilators, diuretics, and positive inotropes) will result in reduction of the pressure gradient between the left ventricle and the left atrium, and thus decrease the mitral regurgitant volume. Hence it is not surprising to detect variation in the degree of MR in the same patient at different times, since the degree of MR depends on changes in the peripheral vascular resistance and the pharmacological interventions.

The magnitude of the gradual enlargement of the left atrium secondary to chronic MR depends on the degree of regurgitation and the compliance of the left atrium. In the majority of patients the left atrium is compliant (27), thus it will dilate progressively, accommodating the increased regurgitant flow with no significant increase in left atrial pressure.

The pulmonary capillary wedge (PCW) and the pulmonary artery pressure may remain normal or only slightly elevated despite severe MR. This explains why pulmonary hypertension and right ventricular failure are seen less commonly in MR than in MS. In the latter, and in a small group of patients with chronic MR, the left atrium is not compliant (29). Thus there will be only a slight enlargement in left atrial size and the increased regurgitant volume will cause marked elevation of the left atrial pressure, leading to early pulmonary hypertension. The latter changes also occur in acute MR; here the left atrium has not time to dilate, and the systolic regurgitant pressure is transmitted directly to the pulmonary capillaries, causing early acute pulmonary edema, and may progress rapidly to pulmonary hypertension (refer to Chapter 11).

Despite the increased LV total stroke volume in chronic MR, the LV workload is initially reduced due to the runaway of the regurgitant flow into a low-pressure chamber, the left atrium. The mitral regurgitant volume can be up to 20% of the total LV stroke volume (30). This will enable the left ventricle to sustain a large volume for a prolonged period of time before increase in the wall stress (31). During this period the indices of myocardial function, such as ejection fraction, may remain normal or even above the normal range. With the progression of the disease, however, the LV function will slowly deteriorate, though the extent of the LV dysfunction may be masked and appear only after surgery. Before surgical correction, the left atrium acts as a low-resistant conduit for ejection and allows the left ventricle to empty completely, resulting in reduction of the late systolic ventricular pressure and dimension (27). The latter changes will increase the contractile shortening and ejection fraction.

In contrast, after eliminating the regurgitant flow into the left atrium by corrective surgery, the left ventricle will then start to pump against the high peripheral vascular resistance of the aorta. At this point the occult LV dysfunction will be unmasked. In general, the ejection fraction usually drops following surgery, once the mitral valve is rendered competent (32,33). Therefore, normal myocardial indices in patients with severe MR may actually reflect mildly impaired LV function, with moderately reduced values signifying severe impairment.

IV. CLINICAL FEATURES

A. Symptoms

In patients with chronic MR, symptoms are related principally to the degree of regurgitation and the status of the underlying function of the left ventricle and atrium. Patients with insidious onset and gradual progression of MR are usually asymptomatic for a long period of time. During this time the left atrium gradually enlarges to accommodate the regurgitant volume. Such an indolent course may be misleading, since the onset of symptoms may herald irreversible LV dysfunction.

As the regurgitant volume increases and the forward stroke volume decreases, there will be a fall in forward cardiac output. The symptoms of low output are usually vague, mainly in the form of fatigue and tiredness. Eventually, with onset of LV impairment, effort dyspnoea, orthopnoea, and paroxysmal nocturnal dyspnoea appear.

Palpitation is a common symptom, which is either due to subjective sensation of the forceful LV contractions or may be related to the onset of atrial fibrillation—which occurs in 75% of patients with significant MR (19). Systemic embolization may occur, especially in patients with a large left atrium and atrial fibrillation (34).

This insidious course of chronic MR may be interrupted by an acute exacerbation if complicated by chordal rupture, infective endocarditis, or sudden increase in the left ventricle afterload, i.e., uncontrolled hypertension. All these conditions would produce acute symptoms of pulmonary congestion.

Patients with mitral valve prolapse may complain of atypical chest pain, palpitations, and may suffer from undue anxiety. These symptoms may be out of proportion to the degree of MR and may be due to dysfunction of the autonomic nervous system (35). The cause of the chest pain is unclear but may be due to focal myocardial ischemia in the papillary muscle (36). Palpitation is common in this group of patients, since they are more likely to develop ventricular or supraventricular tachyarrhythmias and have a high incidence of accessory pathway (37). Also, transient ischemic attack or systemic embolization is more common in this group (38–40). (Refer to Chapters 1 and 12 for further details regarding mitral valve prolapse.)

The clinical picture in acute MR is usually different from that seen in chronic MR (see Chapter 9). The most common causes of acute MR are idiopathic spontaneous chordal rupture, infective endocarditis, and acute myocardial infarction with papillary muscle dysfunction. In such patients, symptoms of severe pulmonary congestion predominate, since the left atrium will have no time to dilate and accommodate the large regurgitant volume, thus the left atrial pressure will increase dramatically. In such patients there are usually other features of the underlying pathology causing the acute MR, i.e., peripheral signs of infective endocarditis or a pattern of acute myocardial infarction. Idiopathic rupture of the chordae is the most common cause of acute MR in otherwise healthy individuals.

B. Physical Examination

In general, the patient's physical appearance is normal. In a minority of patients some features of body habitus may suggest the underlying etiological disorder, for example, Marfan's syndrome. Stigmata of infective endocarditis should be sought, particularly when acute exacerbation of chronic MR occurs.

The peripheral pulse is usually normal or brisk in character. This is helpful to differentiate from aortic stenosis, as both entities exhibit a systolic murmur. In patients with long-standing severe MR, the cardiac rhythm is usually atrial fibrillation. Blood pressure is usually normal. Jugular venous pressure is not elevated except in a few patients with long-standing disease accompanied by right ventricular failure and tricuspid regurgitation. The jugular venous pressure is then elevated, with predominant V waves.

The cardiac impulse is usually hyperdynamic and displaced laterally, reflecting a dilated left ventricle. The hyperdynamic apex can be felt as a strong "punch" that disappears almost immediately after its appreciation. In contrast, the apical impulse in aortic stenosis is sustained, indicating LV hypertrophy. In hypertrophic cardiomyopathy, it is bifid or may even be in the form of triple thrust.

Some patients may have left parasternal lift due to either systolic expansion of the left atrium or pulmonary hypertension with right ventricular hypertrophy. The second heart sound may be palpable in patients with pulmonary hypertension. An apical systolic thrill in chronic MR is uncommon, but when it is present, it indicates severe MR.

The first heart sound is usually normal. If concomitant MS is present, however, it may be accentuated. The first heart sound is soft when MR is due to fibrosis of the mitral valve because of restricted leaflet mobility. The second heart sound is usually normal. An accentuated pulmonary component of the second heart sound (P2) indicates pulmonary hypertension. The early occurrence of the aortic component of the second heart sound (A2) is due to the shortening of the LV ejection period, thus leading to wide splitting of the second heart sound.

A third heart sound may be present in moderate and severe MR due to the rapid filling of the ventricle; it generally occurs 120 to 240 ms after the second heart sound and must be distinguished from an opening snap which occurs earlier, after 60–90 ms. In mixed mitral valve disease, the presence of a third heart sound indicates predominant regurgitation, and stenosis is unlikely to be severe. A fourth heart sound is heard in acute MR.

The pansystolic murmur is the leading clinical feature of MR. It is usually holosystolic, begins with the first heart sound, continues throughout systole, and may outshine the second heart sound. The murmur is high-pitched, with its maximum intensity heard at the apex, and usually propagates along the direction of the regurgitant flow, thus radiating toward the axilla. In contrast, the murmur caused by ruptured chordae or flail leaflets radiates toward the left parasternal area and may also reach the root of the neck in the case of posterior leaflet dysfunction. Alternatively, it may be heard over the spine and near the left scapula when the anterior leaflet is involved.

The intensity of the murmur does not correlate with the severity of the MR. The murmur intensity tends to be constant regardless of the variation in the RR interval (cardiac cycle), as in atrial fibrillation (41). This may help to differentiate it from the murmur of aortic stenosis, the intensity of which is affected by ectopies. The murmur also tends to increase with increased afterload, i.e., squatting and isometric exercise, and decreases with decreased afterload, as with amyl nitrate inhalation. In contrast, such maneuvers will result in an opposite effect on the intensity of the murmur of aortic stenosis.

In acute MR the murmur is variable; it may be short and loud, soft or even absent, and the diagnosis may be difficult (refer to Chapter 11). As the left atrial pressure is markedly elevated in acute MR, the systolic gradient across the incompetent mitral valve is diminished, thus the murmur is short and may be soft. In mitral valve prolapse the murmur may occur in late systole, and clicks may be heard. If the prolapse is severe, however, the murmur may become holosystolic. The murmur of papillary muscle dysfunction is variable and may be transient during attacks of ischemia.

A mid-diastolic rumbling murmur may sometimes be present in patients with severe MR without concomitant organic MS. This is caused by the increased diastolic flow across the mitral valve. The diastolic murmur usually starts after the third heart sound and should be differentiated from organic MS by the absence of a loud first heart sound or opening snap, and with the presence of the loud third heart sound.

In the differential diagnosis of MR, other conditions that produce systolic murmurs should be considered, principally tricuspid regurgitation, aortic stenosis, ventricular septal defect, and hypertrophic cardiomyopathy.

The murmur of MR may frequently be confused with tricuspid regurgitation murmur, especially in patients with MS and severe pulmonary hypertension. In such patients the right ventricle may be hypertrophic and dilated, and may in fact form the cardiac apex, producing forceful apical impulse. Thus, in patients with tricuspid regurgitation, the murmur may be wrongly interpreted as that of MR and the right ventricular impulse could be confused with LV impulse. Nevertheless, the presence of an elevated jugular venous pressure with a prominent V wave, a pulsating liver, a loud P2, a systolic murmur that is increasing with inspiration (Carvallo's sign), and the presence of auscultatory features of concomitant significant MS should help in the differential diagnosis.

Aortic stenosis may be confused with MR, especially when MR is due to posterior leaflet dysfunction. In both conditions the murmur is directed toward the base of the heart. The two lesions can be differentiated by the character of the carotid pulse, the LV apical impulse, and the pansystolic or holosystolic feature of the murmur in MR—whereas in aortic stenosis it is ejection in nature. The murmur of MR is constant, whereas the aortic stenosis murmur varies with ectopies; the MR murmur decreases with reduced afterload, whereas the aortic murmur increases.

Differentiating acute MR from ventricular septal rupture is difficult in the context of an acute myocardial infarction with the appearance of a new systolic murmur. Both groups of patients will usually present with severe pulmonary edema and a new systolic murmur toward the end of the first week after myocardial infarction. The murmur of ventricular septal rupture is usually loud at the parasternal area and is more commonly associated with thrill, whereas the MR murmur is usually short and located at the apex, and thrill is rare. Echocardiographic examination with color Doppler, and a Swan Ganz catheter insertion, with an oximetry series at the bedside, will differentiate between these two different complications of acute myocardial infarction.

V. LABORATORY INVESTIGATIONS

A. Electrocardiogram

Patients with MR and normal sinus rhythm nearly always have evidence of left atrial enlargement. However, the majority of patients with significant chronic MR will be in atrial fibrillation. Evidence of LV hypertrophy is present in about one-third of patients (42). Right ventricular hypertrophy is uncommon, and when it is present it indicates significant pulmonary hypertension.

Patients with acute MR due to idiopathic chordae rupture may have a normal ECG. On the other hand, a pattern of acute infarction or acute ischemia is usually present if MR is caused by acute ischemic syndrome.

B. Chest X-Ray

Radiologically, enlargement of the left ventricle and atrium is the main abnormal finding in patients with chronic significant MR (refer to Chapter 4). The atrium may reach gigantic size and is usually larger than those seen in patients with predominant MS. The pulmonary vasculature is usually normal, but it may show some congestion in the late stages of the disease.

In acute MR, however, the cardiac size may be normal and the lung fields exhibit severe congestion.

Calcification of the mitral valve is better detected by fluoroscopy and is less common in MR compared with MS. Mitral annular calcification—which may cause MR in the elderly—may be seen as a dense C-shaped opacity.

C. Echocardiography

Full noninvasive evaluation by echocardiography and Doppler examination will yield essential information regarding: (1) severity of MR, (2) underlying etiology, (3) morphology of the mitral valve apparatus, (4) LV function, and (5) concomitant valvular pathology.

The only relevant information that can be obtained by M-mode echocardiography is the measurement of the dimensions of the left ventricle at end-diastole and end-systole, and the percentage diameter shortening. Precise measurement of the LV dimension at the same level of the LV cavity, as guided by two-dimensional echocardiography, is important for optimal comparison of results of serial echo examinations. The latter is the method of choice for follow-up of patients with chronic MR to determine the time of surgery. Changes in these parameters are recognized guidelines in the management of patients with MR (refer to Chapters 16 and 17).

Two-dimensional echocardiography is the preferred method for studying the morphology of the mitral valve apparatus and determining the etiology of the MR. The rheumatic mitral valve appears thickened, domed, and with restricted mobility. There may be additional involvement of other valves, notably the aortic. Valves with myxomatous degeneration may show thickening, excessive mobility, and flail, or prolapse leaflet with redundant or ruptured chordae. In endocarditis the vegetations may be seen if they measure more than 2 mm in size.

Doppler examination confirms the clinical diagnosis of MR and semiquantitates its severity. MR is diagnosed by demonstrating systolic flow in the atrial side of the mitral valve. Using pulse Doppler, the regurgitant jet can be mapped in the left atrium. With the advent of color Doppler, real-time visualization of the regurgitant jet is possible. The regurgitant jet correlates with the angiographic severity of the MR (43–45).

It must be remembered, however, that Doppler examination provides information on velocity rather than volume of flow. Velocity is dependent on the gradient between the left ventricle and the left atrium. The LV pressure is influenced by changes in the systolic arterial pressure. Thus systemic hemodynamic changes could influence the velocity profile of the MR, hence affecting the assessment of the severity of MR. This may explain some of the discrepancies between the assessment of the degree of MR by cardiac catheterization and Doppler examination.

In acute myocardial infarction with a new systolic murmur, echo Doppler study is very useful in differentiating MR from ventricular septal rupture. In a recent study investigating patients with new systolic murmur with the context of myocardial infarction, all cases due to ventricular septal rupture were clearly established, and the sensitivity of the procedure to detect MR was very high (46). However, in acute MR, Doppler studies tend to underestimate the severity of the MR when compared with angiography. This is due to the high systolic pressure in the left atrium, which diminishes the gradient between the left ventricle and atrium, thus lowering the velocity profile.

In summary, echo Doppler can be used to define morphology of the valves, the cause and severity of the MR, and the LV dimension and function. It is the method of choice to: (1) determine the timing of surgery in the follow-up of patients with significant chronic MR, and (2) help in patient selection for mitral surgical repair (see Chapter 3).

D. Radionuclide Angiography

Radionuclide angiography can be used to calculate the mitral regurgitant fraction (47) and the LV ejection fraction (48). The latter can be measured by the difference in stroke volume between the left and the right ventricles. This method can be used for follow-up examination, since it provides a serial noninvasive means for estimating the ejection fraction and the LV volume. Serial studies will help in deciding the time for surgical intervention by early detection of any changes in the LV function or increase in the end-systolic volume (refer to Chapters 16 and 17).

E. Cardiac Catheterization

In young patients with MR, clinical examination and noninvasive tests—namely, ECG, echocardiography, and isotopic studies—should provide all the necessary information to assist in management, making cardiac catheterization unnecessary. However, cardiac catheterization is indicated in patients with chest pain or in those who are above the age of 40 years, to determine the presence or absence of coronary artery disease. It is indicated in patients in whom LV dysfunction is out of proportion to the degree of MR. This is particularly important in middle-aged patients when asymptomatic coronary artery disease should be excluded. Cardiac catheterization may also be done in patients whose symptoms are out of proportion to the severity of MR.

At cardiac catheterization, the hemodynamic sequelae of MR are assessed by measuring the pressure of the right and left sides of the heart. The left atrial V wave, measured directly by transeptal puncture or indirectly from the pulmonary wedge, may reflect the degree of MR. Although a V wave that is more than twice the mean wedge pressure suggests moderate to severe MR (49), the absence of a prominent V wave does not exclude severe regurgitation. This is due to high compliance of the dilated left atrium. Cardiac output tends to decrease in patients with severe MR and LV dysfunction. As mentioned previously, pulmonary hypertension is less common in patients with MR than in patients with MS.

The severity of MR can be determined by LV angiography. The assessment of the severity of MR is subjective, depending on the degree of opacification of the left atrium by the regurgitant dye. The severity is graded from 1 to 4, with 1 being mild and 4 being severe (50). Angiographic quantitative assessment of the mitral regurgitant volume can be done by subtracting the forward stroke volume (volume ejected into the aorta), as calculated from the cardiac output using the Fick or thermodilution method from the total left ventricle stroke volume, as determined by angiography. The mitral regurgitant fraction is derived by dividing the regurgitant volume by the total stroke volume. In severe MR, the regurgitant fraction can be more than 60%; in mild cases it is usually less than 20%.

VI. NATURAL HISTORY

The natural history and the survival of patients with chronic MR is influenced by the etiology and severity of MR, and the symptomatic status of the patient at time of diagnosis. The underlying pathological etiology may play an important role in the survival of patients with chronic MR, for example, Marfan's syndrome, infective endocarditis, and coronary artery disease. Each one of these diseases may carry a worse prognosis than chronic MR per se.

Although acute MR has a dramatic clinical course, patients with chronic rheumatic MR may remain asymptomatic for a long period of time, as described earlier. Symptoms usually appear 20 years after an attack of acute rheumatic fever, and thereafter progress fairly rapidly. The natural history of the nonrheumatic chronic MR, however, has been ill-defined, because of the lack of follow-up studies in this subgroup of patients. In an unselected group of patients with chronic MR treated medically, 80% were alive 5 years after establishing the diagnosis, and 60% were alive after 10 years (51). In contrast, in patients with severe symptoms, only 45% survived 5 years (52). Patients with combined MS and regurgitation also have a relatively poor prognosis, with 67% survival at 5 years, and 30% at 10 years (51).

Acute MR results in severe, rapidly progressing symptoms of pulmonary congestion. Prognosis is usually very poor in the medically treated patients, and surgery is the optimal choice of therapy (53,54) (refer to Chapter 11).

VII. TREATMENT

A. Medical Treatment

Patients with chronic rheumatic MR should receive prophylactic antibiotic therapy to prevent a further attack of acute rheumatic fever. All patients with MR should also receive prophylactic antibiotics against infective endocarditis if they are expected to be exposed to bacteremia during a medical or dental procedure. Prophylaxis against endocarditis is done according to the recommendation of the American Heart Association (55).

Patients with mild MR are usually asymptomatic and require no cardiac medication other than the above-mentioned prophylaxis. If atrial fibrillation develops, cardioversion to sinus rhythm may be required; This can be achieved electrically, or pharmacologically using digoxin and quinidine. However, it may be justifiable to avoid cardioversion, since (1) the left atrium tends to be markedly enlarged in severe chronic MR, and it may be difficult to maintain sinus rhythm for a long period; and (2) maintaining sinus rhythm is not so important hemodynamically in patients with MR as, for example, in those with MS. Patients then should be treated with digoxin and long-term oral anticoagulation. Anticoagulation is always recommended before any cardioversion, and preferably should be given for a few weeks.

Mild symptoms are usually controlled by digoxin, diuretics, and peripheral vasodilators. The mechanisms by which improvement of symptoms occur have been discussed previously. One has to be careful not to ignore the fact that irreversible LV dysfunction may develop with the onset of symptoms. Thus, careful assessment of the LV function must be made while controlling the symptoms medically.

Patients with significant MR and prominent symptoms should be offered surgery. Timing of surgical intervention is the most important decision in the medical management of a patient with chronic MR. Surgical intervention must be done before irreversible LV dysfunction develops. The indication for surgery is simple in symptomatic patients with mild LV dysfunctions. However, asymptomatic patients who have significant MR and mild LV dysfunction on the one hand, and symptomatic patients with severe LV dysfunction on the other, require careful consideration.

Ross (56) recommended surgery to preserve LV function in patients who are asymptomatic or with mild symptoms—if ejection fraction is less than 55% and diameter shortening is less than 30%, with the LV end-diastolic diameter approaching 75 mm and end-systolic diameter of 50 mm. (Refer also to the discussion in Chapters 16 and 17.) If the preoperative LV ejection function is less than 30%, surgery will have increased risk and the benefit of operation is limited. This is due to the potential worsening of LV function after the operation, as mentioned above, hence persistence of symptoms.

The treatment of patients with acute MR differs from those with chronic regurgitation, and is usually influenced by the underlying etiology, e.g., infective endocarditis or ischemia. The management of such patients is surgical (see Chapter 11).

B. Timing of Surgery

This important topic is covered extensively and general guidelines are suggested in Chapters 16 and 17.

C. Surgical Treatment

Mitral valve repair or mitral valve replacement (MVR) are the two available surgical techniques for the treatment of MR.

Operative mortality for has been reported to be 5–12% (57,58). However, this is mainly affected by the patient's age, preoperative LV function, and concomitant surgical procedures, e.g., coronary bypass surgery or other valve procedures. Long-term survival after valve replacement was shown to be 70% at 5 years, 50% at 10 years, and 40% at 15 years (59). This is also influenced by the underlying etiology for chronic MR. Postoperative 5-year survival in ischemic heart disease is 30%, whereas in rheumatic heart disease it is 70% (60).

The surgical risk is usually higher in patients above the age of 60 and in those with a reduced cardiac index and reduced LV ejection fraction. In elective isolated MVR or surgical repair of chronic MR, the postoperative course depends mainly on the preoperative degree of LV dysfunction. The ejection fraction tend to fall by 10–20% after successful surgery (32).

In a comparative study between valve repair and MVR, it was shown that patients with repair have better short- and long-term survival (61).

(Refer to surgical chapters for detailed discussion.)

REFERENCES

1. Roberts WC, Perloff JK. Mitral valvular disease: a clinicopathologic survey of the conditions causing the mitral valve to function abnormally. Ann Intern Med 1972; 77:939.
2. Zimmerman J, Baily CP. The surgical significance of the fibrous skeleton of the heart. J Thorac Cadiovasc Surg 1962; 44:701.
3. Chandraratna PA, Aronow WS. Mitral valve ring in normal vs dilated left ventricle. Cross-sectional echocardiographic study. Chest 1981; 79:151.
4. Roberts WC, Cohen LS. Left ventricular papillary muscles. Description of the normal and a survey of conditions causing them to be abnormal. Circulation 1972; 46:138.
5. Estes EH Jr, Dalton FM, Entman ML, Dixon HB 2d, Hackel DB. The anat-

omy and blood supply of the papillary muscles of the left ventricle. Am Heart J 1966; 71:356.

6.   Waller BF. Rheumatic and non-rheumatic conditions producing valvular heart disease. In Frankel WS, Brest AN, eds. Valvular Heart Disease: Comprehensive Evaluation and Management. Philadelphia: Cardiovascular Clinics, F.A. Davis, 1986:8.

7.   Roberts WC. Morphologic features of the normal and abnormal mitral valve. Am J Cardiol 1983; 51:1005.

8.   Waller BF, Morrow AG, Maron BJ, Del-Negro AA, Kent KM, McGrath FJ, Wallace RB, McIntosh CL, Roberts WC. Etiology of clinically isolated, severe, chronic, pure mitral regurgitation: analysis of 97 patients over 30 years of age having mitral valve replacement. Am Heart J 1982; 104:276.

9.   Vlodaver Z, Edwards JE. Mitral insufficiency in subjects 50 years of age or older. Cardiovasc Clin 1973; 5:149.

10. Pomerance A. Pathological and clinical study of calcification of the mitral valve ring. J Clin Pathol 1970; 23:354.

11. Edwards JE. Pathology of mitral incompetence. In: Silver MD, ed. Cardiovascular Pathology. Vol 1. New York: Churchill Livingstone, 1983:575.

12. Wenger NK. Valvular heart disease in the elderly. Cardiol Clin 1986; 4:263.

13. Kaul S, Spotnitz WD, Glasheen WP, Touchstone DA. Mechanism of ischemic mitral regurgitation. An experimental evaluation. Circulation 1991; 84:2167.

14. Aronow WS, Schwartz KS, Koenigsberg M. Correlation of serum lipids, calcium and phosphorus, diabetes mellitus, aortic valve stenosis and history of systemic hypertension with presence or absence of mitral annular calcium in persons older than 62 years in a long-term health care facility. Am J Cardiol 1987; 59:381.

15. Forman MB, Virmani R, Robertson RM, Stone WJ. Mitral anular calcification in chronic renal failure. Chest 1984; 85:367.

16. Roberts WC, Honig HS. The spectrum of cardiovascular disease in the Marfan syndrome: a clinico-morphologic study of 18 necropsy patients and comparison to 151 previously reported necropsy patients. Am Heart J 1982; 104: 115.

17. Hammer WJ, Roberts WC, deLeon AC. "Mitral stenosis" secondary to combined "massive" mitral annular calcific deposits and small, hypertrophied left ventricles. Hemodynamic documentation in four patients. Am J Med 1978; 64:371.

18. Osterberger LE, Goldstein S, Khaja-F S, Lakier JB. Functional mitral stenosis in patients with massive mitral annular calcification. Circulation 1981; 64:472.

19. Selzer A, Katayama F. Mitral regurgitation: clinical patterns, pathophysiology and natural history. Medicine—Baltimore 1972; 51:337.

20. Inoue K, Owaki T, Kitamura F, Miyamoto N. Clinical application of transvenous mitral commissurotomy by a new balloon catheter. J Thorac Cardiovasc Surg 1984; 87:394.

21. Al-Zaibag M, Ribeiro PA, Al-Kasab S, Al-Fagih MR. Percutaneous double-

balloon mitral valvotomy for rheumatic mitral-valve stenosis. Lancet 1986; 1:757.
22. Al Zaibag M, Ribeiro PA. The future of balloon valvotomy. In: Topol EJ, ed. Textbook of Interventional Cardiology. Philadelphia: Saunders, 1990: 912.
23. Davies JJ. Pathology of Cardiac Valves. London: Butterworth, 1980.
24. Becker AE, Anderson RH. Mitral insufficiency complicating acute myocardial infarction. Eur J Cardiol 1975; 2:351.
25. Gahl K, Sutton R, Pearson M, Caspari P, Lairet A, McDonald L. Mitral regurgitation in coronary heart disease. Br Heart J 1977; 39:13.
26. Izumi S, Miyatake K, Beppu S, Park YD, Nagata S, Kinoshita N, Sakakibara H, Nimura Y. Mechanism of mitral reguigitation in patients with myocardial infarction: a study using real-time two-dimensional Doppler flow imaging and echocardiography. Circulation 1987; 76:777.
27. Braunwald E. Mitral regurgitation: physiologic, clinical and surgical considerations. N Engl J Med 1969; 281:425.
28. Braunwald E, Welch GH Jr, Sarnoff SJ. Hemodynamic effects of quantitatively varied experimental mitral regurgitation. Circ Res 1957; 5:539.
29. Braunwald E, Swe WC. The syndrome of severe mitral regurgitation with normal left atrial pressure. Circulation 1963; 27:29.
30. Eckberg DL, Gault JH, Bouchard RL, Karliner JS, Ross J Jr. Mechanics of the left ventricular contraction in chronic severe mitral regurgitation. Circulation 1973; 47:1252.
31. Sasayama S, Kubo S, Kusukawa R. Hemodynamic and angiocardiographic studies on cardiodynamics. Experimental mitral insufficiency. Jpn Circ J 1970; 34:513.
32. Boucher CA, Bingham JB, Osbakken MD, Okada RD, Strauss HW, Block PC, Levine FH, Phillips HR, Pohost GM. Early changes in left ventricular size and function after correction of left ventricular volume overload. Am J Cardiol 1981; 47:991.
33. Wisenbaugh T, Spann JF, Carabello BA. Differences in myocardial performance and load between patients with similar amounts of chronic aortic versus chronic mitral regurgitation. J Am Coll Cardiol 1984; 3:916.
34. Coulshed N, Epstein EJ, McKendrick CS, Galloway RW, Walker E. Systemic embolism in mitral valve disease. Br Heart J 1970; 32:26.
35. Gaffney FA, Karlsson ES, Campbell W, Schutte JE, Nixon JV, Willerson JT, Blomqvist CG. Autonomic dysfunction in women with mitral valve prolapse syndrome. Criculation 1979; 59:894.
36. Barlow JB, Pocock WA, Obel IW. Mitral valve prolapse: primary, secondary, both or neither? Am Heart J 1981; 102:140.
37. Josephson ME, Horowitz LN, Kastor JA. Paroxysmal supraventricular tachycardia in patients with mitral-valve prolapse. Circulation 1978; 57:111.
38. Barnett HJ, Boughner DR, Taylor DW, Cooper PE, Kostuk WJ, Nichol PM. Further evidence relating mitral valve prolapse to cerebral ischemic events. N Engl J Med 1980; 302:139.
39. Walsh PN, Kansu TA, Corbett JJ, Savion PJ, Goldburgh WP, Schatz NJ.

Platelets, thromboembolism and mitral valve prolapse. Circulation 1981; 63: 552.

40. Hanson MR, Conomy JP, Hodgman JR. Brain events associated with mitral valve prolapse. Stroke 1980; 11:499.

41. Karliner JS, O'Rourke RA, Kearney DJ, Shabetai R. Haemodynamic explanation of why the murmur of mitral regurgitation is independent of cycle length. Br Heart J 1973; 35:397.

42. Bentivoglio LG, Uricchio JF, Waldow A. An electrocardiographic analysis of sixty-five cases of mitral regurgitation. Circulation 1958; 18:572.

43. Quinones MA, Young JB, Waggoner AD, Ostojic MC, Ribeiro LG, Miller RR. Assessment of pulsed Doppler echocardiography in detection and quantification of aortic and mitral regurgitation. Br Heart J 1980; 44:612.

44. Miyatake K, Izumi S, Okamoto M, Kinoshita N, Asonuma H, Nakagawa H, Yamamoto K, Takamiya M, Sakakibara H, Nimura Y. Semiquantitative grading of severity of mitral regurgitation by real-time two-dimensional Doppler flow imaging technique. J Am Coll Cardiol 1986; 7:82.

45. Yoshida K, Yoshikawa J, Yamaura Y, Hozumi T, Akasaka T, Fukaya T. Assessment of mitral regurgitation by biplane transesophageal color Doppler flow mapping. Circulation 1990; 82:1121.

46. Smyllie JH, Sutherland GR, Geuskens R, Dawkins K, Conway N, Roelandt JR. Doppler color flow mapping in the diagnosis of ventricular septal rupture and acute mitral regurgitation after myocardial infarction. J Am Coll Cardiol 1990; 15:1449.

47. Rigo P, Alderson PO, Robertson RM, Becker LC, Wagner HN Jr. Measurement of aortic and mitral regurgitation by gated cardiac blood pool scans. Circulation 1979; 60:306.

48. Green MV, Brody WR, Douglas MA, Borer JS, Ostrow HG, Line BR, Bacharach SL, Johnston GS. Ejection fraction by count rate from gated images. J Nuclear Med 1978; 19:880.

49. Grossman W. Profiles in valvular heart disease. In: Grossman W, ed. Cardiac Catheterisation and Angiography. 3d ed. Philadelphia: Lea & Febiger, 1991: 564.

50. Sellers RD, Levy MJ, Amplatz K, Lillehei CW. Left retrograde cardioangiography in acquired cardiac disease: technic, indications and interpretations in 700 cases. Am J Cardiol 1964; 14:437.

51. Rapaport E. Natural history of aortic and mitral valve disease. Am J Cardiol 1975; 35:221.

52. Munoz S, Gallardo J, Diaz-Gorrin JR, Medina O. Influence of mitral commissurotomy: ten year follow-up study of 202 patients. Am J Cardiol 1981; 47: 821.

53. Sanders RJ, Newbuerger KT, Lavin A. Rupture of papillary muscles: occurrence of rupture of the posterior muscle in posterior myocardial infarction. Dis Chest 1957; 31:316.

54. Radford MJ, Johnson RA, Buckley MJ, Daggett WM, Leinbach RC, Gold HK. Survival following mitral valve replacement for mitral regurgitation due to coronary artery disease. Circulation 1979; 60(suppl I):39.

55. Prevention of bacterial endocarditis: special report. Circulation 1991; 83: 1174.

56. Ross J Jr. Afterload mismatch in aortic and mitral valve disease: implications for surgical therapy. J Am Coll Cardiol 1985; 5:811.

57. Dalby AJ, Firth BF, Forman R. Preoperative factors affecting the outcome of isolated mitral valve replacement: a 10 year review. Am J Cardiol 1981; 47:826.

58. Cohn LH, Allred EN, Cohn LA, Austin JC, Sabik J, DiSesa VJ, Shemin RJ, Collins JJ Jr. Early and late risk of mitral valve replacement. A 12 year concomitant comparison of the porcine bioprosthetic and prosthetic disc mitral valves. J Thorac Cardiovasc Surg 1985; 90:872.

59. McGoon MD, Fuster V, McGoon DC, Pumphrey CW, Pluth JR, Elveback LR. Aortic and mitral valve incompetence: long-term follow-up (10 to 19 years) of patients treated with the Starr-Edwards prosthesis. J Am Coll Cardiol 1984; 3:930.

60. Bonchek LI. Current status of cardiac valve replacement: selection of a prosthesis and indications for operation. Am Heart J 1981; 101:96.

61. Cohn LH, Kowalker W, Bhatia S, DiSesa VJ, St-John-Sutton M, Shemin RJ, Collins JJ Jr. Comparative morbidity of mitral valve repair versus replacement for mitral regurgitation with and without coronary artery disease. Ann Thorac Surg 1988; 45:284.

6

Mitral Valve Stenosis

Muayed Al Zaibag
Armed Forces Hospital, Riyadh, Saudi Arabia, and Loma Linda University Medical Center, Loma Linda, California

Murtada A. Halim
Armed Forces Hospital, Riyadh, Saudi Arabia

I. ETIOLOGY AND PATHOLOGY

Mitral valve stenosis (MS) is nearly always caused by acute rheumatic fever; other etiological causes are rare. In patients with rheumatic heart disease, mitral valve involvement occurs in 65–90% (1,2), and such a high prevalence was initially observed at the beginning of the century (3). Pure MS was detected in 25% of the patients with rheumatic mitral valve disease (1).

The pathogenesis of MS is still not well understood. Conceivably, the severity of the pathological changes are secondary to the high recurrence and/or the severity of the acute rheumatic fever process; this pattern is observed in children and adolescents in the developing countries (4,5). In these countries, 70% of patients may develop symptomatic MS after a latent period of less than 5 years following the episode (4).

Alternatively, the pathogenesis of MS could be due to progressive fibrosis caused by the continuous blood turbulence, which increases the initial mitral valve deformity (6,7). The latter mechanism is similar to that observed in the development of severe aortic stenosis in patients with congenital bicuspid valve, who initially had no significant hemodynamic obstruction (8). In contrast to the developing countries, two-thirds of the children in the developed Western countries do not have clinical features of MS 10 years after an attack of acute rheumatic fever (2). It is likely that both of these mechanisms may be responsible for the increasing fibrosis and deformity, causing progressively worsening mitral stenosis.

The components of the mitral valve—leaflets, chordae, and papillary muscles—may be involved in the process of chronic rheumatic mitral valve disease. The pathological hallmark of MS is commissural fusion, with thickening of the leaflets (9). The process may extend to the chordae, causing thickening, shortening, and fusion, i.e., subvalvular matting (9). The leaflets fibrose and may retract, and even calcify. The valve will eventually exhibit an inverted-funnellike appearance, with the annulus as the base.

The resultant dysfunction of the mitral valve, whether stenosis, regurgitation, or a combination of both, is determined by the nature and degree of the pathological changes. Pure or predominant MS is more likely to occur if commissural fusion is the only, or the main, pathological change. Pure or predominant mitral regurgitation (MR), on the other hand, is the result of shrinkage, fibrosis, and contraction of the leaflets and/or chordeae (9,10). In contrast to pure MS, regurgitant valves have minimal calcification and chordal fusion, with minimal or no commissural fusion (10).

II. PATHOPHYSIOLOGY

The hemodynamic changes that are present in patients with mitral stenosis are all secondary to obstruction of blood flow at the level of the stenotic mitral valve. The length of the diastolic period in patients with MS is of critical importance in the development of symptoms.

In MS, the left atrial pressure increases and propels blood across the narrowed valve. The elevated left atrial pressure is passively reflected into the pulmonary venous circulation. Later, the pulmonary artery pressure will rise, principally due to the back pressure from the venous circulation. In addition, there is an element of pulmonary arterial vasoconstriction (reactive hypertension). While this may initially protect the lungs from pressure overload and congestion, eventually fixed pulmonary hypertension due to intimal and medial hyperplasia and hypertrophy will develop. The degree of pulmonary hypertension that subsequently develops is related to the severity and duration of MS. The resulting high pressure is reflected into the right ventricle, which dilates, hypertrophies, and later may fail—causing right-sided heart failure. Right-sided failure may be compounded by concomitant tricuspid regurgitation secondary to right ventricular dilatation (see Chapter 7).

The normal mitral valve orifice is around 4–6 cm^2. This area must be decreased by more than half, i.e., <2 cm^2, for symptomatic MS to develop. In a normal subject, with a mobile mitral valve, the increase in cardiac output during exercise was shown to be due to tachycardia and to a 30% increase in the mitral valve orifice (11). This observation has an implication for patients with conditions such as MS, where the mitral valve is thickened and its mobility is reduced.

In mild or moderate MS, the left atrial pressure will be markedly increased in response to exercise, thereby increasing the mitral blood flow across the narrowed valve, and thus maintaining cardiac output. On the other hand, in severe MS, with a valve area of 1.0 cm² or less, further increase in the left atrial pressure and mitral gradient during exercise will hardly lead to an increase in the blood flow through the stenotic mitral valve (12), thus causing severe symptoms of pulmonary venous congestion without concomitant increase in cardiac output.

The high left atrial pressure causes pulmonary venous congestion, leading to shortness of breath. Pulmonary edema may develop when the capillary pressure exceeds the plasma oncotic pressure. Such a complication is more likely to occur in the presence of tachycardia, especially fast atrial fibrillation, due to shortening of diastolic filling time (Figs. 1A and 1B). In atrial fibrillation, the loss of the atrial contraction will jeopardize ventricular filling, and further increases the left atrial pressure. Therefore, all causes of tachycardia or increased body fluid may aggravate the symptoms in patients with MS; this includes patients with fever, excessive fluid overload, and exercise, and particularly in pregnancy, with its associated sinus tachycardia and volume overload.

The development of pulmonary hypertension causes a decrease in forward cardiac output, which tends to protect the patient from developing pulmonary edema—but at the expense of a low cardiac output and right-sided failure. This is probably why 78% of patients with severe MS and high pulmonary vascular resistance had no orthopnea or paroxysmal nocturnal dyspnea (13). In these circumstances the patient will complain less of attacks of dyspnea and orthopnea, but will develop clinical features of low cardiac output—excessive fatigue, tiredness, and eventually lower-limb edema and ascitis due to right heart failure.

In MS, the left ventricle is usually normal in size and function. However, 25–50% of patients with MS have some degree of left ventricular (LV) dysfunction (14–17). The LV function is influenced by LV contractility and compliance, preload, and afterload. Thus LV dysfunction may be caused by: chronically underfilled LV (decreased preload) (14); increased LV systolic wall stress (increased afterload) (14,16); impaired contractility due to severe rheumatic carditis (15,16); or concomitant coronary artery disease (18). The increased systolic wall stress that causes LV dysfunction (14,16) is thought to be due to LV wall thinning (14) (wall stress = LV pressure × LV radius/2 × wall thickness). Localized hypokinesis of the

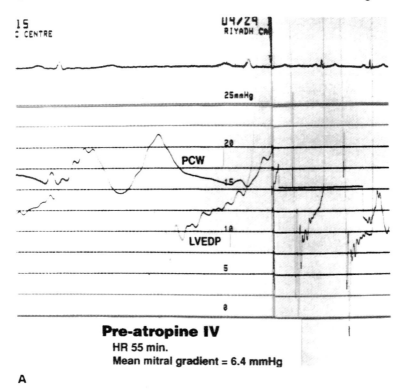

Pre-atropine IV
HR 55 min.
Mean mitral gradient = 6.4 mmHg

A

Figure 1 Pressure tracing recordings in a patient with severe mitral stenosis showing a marked increase of the pulmonary capillary wedge (PCW) pressure and transmitral diastolic gradient after atropine challenge. Note that the heart rate increase from 55 (A) to 102 per minute (B) led to an increase of PCW from 15 to 25 mmHg and an increase in the mean mitral gradient from 6.4 to 10.4 mmHg.

posterior basal segment of the LV wall is common (19), probably caused by extension of the mitral valve scarring process.

The obstruction to blood flow at the mitral valve will result in some degree of left atrial dilatation, which, in association with a fall in the cardiac output, leads to sluggishness of blood flow through the left atrium. In addition, dilatation of the left atrium renders it prone to atrial fibrillation—which occurs in about 70% of patients with mitral stenosis above

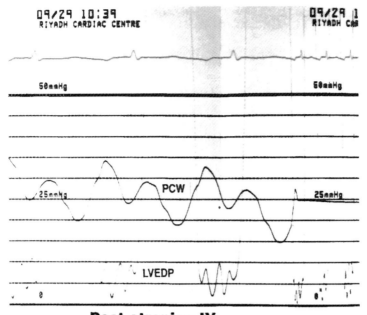

Post-atropine IV
HR 102 min.
Mean mitral gradient = 10.4 mmHg

B

the age of 40 (20). These factors—low cardiac output, sluggishness of flow in the left atrium, dilatation of the left atrium, and atrial fibrillation—may lead to the formation of thrombus. Atrial fibrillation was present in two-thirds of patients with a history of systemic embolization. Left atrial thrombus, however, was found in only 20% of the patients who underwent closed surgical valvotomy (13). Thrombus is most commonly found in the left atrial appendage, but it may also occur in the body of the left atrium (21). This may result in systemic embolization, which is a major cause of mortality and morbidity in mitral stenosis. In contrast to MS, patients with pure MR are unlikely to have thrombus in the body of the left atrium, with or without the presence of atrial fibrillation (Chapter 1). Thrombus formation in the left atrial appendage can occur in any condition with a low cardiac output state—including severe MS.

III. CLINICAL FEATURES

A. Symptoms

Patients with MS may present with symptoms reflecting the hemodynamic changes caused by obstruction of flow at the mitral level or by complication of the disease, such as atrial fibrillation or systemic embolization.

As explained above, the increased left atrial pressure leads to pulmonary congestion and interstitial edema. This, in turn, causes reduction in lung compliance (22), with shortness of breath being the most common symptom.

Orthopnea and paroxysmal nocturnal dyspnea are caused by the redistribution of blood volume when lying supine, resulting in increased volume delivery to the heart and lungs.

Hemoptysis is a significant symptom in MS and could be due to one of the following factors: (1) rupture of bronchial vein, causing severe hemoptysis (though profuse, it is rarely life threatening); (2) rupture of small alveolar capillaries, causing pink frothy sputum accompanying pulmonary edema; (3) blood-streaked sputum associated with attacks of nocturnal dyspnea; and (4) recurrent attacks of bronchitis, which are more common in patients with MS (13).

The symptoms of MS in general tend to progress gradually, with exacerbration precipitated by increased physical and emotional stress, fever, pregnancy, atrial fibrillation, and pulmonary embolism. The development of pulmonary hypertension may protect the patient from developing pulmonary edema; however, this will eventually lead to right ventricular failure, tricuspid regurgitation, hepatic congestion, and lower-limb edema. At this time the patient will usually have manifestation of low cardiac output, causing fatigue and easy tiredness.

Another mode of presentation in patients with MS is systemic embolization. This is one of the most serious complications and will occur in 10–25% of patients (6,23,24). Before the era of anticoagulation, 20% of fatalities from MS were due to systemic embolization (6,25). There is no direct correlation between the frequency of embolization and severity of the stenosis. Systemic embolization may be the first symptom in patients with mild MS. It tends to be more common in patients with atrial fibrillation (26), who are over age of 40 (27), have a large left atrium (28) and mitral calcification (29). Any condition with low cardiac output will also predispose left atrial thrombus formation.

The two factors most closely associated with systemic embolization are age and the presence of atrial fibrillation (26,27). The incidence is usually less than 10% in patients less than 35 years old, but increases to 24% in older patients (27). Eighty percent of patients who develop systemic embolization are in atrial fibrillation (26). Large left atria may contribute directly to clot formation or indirectly by increasing the incidence of atrial fibrillation (28). In severely calcific valves, surface ulceration and subsequent thrombus formation may result in systemic embolization (29).

Other symptoms of MS include anginal chest pain (13), hoarseness of voice caused by compression of the recurrent laryngeal nerve by the dilated left atrium or left main pulmonary artery (Ortner's syndrome), frequent chest infection due to chronic pulmonary congestion, and partial obstruction to the left bronchus that is occasionally caused by the dilated left atrium. Infective endocarditis is a very rare complication in patients with MS.

B. Physical Examination

The general appearance of patients with MS is usually normal. Patients with advanced disease may exhibit the classical features of the so-called mitral facies, with its characteristic purple discoloration of the cheeks.

The peripheral pulse is usually small in volume but may be normal in mild cases. Atrial fibrillation frequently develops. The jugular venous waves are variable: (1) normal, (2) exhibit a large A wave in the presence of pulmonary hypertension and a stiff right ventricle, (3) show elevated A and V waves because of right ventricular failure, or (4) reveal a giant V wave in the case of severe tricuspid regurgitation. The cardiac impulse is usually tapping, which is caused by a palpable first heart sound (S1). There may be a palpable second heart sound (S2) and left parasternal lift in patients with pulmonary hypertension and right ventricular hypertrophy.

A diastolic thrill may be present at the apex. In some patients the right ventricle may be largely dilated, pushing the left ventricle posteriorly, producing a prominent apical beat which may be confused with the left ventricular impulse. Examining the patient in the left lateral decubitus position may be the only way to feel this thrill. This maneuver is also important to appreciate the auscultatory signs.

The classic auscultatory findings in patients with pliable MS are a loud S1, opening snap (OS), and a mid-diastolic rumbling murmur. The accentuation of S1 is due to a rapid closure rate of the valve, which is due to the elevated left atrial pressure. The loud S1 usually indicates a pliable leaflet, and its intensity is reduced in the presence of marked thickening or calcification.

The opening snap (OS) is a classic feature of pliable MS and is due to abrupt termination of the rapid opening movement of the thickened fused mitral valve. It is best heard at the cardiac apex and lower left sternal border, and with the diaphragm of the stethoscope because of its high frequency. The OS occurs after the pulmonary component of the second heart sound (P2), and the short duration of the A2–OS interval reflects the severity of the MS (Fig. 2).

Factors apart from MS may also influence the A2–OS period. For instance, with similar degrees of MS and concomitant aortic valve disease or tachycardia, the time interval is decreased. In contrast, systemic hypertension may prolong it. The duration of A2–OS depends on: (1) the severity of the left atrial pressure, and (2) the closing pressure of the aortic valve, i.e., left ventricular-left atrial crossover dynamics (30–34). An A2–OS interval of more than 90 ms (milliseconds) usually reflects mild MS: an interval of less than 60 ms indicates severe MS (30,31) (Fig. 2).

The mid-diastolic murmur of mitral stenosis is usually low-pitched and rumbling, located at the apex. In some cases of mild MS the murmur may be heard only after exercising and turning the patient to the left lateral side. The murmur commences after the mitral opening snap and has a presystolic accentuation due to atrial contraction. Therefore the presys-

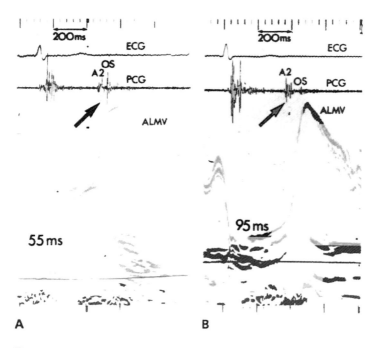

Figure 2   M-mode echocardiography and phonocardiography study (A) before and (B) after balloon valvotomy. Note the marked increase in A2–OS duration following successful valvotomy (B) from 55 to 95 ms (arrows).

tolic murmur will not be heard in patients with atrial fibrillation. The duration of the murmur rather than its intensity correlates with the severity of MS. In patients with severe pulmonary hypertension and low cardiac output, the diastolic murmur may not be audible, the so-called silent MS. In such patients, a loud first heart sound and opening snap may be the only clues to the presence of MS.

When pulmonary hypertension is present, P2 is usually accentuated and widely transmitted and can be heard all over the precordium. With progression of pulmonary hypertension, the A2–P2 duration narrows and the second heart sound eventually may become single. In extreme cases of pulmonary hypertension, the murmur of pulmonary regurgitation (Graham Steel) may develop. Functional tricuspid incompetence, which may cause a systolic murmur and a right ventricular third heart sound (S3), heralds the development of right ventricular failure.

In some patients, the dilated right ventricle displaces the left ventricle posteriorly and the apical impulse will then be formed by the right ventricle. When a pansystolic murmur of tricuspid regurgitation is detected upon ausculation, the clinical diagnosis may be confused with left ventricular hypertrophy and MR.

IV. LABORATORY INVESTIGATIONS

A. Electrocardiogram

The electrocardiogram (ECG) changes of left atrial enlargement found in 90% of patients with severe MS (35) include: (1) a bifid P wave with a duration of more than 120 ms in lead II, and (2) a biphasic P wave with a negative terminal deflection in lead V1.

The P-wave changes have been shown to correlate more closely with left atrial volume than with left atrial pressure (36). These ECG features may regress after successful surgical valvotomy (13). In our experience, despite a marked reduction of the left atrial pressure, there is little change in its size after successful balloon mitral valvotomy.

Atrial fibrillation is commonly present in patients over the age of 40 with chronic MS (37–39) and is related to the degree and duration of left atrial enlargement (36,37). In children and teenagers with MS, atrial fibrillation is present in only 6%, despite the fact that 80% of patients are symptomatic and 45% of patients are in cardiac failure (4). In symptomatic patients with severe MS and who underwent percutaneous balloon mitral valvotomy, atrial fibrillation was present in 13% and 37% of those in the third and fourth decades of age, respectively (38,39). New-onset atrial fibrillation has been shown to develop in 14% of patients with chronic MS over a period of 10 years, and in 22% at 20 years' follow-up (6).

The ECG changes of right ventricular hypertrophy are usually present if the systolic right ventricular pressure exceeds 70 mmHg, with right axis deviation being the most common finding (35,40). (For further discussion, refer to Chapter 14.)

B. Radiological Findings

The chest X-ray may show changes in the cardiac silhouette and lung fields. In patients with severe MS, the left atrium is mildly to moderately enlarged. A giant left atrium is rarely seen in pure mitral stenosis, and its presence usually indicates concomitant severe MR (41,42). When pulmonary hypertension is present, the pulmonary artery may be dilated and the right ventricle enlarged. With the presence of tricuspid regurgitation, the right atrium may also become prominent.

Changes in the lung fields are usually due to high pulmonary venous pressure. The initial changes of upper-lobe venous diversion usually reflect a mild pulmonary venous congestion. The development of Kerly-B lines usually reflect a pulmonary venous pressure of 20–25 mmHg. As pulmonary venous pressure increases to more than 25 mmHg, the radiological features of pulmonary edema may be detected. However, in some cases with long-standing severe MS, we have not observed a good correlation between the radiological changes in the lung fields and the level of the pulmonary wedge pressure.

Another important radiological finding is calcification of the mitral valve, which can be better assessed by fluoroscopy. Rarely, the calcification of the left atrial wall may occur.

(Refer to Chapter 4 for detailed radiological findings in MS.)

C. Echocardiography

Echocardiography is the main diagnostic tool in assessing patients with MS. This technique enables quantification of the mitral valve area and evaluates the suitability of the valve for valvotomy. In addition, it detects natural complications of the disease or those arising from its treatment by balloon or surgical valvotomy. These may include left atrial thrombi, severe pulmonary hypertension, leaflet and chordae rupture, severe MR, and LV perforation. Two-dimensional echocardiography (2-DE) is the gold-standard method in studying the morphology of the valve and the subvalvular apparatus. It obviates the need for diagnostic cardiac catheterization.

The mitral valve area (MVA) can be measured in the short axis by

planimetry (Fig. 3), and a good correlation with the valve area estimated
at surgery (43) and at cardiac catheterization (44) were reported. In
15–20% of patients, technically suboptimal echocardiographic studies or
the presence of calcification and subvalvular stenosis may jeopardize the
accurate estimation of the effective MVA. In these cases Doppler examination is the only reliable noninvasive method to calculate the MVA.

Doppler was added to the noninvasive armament for diagnosis and
assessment of the severity of MS. Doppler can be used to quantitate the
gradient between the left atrium and ventricle by recording the maximal
transmitral flow velosity (V) and applying the Bernoulli equation: pressure
gradient $= 4 \times V^2$. The method of using the pressure half-time $(T\frac{1}{2})$ to
calculate the mitral pressure gradient and valve area was initially demonstrated in the cardiac catheterization laboratories (45). Ten years later this
method became a diagnostic tool in the noninvasive laboratories (46). The
pressure half-time is the time needed for the initial maximum pressure to
drop to half its value (47). The normal pressure half-time is 20 to 60 ms

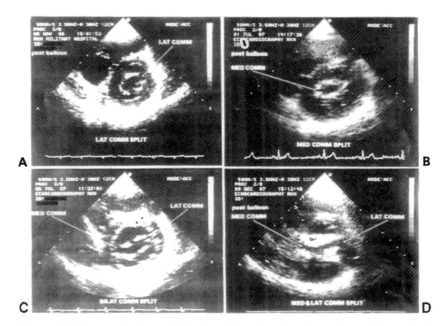

Figure 3 Short-axis view of the two-dimensional echocardiographic study in
four different patients after successful mitral valvotomy. Note the splitting of the
lateral commissure (A), medial commissure (B), bilateral commissures (C), and
bilateral commissures in a heavy calcified mitral valve (D).

(47). In MS the pressure half-time exceeds 100 ms. The MVA can then be calculated by dividing 220 by the pressure half-time (47).

There is a good correlation between the mitral valve pressure gradient measured simultaneously by cardiac catheterization and Doppler (46,47). The pressure half-time method was shown to be independent of the heart rate, cardiac output, and severity of MR (46–48). These factors may interfere with MVA calculation using the Gorlin formula. In patients with severe mitral or tricuspid regurgitation, and low cardiac output, the pressure half-time method may be more accurate than cardiac catheterization in calculating the MVA (45–49).

Color Doppler examination can be used to detect and quantify the degree of MR. This information is essential in determining suitability for valvotomy. Color Doppler is also useful during percutaneous balloon mitral valvotomy as a guide to further balloon inflations and for detection of potential complications. It is used on a routine basis for postoperative evaluation and follow-up.

The development of transesophageal echocardiography (TEE) has proved particularly useful in determining the presence or absence of thrombi in the left atrial body and appendages (21,50). This has important clinical implications in the selection of patients for percutaneous mitral balloon valvotomy.

(Refer to Chapter 3 for comprehensive discussion on echocardiography and mitral valve disease.)

D. Cardiac Catheterization

With the advent of the echo/Doppler technique, young patients with predominant MS do not need diagnostic cardiac catheterization. It is indicated if there is discrepancy between the patient's symptoms and clinical findings, and to rule out the presence of coronary artery disease in elderly patients or those with a history of angina.

The mitral valve gradient is estimated by simultaneous measurement of the pulmonary capillary wedge (PCW) and the left ventricle diastolic pressure. In most patients there is no need for direct left atrial pressure measurement, provided a true PCW pressure is measured accurately (51). This can be achieved by using a stiff, wide-bore catheter, confirming correct position in the PCW by oximetry, and correcting for the time delay in recording the wedge pressure. In patients for whom a true wedge is difficult to achieve, direct left atrial pressure by transseptal technique should be obtained. Transseptal puncture requires skill; otherwise it carries some risk. The MVA is calculated by using the Gorlin formula:

$$\text{Valve area} = \frac{\text{Blood flow (mL/s)}}{44.3C \text{ mean pressure gradient}}$$

$$MVA = \frac{CO/(DFP)(HR)}{37.7 \text{ mean P}}$$

where

CO = cardiac output, mL/min
DFP = seconds/beat
HR = beats/minute
C = empirical constant, = 0.85 for mitral valve
and 1 for aortic valve
P = mean diastolic pressure gradient

V. NATURAL HISTORY

After an attack of acute rheumatic fever, there is a latent period of 20–25 years before symptoms of mitral valve involvement develop in patients residing in the Western countries (6,52). The natural history of the disease is more aggressive in developing countries (4,5,53), with the onset of symptoms occurring on average 10 years earlier than in the West (53). After the onset of symptoms, the course of the disease is progressive, with episodes of sudden deterioration precipitated by the onset of atrial fibrillation, pregnancy, or increased emotional and physical stress.

Follow-up studies of patients with MS showed markedly variable overall mortality rates, i.e., 7–70% at 10 years (5,6,25,54). These differences can be explained by the heterogenous population of patients included in the studies. However, the mortality of patients in NYHA functional class III was at 62–85% at 10 years follow-up, and 100% for class IV patients (24,25). The overall mortality at 5 years was 20% (6), around 40–70% at 10 years (6,7,25), and 83% at 20 years (6); of the latter group, 62% of patients had cardiac failure and 21% had thrombo-embolic complications (6).

VI. TREATMENT

A. Medical Treatment

Patients with mitral stenosis should receive prophylaxis with long-acting penicillin against acute rheumatic fever. This treatment must be continued up to the age of 30 years, or 5 years after an attack of rheumatic fever. Although infective endocarditis is a rare complication in pure MS, prophylaxis against endocarditis is advisable.

Mild symptoms are usually controlled with diuretics and reduced salt intake. The importance of prolonging the diastolic filling period in patients with mitral stenosis was discussed in the pathophysiology section. In patients with atrial fibrillation, digoxin is useful to gradually reduce the ventricular rate, but it is of no value in patients with sinus rhythm. In contrast, beta blockers are effective in controlling the heart rate in patients with atrial fibrillation and in particular those in sinus rhythm. In our experience, beta blockers are the cornerstone therapy in the management of patients with mitral stenosis. Recently we have demonstrated its valuable role in the treatment of pregnant patients with severe symptomatic mitral stenosis (55), reducing the need for surgical intervention during pregnancy, which is known to have a high complication rate. In our study, no adverse effect of beta blockers on the fetus was detected.

The aim of the treatment of acute atrial fibrillation is to control the rapid ventricular response, restore sinus rhythm, and attempt to prevent relapse. The rapid ventricular rate may be controlled with intravenous (IV) digoxin and/or propranolol. Digoxin alone will take several hours to produce significant reduction of the ventricular rate, and may not be useful in acute pulmonary edema and severe MS.

Oral and IV calcium channel blockers—for example, verapamil or diltiazem—have been shown to control the rapid ventricular rate in both chronic and acute atrial fibrillation (56,57). Intravenous diltiazem was also found to control acute-onset rapid ventricular rate adequately in patients with already compromised left ventricle function and congestive cardiac failure; no significant negative adverse effect on myocardium was detected (58).

In patients with MS, tachycardia, and acute pulmonary edema, urgent two-dimensional echocardiography is mandatory to assess left ventricular function. Thus, appropriate treatment to control heart rate and reduce mitral diastolic gradient can be commenced promptly (Fig. 1). Beta blockers and calcium channel blockers should be used to treat patients with pulmonary edema secondary to MS, tachycardia, and good left ventricular function; these drugs should be used judiciously in patients with left ventricular dysfunction.

Amiodarone is the most effective drug in converting and maintaining atrial fibrillation to sinus rhythm (59), but its efficacy in patients with chronic mitral valve disease has not been encouraging (60,61). In patients with chronic rheumatic valve disease, amiodarone maintained sinus rhythm in 55% of patients at 12 months' follow-up, and only 30% at 36 months' (62). However, patients who continue to be in sinus rhythm at 2 years' follow-up remain so at their 4 years' examination (62). The side effects of this drug during long-term therapy should be taken into consideration. Therefore, amiodarone should be used judiciously and only in patients for whom adequate ventricular rate cannot be maintained with conventional drugs.

As mentioned, sinus rhythm is difficult to maintain in patients with rheumatic mitral valve disease and chronic atrial fibrillation. Cardioversion should not be attempted repeatedly, as such a process may precipitate systemic embolization and/or serious ventricular arrythmias. Patients with long-lasting atrial fibrillation should receive oral anticoagulation for 3–4 weeks prior to cardioversion. Intravenous heparin is indicated in patients with new-onset atrial fibrillation.

As thrombo-embolism remains the most serious complication of mitral stenosis, anticoagulation therapy is mandatory unless there is a major contraindication. A recent randomized study demonstrated the advantages of low doses of warfarin (coumadin), keeping the prothrombin time ratio at 1.5 (or the international normalized ratio at 2.65) (63). Using the latter ratio, a similar rate of thrombo-embolic events was reported, with fewer bleeding complications, when compared to the use of the conventional prothrombin time ratio of 2.5.

B. Balloon Mitral Valvotomy

Mitral stenosis had been traditionally treated using surgical techniques until the advent of balloon mitral valvotomy. The potential benefit of surgical valvotomy for MS was first reported way back in 1923 by Cuttler and Levine (64), and 60 years later balloon catheters (65) achieved a similar result, namely, splitting of the fused commissures.

1. Mechanism

The pathological hallmark of rheumatic MS is commissural fusion with fibrosis and leaflet thickening; there is also a wide spectrum of subvalvular involvement (q.v. pathology section and Chapter 1).

Postmortem, in-vivo and in-vitro studies (66–69) confirmed the surgically observed (70) mechanism by which mitral valve area increases after balloon valvotomy. This is similar to that of surgical valvotomy, that is, commissural splitting. These studies have also demonstrated that the rarely observed splitting of fused chordae during balloon valvotomy is not the mechanism by which MVA increases (66–69). These findings have important clinical implications in the selection of patients for this therapeutic intervention. The best results after valvotomy are achieved in patients with severe commissural fusion, pliable leaflets, and minimal sub-valvular involvement (71–76).

We, and others, observed that the degree of MS is not the sole predictor for the extent of splitting of the fused commissures after balloon val-votomy (66,67,71–77). The status of the subvalvular disease and the texture of the mitral leaflets are also important; the latter is presently difficult to characterize in vivo. Tissue characterization using echocardiography may in the future enable the selection of patients with the best valve texture for the procedure. The importance of leaflet thickening has been highlighted in most studies and correlates well with the valve area achieved after valvotomy (75,76).

Several studies have emphasized the importance of the echocardiographic findings of the severity of valvular and subvalvular involvement (72–77). These parameters are leaflet thickening and mobility, the presence of calcification, and the degree of subvalvular pathology. The severity of involvement of these valvular structures were each scored on scale 1 to 4—the so-called Boston total echocardiographic score (71).

For patients with high echocardiographic score (>8), less optimal results immediately after balloon valvotomy may be predicted; i.e., in 56% of patients the procedure achieved a MVA of less than 1.5 cm^2 (74). A high score is also associated with a high and early restenosis rate up to 70% in the 9-month period following the procedure (74) (see pitfalls, in restenosis section, later). Twenty percent of these patients, however, underwent balloon valvotomy using a single balloon catheter of 20 mm in diameter. Using in-vitro and in-vivo studies, we demonstrated that the outcome of the single-balloon technique is markedly inferior to that using a double-balloon method—two, each 20 mm in diameter (67,78) (Fig. 4).

Whereas valvular thickening was the strongest parameter to correlate with MVA achieved after valvotomy, there was no unanimous agreement on the other echocardiographic criteria (72,75–77). The above reports support our belief that these echocardiographic findings are very subjective, with high intra- and interobserver variability, and consequently cannot predict outcome precisely.

Valve calcification was shown to be a less important predictor of immediate outcome after balloon valvotomy (72,75,77), though the reported incidence of early restenosis is very high (74,79) (see pitfalls, in restenosis section, later). In-vitro (67) and postmortem (69) studies of balloon mitral valvotomy using either single- or double-balloon techniques have also revealed that inflated balloon catheters split fused, heavily calcified commissures (Figs. 5 and 6). In one study, commissural splitting occurred preferentially in calcific as opposed to noncalcific commissures (67). Thus

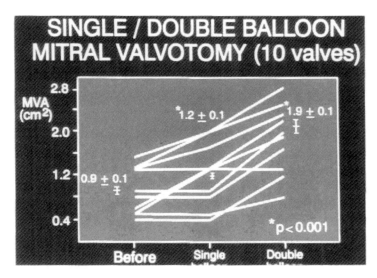

Figure 4 In-vitro balloon mitral valvotomy showing the mean valve area achieved of 1.2 cm² after single-balloon valvotomy (20-mm diameter) and further increase of the MVA to 1.9 cm² after double-balloon valvotomy (20 mm and 20 mm).

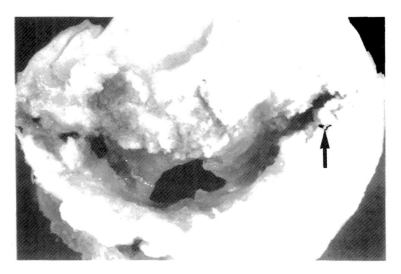

Figure 5 In-vitro double-balloon valvotomy of a heavily calcified stenotic mitral valve. Note splitting of both calcified commissures (arrow).

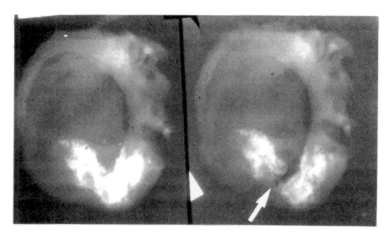

Figure 6   Radiological studies before and after in-vitro balloon mitral valvotomy. Note splitting of the heavily calcified commissure (arrow).

balloon valvotomy is not contraindicated in patients with calcific mitral stenosis, particularly when calcification is not severe (77,80).

Based on the above findings, it is justifiable to offer balloon valvotomy to all patients with high and low total echo scores (80). This is in particular when balloon valvotomy can be done percutaneously and with minimal risk by experienced operators. We and others managed to achieve a good MVA with this procedure in many patients who initially were judged not to be suitable for balloon valvotomy (77).

Two potential complications related to balloon mitral valvotomy emerged from the in-vitro studies (67). First, the detachment of small calcium debris is a potential source for systemic embolization. Second, a tear induced in the mitral valve leaflet would cause severe MR (Fig. 7). These finding have been confirmed in clinical series (81,82).

2. Technique

Since Inoue described balloon mitral valvotomy in 1984 (65), several different techniques have been introduced (70,83–85). We developed the technique of double-balloon mitral valvotomy at the time when there was no commercially available balloon catheter with an adequate size to achieve successful valvotomy (70) (Fig. 8).

Inoue described the technique of mitral valvotomy using a rubber-mesh balloon catheter. This technique requires only a single transseptal puncture. The main advantage of this technique is that it allows calibrated stepwise dilatation, using different degrees of balloon inflation. This de-

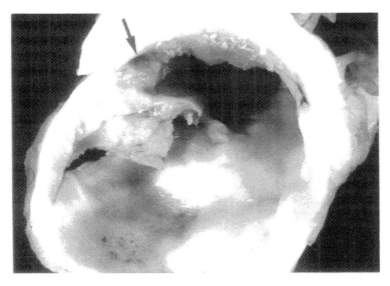

Figure 7 Surgically excised mitral valve showing leaflet tear (arrow) following balloon mitral valvotomy causing severe mitral regurgitation.

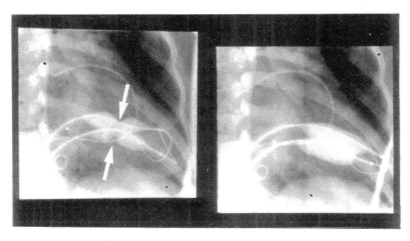

Figure 8 Double-balloon mitral valvotomy showing balloon indentation (arrows) during inflation (left panel) and disappearance of the indentation after successful valvotomy.

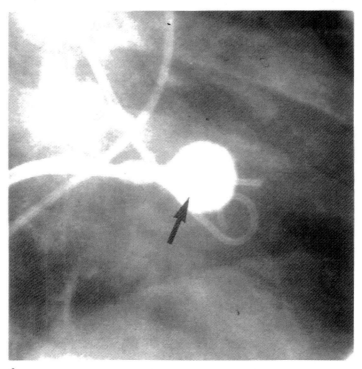

A

Figure 9 Balloon mitral valvotomy using the Inoue balloon catheter. Note inflation of the distal portion of the balloon (arrow) and its anchoring with the mitral
valve (A), and finally during complete inflation (B).

vice crosses the mitral valve orifice without the need for a prepositioned
guidewire in the left ventricular cavity. The inflation/deflation time is very
rapid, and therefore it is unlikely that balloon inflation will cause any
hemodynamic disturbances. Another unique feature of this device is that
of inflation of the distal portion of the balloon, which anchors the device
in position during full balloon inflation (Fig. 9); this prevents the slippage
of the balloon from the mitral annulus during inflation. In pregnant patients, the Inoue balloon catheter should be used preferentially, in view
of the marked reduction of fluoroscopy time using this technique (38,86).
The main disadvantage of this method is the high cost of the balloon
catheter.

Our original double-balloon technique used two Mansfield balloon catheters (70). The procedure has been described extensively (80,87). Both

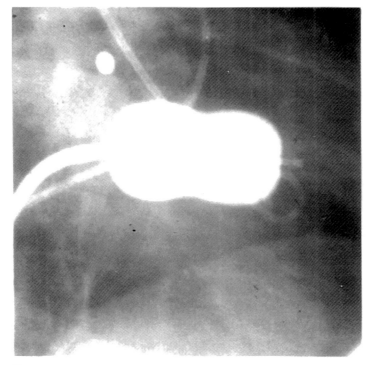

B

balloon catheters are advanced over two prepositioned guidewires in the left ventricular cavity. We relied on two long 14 French transseptal sheaths to deliver the balloon catheters across the mitral valve (Fig. 10). The advantage of these large transseptal sheaths are to enable (1) better stabilization of the balloon across the mitral valve during inflation, (2) rapid exchange of the balloon if a larger size is required, and (3) for more accurate hemodynamic pressure recording and cardiac output measurement immediately after valvotomy. Using oximetry, no iatrogenic atrial septal defect could be detected 6 weeks after the procedure (80). The main disadvantage of this technique is the requirement for two transseptal punctures, which requires greater experience in the transseptal technique and relatively longer fluoroscopy time (38,86). The double-balloon technique is also associated with frequent transient ventricular arrhythmias during stabilization of the balloon catheter across the mitral valve. However, we did not encounter any serious adverse effect, and no procedure was dis-

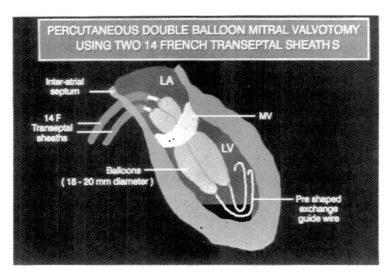

Figure 10 Diagramatic representation of the original technique of balloon mitral valvotomy using two 14F long transseptal sheaths, through which the balloons are advanced over two prepositioned, preshaped, exchange guidewires.

continued because of this problem. Economically, this technique is less expensive when compared to the Inoue technique (38,86).

The modified double-balloon technique (84), which has been used widely in the United States, is technically simpler to perform. It produces a similar result to our original technique, but the incidence of significant iatrogenic atrial septal defect (ASD) is higher (69,80,88). This is due to (1) the need to dilate the atrial septum before valvotomy with a balloon catheter 6 to 8 mm in diameter; (2) accidental dilatation of the septum during simultaneous balloon inflation (Fig. 11); and (3) trauma to the atrial septum during withdrawal of the deflated balloon catheter (Fig. 12). The effect of the iatrogenic ASDs appears to be benign, and they close spontaneously in the majority of cases (79). However, one study showed that only 59% of ASDs were closed at 2-year follow-up (89). The main disadvantage of this technique is that the balloon catheter may be forcibly ejected, either toward the LV apex, causing possible LV perforation, or toward the left atrium. The latter will require restabilization of the guidewires, across the valve, into the LV cavity for further inflation.

The improvements in the new modified Mansfield balloon catheters include the pigtail at the tip of the balloon catheter, which prevents left ventricular perforation (Fig. 12); and the relatively short length of the

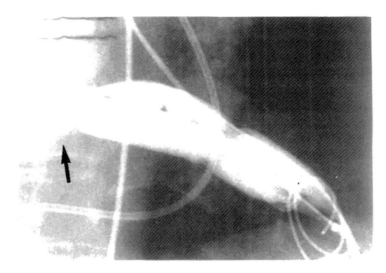

Figure 11 Balloon mitral valvotomy using 5.5-cm-long balloons (without the 14F long sheath). Note the potential complication of dilating the interatrial septum (arrow) with these large balloons (20-mm diameter).

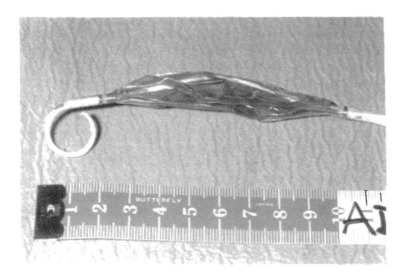

Figure 12 Note the large balloon profile after deflation of the balloon immediately after valvotomy. This may contribute to the increase in the size of the iatrogenic ASD and hence the potential advantage of the use of the 14F transseptal sheath. Note the technical improvement in the balloon catheter design with pigtailed distal end to minimize the potential complication with this technique.

balloon, i.e., 4 cm, which minimizes accidental dilatation of the atrial septum (Fig. 12).

We believe that the Inoue and double-balloon techniques will continue to be used for the treatment of mitral stenosis. The final mitral valve area results appeared to be similar to those of any of the above-discussed techniques, though some differences have been reported occasionally (38,81,86,88,90–92).

3. Indications

In our opinion, percutaneous balloon mitral valvotomy is the procedure of choice for patients with severe pliable valvular stenosis and suitable mitral valve anatomy for this procedure.

We nevertheless offer this procedure to any patient with severe MS, even in the presence of calcification or extensive subvalvular fibrosis. Our approach is based on learning that: (1) in in-vitro studies the balloon catheter achieved good commissural splitting of the severely narrowed valve with or without calcification; (2) there is lack of unanimity in predicting successful results with the present method of assessing mitral valvular pathology; and (3) a good MVA can still be achieved in patients with high echocardiographic scores.

4. Contraindications

The presence of moderate or severe MR (grade 3 or 4 out of 4) and left atrial clot, particularly in the body of the atrium, constitute the only contraindications for balloon mitral valvotomy.

In rare instances, a long-standing organized thrombus in the left atrial appendage may be detected by transesophageal echocardiography (21,50). Although we and others have performed percutaneous balloon valvotomy despite the presence of such a clot, one has to be discriminating in doing so. The presence of severe pulmonary hypertension, renal insufficiency, pregnancy, or other concomitant valvular stenosis that can be treated by a similar method are not contraindications, though each case has to be assessed individually.

5. Results

As with any new therapeutic intervention, the results of mitral balloon valvotomy have to be compared with those of the established surgical technique. The mechanisms of closed surgical and balloon valvotomy have been shown to be similar; thus the expected results after these procedures should be comparable.

As yet, insufficient time has elapsed since the introduction of balloon mitral valvotomy to compare the long-term results with surgical valvotomy. Randomized studies in a homogenous group of patients with severe mitral stenosis showed that the immediate and short-term results of balloon valvotomy were equivalent to those of closed surgical valvotomy, and were also comparable to the results of opened valvotomy (93–95).

Turi and his colleagues showed that the overall cost of the balloon technique was half of that of surgery in the United States (93). In contrast, balloon valvotomy was six times more expensive when compared to closed valvotomy in some of the Third World countries (93), in which mitral stenosis is prevalent. This finding indicates that closed surgical valvotomy may continue to be a therapeutic alternative for the treatment of mitral stenosis in these countries.

The overall results of both the Inoue and the double-balloon technique are similar (38,86), apart from one study which favored the latter (39). On an individual basis, however, there is a wide spectrum of results of mitral valve area achieved after balloon or closed surgical valvotomy. These differences reflect the heterogenicity of patients included in these studies, with different texture of the mitral valve and morphological features, including the subvalvular apparatus.

In our series, using the double-balloon technique, the overall mean MVA achieved was 1.9 cm^2, with an 11% rate of inadequate valvotomy—defined as a MVA less than 1.5 cm^2 (80). The latter may reflect the facts that: (1) we did not exclude any patient based on echocardiographic morphological and functional features; and (2) small-sized balloon catheters were used during our initial experience. The mean MVA achieved is similar to that reported by Block, Vahanian, and Ruiz, also using the double-balloon technique (93–95) (Tables 1 and 2).

During the development of the double-balloon mitral valvotomy technique, we were not confident of how to choose the balloon size combination. Therefore we prospectively used various balloon size combinations in 77 patients, in increasing increments. This was to ascertain the best valve area achieved after balloon valvotomy with least increase in mitral regurgitation. We demonstrated that the size combination of 18 mm with 20 mm, and two 20-mm balloon diameters produced adequate MVA ($>$1.5 cm^2) in 87% of patients (88,96). A third of these patients developed mild MR. Thus we consider these balloon size combinations are the most suitable for adult patients. Interestingly, there is still no general agreement on the best way of choosing the optimal balloon size combination with the double-balloon technique.

Other authors, using the double-balloon technique, have reported comparable degrees of increase in MR after valvotomy (Table 2). The degree of increase in MR after the Inoue or double-balloon technique was comparable (38,86), apart from one study (39). The latter showed that moderate MR occurred more frequently after the Inoue technique ($p < 0.001$).

Table 1 Patient Characteristics

| | Mean age (yr) | AF[a] | CA^{2+}[b] | Incidence of MR#[c] | | Restenosed valve |
				1/4	2/4	
Inoue (90) n = 27	50	58%	—	28%	—	10%
Block (91) n = 311	54	50%	46%	29%	4%	21%
Ruiz (92) n = 285	44	30%	38%	36%	12%	16%
Vahanian (81) n = 200	43	34%	34%	31%	1%	21%
Al Zaibag[d] n = 179	30	17%	13%	40%	7%	10%

[a] AF = atrial fibrillation.
[b] Ca^{2+} = mitral valve calcification.
[c] MR = mitral regurgitation; # = Grossman scale 0–4.
[d] Unpublished series.

6. Balloon Versus Closed Versus Opened Mitral Valvotomy

Closed mitral valvotomy requires no advanced technology of cardiopulmonary bypass, though the surgeon must assert special skill to achieve adequate commissural splitting and minimal iatrogenic MR. It is a popular surgical method of treatment for severe rheumatic MS, particularly in the developing countries.

Open surgical valvotomy, on the other hand, demands more technical support, and cardiac surgeons claim far superior results with this technique, although randomized studies have only recently been reported

Table 2 Results After PBMV

	Mean MVA	Percent MR increase	Inadequate valvotomy
Inoue (90)	1.9 cm^2	21%	—
Block (107)	2.1 cm^2	—	23%
Ruiz (92)	2.4 cm^2	51%	—
Vahanian (81)	2.2 cm^2	35%	11%
Al Zaibag[a]	1.8 cm^2	—	11%

[a] Unpublished series.

(95,97). All previously published studies were based on subjective clinical follow-up results.

A recently published randomized study revealed that open surgical valvotomy, for pure noncalcific mitral valve stenosis, is far superior than the closed technique (97). Results were judged by calculating the MVA, using the Gorlin formula, shortly after surgery. The MVAs achieved were 1.4 cm^2 and 2.1 cm^2 after closed and opened valvotomy, respectively. Both induced a similar rate of MR, 12% and 13%, respectively. A similar randomized study between balloon, closed, and open surgical valvotomies was performed in 90 patients (95). This showed that balloon and open surgical valvotomies achieved similar mitral valve areas; and both were superior to the closed surgical technique—the MVAs were 2.2 cm^2 and 1.7 cm^2, respectively.

We compared the results of balloon valvotomy (sizes 20-mm and 20-mm diameter) with that of opened surgical valvotomy in 122 consecutive patients who had MS (98). The study was retrospective, but both groups had similar baseline characteristics. The MVAs achieved, as calculated by Doppler method, were 1.9 cm^2 and 2.2 cm^2 after balloon and opened surgical valvotomy, respectively.

Another two randomized studies (93,94), comparing balloon versus closed surgical mitral valvotomy, not only produced a similar trend, but one study (94) also favored balloon valvotomy over surgery.

These findings corroborate our conclusion regarding the good results of balloon mitral valvotomy, using optimal-sized balloon combinations. In summary, balloon mitral valvotomy is probably superior to closed surgical valvotomy, and produces comparable results as open surgical valvotomy.

7. Restenosis

The rate of early restenosis (12 months after valvotomy) has been reported to range from zero to 70% (74,79,99). The variability in the reported restenosis rate may be due to patients selected or secondary to inaccurate calculation of MVA immediately after balloon valvotomy.

We believe that the very high rate of early restenosis of 24% at 6 months (79), and 70% at 1 year in patients with high echocardiographic score (74), is not genuine. This is supported by pathological studies (100,101), hemodynamic studies that were performed before and after closed surgical valvotomy (102,103), and our 1-year follow-up study that showed zero restenosis compared to the MVA achieved at 4–6 weeks after valvotomy (99).

We, and others, observed the apparent discrepancy between the MVA calculation by Doppler and Gorlin immediately after balloon valvotomy (104,105). Therefore, we always measured the final MVA at 4 weeks follow-up study, disregarding the immediate result after balloon valvotomy (70,80). Iatrogenic ASD, which is present in nearly all cases, also hinders the accurate calculation of Gorlin MVA. This is crucial in estimating the true MVA after valvotomy. The inherent methodological limitation of both the Gorlin formula and the Doppler mitral valve area calculation immediately after the procedure may overestimate MVA, and result in mistaking residual stenosis for early restenosis. A critical evaluation of the method used to calculate MVA, and its limitation, is of paramount importance.

Pathological studies, up to 1 year after closed surgical valvotomy, demonstrated no evidence of mitral restenosis or even epithelization of the incised fused mitral commissures by the cardiac surgeon (100,101).

Hemodynamic studies showed that the cause of recurrence of symptoms after surgical valvotomy is usually inadequate valvotomy with residual stenosis, or development of MR or concomitant valvular lesions (102). In patients who proved to have no residual MS shortly after surgery, restenosis was detected in 28% at 10 to 14 years follow-up (103); in only 50% of patients with symptoms was mitral restenosis a contributing factor (103).

8. Complications

The report from the National Heart, Lung, and Blood Institute on valvoplasty showed a high rate of complications: 12% of patients with serious complications and 1% death (106). These results are in contrast with the low complications rate reported in several medical centers from the Middle East, the Far East, Europe, and selected centers in the United States. The difference in the complication rates might be explained on the basis of the patients' baseline clinical characteristics and selection criteria. Alternatively, it may reflect the high complication rate in institutions with a low volume of cases. The latter explanation is corroborated by the difference in the overall complication rate observed between the Registry and that reported in U.S. institutions with more extensive experience.

Severe MR occurs in less than 5% of patients (Table 3). It has been found to relate to balloon size used (88,91) and morphological features of the valve as assessed by echocardiography (77). Contrary findings have been reported (107). We believe that the size of the balloon selected for the procedure is of prime importance. Incorrect positioning of balloon catheters through the chordae may cause its rupture, resulting in severe MR.

Our in-vitro study showed that in some fibrotic valves the inflated balloon induces a tear rather than a split of the fused commissure (67). This complication has been confirmed at surgery (Fig. 7).

The reported incidence of iatrogenic ASD following balloon valvotomy

Table 3 Procedure-Related Complications

	Mortality	Cardiac tamponade	Thrombo-embolism	Severe MR, needed surgery	Oximetry ASD
Inoue (90)	0%	1.5%	0.6%	1.7%	12%
Block (91)	2%	1%	1.2%	1%	19%
Ruiz (92)	1%	3%	1.5%	1.2%	14%
Vahanian (81)	0%	1%	4%	4%	8%
Al Zaibag[a]	0%	2.5%	0%	1.3%	0% at 6/52

[a] Unpublished series.

is variable (Table 3), and depends on the technique used. More important, the rate of this complication depends on the method of detection. The oximetry series detects only large ASD, whereas transesophageal color Doppler can detect tiny ASD. The incidence of iatrogenic ASD with the Inoue method is 10–12% (93,108). In the double-balloon technique it is reported to be 8–19%. In our technique, where 14F transseptal sheaths are used during the procedure to protect the atrial septum, ASD was not detected (using oximetry) at 6 weeks' follow-up. Regardless of the method used for balloon valvotomy, these ASD were shown to close sponta-neously (79,89,108).

C. Surgical Treatment

1. Surgical Mitral Valvotomy

Open surgical valvotomy is more commonly used than the closed tech-nique in centers where open-heart surgical programs exist. The commis-sures are split under direct vision, and the subvalvular apparatus may be repaired if necessary. Thrombi in the left atrium and appendage can be removed during the procedure (see Chapter 18).

2. Mitral Valve Replacement

In patients who have severely deformed calcific valves where the subval-vular apparatus is extremely fused, open valvotomy may not be feasible. In these patients, mitral valve replacement (MVR) is the treatment of choice.

If MVR is indicated in females of child-bearing age, we recommend the use of a bioprosthetic valve. This is particularly important in developing countries, where pregnancy rates are high. A metallic valve may be recommended in the Western developed countries if good control of anticoagulation therapy can be assured.

As mentioned in the section on medical treatment, in patients with prosthetic valves, low-dose warfarin (coumadin) therapy has a lower complication rate and is as effective as full anticoagulation. The recommended prothrombin time ratio is 1.5 (INR 2.65).

(For further details on mitral valve replacement and prosthetic valve complications, refer to the surgical chapters.)

REFERENCES

1. Kumar A, Sinha M, Sinha DN. Chronic rheumatic heart diseases in Ranchi. Angiology 1982; 33:141.
2. Bland EF, Jones TD. Rheumatic fever and rheumatic heart disease. A twenty year report on 1000 patients followed since childhood. Circulation 1951; 4:836.
3. Cabot RC. In: Cabot RC, ed. Facts on the Heart. Philadelphia: Saunders, 1926:30.
4. Roy SB, Bhatia ML, Lazaro EJ, Ramalingaswami V. Juvenile mitral stenosis in India. Lancet 1963; 2:1193.
5. Al-Bahrani IR, Thamer MA, Al-Omeri MM, Al-Naaman YD. Rheumatic heart disease in the young in Iraq. Br Heart J 1966; 28:824.
6. Rowe JC, Bland EF, Sprague HB, White PD. The course of mitral stenosis without surgery: ten and twenty-year perspectives. Ann Intern Med 1960; 52:741.
7. Rapaport E. Natural history of aortic and mitral valve disease. Am J Cardiol 1975; 35:221.
8. Edwards JE. The congenital bicuspid aortic valve. Circulation 1961; 23: 485.
9. Roberts WC. Morphologic features of normal and abnormal mitral valve. Am J Cardiol 1983; 51:1005.
10. Waller BF. Rheumatic and non-rheumatic conditions producing valvular heart disease. In: Frankl WS, Brest AN, eds. Valvular Heart Disease: Comprehensive Evaluation and Management. Philadelphia: Cardiovascular Clinics, Davis, 1986:8.
11. Rassi A Jr, Crawford MH, Richards KL, Miller JF. Differing mechanisms of exercise flow augmentation at the mitral and aortic valves. Circulation 1988; 77:543.
12. Wallace AG. Pathophysiology of cardiovascular disease. In: Smith LH Jr, Thier SO, eds. Pathophysiology: The Biological Principles of Disease, The International Textbook of Medicine. Philadelphia: Saunders, 1981:1192.
13. Wood P. An appreciation of mitral stenosis, Part I, Clinical features. Br Med J 1954; 1:1051.
14. Gash AK, Carabello BA, Cepin D, Spann JF. Left ventricular ejection per-

formance and systolic muscle function in patients with mitral stenosis. Circulation 1983; 67:148.

15. Harvey RM, Ferrer MI, Samet P, Bader RA, Bader ME, Cournand A, Richards DW. Mechanical and myocardial factors in rheumatic heart disease in mitral stenosis. Circulation 1955; 11:531.

16. Mohan JC, Khalilullah M, Arora R. Left ventricular intrinsic contractility in pure rheumatic mitral stenosis. Am J Cardiol 1989; 64:240.

17. Hildner FJ, Javier RP, Cohen LS, Samet P, Nathan MJ, Yahr WZ, Greenberg JJ. Myocardial dysfunction associated with valvular heart disease. Am J Cardiol 1972; 30:319.

18. Reis RN, Roberts WC. Amounts of coronary arterial narrowing by atherosclerotic plaques in clinically isolated mitral valve stenosis: analysis of 76 necropsy patients older than 30 years. Am J Cardiol 1986; 57:1117.

19. Heller SJ, Carleton RA. Abnormal left ventricular contraction in patients with mitral stenosis. Circulation 1970; 42:1099.

20. Deverall PB, Olley PM, Smith DR, Watson DA, Whitaker W. Incidence of systemic embolism before and after mitral valvotomy. Thorax 1968; 23:530.

21. Bansal RC, Heywood JT, Applegate PM, Jutzy KR. Detection of left atrial thrombi by two-dimensional echocardiography and surgical correlation in 148 patients with mitral valve disease. Am J Cardiol 1989; 64:243.

22. Wilhelmsen L. Lung mechanics in rheumatic valvular disease. Acta Med Scand 1968; (suppl) 489:3.

23. Ellis LB, Harken DE. Arterial embolization in relation to mitral valvuloplasty. Am Heart J 1961; 62:611.

24. Neilson GH, Galea EG, Hossack KF. Thromboembolic complications of mitral valve disease. Austral NZ J Med 1978; 8:372.

25. Olesen KH. The natural history of 271 patients with mitral stenosis under medical treatment. Br Heart J 1962; 24:349.

26. Bannister RG. The risks of deferring valvotomy in patients with moderate mitral stenosis. Lancet 1960; 2:329.

27. Coulshed N, Epstein EJ, McKendrick CS, Galloway RW, Walker E. Systemic embolism in mitral valve disease. Br Heart J 1970; 32:26.

28. Sherrid MV, Clark RD, Cohn K. Echocardiographic analysis of left atrial size before and after operation in mitral valve disease. Am J Cardiol 1979; 43:171.

29. Wooley CF, Baba N, Kilman JW, Ryan JM. Thrombotic calcific mitral stenosis: morphology of the calcific mitral valve. Circulation 1974; 49:1167.

30. Craige E. Phonocardiographic studies in mitral stenosis. N Engl J Med 1957; 257:650.

31. Kalmanson D, Veyrat C, Bernier A, Witchitz S, Chiche P. Opening snap and isovolumic relaxation period in relation to mitral valve flow in patients with mitral stenosis. Significance of A2-OS interval. Br Heart J 1976; 38: 135.

32. Ebringer R, Pitt A, Anderson ST. Haemodynamic factors influencing opening snap interval in mitral stenosis. Br Heart J 1970; 32:350.

33. Wooley CF, Klassen KP, Leighton RF, Goodwin MS, Ryan JM. Left atrial

and left ventricular sound and pressure in mitral stenosis. Circulation 1968;
38:295.

34. Craige E. On the genesis of heart sounds. Contributions made by echocardiographic studies. Circulation 1976; 53:207.

35. Cooksey JD, Dunn M, Massie E. Clinical vectorcardiography and electrocardiography. 2d ed. Chicago: Year Book Medical Publishers, 1977:272.

36. Kasser I, Kennedy JW. The relationship of increased left atrial volume and pressure to abnormal P waves on the electrocardiogram. Circulation 1969; 39:339.

37. Probst P, Goldschlager N, Selzer A. Left atrial size and atrial fibrillation in mitral stenosis: factors influencing their relationship. Circulation 1973; 48:1282.

38. Abdullah M, Halim M, Rajendran V, Sawyer W, Al-Zaibag M. Comparison between single (Inoue) and double balloon mitral valvuloplasty: immediate and short-term results. Am Heart J 1992; 123:1581.

39. Ruiz CE, Zhang HP, Macaya C, Aleman EH, Allen JW, Lau FY. Comparison of Inoue single-balloon versus double-balloon technique for percutaneous mitral valvotomy. Am Heart J 1992; 123:942.

40. Cueto J, Toshima H, Armijo G, Tuna N, Lillehei CW. Vectorcardiographic studies in acquired valvular disease with reference to the diagnosis of right ventricular hypertrophy. Circulation 1966; 33:588.

41. Desanctis RW, Dean DC, Bland EF. Extreme left atrial enlargement. Circulation 1964; 29:14.

42. Plaschkes J, Borman JB, Merin G, Milwidsky H. Giant left atrium in rheumatic heart disease: a report of 18 cases treated by mitral valve replacement. Ann Surg 1971; 174:194.

43. Henry WL, Griffith JM, Michaelis LL, McIntosh CL, Morrow AG, Epstein SE. Measurement of mitral orifice area in patients with mitral valve disease by real-time two-dimensional echocardiography. Circulation 1975; 51:827.

44. Nichol PM, Gilbert BW, Kisslo JA. Two-dimensional echocardiographic assessment of mitral stenosis. Circulation 1977; 55:120.

45. Libanoff AJ, Rodbard S. Atrioventricular pressure half-time. Circulation 1968; 38:144.

46. Hatle L, Brubakk A, Tromsdal A, Angelsen B. Non-invasive assessment of pressure drop in mitral stenosis by Doppler ultrasound. Br Heart J 1978; 40:131.

47. Hatle L, Angelsen B, Tromsdal A. Non-invasive assessment of atrioventricular pressure half-time by Doppler ultrasound. Circulation 1979; 60:1096.

48. Holen J, Aaslid R, Landmark K, Simonsen S. Determination of pressure gradient in mitral stenosis with a non-invasive ultrasound Doppler technique. Acta Med Scand 1976; 199:455.

49. Fredman CS, Pearson AC, Labovitz AJ, Kern MJ. Comparison of hemodynamic pressure half-time method and Gorlin formula with doppler and echocardiographic determinations of mitral valve area in patients with combined mitral stenosis and regurgitation. Am Heart J 1990; 119:121.

50. Aschenberg W, Schluter M, Kremer P, Schroder E, Siglow V, Bleifeld W. Transesophageal two-dimensional echocardiography for the detection of left atrial appendage thrombus. J Am Coll Cardiol 1986; 7:163.
51. Lange RA, Moore DM, Cigarroa RG, Hillis LD. The use of pulmonary capillary wedge pressure to assess the severity of mitral stenosis: is a true left atrial pressure needed in these patients? J Am Coll Cardiol 1989; 13: 825.
52. Kloster FE, Morris CD. Natural history of valvular heart disease. Circulation 1982; 65:1283.
53. Joswig BC, Glover MU, Handler JB, Warren SE, Vieweg WVR. Contrasting progression of mitral stenosis in Malayans versus American-born Caucasians. Am Heart J 1982; 104:1400.
54. Wilson MG, Lim WN. The natural history of rheumatic heart disease in the third, fourth, and fifth decades of life—1. Prognosis with special references to survivorship. Circulation 1957; 16:700.
55. Al Kasab SA, Sabag T, Al-Zaibag MA, Awaad M, Al-Bitar I, Halim MA, Abdullah MA, Shahed M, Rajendran V, Sawyer W. B-adrenergic receptor blockade in the management of pregnant women with mitral stenosis. Am J Obstet Gyn 1990; 163(1):37.
56. Waxman HL, Myerburg RJ, Appel R, Sung RJ. Verapamil for control of ventricular rate in paroxysmal supraventricular tachycardia and atrial fibrillation or flutter. Ann Intern Med 1981; 94:1.
57. Salerno DM, Dias V, Kleiger R, Sami M, Sung R, Tschida V, Giorgi L. Efficacy and safety of intravenous diltiazem for treatment of atrial fibrillation and flutter, The Diltiazem-Atrial Fibrillation/Flutter Study Group. Am J Cardiol 1989; 63:1046.
58. Heywood JT, Graham B, Marais GE, Jutzy KR. Effects of intravenous diltiazem on rapid atrial fibrillation accompanied by congestive heart failure. Am J Cardiol 1983; 67:1347.
59. Haffajee CI, Love JC, Canada AT, Lesko LJ, Asdourian G, Alpert JS. Clinical pharmacokinetics and efficacy of amiodarone for refractory tachyarrhythmias. Circulation 1983; 67:1347.
60. Rodsky MA, Allen BJ, Capparelli EV, Luckett CR, Morton R, Henry WL. Factors determining maintenance of sinus rhythm after chronic atrial fibrillation with left atrial dilatation. Am J Cardiol 1989; 63:1065.
61. Crijns HJ, Van-Gelder IC, Van-Gilist WH, Hillege H, Gosselink AM, Lie KI. Serial antiarrhythmis drug treatment to maintain sinus rhythm after electrical cardioversion for chronic atrial fibrillation or atrial flutter. Am J Cardiol 1991; 68:335.
62. Gonazales R, Liancaqueo A, Giardina P. Efficacy of amiodarone in the management of atrial fibrillation related to rheumatic heart disease. J Arrythmias Management 1991; Fall:33.
63. Saour JN, Sieck JO, Mamo LA, Gallus AS. Trial of different intensities of anticoagulation in patients with prosthetic heart valves. N Engl J Med 1990; 322:428.

64. Cutler EC, Levine SA. Cardiotomy and valvulotomy for mitral stenosis: experimental observations and clinical notes concerning an operated case with recovery. Boston Med Surg J 1923; 188:1023.

65. Inoue K, Owaui T, Nakamura T, Kitamura F, Miyamoto N. Clinical application of transvenous mitral commissurotomy by a new balloon catheter. J Thorac Cardiovasc Surg 1984; 87:394.

66. Kaplan JD, Isner JM, Karas RH, Halaburka KR, Konstam MA, Hougen TJ, Cleveland RJ, Salem DN. In vitro analysis of mechanisms of balloon valvuloplasty of stenotic mitral valves. Am J Cardiol 1987; 59:318.

67. Ribeiro PA, Zaibag MA, Rajendran V, Faraidi Y, Halim M, Abdullah M, Fagih MR. Mechanism of mitral valve area increase by in vitro single and double balloon mitral valvotomy. Am J Cardiol 1988; 62:264.

68. Sadee AS, Becker AE. In vitro balloon dilatation of mitral valve stenosis: the importance of subvalvular involvement as a cause of mitral valve insufficiency. Br Heart J 1991; 65:277.

69. McKay RG, Lock JE, Safian RD, Come PC, Diver DJ, Baim DS, Berman AD, Warren SE, Mandell VE, Royal HD, Grossman W. Balloon dilatation of mitral stenosis in adult patients postmortem and percutaneous mitral valvuloplasty studies. J Am Coll Cardiol 1987; 9:723.

70. Al-Zaibag MA, Ribeiro PA, Al-Kasab SA, Al-Fagih MR. Percutaneous double balloon mitral valvotomy for rheumatic mitral stenosis. Lancet 1986; 1: 757.

71. Abascal VM, Wilkins GT, Choong CY, Thomas JD, Block PC, Palacios IF, Weyman AE. Echocardiogrpahic evlauation of mitral valve structure and function in patients followed for at least six months after percutaneous balloon mitral valvuloplasty. J Am Coll Cardiol 1988; 12:606.

72. Wilkins GT, Weyman AE, Abascal VM, Block PC, Palacios IF. Percutaneous mitral valvotomy: an analysis of echocardiographic variables related to outcome and the mechanism of dilatation. Br Heart J 1988; 60:299.

73. Mobuyoshi M, Hamasaki N, Kimura T, Nosaka H, Yokoi H, Yasumoto H, Horiuchi H, Shindo T, Mori T, Miyamoto AT, Inoue K. Indications, complications, and short-term clinical outcome of percutaneous transverse mitral commissurotomy. Circulation 1989; 80:782.

74. Palacios IF, Block PC, Wilkins GT, Weyman AE. Follow-up of patients undergoing percutaneous mitral balloon valvotomy: analysis of factors determining restenosis. Circulation 1989; 79:573.

75. Reid CL, Chandraratna AN, Kawanishi DT, Kotlewski A, Rahimtoola SH. Influence of mitral valve morphology on double-balloon catheter balloon valvuloplasty in patients with mitral stenosis. Circulation 1989; 80:515.

76. Abascal VM, Wilkins GT, O'Shea JP, Choong CY, Palacios IF, Thomas JD, Rosas E, Newill JB, Block PC, Weyman AE. Prediction of successful outcome in 130 patients undergoing percutaneous balloon mitral valvotomy. Circulation 1990; 82:448.

77. Chen C, Wang X, Wang Y, Lan Y. Value of two-dimensional echocardiography in selecting patients and balloon sizes for percutaneous balloon mitral valvuloplasty. J Am Coll Cardiol 1989; 4:1651.

78. Al-Kasab S, Ribeiro P, Al-Zaibag M, Bitar I, Idris M, Shahed M, Sawyer W. Comparison of results of percutaneous balloon mitral valvotomy using single and double balloon technique. Am J Cardiol 1989; 63:135.
79. Cequier A, Bonan R, Serra A, Dyrda I, Crepaeau J, Dethy M, Water D. Left-to-right shunting after percutaneous mitral valvuloplasty: incidence and long-term haemodynamic follow-up. Circulation 1990; 81:1190.
80. Al-Zaibag M, Halim M. Balloon valvotomy in atrioventricular valve stenosis. In: Rao PS, ed. Transcatheter Therapy in Pediatric Cardiology. New York: Wiley (1993).
81. Vahanian A, Michel PL, Cormier B, Vitous B, Michael X, Siama M, Sarano LE, Trabelsi S, Ismail MB, Acar J. Results of percutaneous mitral commissurotomy in 200 patients. Am J Cardiol 1989; 63:847.
82. Acar C, Deloche A, Tibi PR, Jebara V, Chachques JC, Fabiani JN, Carpentier A. Operative findings after percutaneous mitral dilation. Ann Thorac Surg 1990; 49:959.
83. Lock JE, Khalilullah M, Shrivastava S, Bahl V, Keane JF. Percutaneous catheter commissurotomy in rheumatic mitral stenosis. N Engl J Med 1985; 313:1515.
84. Palacios IF, Block PC, Brandi-Pifano S, Blanco P, Casal H, Pulido JI, Munoz S, D'Empaire G, Ortega MA, Jacobs M, Vlahakes G. Percutaneous balloon valvotomy for patients with severe mitral stenosis. Circulation 1987; 75:778.
85. Babic UU, Dorros G, Pejcic P, Djurisic Z, Vucinic M, Lewin R, Grujicic SN. Percutaneous mitral valvuloplasty: retrograde, transarterial double-balloon technique utilizing the transseptal approach. Cathet Cardiovasc Diagn 1988; 14:229.
86. Ribeiro PA, Fawzy ME, Arafat MA, Dunn B, Sriram R, Mercer E, Duran CG. Comaprison of mitral valve area results of balloon mitral valvotomy using the inoue and double balloon techniques. Am J Cardiol 1991; 68:687.
87. Al-Zaibag M. Percutaneous mitral valvotomy: the double balloon technique. In: Vogel JHK, King SB III, eds. International Cardiology: Future Direction. St. Louis: Mosby, 1988:194.
88. Al-Zaibag M, Ribeiro PA. The future of balloon valvotomy. In: Topol EJ, ed. Textbook of Interventional Cardiology. Philadelphia: Saunders, 1990: 912.
89. Casale P, Block PC, O'Shea JP, Palacios IF. Atrial septal defect after percutaneous mitral balloon valvuloplasty: immediate results and follow-up. J Am Coll Cardiol 1990; 15:1300.
90. Inoue K, Hung JS. Percutaneous transvenous mitral commissurotomy—the Far East experience. In: Topol EJ, ed. Textbook of Interventional Cardiology. Philadelphia: Saunders, 1990:887.
91. Block PC, Palacios IF. Aortic and mitral balloon valvuloplasty: the United States experience. In: Topol EJ, ed. Textbook of Interventional Cardiology. Philadelphia: Saunders, 1990:831.
92. Ruiz CE, Allen JW, Lau F. Percutaneous double balloon valvotomy for severe rheumatic mitral stenosis. Am J Cardiol 1990; 65:473.

93. Turi ZG, Reyes VP, Raju BS, Raju AR, Kumar DN, Rajagopal P, Sathya-
narayana PV, Rao DP, Srinath K, Peters P, Connors B, Fromm B, Farkas
P, Wynne J. Percutaneous balloon versus surgical closed commissurotomy
for mitral stenosis: a prospective randomized trial. Circulation 1991; 83:
1179.

94. Patel JJ, Shama D, Mitha AS, Blyth D, Hassen F, LeRoux BT, Chetty
S. Balloon valvuloplasty versus closed commissurotomy for pliable mitral
stenosis: a prospective hemodynamic study. J Am Coll Cardiol 1991; 18:
1318.

95. Ayari M, Farhat MB, Chouaieb A, Maatoug F, Jarrar M, Sghairi K, Fendri
A. Two-dimensional echocardiographic and hemodynamic assessment of
surgical valvulotomies versus percutaneous balloon mitral commissurotomy. Eur Heart J 1991; 144:172.

96. Al-Zaibag MA, Ribeiro PA, Al-Kasab SA, Halim M. Percutaneous double
balloon mitral valvotomy: results using different sized balloon catheters
(abstr). J Am Coll Cardiol 1987; 9(suppl A):83A.

97. Farhat MB, Boussadia H, Gandjbakhch I, Mzali H, Chouaieb A, Ayari M,
Salah KB. Closed versus open mitral commissurotomy in pure non-calcific
mitral stenosis: hemodynamic studies before and after operation. J Thorac
Cardiovasc Surg 1990; 99:639.

98. Shahed MS, Al-Zaibag M, Al-Kasab S, Al-Fagih MR, Ribeiro PA. Comparison of results of percutaneous double balloon mitral valvotomy with open
surgical valvotomy (abstr). Eur Heart J 1989; 10(suppl):373.

99. Al-Zaibag M, Ribeiro P, Al-Kasab S, Halim M, Idris M, Habbab M, Shahed
M, Sawyer W. One-year follow-up after percutaneous double balloon mitral
valvotomy. Am J Cardiol 1989; 63:126.

100. Glover RP, Davila LD, O'Neill JJ, Jamon OH. Does mitral stenosis recur
after commissurotomy? Circulation 1955; 11:14.

101. Koiwai EK, Sokol DM, Mirikitani CK. The study of the incised commissure
in mitral stenosis. J Thorac Cardiovasc Surg 1964; 47:205.

102. Higgs LM, Glancy DL, O'Brien KP, Epstein SE, Morrow AG. Mitral restenosis: an uncommon cause of recurrent symptoms following mitral commissurotomy. Am J Cardiol 1970; 26:34.

103. Heger JJ, Wann LS, Weyman AE, Dillon JC, Feigenbaum H. Long-term
changes in mitral valve area after successful mitral commissurotomy. Circulation 1979; 59:443.

104. Thomas JD, Wilkins GT, Choong CY, Abascal VM, Palacios IF, Block PC,
Weyman AE. Inaccuracy of mitral pressure half-time immediately after
percutaneous mitral valvotomy. Dependence on transmitral gradient and
left atrial and ventricular compliance. Circulation 1988; 78:980.

105. Chen C, Wang Y, Guo B, Lin Y. Reliability of the Doppler pressure half-
time method for assessing effects of percutaneous mitral balloon valvuloplasty. J Am Coll Cardiol 1989; 13:1309.

106. The National Heart, Lung, and Blood Institute Balloon Valvuloplasty Registry Participants. Multicenter experience with balloon mitral commissurot-

omy: NHLBI balloon valvuloplasty registry report on immediate and 30-day follow-up results. Circulation 1992; 85:448.

107. Abascal VM, Wilkins GT, Choong CY, Block P, Palacios IF, Weyman A. Mitral regurgitation after percutaneous balloon mitral valvuloplasty in adults: evaluation by Doppler echocardiography. J Am Coll Cardiol 1988; 11:257.

108. Yoshida K, Yoshikawa J, Akasaka T, Yamura Y, Shakudo M, Hozumi T, Fukaya T. Assessment of left to right shunting after percutaneous mitral valvuloplasty by transoesophageal colour Doppler flow-mapping. Circulation 1989; 80:1521.

7

Aortic Valve Regurgitation

Muayed Al Zaibag
Armed Forces Hospital, Riyadh, Saudi Arabia, and Loma Linda University Medical Center, Loma Linda, California

I. ETIOLOGY AND PATHOLOGY

Rheumatic aortic regurgitation (AR) is common in the developing countries. In the developed industrialized countries, however, rheumatic AR was common half a century ago, accounting for three-quarters of the cases of AR (1–4). Today, aortic wall disorders, particularly idiopathic dilatation of the aortic root, have become the most common etiology. In patients undergoing aortic valve replacement (AVR) for AR, 50% of the procedures are now due to aortic root dilatation and only 25% are secondary to rheumatic valvular disease (2–4).

A high incidence of systemic hypertension has been detected in patients with aortic root dilatation (4). Other studies have shown idiopathic myxoid degeneration of the aortic valve cusps in 35% to 54% of the excised valves (5,6); systemic hypertension was present in 77% of these patients (6). There is a large number of patients who may have undiagnosed systemic hypertension before the onset of AR. As aortic root dilatation can result in secondary structural changes of the aortic valve cusps, and vice versa, one may not be able to define precisely the primary etiology of AR in the presence of these different but interrelated pathological processes, i.e., hypertension, idiopathic aortic root dilatation, and idiopathic myxoid degeneration of the aortic valve cusps.

Ten percent of patients with systemic hypertension have been shown to develop AR (7,8). It is conceivable that hypertension may be the most common etiological cause of AR, particularly in Western countries. This is derived from an estimate that more than 60 million Americans have

Table 1 Causes of Aortic Regurgitation

I. Aortic cusp abnormalities
    A. Rheumatic heart disease
    B. Infective endocarditis
    C. Congenital heart disease, e.g., bicuspid aortic valve, VSD, and rupture of congenitally fenestrated valve
    D. Traumatic, e.g., balloon aortic valvotomy, external chest trauma
    E. Connective tissue disorders, e.g., SLE and rheumatoid arthritis
II. Aortic root abnormalities
    A. Aortic root dilatation
        1. Idiopathic
        2. Secondary to systemic hypertension, myxomatous degeneration, connective tissue disorders, and syphilis
            (a) Myxomatous degeneration, e.g., Marfan syndrome, Ehler-Danlos syndrome, and osteogenesis imperfecta
            (b) Connective tissue disorders, e.g., ankylosing spondylitis, rheumatoid arthritis, Reiter's syndrome, sacroiliitis with HLA B27, and giant cell aortitis
    B. Dissecting aneurysm, e.g., traumatic, hypertension, Marfan syndrome, pregnancy, etc.
    C. Rupture of sinus of Valsalva

---

systemic hypertension, of whom 46% are unaware of the disease, 67% are on no treatment, and 22% of patients are on inadequate medical therapy (9). Therefore, the true incidence of AR secondary to systemic hypertension may be underestimated.

The most common causes of acute AR differ from those responsible for chronic AR. Infective endocarditis, dissecting aortic aneurysm, and chest trauma are the principal causes of acute AR (Chapter 9).

For detailed pathological description, refer to Chapter 1. Aortic regurgitation may be caused primarily by aortic valve leaflet and/or aortic root abnormalities (Table 1).

A. Aortic Cusp Abnormalities

The etiology of pathological aortic cusp abnormalities is variable—with rheumatic fever, infective endocarditis, and chest trauma in the vast majority. Rheumatic heart disease almost never affects the aortic valve alone (Chapter 1), being usually associated with mitral valve involvement; the latter may vary from mild leaflet thickening to severe mitral stenosis.

Congenital heart disease is a rare cause of AR resulting from aortic cusp abnormality, except for the bicuspid aortic valve which typically can cause aortic stenosis in adult life. Bicuspid aortic valve is present in 1% at birth (Chapter 1). Aortic regurgitation is a well-recognized consequence of bicuspid valve in the elderly, even in the absence of stenosis and, less commonly, during early adulthood (10). Bicuspid aortic valves are more prone to infection; however, most patients with infective endocarditis have tricuspid (trileaflet) aortic valves (Chapter 1). Tricuspid aortic valve is far more common in the general population than bicuspid aortic valve.

Aortic regurgitation can occur secondary to other congenital heart defects. It has been detected in 5%–8% of young patients with ventricular septal defect in which the unsupported aortic cusp lies above the VSD (11). This may result in prolapse of the noncoronary cusp into the membranous VSD, or the right coronary cusp into the left ventricle outflow tract in supracristal (subpulmonic) VSD. Another rare form of congenital AR is the spontaneous rupture of a congenitally fenestrated aortic valve (12).

Connective tissue diseases such as systemic lupus erythematosus (13) and rheumatoid arthritis (14) may cause cusp damage leading to AR.

B. Aortic Root Abnormalities

Aortic root abnormalities can produce a marked dilatation of the ascending aorta and of the aortic annulus. The aortic valve cusps will then not coapt properly and will cause AR. Dilatation of the aortic root may also cause secondary structural changes in the cusps of the aortic valve. This will result in thickening, retraction, and possibly shortening of the cusps, thus preventing them from coapting fully. This will further deteriorate the preexisting AR secondary to the aortic root dilatation.

Idiopathic dilatation of the aortic root (aortic annulus ectasia) comprised up to 40% of the patients with severe AR requiring AVR (2,3). This has become a well-recognized cause of pure AR and usually leads to significant AR in middle-aged or elderly patients. Patients with idiopathic dilatation of the aortic root may exhibit various degrees of elastic and muscle fiber destruction in the media (cystic medial necrosis of the aortic wall), despite the absence of features of Marfan's syndrome or systemic hypertension. Similar histological abnormalities may also be seen in the very elderly and in patients with systemic hypertension.

Marfan's syndrome, though uncommon, is considered the second most common disease causing isolated aortic incompetence due to aortic wall pathology. (Marfan's syndrome is discussed in detail in Chapter 1.) Typically, the sinus of Valsalva is the main site of marked dilatation, with fusiform aneurysms of the ascending aorta. Other myxomatous degenerative disorders, i.e., Ehlers-Danlos syndrome and osteogenesis imperfecta, can also result in AR (15).

Syphilis causes destructive inflammation of the media. It results in AR when the disease process involves the aortic edges of the sinus of Valsalva, with secondary dilatation. AR occurs in 30% of patients with cardiovascular syphilis, but at present it is rare in Western countries (Chapter 1).

The inflammatory connective tissue disorders can result in AR, particularly ankylosing spondylitis (16), and may be associated with various degrees of heart blocks with involvement of the mitral valve. Similar involvement has been reported in Reiter's syndrome (17), rheumatoid arthritis (14), giant cell aortitis (18), and sacroiliitis with HLA B27 (19).

II. PATHOPHYSIOLOGY

In brief, regurgitant blood from the aorta into the left ventricle cavity results in various degrees of dilatation and hypertrophy of that chamber. In AR, the entire forward ventricular stroke volume is ejected into a higher-pressure chamber—the aorta. In contrast, in mitral regurgitation, a substantial amount of regurgitant blood volume is ejected into a low-pressure chamber—the left atrium.

Unlike those patients with chronic advanced mitral regurgitation, patients with long-standing AR (with a comparable degree of left ventricular (LV) dilatation or dysfunction) can maintain better cardiac output at rest and on exercise. During exercise, the systemic vascular resistance decreases, and the diastolic period shortens and results in less regurgitation. Both these changes will help to increase forward cardiac output (20,21).

As mentioned in Chapters 16 and 17, whereas LV function can be demonstrated to be normal by using a crude method, i.e., ejection fraction, the LV systolic function may be revealed already impaired when it is assessed by a more sophisticated test, e.g., the end-systolic pressure–volume curve. In the early phase of LV impairment, calculated ejection fraction may be normal at rest, but it may decrease with exercise. The measurement of end-systolic LV volume (by angiography) and dimension (by M-mode echocardiography) have both been shown to be sensitive and reliable indices for monitoring the progression of the disease.

The severity of the aortic valve regurgitation depends on the size of the valvular orifice area in diastole, systemic vascular resistance, diastolic period, i.e., heart rate, and diastolic pressure gradient across the aortic valve. Left ventricular end-diastolic pressure (LVEDP) may remain within normal limits until late stage of the disease, when LVEDP is markedly increased, and may equalize with diastolic aortic pressure. The LV filling period will be shortened and limited to the early phase of diastole, and the decrescendo murmur of AR will shorten.

See Chapters 11, 16, and 17 for detailed description of the pathophysiology, the changes in the left ventricle size and function in chronic AR, and its comparison to acute AR.

III. CLINICAL FEATURES

A. Symptoms

Symptoms of AR are uncommon until the advanced stage of disease is reached. The time interval between the episode of acute rheumatic fever and the onset of symptoms is variable, depending on the degree of the LV dysfunction. The development of symptoms in chronic AR constitutes an ominous sign, heralding the presence of irreversible LV dysfunction.

Commonly, the AR murmur is detected on routine physical examination. However, patients may notice or be aware of the vigorous pulsations in the precordium or the neck, especially in the lying position. This is due to the marked increase in the LV stroke volume (including the forward and the regurgitant fraction), which can reach up to 20 L/min. In severe chronic AR, the degree of cardiac enlargement can be substantial, hence the term "cor bovinum."

In advanced cases, severe palpitation and pounding of the head are other symptoms experienced by the patient. The tachycardia induced by exertion may produce a more forceful palpitation and head pounding due to marked increase in stroke volume. Premature ventricular contractions may be particularly distressing in aortic incompetence.

This uncomfortable awareness of the heart beat in these patients may become accentuated after treatment with arterial vasodilators. These symptoms may be present for many years, perhaps up to 10–30 years, before the development of symptoms of LV dysfunction, such as exertional shortness of breath and orthopnea. Half of patients who developed angina were dead after 5 years, but half of those with NYHA class III–IV were dead after only 2 years (22,23).

Less common symptoms include dizziness, syncope, and anginal pain, particularly during sleep. Anginal pain in these circumstances is due to decreased coronary blood flow and decreased myocardial oxygen supply, and increased myocardial oxygen demand secondary to increased LV mass and wall tension. Elevated LVEDP and increased wall tension impair subendocardial perfusion.

Coronary blood flow depends on the aortic diastolic pressure, since the flow occurs in diastole. Thus the marked decrease in diastolic pressure in patients with severe AR compromises coronary blood flow. The heart rate slows during sleep and further increases the degree of AR. This also jeopardizes coronary blood flow. Angina at night is usually associated with hot flushes and sweating.

Excessive perspiration is also a rare late symptom. The mechanism of this symptom is not well understood, but it has been postulated to be related to changes in the autonomic nervous system.

In contrast, acute AR is almost always associated with a dramatic clinical presentation of severe shortness of breath and pulmonary edema (Chapter 11). In those patients who develop chronic AR, the onset of exertional shortness of breath in the early years of life may well be due to associated mitral valve disease. The latter usually dominates the clinical picture in patients with concomitant AR.

B. Physical Examination

The systolic blood pressure—which is usually elevated because of the marked increase of the stroke volume—will be reduced if the left ventricle fails. Clinically, the true diastolic blood pressure correlates well with the severity of AR. Although the true diastolic arterial pressure is usually maintained above 30–40 mmHg, the cuff recorded diastolic pressure can fall to zero if it is measured at the disappearance of the Korotkoff sounds, i.e., phase V. The true diastolic pressure is more accurately recorded at phase IV—the change of intensity or muffling of Korotkoff sounds. In the elderly, and particular in those with systemic hypertension, the already increased diastolic pressure may not reflect the severity of AR.

Chronic AR can produce characteristic physical signs that have been described over the years (Table 2). In the early stages of AR, an early diastolic murmur may be detected in the absence of peripheral signs. As the disease progresses, the peripheral signs (Table 2) dominate the physical examination. The pulse is characteristically of large volume and falls quite quickly—The so-called collapsing pulse. It also has been described as a "water-hammer" pulse, which can be well appreciated if the patient's forearm is grasped with the whole hand while the arm is elevated. Such typical pulse abnormalities, however, are more striking in the carotid arteries, where a thrill can also be felt. The large pulse pressure is not diagnostic for AR; it can be detected in other conditions that result in hyperdynamic circulation, such as beri beri, severe anemia, thyrotoxicosis, and patent ductus arteriosus. The character of the pulse will change in the presence of aortic stenosis or with the onset of cardiac failure.

Table 2 The Classic Physical Signs of Severe Aortic Regurgitation

Signs Detected by Inspection and Palpitation	
de Musset's sign	Head nodding synchronous with each systole. This is due to marked arterial pulsation.
Muller's sign	Bobbing or visible pulsation of the uvula.
Quincke's sign	Visible capillary pulsations in the nail beds. This can be demonstrated by translumination of the fingertip.
Corrigan's sign	Collapsing pulse or water-hammer pulse. This can been detected by sudden and brisk distension of the vessel and then quick collapse.
Signs Detected by Auscultation	
Hill's sign	This is a marked systolic pressure difference between the popliteal cuff and the brachial cuff pressure of more than 60 mmHg. Normally it is less than 10–20 mmHg.
Traube's sign	Booming systolic and diastolic sounds over the femoral artery—so-called pistol shot sounds.
Duroziez's sign	This is a to-and-fro bruit produced during mild compression of the femoral artery by stethoscope.
Bruit de tambour	A very loud S2 with ringing character. It can be elicited in syphilitic aortic regurgitation.

With mild AR the apical impulse is normal. However, with severe regurgitation it becomes vigorous, heaving, diffuse, and displaced downward and outward. A systolic basal thrill may be detected in the absence of aortic stenosis; this is due to increased stroke volume with disturbance of flow across the valve. In rare instances a diastolic thrill can be felt, but this usually occurs with ruptured or perforated aortic valve cusps. The latter may cause a musical murmur. In this context, other signs of infective endocarditis should be carefully sought, since it is the most common cause of perforated/ruptured cusps and usually causes acute severe AR.

In chronic AR the first heart sound is soft; however, in very advanced stages of the disease or in acute severe cases with premature closure of the mitral valve, it may be absent. This is due to the partial closure of the mitral valve before the onset of systole. The second heart sound is variable and may be obscured by the early diastolic murmur. In syphilitic AR the second heart sound may be quite loud and has a ringing character (bruit de tambour); this is due to dilatation of the aortic root and the proximity of the aorta to the chest wall.

In advanced cases with pulmonary hypertension, P2 may be accentuated. A systolic ejection sound or click may be detected, particularly with congenital bicuspid valve. A third heart sound usually correlates with LV dysfunction. This is due to rapid early diastolic filling of the left ventricle from both transmitral and aortic regurgitant flow.

The high-pitched murmur of AR occurs typically in early diastole and has a decrescendo shape. It is usually soft, exhibiting a "blowing" character, and therefore can be missed. The AR murmur starts immediately after A2, but the pulmonary regurgitation murmur starts after P2. The presence of other peripheral signs of AR, intensity of P2, chest X-ray, and EKG will help to differentiate between the two murmurs. In most cases the aortic murmur is best heard if the patient is sitting, standing upright, or leaning forward with the breath held in full expiration. It can be heard maximally over the left side of the sternum at the third or fourth intercostal space and rarely over the apex. The presence of the murmur on the right side of the sternum usually suggests severely dilated aortic root or rupture of aortic sinus of Valsalva into the right-sided cardiac chambers. A seagull type or musical quality of such a murmur is usually due to perforation of the aortic cusp.

Maneuvers that elevate the blood pressure, e.g., squatting and isometric exercise, will increase the pressure gradient across the aortic valve in diastole, thus accentuating the murmur. In contrast, the murmur can be reduced by lowering blood pressure, e.g., using amyl nitrite inhalation and during Valsalva maneuver.

As the degree of AR increases, the duration of the early diastolic murmur also increases, though in severe AR the late phase of the murmur may be abolished and exhibit an early peak. This is due to equalization of diastolic pressures between the left ventricle and aorta. Therefore the duration of the murmur, rather than its intensity, correlates with the severity of the regurgitation, until the very late stage of the disease.

A mid- and late-diastolic apical rumble is commonly heard in severe AR, the so called Austin-Flint murmur. It occurs without pathological involvement of the mitral valve. The diastolic rumble may be indistinguishable from the rumble of mitral stenosis. A loud S1 together with the opening snap and occasionally a diastolic thrill are helpful in diagnosing mitral stenosis. Inhalation of amyl nitrite reduces the afterload and increases the heart rate, and thus the intensity of Austin-Flint murmur will be decreased while that of mitral stenosis will be accentuated.

Austin-Flint murmur has been shown not to be caused by the fluttering/vibration of the anterior mitral leaflet. The latter develops in the early diastole, while Austin-Flint murmur occurs in the mid-late diastole. It has been suggested that the Austin-Flint murmur is due to "functional mitral stenosis" caused by the antegrade blood flow through closing mitral valve during mid-late diastole (24). The late diastolic phase of the Austin-Flint murmur has also been demonstrated to be abolished with the premature closure of the mitral valve in the presence of high end-diastolic pressure (LVEDP) (24).

IV. LABORATORIES INVESTIGATIONS

The 12-lead electrocardiogram may be normal in the early stage of AR; as regurgitation progresses, LV hypertrophy may develop, with increase in the LV voltage and a strain pattern. Atrial arrhythmias are uncommon in the absence of concomitant mitral valve disease, and atrial fibrillation is rare. Ventricular arrhythmias are uncommon, and usually occur in the form of premature ventricular complexes.

Chest X-ray shows cardiac enlargement with LV configuration (Chapter 4). With the onset of LV failure, pulmonary venous congestion develops. The aorta is dilated in many cases with AR, but severe dilatation suggests aortic wall disease (Chapter 1). Linear calcification in the wall of the ascending aorta has been considered to be a characteristic feature of syphilitic aortitis, though it has also been described in other diseases.

The echocardiographic examination is the most important diagnostic tool in the management of AR, not only for initial assessment, but more important, in the follow-up and timing of surgery (refer to Chapters 3, 16, and 17).

Angiographic assessment of the degree of AR is presently not necessary, since all of the required information can be extrapolated from echo/ Doppler examination. However, in middle-aged and elderly patients, coronary angiogram is indicated to detect the possible coexistence of significant coronary artery disease.

V. NATURAL HISTORY AND PROGNOSIS

Patients with mild to moderate AR may remain asymptomatic for 10–30 years, with a 10-year mortality rate of only 5–15% without surgery. For those patients with severe AR, mortality was reported at 30% at 10 years and 50% at 20 years (25–27).

Patients with severe AR but with normal diastolic blood pressure, no EKG changes of LV hypertrophy, no LV enlargement, and preserved LV systolic contractility have a good prognosis (28). In patients with severe AR and normal LV function at rest, only 1% of them developed LV dysfunction without symptoms during the follow-up period of 7 years (29). There were no deaths during the same period. Patients who carry an unfavorable prognosis are those with severe AR and impaired systolic LV function. These patients will develop heart failure and die within a few years. Therefore the development of symptoms with severe AR carries a poor prognosis (23,26,30). The mortality of patients with severe AR and angina pectoris is 50% at 5 years. However, in those patients with severe impairment of LV function, 50% are dead in 2 years, and 96% at 10 years' follow-up.

Previous studies have attempted to use crude methods and criteria as a means for choosing the optimum timing for surgery: These parameters include serial ECG, chest X-ray, diastolic blood pressure recordings, and symptoms (30). With the availability of more sensitive diagnostic tests and with better knowledge of the natural history of chronic AR, the timing of surgery in such patients can be more accurately assessed before the onset of LV impairment. These diagnostic parameters include measurement of LV function at rest and after exercise, LV end-systolic and end-diastolic volume indices, and LV wall stress calculation. Since the deterioration of LV function may occur despite the lack of symptoms, serial measurements of these indices should be performed regularly, i.e., at 4- to 6-month intervals. Chapters 16 and 17 discuss in detail the importance of LV function and the various methods of its evaluation that should be done serially to assess the timing of surgery in severe AR. In summary, a patient is eligible for cardiac surgery when:

1. Left end-systolic dimension approaches 55 mm (echo).
2. Fractional shortening decreases towards 25% (echo).
3. LV peak systolic wall stress is <600 mmHg (echo).
4. LV end systolic wall stress is <235 mmHg (echo).
5. LV end systolic volume index is <90 c/m^2 (angio).
6. Ejection fraction decreases on serial examinations to 50% (echo or angio).
7. Exercise capacity decreases.

Aortic valve replacement should be advised even in asymptomatic patients, if more than one criterion of the above list has been be met on serial studies.

In developing countries, significant LV dysfunction can occur despite the presence of only mild to moderate chronic AR; acute rheumatic fever with severe carditis has been suggested to be the underlying etiology. Although there are no studies to indicate what is the optimal time for surgery for this subgroup of patients, in clinical practice they have been managed similarly to those with severe AR and LV dysfunction. A long-term follow-up study is required to identify the natural history of such patients, particularly the response to the administration of vasodilators in delaying cardiac surgery.

Acute clinical deterioration in patients with chronic AR is usually due to the development of infective endocarditis or, more commonly, coexisting mitral valve disease.

VI. TREATMENT

A. Asymptomatic Patients

Patients with AR require antibiotic prophylaxis for endocarditis. Preventing further attack of acute rheumatic fever is essential in patients up to the age of 30 years. This goal is accomplished with long-acting intramuscular penicillin injection or oral erythromycin for patients with penicillin sensitivity.

For those patients with asymptomatic AR and LV dilatation, Digoxin may be appropriate. In a small study of 10 patients with 1-month follow-up, comparing the effect of digoxin, nifedipine, and hydralazine on LV function at rest and exercise, digoxin was shown to be superior (31). Diuretics together with digoxin should be used to treat LV failure.

Control of systemic hypertension is essential, since it can exacerbate the degree of AR. Hypertension can also play a role in precipitating aortic dissection in patients with aortic root disorders. Eighty percent of patients with aortic dissection have elevated systemic blood pressure (32).

The use of oral vasodilators in asymptomatic AR in an attempt to delay/prevent the dilatation and deterioration of the LV systolic function and postponing AVR has recently been investigated (33–35). Although it was as early as 1970 (36) when the short-term beneficial effect of the arterial vasodilators was demonstrated—then the amyl nitrates—it was not until the late 1980s (34) that the value of the longer-acting vasodilators was appreciated.

In a double-blind, placebo-controlled trial (n = 80) lasting 24 months, hydralazine has been shown to reduce LV end-diastolic volume (LVEDV) by 18%, and end-systolic volume (LVESV) by 28% (34). Correlations were highly significant between baseline levels of LVEDV, LVESV, and ejection fraction and the subsequent reduction in these parameters after therapy with hydralazine. Also during this period of follow-up, deterioration of LV function was noted in 17% of the placebo group and in only 2% of patients on hydralazine. This study showed that those with the largest hearts were the most likely to benefit from hydralazine. Since 9% of those patients treated with hydralazine had to discontinue this drug during the follow-up period of 24 months, because of the development of lupuslike syndrome, ACE inhibitors may prove to be useful as an alternative.

In a recent randomized, double-blind, placebo-controlled study, the result of the use of calcium channel blockers in 72 asymptomatic patients with severe chronic AR and normal LV function has been evaluated (37). This study showed that short-term therapy with nifedipine during a 12-month period reverses both LV dilatation and hypertrophy.

At present—and despite the above—asymptomatic patients with severe cardiomegaly and LV dysfunction should be advised to undergo AVR until there is further evidence to support the contrary. This is because the study discussed above randomized only a small number of patients and therefore was not designed to assess the long-term effect on the clinical course of chronic AR.

Asymptomatic patients with severe AR and normal LV function should not be advised to undergo surgery as a prophylactic measure to prevent irreversible LV dysfunction. Early detection of LV dysfunction, by serial echocardiography and/or radionuclide cardiac scintigraphy, is adequate for timing the surgery. In all such patients, who are regularly examined and develop parameters indicating LV dilatation or dysfunction, aortic valve replacement is rewarded by reduction of the LV dilatation and reversal of the LV dysfunction (29).

B. Symptomatic Patients

There is no indication, with the presently available data, to delay surgery in symptomatic patients with the use of various medications.

REFERENCES

1. Campbell M. Aortic valvular disease. Br Heart J 1932; 1:328.
2. Davies MJ. In: Pathology of cardiac valves. London: Butterworths, 1980.
3. Olson LJ, Subramanian R, Edwards WD. Surgical pathology of pure aortic insufficiency: a study of 225 cases. Mayo Clin Proc 1984; 59:835.
4. Roman MJ, Devereaux RB, Niles NW, Hochreiter C, Kligfield P, Sato N, Spitzer MC, Borer JS. The aortic root dilatation as a cause of isolated, severe aortic regurgitation. Prevalence, clinical and echocardiographic patterns, and relation to left ventricular hypertrophy and function. Ann Intern Med 1987; 106:800.
5. Lakier JB, Copans H, Rosman HS, Lam R, Fine G, Khaja F, Goldstein S. Idiopathic degeneration of the aortic valve: a common cause of isolated aortic regurgitation. J Am Coll Cardiol 1985; 5:347.
6. Allen WM, Matloff JM, Fishbein MC. Myxoid degeneration of the aortic valve and isolated severe aortic regurgitation. Am J Cardiol 1985; 55:439.
7. Moran SV, Casanegra P, Maturana G, Dubernet J. Spontaneous rupture of

a fenestrated aortic valve. Surgical treatment. J Thorac Cardiovasc Surg 1977; 73:716.

8. Waller BF, Kishel JC, Roberts WC. Severe aortic regurgitation from systemic hypertension. Chest 1982; 82:365.

9. Barlow J, Kincaid-Smith P. The auscultatory findings in hypertension. Br Heart J 1960; 22:505.

10. American Heart Association, National Center for Health Statistics, 1991.

11. Frahn CJ, Braunwauld E, Morrow AG. Congenital aortic regurgitation. Clinical and haemodynamic findings in four patients. Am J Med 1961; 31:63.

12. Tatsuno K, Konno S, Sakakibara S. Ventricular septal defect with aortic insufficiency. Angiocardiographic aspects and a new classification. Am Heart J 1973; 85:13.

13. Bernhard GC, Lange RL, Hensley GT. Aortic disease with valvular insufficiency as the principal manifestation of systemic lupus erythematosus. Ann Intern Med 1969; 71:81.

14. Roberts WC, Kehoe JA, Carpenter DF, Golden A. Cardiac valvular lesions in rheumatoid arthritis. Arch Intern Med 1968; 122:141.

15. Heppner RL, Babitt HI, Bianchine JW, Warbasse JR. Aortic regurgitation and aneurysm of sinus of Valsalva associated with osteogenesis imperfecta. Am J Cardiol 1973; 31:654.

16. Bulkley BH, Roberts WC. Ankylosing spondylitis in aortic regurgitation. Description of the characteristic cardiovascular lesion from study of eight necropsy patients. Circulation 1973; 48:1014.

17. Paulus HE, Pearson CM, Pitts W Jr. Aortic insufficiency in five patients with the Reiter's syndrome. A detailed clinical and pathologic study. Am J Med 1972; 53:464.

18. Gula G, Pomerance A, Bennet M, Yacoub MH. Homograft replacement of aortic valve and ascending aorta in a patient with non-specific giant cell aortitis. Br Heart J 1977; 39:581.

19. Hollingworth P, Hall PJ, Knight SC, Newman R. Lone aortic regurgitation, sacroiliitis, and HLA B27. Case history and frequency of association. Br Heart J 1979; 42:229.

20. Firth BG, Dehmer GJ, Nicod P, Willerson JT, Hillis LD. Effect of increasing heart rate in patients with aortic regurgitation. Effect of incremental atrial pacing on scintigraphic, hemodynamic and thermodilution measurements. Am J Cardiol 1982; 49:1860.

21. Steingart RM, Yee C, Weinstein L, Scheuer J. Radionuclide ventriculographic study of adaptations to exercise in aortic regurgitation. Am J Cardiol 1983; 51:483.

22. Hegglin R, Scheu H, Rothlin M. Aortic insufficiency. Circulation 1968; 38(suppl 5):77.

23. Segal J, Harvey WP, Hufnagel C. A clinical study of 100 cases of severe aortic insufficiency. Am J Med 1956; 21:200.

24. Fortuin NJ, Craige E. On the mechanism of the Austin Flint murmur. Circulation 1972; 45:558.

25. Rapaport E. Natural history of aortic and mitral valve disease. Am J Cardiol 1975; 35:221.
26. Hegglin R, Scheu H, Rothlin M. Aortic insufficiency. Circulation 1968; 38(suppl 5):77.
27. Bland EF, Wheeler EO. Severe aortic regurgitation in young people: a long-term perspective with reference to prognosis and prosthesis. N Engl J Med 1957; 256:667.
28. Friedberg CK, ed. Diseases of the Heart. 3d ed. Philadelphia: Saunders, 1966.
29. Bonow RO, Rosing DR, McIntosh CL, Jones M, Maron BJ, Lan KK, Lakatos E, Bacharach SL, Green MV, Epstein SE. The natural history of symptomatic patients with aortic regurgitation and normal left ventricular function. Circulation 1983; 68:509.
30. Spagnuolo M, Kloth H, Taranta A, Doyle E, Pasternack B. Natural history of rheumatic aortic regurgitation. Criteria predictive of death, congestive heart failure, and angina in young patients. Circulation 1971; 44:368.
31. Crawford MH, Wilson RS, O'Rourke RA, Vittitoe JA. Effect of digoxin and vasodilators on left ventricular function in aortic regurgitation. Int J Cardiol 1989; 23:385.
32. Roberts WC. The hypertensive diseases. Evidence that systemic hypertension is a greater risk factor to the development of other cardiovascular diseases than previously suspected. Am J Med 1975; 59:523.
33. Greenberg BH, DeMots H, Murphy E, Rahimtoola SH. Mechanism for improved cardiac performance with arteriolar dilators in aortic insufficiency. Circulation 1981; 63:263.
34. Greenberg B, Massie B, Bristow JD, Cheitlin M, Siemienczuk D, Topic N, Wilson RA, Szlachcic J, Thomas D. Long-term vasodilator therapy of chronic aortic insufficiency. A randomized double-blinded, placebo-controlled clinical trial. Circulation 1988; 78:92.
35. Rahimtolla SH. Vasodilator therapy in chronic severe aortic regurgitation. J Am Coll Cardiol 1990; 16:430.
36. Delius W, Enghoff E. Studies of the central and peripheral hemodynamic effects of amyl nitrite in patients with aortic insufficiency. Circulation 1970; 42:787.
37. Scognamiglio R, Fasoli G, Ponchia A, Dalla-Volta S. Long-term nifedipine unloading therapy in asymptomatic patients with chronic severe aortic regurgitation. J Am Coll Cardiol 1990; 16:424.

8

Aortic Valve Stenosis

Jeffrey M. Isner
*Tufts University School of Medicine
and St. Elizabeth's Medical Center
Boston, Massachusetts*

I. ETIOLOGY AND PATHOLOGY

Isolated aortic stenosis rarely occurs as the result of rheumatic heart disease (1); a congenitally bicuspid aortic valve (Fig. 1) is the most common cause of isolated aortic stenosis in adults (aged 15–65) (2), while calcification of a congenitally normal three-cuspid aortic valve (Fig. 2) accounts for most older patients with aortic stenosis (3). Development of stenosis in a bicuspid valve is thought to result from leaflet asymmetry, which is characteristic of these valves. Calcification of a three-cuspid valve may on occasion have an obvious etiology such as ochronosis (4), lupus, or hypercholesterolemia (5), but in most cases the etiology is obscure.

We evaluated the histoarchitecture of calcific deposits in 30 operatively excised aortic valves (6). Light microscopic sections taken through the calcified aortic valve leaflets disclosed two principal types of histoarchitecture (Fig. 3). In 11 aortic valves nodular calcific deposits were superimposed on an underlying fibrotic aortic valve leaflet (type A); in 17 valves calcific deposits were distributed diffusely throughout the body (spongiosa) of the aortic valve leaflets (type B). Two aortic valves could not be classified histologically.

These histologic subtypes were *not* randomly distributed with regard to gross valvular morphology. All 14 bicuspid valves (100%) were type B; in contrast, 11 (69%) of 16 tricuspid valves were type A, and only 3 (19%) of 16 tricuspid valves were type B ($p < 0.01$). Both valves with nonclassifiable histological features were tricuspid on the basis of gross

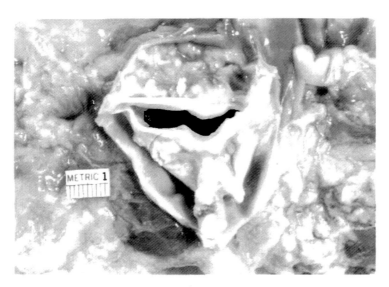

Figure 1 Classic congenitally bicuspid aortic valve, as viewed from aorta at necropsy. Both leaflets contain extensive calcific deposits, including centrally disposed median raphe of conjoined (bottom) leaflet.

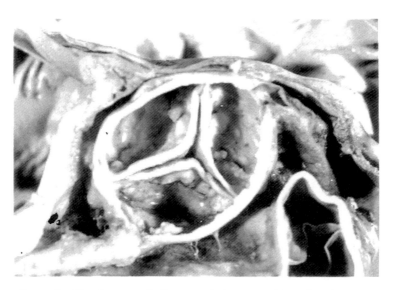

Figure 2 Classic congenitally normal, three-cuspid aortic valve, as viewed from aorta at necropsy. Each of three leaflets contains extensive calcific deposits. There is no commissural fusion.

AORTIC VALVULAR CALCIFIC DEPOSITS

TRICUSPID

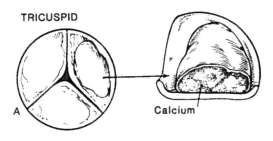

BICUSPID (Congenital)

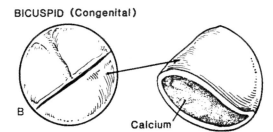

Figure 3 Contrasting distribution of calcific deposits in three-cuspid (A) versus bicuspid (B) aortic valve. Calcific deposits are often confined to the aortic aspect of the three-cuspid valve; in contrast, calcific deposits are routinely distributed throughout the entire thickness of the bicuspid valve leaflets.

examination. Thus the histoarchitectural distribution of calcific deposits is different for bicuspid than for tricuspid stenotic aortic valves.

Distribution of calcific deposits according to the pattern arbitrarily designated as type A implies that a cleavage plane may be established between the calcific nodule and underlying fibrotic leaflet. Accordingly, such valves would be expected to be amenable to intraoperative manual or ultrasonic debridement. In contrast, the calcific deposits in a type B valve are distributed as such an integral part of the valve leaflet that attempts to remove the calcific deposits necessarily violate the integrity of the valve leaflet. The fact that *all* bicuspid valves in our study were type B suggests that few exceptions regarding debridement opportunities will be found. The distribution of type A versus type B among tricuspid valves suggests that although most tricuspid valves will prove appropriate for intraoperative debridement, there will be some in which debridement will not be possible.

A second potential implication of these findings is the possibility that the pattern by which the calcific deposits are distributed within the valve leaflet determines whether or not such a valve will prove amenable to balloon valvuloplasty. It is possible, but as yet unproved, that fracture of calcific deposits may be more readily accomplished when the calcium is deposited in nodular form on an underlying leaflet rather than distributed throughout the full thickness of the leaflet. Perhaps this explains the apparent increased refractoriness of the bicuspid valve to balloon dilation.

The basis for these differing histoarchitectural patterns remains enigmatic. One possible explanation relates to the duration of the degenerative process. Because the bicuspid valve has been considered to be subject to accelerated degeneration as a result of stresses imposed by asymmetric leaflet motion (7), the onset of calcification at a relatively earlier age may ultimately lead to more thorough leaflet involvement than in the case of a normally functioning tricuspid valve. Alternatively, these two patterns could conceivably be related to sites of maximal stress. For example, a heteromerous bileaflet valve in the aortic position may open and close in such a manner that all aspects of the leaflet are stressed to an abnormal and equivalent degree. In a normal valve the finding of calcium distributed primarily on the aortic (versus ventricular) surface of the valve leaflet suggests that stress may be predominant along the aspect of the valve leaflet subjected over long periods to the closing pressure of the systemic circulation.

Acquired aortic stenosis can, of course, also result from rheumatic heart disease; in such cases the mitral valve is typically also pathological. Unlike bicuspid and calcific three-cuspid aortic stenosis, in which obstruction results from leaflet immobilization by calcific deposits, aortic stenosis due to a rheumatic etiology results from leaflet immobilization by commissural fusion; extensive calcific deposits are *not* characteristic of rheumatic, stenotic aortic valves. The "fixed" orifice resulting from commissural fusion and leaflet retraction typically renders such a rheumatic valve regurgitant as well as stenotic.

Diagnosis of valvular morphology: Identification of congenital valvular morphology is more problematic in adults than in children. The extensive calcific deposits characteristic of adult-type aortic stenosis obviate clinical signs of congenital deformity, such as an early systolic ejection sound, and obscure demonstration of cusp morphology by conventional transthoracic ultrasound. Nanda et al. (8), for example, studied the M-mode echocardiograms of 21 patients with a congenitally bicuspid aortic valve and noted that the echocardiogram in each case disclosed eccentric displacement of the aortic valve during diastole; because ". . . deposits of calcium in the aortic valve [were found to] produce confusing echo patterns. . . "; however, patients with aortic valve calcification were excluded from the study. Brandenburg et al. (9) subsequently evaluated two-dimensional echocardiograms recorded preoperatively from 115 patients in whom aortic valve morphology was documented by the operating surgeon, pathologist, or both. Two-dimensional echocardiography proved useful for identifying congenitally bicuspid valves in young individuals, particularly those with isolated or predominant aortic insufficiency; in heavily calcified valves, however, extensive calcific deposits precluded identification of either the number of aortic valve cusps or the presence of a median raphe. More recently, analysis of trans-thoracic two-dimensional echocardiograms recorded specifically from patients with calcific aortic stenosis demonstrated that trans-thoracic ultrasound was a poor predictor of the congenital morphology of the operatively excised aortic valve specimen (10).

Aortic root angiography has also been previously employed to determine aortic valve morphology in patients with aortic stenosis and/or insufficiency. Because the aortic sinus related to the conjoined cusp is divided by the median raphe into two distinct angiographic subdivisions, the angiographic demonstration of three apparent sinus formations does not exclude the presence of a congenitally bicuspid valve (11). While trans-esophageal echocardiography (12), aortic root angioscopy (13), and ultrafast computed tomography (14,15) have been suggested as potential means of distinguishing bicuspid from tricuspid aortic valvular morphology, experience with these modalities for this particular application remains limited.

We have previously investigated the possibility that an intravascular catheter-mounted ultrasound probe could be used to identify aortic valve morphology in adult patients with calcific aortic stenosis (16). The intravascular ultrasound catheter (Boston Scientific) consists of a braided polyethylene outer shell enclosing a rotary drive shaft with a single element transducer at its tip (Fig. 4). The outer dimension of the catheter is 6.6F, and the total catheter length is 95 cm. An integral sonolucent window permits ultrasound transmission at <7 dB attenuation while still providing sufficient mechanical strength for catheter manipulation.

A satisfactory examination was accomplished in each of the 15 patients studied by intravascular ultrasound in vivo. Among 10 patients undergoing diagnostic catheterization for suspected aortic stenosis, the images recorded in 5 were similar to those recorded in vitro from calcified but congenitally normal tricuspid valves: Three cusps, each of which contained highly echogenic, presumably calcific, foci were identified (Fig. 5).

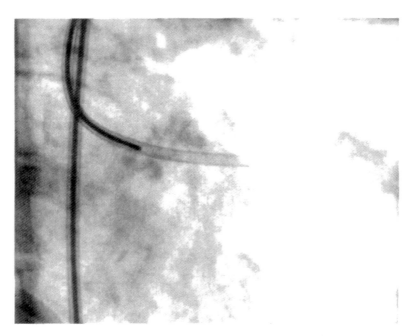

Figure 4 Intravascular ultrasound (IVUS) examination of aortic valve. A long sheath has been advanced across aortic valve into the left ventricle. IVUS catheter is positioned within long sheath at the site of heavily calcified aortic valve.

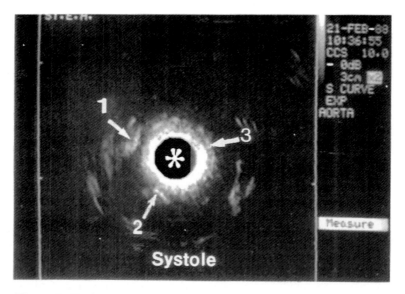

Figure 5 Typical IVUS appearance of congenitally normal, three-cuspid aortic valve; three highly echogenic leaflets are seen abutting IVUS catheter (asterisk).

266

Furthermore, the mobility of the aortic valve leaflets in these 5 patients was typically severely diminished. Diminution in leaflet mobility was often asymmetrical, however, frequently limiting the mobility of two leaflets more severely than the third. Similar findings indicative of a calcified but congenitally normal tricuspid aortic valve were observed in 4 of 5 patients undergoing balloon aortic valvuloplasty.

In the remaining 5 patients undergoing diagnostic catheterization and in 1 patient undergoing balloon valvuloplasty, intravascular ultrasound examination disclosed one or both findings observed in vitro for calcified congenitally bicuspid aortic valves; in all 6 patients, intravascular ultrasound identified two leaflets (Fig. 6), and in 4 of the 6 patients identified a high-intensity linear echo corresponding to the calcified median raphe (Fig. 7). The mobility of both leaflets of the bicuspid valves was observed to be diminished; the mobility of the leaflet containing the median raphe, however, generally appeared disproportionately reduced in comparison to the complementary leaflet.

The ability to discriminate bicuspid from tricuspid morphology in heavily calcified aortic valves of patients undergoing diagnostic catheterization has potential therapeutic implications. Heavily calcified, stenotic tricuspid valves, in which the calcific deposits are distributed in nodular form, superimposed on an underlying fibrotic leaflet, have proved amenable to

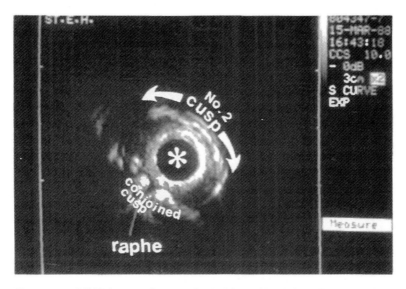

Figure 6 IVUS image of congenitally bicuspid aortic valve. In this case, two distinct leaflets are easily appreciated and median raphe is less obvious.

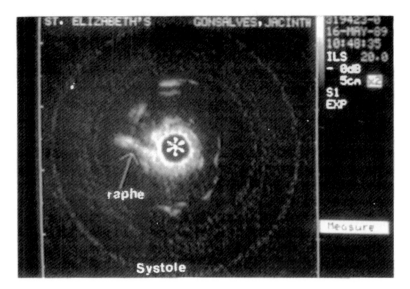

Figure 7 IVUS image of congenitally bicuspid aortic valve in different patient from that whose valve was illustrated in Fig. 6. In this case, median raphe is prominent.

intraoperative debridement using manual (17,18) or ultrasound (19,20) techniques. In contrast, heavily calcified, congenitally bicuspid valves, because the calcific deposits are distributed throughout the body of the leaflet and thereby prohibit identification of a potential cleavage plane, have proved refractory to such therapy (21,22).

II. CLINICAL FEATURES

A. Symptoms and Natural History

Patients with aortic stenosis exhibit an insidious clinical course and are often asymptomatic for many years (23). The progression of aortic stenosis has been shown to be slower in rheumatic and congenital aortic stenosis than in degenerative calcific stenosis when compared by serial hemodynamic studies (24).

The onset of symptoms in patients with aortic stenosis is related to the severity of the stenosis and the underlying pathology. Patients with rheumatic tricuspid and congenital bicuspid aortic stenosis present at an earlier age than patients with degenerative calcific stenosis. The study of Horstkotte and colleagues showed that the mean age of patients at onset of symptoms was 39 years for the rheumatic, 48 years for the congenital bicuspid, and 66 years for degenerative calcific aortic stenosis (25). Younger patients tolerate more severe degree of stenosis compared to elderly patients, who are rarely asymptomatic when aortic stenosis is severe (26).

The development of symptoms in patients with aortic stenosis constitutes an ominous sign; 60% of patients are dead 5 years after the onset of symptoms, and 90% in 10 years (27). In another study, all symptomatic patients with aortic stenosis who refused surgery died within 12 years (25). Interestingly, the literature emphasizes that the onset of symptoms in patients with aortic stenosis carries the worst prognosis compared to other valvular diseases. The onset of symptoms in patients with severe aortic regurgitation usually indicates irreversible left ventricular dysfunction. With the availability of cardiac surgery, the long-term prognosis of symptomatic aortic stenosis has markedly improved. In contrast, the long-term benefit after surgery for symptomatic patients with aortic regurgitation is not as dramatic.

The characteristic symptoms of hemodynamically severe aortic stenosis (valve area of less than 0.7 cm^2) are dyspnea, angina pectoris, and dizziness/syncope on exertion. Mild dyspnea on exertion has been shown to be the most common symptom, while left ventricular failure occurs late in the course of the disease. In one prospective study, dyspnea was 2.5 times and 4.8 times more common than angina pectoris and syncope, respectively (28). Dyspnea due to cardiac failure also carries the worst prognosis, with an average life expectancy of 1 to 2 years (25,27). Hence, in patients with aortic stenosis, a long history of moderate to severe dyspnea on exertion may indicate a concomitant medical problem such as mitral valve disease. The life expectancy after the onset of syncope and angina is 3 to 5 years (27,29).

Patients with aortic stenosis and congestive heart failure are not a homogenous group. Only 40% of these patients have depressed left ventricular ejection fraction (30). Dyspnea in patients with aortic stenosis is due to systolic and/or diastolic left ventricular dysfunction. Conceivably, the prognosis and the natural history of these two different types of dysfunction may be different.

While acute myocardial infarction is rare, angina pectoris, caused by hemodynamically significant aortic stenosis, is a common symptom. It is the earliest symptom in 34% of patients (31). The mechanism of angina is due to an unbalanced myocardial oxygen supply/demand ratio. The underlying factors are the inability to increase the coronary blood flow with the increased muscle mass, and the increased diastolic left ventricular pressure. Concomitant coronary artery disease is also common and present in 50% of elderly patients with aortic stenosis (32). In patients with severe aortic stenosis, the absence of angina pectoris and coronary risk factors markedly reduce the probability of significant coronary artery disease, i.e., less than 4% (33,34). In contrast, Selzer found no difference in the incidence of angina pectoris in patients who had normal, mild or significant coronary disease (35).

Syncope occurs in 20% of the patients with aortic stenosis and is classically exercise induced. It is the earliest symptom in 15% of patients (31). Although arrhythmias are an important cause of syncope in aortic stenosis, particularly those occurring at rest, hemodynamic abnormalities that are associated with aortic stenosis have been shown to be another possible mechanism. Stimulation of left ventricular baroreceptors, causing arterial hypotension followed by gradual bradycardia and reduced venous return, has been demonstrated in patients experiencing syncope or severe dizziness on exercise (36). No arrhythmias were detected during exercise. Alternatively, decreased systemic vascular resistance during exercise, in the presence of a fixed stenotic aortic valve, is another possibility.

Sudden cardiac death, though rare in asymptomatic patients with aortic stenosis, may be the first clinical presentation. Based on a summary of seven retrospective postmortem studies, sudden death occurred in 5% of asymptomatic patients with aortic stenosis (27). Nonetheless, in two other prospective studies, with 24- and 17-month follow-ups, sudden death did not occur in asymptomatic patients (37,38). The 2% of patients who had sudden cardiac death had warning symptoms of angina or heart failure prior to the episode of sudden death (37). In contrast, sudden death is common in symptomatic patients with aortic stenosis, i.e., 13% at 1-year follow-up (28) and 34% to 50% at 2 years (38,39).

Other rare symptoms include cerebral calcium emboli from the calcific aortic valve. Gastrointestinal bleeding, due to colonic idiopathic angiodysplasia, may complicate the clinical picture.

B. Physical Examination

The systolic murmur constituted the *sine quan non* of the physical examination in patients with aortic stenosis. While the physical examination may leave undecided the magnitude of physiological dysfunction represented by a systolic murmur, it may nevertheless be adequate to identify the *source* of the murmur when considered in the context of the remainder of the physical examination.

Examination of the carotid pulses may be extremely helpful: The classic "parvus et tardus," bilaterally symmetrical carotid upstroke is typical of critical aortic stenosis. In the elderly patient, the contour of the pulse is more useful than auscultation of the pulse, inasmuch as the latter may be more unduly influenced by local carotid vascular disease. A "spike-and-dome" contour to the carotid pulse is the classic physical finding of hypertrophic cardiomyopathy. Mitral regurgitation classically produces a bounding pulse with a fast descent. In a younger patient, particularly if carotid disease is excluded, the finding of a bruit in association with an abnormal carotid examination is a clue that the systolic murmur is due to left ventricular outflow tract obstruction.

Examination of jugular venous pulse is more useful in the evaluation of systolic murmurs generated on the right side of the heart than on the left side of the heart. The finding of large V waves in the jugular venous pulse is typical of tricuspid regurgitation. The finding of a well-defined, double-impulse (A- and V-wave) jugular venous contour is more typical of pulmonary outflow tract obstruction.

Palpation of the precordium is an often-neglected examination that is crucial to the evaluation of the systolic murmur. Palpation of a systolic thrill (best performed using the portion of the palm at the base of the digits, with the patient lying in either the left lateral decubitus position or sitting upright) may indicate that the murmur is due to left ventricular outflow tract obstruction when the thrill is palpated along the upper sternal border. In contrast, when the thrill is palpated at the left ventricular apex, the murmur is more likely due to mitral regurgitation. The exception to this is the patient with a recent myocardial infarction in whom a systolic thrill caused by a ruptured ventricular septum may be palpable at any site between the lower left sternal border and left ventricular apex. The finding of a so-called triple ripple, i.e., three distinct precordial palpatory impulses, is typical of hypertrophic cardiomyopathy. A well-localized, protracted precordial impulse generally represents left ventricular outflow tract obstruction; a diffuse, fleeting precordial impulse is more typical of a volume overload lesion such as mitral regurgitation.

While the auscultatory features of S_1 are generally not helpful, detection of two clear components of the S_2 may be extremely helpful: Absence of an aortic component of the second heart sound indicates the presence of valvular aortic stenosis. Prolonged splitting of the second heart sound may be due to pulmonic stenosis. The finding of gallop sounds are nonspecific, although the finding of gallop sounds that augment with inspiration may indicate that the associated systolic murmur is right-sided. Discrete sounds between S_1 and S_2 may be specific for the anatomic basis of the systolic murmur. An ejection sound is typical of a noncalcified, congenitally bicuspid aortic valve. The finding of a systolic click, particularly when it occurs during the latter two-thirds of systole, is typical of mitral valve prolapse. In the rare adult who escapes detection of a congenital right-sided murmur during childhood, an ejection click may be associated with valvular pulmonic stenosis.

Careful attention to the auscultatory features of systolic murmur are critical in determining its origin and importance. A holosystolic closing murmur is almost always due to mitral regurgitation, and is heard best at the left ventricular apex, radiating well to the left anterior axillary line. A harsh, diamond-shaped murmur is generally due to valvular aortic stenosis; it is important to note that in the elderly patient the murmur of valvular aortic stenosis may be heard better at the left ventricular apex than along the left upper sternal border. The murmurs of hypertrophic cardiomyopathy, mitral valve prolapse, and papillary muscle dysfunction are highly variable in configuration, intensity, and quality. As a result, the performance of several maneuvers is mandatory in the evaluation of the undefined systolic murmur. The most useful of these maneuvers, provided the patient is physically able to cooperate, is the standing-squatting maneuver. An increase in the intensity of the murmur going from the squatting to the standing position is typical of patients with hypertrophic cardiomyopathy and mitral valve prolapse. A similar response to the Valsalva maneuver occurs in these two entities; however, the Valsalva maneuver is less reliable than standing-squatting for two reasons. First, it is difficult for many patients to perform the maneuver correctly, particularly if they are told to "bear down as if you are having a bowel movement." It is generally more useful to ask the patient either to purse his lips around his index finger and "blow on your finger as if you are blowing up a balloon; or to ask him to "press your belly against my hand." Second, if the outflow tract obstruction caused by hypertrophic cardiomyopathy is particularly severe, the Valsalva maneuver may result in total obstruction to left ventricular outflow, causing a paradoxical *diminution* in the intensity of the murmur.

One "maneuver" that does not require any active participation on behalf of the patient is evaluation of the systolic murmur in response to a premature beat, or a short cycle followed by a long cycle in patients with atrial fibrillation. The murmur of valvular aortic stenosis typically increases during the long cycle, while the murmur of mitral regurgitation typically remains unchanged.

Whether or not the systolic murmur is accompanied by a diastolic murmur provides an important clue to the site at which the systolic murmur is being generated, and to the morphology of the responsible valve. The diastolic "blowing" murmur of aortic insufficiency, best heard at the lower left sternal border, is common with either rheumatic aortic stenosis and/or valvular aortic stenosis attributable to a congenitally bicuspid aortic valve. On the other hand, aortic insufficiency present in more than "trace" amounts is rare in patients with a calcified congenitally normal, tricuspid aortic valve. The presence of a diastolic murmur is rare in patients with dynamic subaortic left ventricular outflow tract obstruction, although it is common in patients in whom left ventricular outflow tract obstruction is due to a subvalvular discrete membrane. The finding of an opening snap and a diastolic low-frequency rumbling murmur at the left ventricular apex suggests that the systolic murmur of mitral regurgitation is rheumatic in origin. Diastolic rumbles in the absence of an opening snap may be due to torrential mitral regurgitation and/or severe mitral valve annular calcification.

III. LABORATORY INVESTIGATION

Until recently the electrocardiogram was more important in the evaluation of the systolic murmur than it is now with the currently available noninvasive imaging techniques. The absence of any electrocardiographic abnormalities is consistent with a nonorganic basis for the systolic murmur, such as anemia, an alternative high-output state, or innocuous valvular calcification. The most useful positive finding is left ventricular hypertrophy, which favors a diagnosis of left ventricular outflow tract obstruction. It is important to note that in elderly individuals, due to changes in chest wall configuration, voltage criteria for left ventricular hypertrophy may be fulfilled less often than other criteria, such as ST-T wave changes. The finding of a left atrial enlargement may occur in patients with left ventricular outflow tract obstruction caused by a hypertrophied noncompliant left ventricle. Electrocardiographic evidence of myocardial infarction may suggest that papillary muscle dysfunction due to ischemic heart disease is the basis for the systolic murmur. Finally, in any patient with a systolic murmur and a "bizarre" electrocardiogram, the patient should be considered to have hypertrophic cardiomyopathy until proven otherwise.

For radiological findings and echocardiographic examination, refer to Chapters 3 and 4.

IV. TREATMENT

A. Medical Treatment

The role of medical treatment in the management of patients with aortic stenosis is limited.

B. Aortic Valvuloplasty

1. Developmental History

The first recorded attempt to ameliorate the hemodynamic burden of aortic stenosis was by Tuffier (43), who in 1913 performed a commissurotomy by digitally invaginating a portion of the aortic wall through the orifice of a heavily calcified aortic valve. In 1947 Smithy and Parker (44) reported the use of a trans-ventricular approach in a series of operations in which a thin-bladed knife was used to incise one or more of the aortic valve leaflets. Bailey (45) experimented with a similar approach to deliver a uterine dilator to the aortic valve, later switching to a right carotid trans-aortic route and the use of three dilating springs mounted on a straight probe. As a result of these experiments, Bailey felt moved to pronounce that ". . . blind retrograde performance of aortic commissurotomy was inherently unsound and could never be surgically acceptable." Harken et al. devised a "modified" closed commissurotomy via a supravalvular prosthetic pouch which resulted in some hemodynamic improvement and a lower operative mortality (46). Follow-up in the survivors, however, showed evidence of recurrence. Postmortem studies by MacMillan (47) confirmed suspicions that any changes in the valves were quite temporary, and Bailey reiterated, "we do not accomplish much opening of the stenotic valve by any closed method. It is not surprising that many of our surviving patients are beginning to show evidence of recurrence of the stenosis. . . ." He further proposed an exclusively open procedure, "a painstaking technique, somewhat analogous to soap sculpture. . . to remove the extremely. . . calcified layer. Shortly thereafter, Kirklin at the Mayo Clinic (48) and Hufnagel at Georgetown (49) began performing manual debridement of heavily calcified aortic valves. The increased operative time and improved surgical exposure allowed by the development of the pump oxygenator in 1954 permitted these operations to follow the meticulous approach outlined by Bailey. Both of these surgeons documented clinical and hemodynamic improvement after these operations, but the treatment of valvular heart disease was about to change dramatically with the advent of valvular prostheses.

Beginning with the development of a single-leaflet prosthesis, and followed by the ball valve developed by Harken and Starr, by 1960 aortic valvulectomy with prosthetic replacement was firmly established. The efforts of investigators then shifted toward the development of better and more physiological prostheses. With each new device came the hope of a more durable valve, free of the thrombotic, infectious, and hemodynamic problems of its predecessors.

This initial groundswell of enthusiasm was tempered when the reality of artificial valve replacement was revealed by careful scrutiny of the performance of each prosthesis. Reports detailed the limited longevity and unique pathological complications of artificial valves, and led to renewed interest in the preservation of the native aortic valve architecture. Experiments in our laboratory demonstrated that heavily calcified aortic valves could be debrided using carbon dioxide laser irradiation (50). King et al. (17) and Mindich and colleagues (18) continued in their attempts to manually debride aortic valves intraoperatively. At the same time, however, several groups of pediatric investigators were performing ground-breaking experiments that would herald the era of percutaneous treatment of valvular heart disease.

Lock and colleagues created a model of pulmonary branch stenosis in newborn lambs and went on to successfully dilate the stenosis with a balloon catheter (51). Lababidi and Wu (52) and Jan et al. (53) reported successful balloon dilation of pulmonic valve stenosis in children in 1982, and Lababidi et al., in 1984, was the first to report on balloon aortic valvuloplasty in children with congenital aortic stenosis (54).

2. Balloon Valvuloplasty

a. Acute Hemodynamic Results. In 1986, following the example set by these pioneering efforts, Cribier et al. in France (55) and McKay et al. (56) in the United States reported on the use of balloon valvuloplasty in adults with acquired aortic stenosis.

Cribier et al.'s report detailed this experience in three patients who had refused, or were considered poor risks for, aortic valve replacement. The brachial artery approach was used, primarily because of the short length of the balloon catheters, originally designed for use in pediatric congenital valvular disease. Three inflations of 20–60 s each were performed using catheters of 8, 10, and 12 mm diameter in succession. Aortic pressure was monitored continuously in all patients and did not fall below 60 mmHg at any time during balloon inflations. No significant complications occurred, and aortic root angiography performed after the procedure disclosed no significant degree of aortic insufficiency. After the procedure, the peak aortic valve gradient had fallen from 90 to 40, 80 to 30, and 60 to 30 mmHg in the three patients, respectively, with aortic valve area improving from 0.46 to 0.96 and 0.5 to 0.75 cm^2 in the last two patients in whom cardiac output measurements were made.

Similarly, the results reported shortly thereafter by McKay and colleagues suggested this method's potential for treating calcific aortic stenosis percutaneously. After performing a series of postmortem and then intraoperative balloon aortic valvuloplasties (in which the valves were all subsequently excised for pathological examination), two elderly patients who had refused surgical intervention underwent aortic valvuloplasty by a femoral approach. The first patient was treated with three inflations of a 12-mm balloon, while the second patient had serial inflations with 12-, 15-, and 18-mm balloons. Again, neither patient suffered serious complications, and postprocedure aortography revealed only a mild increase in aortic insufficiency in both patients. Peak transvalvular gradients were reduced from 66 to 32 and 44 to 31 mmHg and aortic valve areas increased from 0.4 to 0.6 and 0.5 to 0.7 cm^2 in these two patients.

At the time of these reports, we and others began to accumulate experience with this technique (57). In our laboratories, patients were selected based on either their refusal of or noncandidacy for aortic valve surgery. Patients in the latter group included those for whom surgery posed an inordinate risk, as well as patients whose life expectancy was limited by other conditions (e.g., metastatic carcinoma).

In the first 52 patients treated in our series, the average mean gradient decreased from 48.8 ± 3.0 mmHg (mean $\pm$ SEM) before valvuloplasty to 23.8 ± 2.0 mmHg after valvuloplasty. This was associated with an increase in cardiac output from 3.5 ± 0.2 to 3.9 ± 0.2 L/min and a corresponding increase in aortic valve area from 0.46 ± 0.03 to 0.86 ± 0.06 cm^2. Aortic insufficiency, as assessed by angiography, Doppler echocardiography, and/or physical examination did not increase significantly in the group. This hemodynamic improvement translated into a significant clinical benefit in the majority of patients; 76% of patients were in NYHA class II or III before valvuloplasty, while only 9% remained in these classes after the procedure.

Subsequent studies in hundreds of patients (58,59) confirmed the ability of balloon valvuloplasty to confer immediate hemodynamic and symptomatic improvement in the majority of patients. It is interesting to note that the postvalvuloplasty hemodynamic profiles in all of these reports were still compatible with the diagnosis of severe aortic stenosis in the majority of patients. This seeming incongruity became acceptable by virtue of a series of observations which came to light as data on the results of valvuloplasty began to accumulate. First, the procedure was initially performed in patients for whom it was the sole option, i.e., they were considered poor operative candidates or had refused aortic valve replacement. Second, refinements in the equipment and in operator technique were expected to improve the outcome over time. Finally, the clinical improvement in the patients was irrefutable and occurred regardless of the apparently persistent critical aortic valve obstruction. As some surgeons had noted three decades earlier, ". . . small. . . increase(s) of the effective aortic orifice can bring about considerable clinical improvement" (60).

b. Long-Term Results. Indeed, early reports confirmed that modest hemodynamic improvement was sufficient to accomplish substantial clinical improvement in most patients (39,55–57). The disparity between hemodynamics and clinical status in patients treated with balloon valvuloplasty persisted when patients are followed over time. In several series (61–63) a significant percentage of patients returned toward their baseline, prevalvuloplasty hemodynamics within 6 months, while only a much smaller percentage had a proportionate return of symptoms. The reason(s) for this paradox are unknown, but may involve some recovery of intrinsic left ventricular function which is allowed to occur by the, albeit partial and temporary, amelioration of the stress of obstruction.

In an attempt to improve upon the unsatisfying postvalvuloplasty hemodynamics, a double-balloon technique was employed for a period of time in our laboratory (64). Patients were selected for the dual-balloon approach if single-balloon valvuloplasty resulted in a residual peak gradient of greater than 35 mmHg or a calculated aortic valve area of less than 0.5 cm^2. The dual-balloon procedure was performed immediately after assessing the hemodynamic results of the single-balloon dilation, allowing comparison of results within an individual patient. Peak aortic valve gradient decreased from 79 ± 8 mmHg prevalvuloplasty to 57 ± 7 mmHg after single-balloon dilation and further decreased to 36 ± 4 mmHg after the double-balloon technique. Similarly, mean gradient decreased from 56 ± 5 to 42 ± 5 and then to 27 ± 3 mmHg and aortic valve area increased from 0.45 ± 0.04 to 0.57 ± 0.05 and finally to 0.77 ± 0.05 cm^2, respectively, using the two techniques.

Unfortunately, although these early results were favorable, the incidence of restenosis was not diminished (65). Indeed, the most disheartening aspect of balloon valvuloplasty in adult aortic stenosis has been restenosis. While most of the data on follow-up have been collected using noninvasive techniques, invasive hemodynamic data collected in a few series corroborate the noninvasive findings. In a group of 40 patients followed in our laboratory for 2 to 12 months (mean 6.3 months), echocardiography revealed a return of the ventriculoaortic pressure gradient to near preprocedure levels in 62% of patients. The mean aortic valve gradient in this group of patients was 65 mmHg before valvuloplasty, decreased to 40 mmHg immediately after valvuloplasty, but then increased to 50 mmHg in follow-up. Aortic valve area averaged 0.53 cm^2 prevalvuloplasty, increased to 0.77 cm^2 post-, and fell to an average of 0.63 cm^2.

The clinical outcome in these patients reflected the paradox mentioned previously, with symptomatic improvement seemingly out of proportion to, and more durable than, the hemodynamic benefits. At 6-month follow-up, three patients had died while three others had undergone aortic valve surgery. In the remaining group of 34 patients, 26 were in NYHA functional classes III and IV prevalvuloplasty, while 19 of 21 were class I or II at 6-month follow-up.

    c. Indications. The inability of balloon aortic valvuloplasty to confer a hemodynamic result comparable to that of aortic valve replacement has consigned valvuloplasty to a "second string" position on the list of treatment options for patients with aortic stenosis. This is not to say, however, that it is without some important potential advantages and discrete indications.

    In elderly or debilitated patients who are at high risk for aortic valve surgery, balloon aortic valvuloplasty provides a lower-risk option for relief of symptoms. In many of these patients the lack of durability of the results is less of a concern due to poor overall life expectancy. Letac and colleagues (66) have reported their results in a series of 92 patients aged 80 and older who had balloon aortic valvuloplasty as primary treatment for aortic stenosis. Eighty-two of these patients were in NYHA functional classes III and IV before the procedure. Twenty percent of the patients had associated pathological conditions which made them unacceptable surgical candidates. Peak gradient averaged 71 ± 27 mmHg before the procedure and the calculated aortic valve area averaged $0.48 \pm 0.16 \text{ cm}^2$. After valvuloplasty the aortic valve gradient had decreased to 27 ± 15 mmHg and the valve area rose to $0.91 \pm 0.35 \text{ cm}^2$. The periprocedural mortality was 6.5%, with three deaths occurring in the catheterization laboratory in critically ill patients aged 82, 92, and 98 years. There was no stroke and one case of transient complete heart block treated with temporary pacing. At follow-up among 62 patients who had their procedure an average of 13 months earlier (the other 30 had their procedure within 5 months), late mortality was 29%. Among the 44 survivors, nine were in NYHA functional class III (none in class IV) at follow-up versus 14 in class IV and 24 in class III before valvuloplasty. These results echo those of previous reports: Safian et al. (58) reported a 27% mortality in follow-up of 44 patients over 80 years old, while Block and Palacios (67) reported 28% mortality at 5-month follow-up in a group of 90 patients averaging 79 years old. These results must be viewed in context: In the latter two series patients were selected for valvuloplasty generally because they were considered at extremely high risk for surgery. Balloon aortic valvuloplasty in this setting is performed on a "compassionate" basis for palliation of symptoms that would not be treated otherwise.

    Another niche which has been suggested for aortic valvuloplasty is as a life-saving measure in patients who present in extremis (68). These individuals might otherwise qualify for aortic valve surgery, but enter the hospital in such debilitated condition as to make consideration for aortic valve replacement impossible. In such patients valvuloplasty is proposed as a "bridge" to more definitive therapy. In our initial experience of 52 patients, 2 presented in cardiogenic shock with left ventricular ejection fractions less than 20%, on pressors to maintain systemic perfusion. Aortic balloon valvuloplasty was performed emergently in both patients. In the first, peak transaortic gradient was decreased from 88 to 33 mmHg and cardiac output increased from 2.1 to 3.0 L/min. After 2 days cardiac output had risen further to 4.6 L/min and renal function had returned to a sufficient degree to allow discontinuation of peritoneal dialysis. This particular patient was discharged and remained in NYHA functional class II for several months. Repeat Doppler echocardiography 10 months later revealed return of critical aortic stenosis. This was confirmed at catheterization, as was a marked improvement in LV function with an ejection fraction of 45%. She subsequently underwent uncomplicated aortic valve replacement.

This very discrete patient population represents a setting in which balloon aortic valvuloplasty may be both immediately life-saving and allow for the later performance of more definitive treatment of aortic stenosis.

An analogous indication for valvuloplasty is in patients who require noncardiac surgery. Levine et al. (69) performed aortic valvuloplasty in 7 patients in preparation for noncardiac surgery. The group consisted of 4 men and 3 women, aged 65–83 years (mean 74), with syncope (1 pt.), angina (1 pt.), congestive heart failure (3 pts.) or angina and failure (1 pt.). The conditions requiring surgical procedures included 3 hip fractures and one each of lung carcinoma, colonic carcinoma, gastric bleeding, and urinary obstruction. The mean peak aortic valve gradient of 66 ± 34 was reduced to 28 ± 17 mmHg, with an associated rise in calculated aortic valve area from 0.6 ± 0.2 to 0.9 ± 0.3 cm^2 while cardiac index remained stable. All of the patients in this series underwent the planned surgical procedures, and only one suffered hemodynamic problems during surgery. The remaining 6 were discharged from the hospital in good condition. Hayes and colleagues (70) dilated severely stenotic aortic valves in 15 patients with the idea of improving hemodynamics and reducing the risk of planned noncardiac surgery and diagnostic procedures. None of these patients were considered candidates for aortic valve replacement because concomitant medical conditions either precluded surgery or precluded long-term survival. Palliative balloon valvuloplasty reduced the mean aortic gradient in this group from 58.1 ± 6.0 to 32.2 ± 4.0 mmHg and aortic valve area was increased from 0.5 ± 0.0 to 0.9 ± 0.1 cm^2. There was one procedure-related death. In the remaining 14 patients the planned noncardiac surgical and surgical-diagnostic procedures were performed without complications.

The interpretation of these small series is hampered by the lack of a control group. The increased risk of noncardiac surgical procedures in patients with severe aortic stenosis has been well shown, and for this reason aortic valve replacement has been advocated in certain instances (71). While a reduction in risk could be expected if the hemodynamic burden of aortic stenosis were alleviated in these patients, the additive risk of surgical valve replacement would detract from the overall benefit. Balloon valvuloplasty in these cases offers the attractive possibility of a lower-risk procedure with which to relieve aortic stenosis and therefore lower the risk of noncardiac surgery.

In addition, patients with critical aortic stenosis are known to be at increased risk of complications, including death, from diagnostic cardiac catherization (72). These patients typically enter the hospital in stable condition but deteriorate acutely during catheterization. Standard resuscitative measures generally fail to produce significant hemodynamic improvement in these patients. We have used emergency "bailout" balloon valvuloplasty in three such patients (73). In all three patients severe hypotension developed after left heart catheterization which was refractory to multiple pressor agents; two patients required emergent intubation for pulmonary edema and severe dyspnea. Emergency balloon valvuloplasty was performed successfully in each patient, allowing pressors and ventilatory support to be weaned and discontinued. Two of the patients were well several months later, one after aortic valve replacement and the other after refusing the same. The third patient died of a subsequently discovered bronchogenic carcinoma.

d. Contraindications. It is clear from the above discussion that the set of clinical criteria which define candidates for balloon aortic valvuloplasty is evolving. Better defined are the guidelines for exclusion from consideration. Patients who are good operative candidates and whose prognosis is not limited by comorbid conditions are generally not considered for balloon valvuloplasty.

The significant incidence of coronary artery disease in the generally elderly patient population with calcific aortic stenosis must be considered in any strategy for patient selection for valvuloplasty. In patients for whom surgical risk is not prohibitive, combined aortic valve replacement and coronary artery bypass grafting is the procedure of choice in the presence of coexistent coronary disease. If significant coronary disease is discovered in combination with aortic stenosis in a patient who is not a candidate for surgery, valvuloplasty can be combined with angioplasty in a staged or serial fashion (74–76). McKay et al. (74) reported results in 9 patients who underwent simultaneous valvuloplasty and angioplasty. After successful valvuloplasty (mean aortic valve gradient reduced from 60 ± 19 mmHg to 30 ± 13 mmHg, $p < 0.01$), PTCA was performed in three left anterior descending, three left circumflex, two right coronary, and one right coronary bypass vessels. In this group, 8 of 9 patients had relief of symptoms, with one going on to aortic valve replacement and coronary bypass. At 6-month follow-up, 7 of 8 patients had persistent clinical improvement, with coronary and aortic valve restenosis in the remaining patient.

Another theoretical contraindication to valvuloplasty is an anticipated poor response to balloon dilation. To date no prospective markers have been successfully applied as predictors of outcome after aortic valvuloplasty. Retrospectively, however, one group of patients has emerged which seems to account for a disproportionate number of treatment failures and major complications—those with congenitally bicuspid aortic valves (Fig. 8). In an analysis of over 100 patients treated with balloon aortic valvuloplasty in our laboratories, a total of 5 have failed to achieve any significant hemodynamic improvement from balloon dilation, 2 of

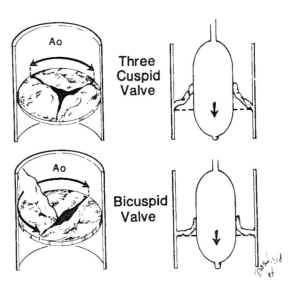

Figure 8 Balloon valvuloplasty and valvular morphology. In case of three-cuspid valve, blood flow persists during balloon inflation through three commissures. In bicuspid valve, inflated balloon tends to occlude residual orifice.

whom experienced sudden and irreversible hypotension as a result of balloon inflation. Four of these patients were later shown to have congenitally bicuspid aortic valves (57,77). Empirically, the resistance of bicuspid aortic valves to balloon dilation should relate to their anatomy. Indeed, both gross and microscopic anatomical considerations could have a role in the behavior of these valves. The greater arc of attachment of the conjoined leaflet of the bicuspid valve may account for part of its resistance to balloon dilation. Microscopically, as indicated above, the histoarchitecture of bicuspid valves has been shown to differ from that of congenitally normal valves (6), and may also contribute to their refractoriness.

   e. Technique. Although the first published series of adult balloon aortic valvuloplasties consisted of cases performed using the brachial artery approach (55), most investigators, including Cribier, now favor the femoral artery approach. This preference reflects the need for an access site capable of accommodating the larger-size balloons now in general use for aortic valvuloplasty. In Cribier's pilot series, balloons were 3 cm in length and ranged from 8 to 12 mm in diameter. These balloons were found to be lacking in two respects: First, their diameter was insufficient to confer maximum hemodynamic benefit; and second, their relatively short length made it difficult to maintain a stable balloon position across the aortic valve. At the present time balloons of a length of approximately 5.5 cm are used, ranging in diameter from 15 to 25 mm, sizes clearly in excess of what could be safely advanced using the brachial artery in most patients.

   At the present time our protocol is as follows: After providing adequate local anesthesia (considering the duration of the procedure and the significant arteriotomy which will come about as the result of balloon passage and removal), an 8F sheath is placed percutaneously in the femoral artery using the Seldinger technique while an 8F sheath is placed in the femoral vein, and a 6F sheath in the femoral artery on the opposite side. After initial right heart catheterization, a 7F pigtail catheter is positioned in the ascending aorta. A 0.038-in. straight guidewire is then used to cross the aortic valve, and the pigtail catheter is positioned within the left ventricle. Hemodynamics are measured, including cardiac output determinations. A 260-cm, J-tipped, multiple-curve exchange wire is then advanced via the pigtail catheter and, leaving the wire in the ventricle, the catheter and 8F sheath are removed. Balloon sizing is estimated according to patient size. An average-sized male will be dilated with a 20-mm balloon initially, while smaller patients, typically female, will be started with an 18-mm or 15-mm balloon. Very rarely, either because of a very restricted valve orifice or tortuous peripheral vasculature making passage of the balloon across the valve difficult, an 8-mm balloon, usually reserved for performing atrial septostomies for mitral valvuloplasties, will be used to create a "pilot hole" for larger balloons. The dilating balloon is centered across the aortic valve and an average of one to three inflations are generally performed. Balloons are inflated with a diluted solution of one part contrast and four parts saline until they are expanded to full width and the presence of any "waist" indenting the midportion of the balloon is eliminated. After this is accomplished, the balloon is fully deflated under negative pressure and removed over an exchange wire. The 8F sheath, which affords some hemostasis (along with manual pressure), and diagnostic catheter are then replaced and complete hemodynamics are repeated. If the residual peak gradient is greater than 35 mmHg or if the calculated valve area remains below 0.5 cm^2, the diagnostic catheter/sheath assembly is once again removed over an exchange wire and the next larger balloon size (23 mm, 25 mm) is implemented as described above. Previously, in the hope of improving both the short- and long-term outcome, a double-balloon technique was used in patients with a less than adequate result after single-balloon inflation. This technique required a duplication of the above-described procedure for single-balloon passage to be performed in the opposite femoral artery, allowing simultaneous positioning of two balloons across the aortic valve. As noted in a previous section, this technique did not result in any improvement in long-term results. We have since found that with due diligence, sometimes requiring multiple inflations, we are able to achieve a reasonable hemodynamic result using a single balloon in most patients, thus avoiding double jeopardy in terms of potential for vascular complications.

When intravascular ultrasound is performed as part of the valvuloplasty procedure, the technique is modified as follows: While maintaining hemostasis at the femoral artery puncture site, an 8F, 85-cm introducer sheath fitted with an 8F pigtail catheter is advanced over the exchange wire and, after positioning the sheath within the left ventricle, the guidewire and pigtail are removed. With the sheath in stable position across the aortic valve, a 6F IVUS catheter is then able to be passed via the sheath to examine the aortic valve. In addition to evaluating aortic valve morphology, IVUS also affords the opportunity to examine the peripheral vasculature before passage of dilating balloons. In some patients the observations of peripheral vascular pathology made with IVUS may lead to changes in strategy, such as using longer introducer sheaths to bypass femoral or iliac stenoses. After completion of the IVUS examination, the ultrasound catheter is removed and an exchange wire is again positioned in the left ventricle. The long sheath is then removed from the ventricle and from the body and the dilating balloon is advanced over the guidewire. After final hemodynamics document a satisfactory result, the 8F, 85-cm sheath is once again positioned across the aortic valve to allow repeat IVUS examination of the aortic valve. In terms of impact on patient management, this follow-up examination is clearly supplementary and may be foregone in certain cases. When it is performed, the results generally confirm improvement in leaflet mobility as well as occasionally demonstrating a "crack" in the aortic valve calcific deposits.

Occasionally, severe peripheral vascular disease will preclude the retrograde femoral approach to aortic valvuloplasty. In these patients the antegrade (trans-septal) approach has been applied. Block and Palacios (78) reported results in a group of 55 patients, 25 of whom underwent antegrade and 30 retrograde aortic valvuloplasty. In this nonrandomized series, those treated by the retrograde approach started with higher transvalvular gradients and lower calculated aortic valve areas. Both groups realized significant improvement in hemodynamics postvalvuloplasty. The antegrade group, however, enjoyed freedom from vascular complications, while 4 thrombectomies were required in the retrograde group. Conversely, in the antegrade group, 2 patients suffered episodes of complete heart block, which did not occur in the retrograde patients. It appears, then, that while the antegrade approach offers some distinct advantages over the retrograde approach in certain patients, the added burden of the trans-septal technique is probably not warranted in most patients.

f. Mechanism. Several mechanisms have been described by which balloon dilation confers hemodynamic benefit in calcific aortic stenosis (79). In their original series, McKay et al. (56) first described the results of balloon dilation in 10 postmortem and intraoperative cases in which the effects could be observed directly. This same group later expanded this experience to include 33 postmortem and 6 intraoperative specimens (80). In both of these series the predominant structural change caused by balloon dilation was fracture or disruption of calcific nodules on the valve leaflets (Fig. 9). In a number of cases these fractures occurred as the "hinge" points of valve leaflets. This was associated with enhanced leaflet mobility and therefore correlates with improved hemodynamics. Another important finding included separation of fused valve commissures, although this is not the principal pathological abnormality which restricts leaflet motion in patients with acquired calcific aortic stenosis. Finally, "microfractures" in valvular calcium were postulated as the mechanism of improved leaflet mobility in cases in which gross fractures were not visible. Other investigators have termed this phenomenon "calcium redistribution" (81). No consistent histological correlate of this phenomenon has been observed, however, and the mechanism of improvement in these cases could be open to speculation. Interestingly, pathological examination of valves several months after valvuloplasty has revealed proliferation

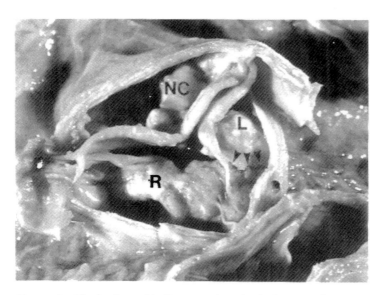

Figure 9 Mechanism of balloon aortic valvuloplasty: A fracture (arrowheads) is seen in calcific portion of left (L) cusp of heavily calcified, congenitally normal, three-cusp aortic valve. NC = noncoronary; R = right.

of granulation tissue in the fracture lines (Fig. 10), presumably the result of balloon dilation, in the aortic valve calcium (82). This may serve as a partial explanation of the restenosis process, as well as verifying the primary mechanism.

A perhaps more interesting and as yet incompletely explained phenomenon is the continued relief of symptoms in patients who experience restenosis. A significant percentage of patients will return to a hemodynamic state which is virtually indistinguishable from their prevalvuloplasty status and yet will retain an improved functional and symptomatic class. While no series of patients has undergone routine follow-up catheterization, some information is available from partial series and noninvasive, i.e., Doppler echocardiography, evaluation. In our laboratory (83), Doppler examinations of 40 patients at a mean of 6.3 months postvalvuloplasty revealed that the ventriculoaortic gradient, which had been reduced significantly at the time of the procedure, was no longer statistically different than the preprocedure gradient in 62% of patients. In this same cohort, while most were in NYHA classes III and IV before valvuloplasty, all but 2 patients were in classes I and II at follow-up.

This discrepancy between clinical and hemodynamic status may be partially explained by results reported by McKay and colleagues (84).

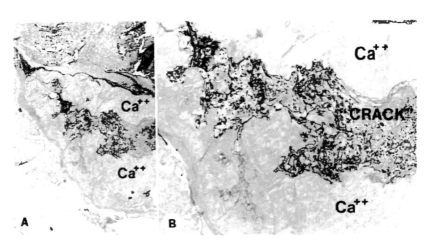

Figure 10 Potential mechanism of restenosis following balloon aortic valvuloplasty. Low-power (A) and high-power (B) light photomicrographs illustrating apparent "sealing in" of fracture created during valvuloplasty of heavily calcified (Ca^{2+}) aortic valve performed 6 months prior to death in this patient.

Using radionuclide angiography and Doppler echocardiography, 32 patients were studied before and after valvuloplasty for severe aortic stenosis. In addition to documenting the usual immediate hemodynamic improvement in terms of reduction in aortic valve gradient and increase in aortic valve area, several new findings came to light. In patients who presented with a depressed left ventricular ejection fraction (<55%), there was a significant improvement in this index after successful valvuloplasty (LVEF 40 ± 13% to 46 ± 12%, $p < 0.03$). In addition, left ventricular end-diastolic volume decreased (138 ± 38 mL/m² to 101 ± 37 mL/m², $p < 0.003$), as did LV ejection time (0.44 ± 0.03 s to 0.42 ± 0.02 s, $p < 0.01$). All of these suggest an improvement in left ventricular function conferred by valvuloplasty. Obviously, the reduced loading conditions play a significant role in altering the metrics employed here, but these observations allude to an important alternative or additional explanation for the clinical improvement in valvuloplasty treated patients. Gradual and progressive deterioration in left ventricular function is an established part of the natural history of aortic stenosis, manifested by chamber dilation, reduction in LVEF, onset of congestive symptoms, and eventuating in death. These changes occur in a relatively brief time span when compared to the hemodynamic criteria for aortic stenosis, which are present in patients for many years before measurable left ventricular dysfunction ensues. Nevertheless, this decline is progressive with time and has been shown to be reversible to some extent by relief of the hemodynamic burden on the left ventricle. This relief was previously accomplished on a more or less permanent basis by timely aortic valve replacement, and it was noted that the natural history of the disease process was halted or significantly curtailed. At some point in the progression of this degenerative process, however, it becomes irreversible despite valve replacement. From these facts it seems reasonable to conclude that aortic stenosis provokes incremental changes in the structure (and, therefore, function) of the left ventricle over time which are reparable for a limited period of time if the aortic stenosis is relieved. If this structural change is, as it must be, related to the duration and severity of the stenosis, it also seems probable that any reduction in the stenosis will allow some reversal to occur. This may, in effect, "turn the clock back" on this degenerative process. Balloon valvuloplasty could act in this manner, by allowing the ventricle to repair itself so that it is better prepared to withstand the hemodynamic burden which returns in so many patients. This would explain the fact that symptomatic benefit is out of proportion to hemodynamic change, measured by the usual parameters, in these patients as well.

   g. Complications.   Previous reports have indicated that the principal morbidity of balloon aortic valvuloplasty in adults (59,74) consists of local vascular trauma at the site of catheter introduction. This particular complication can usually be managed conservatively or with minor surgical repair, resulting in no long-term sequelae. Moreover, availability of lower-profile balloon catheters has further reduced the incidence of local vascular morbidity.

   In contrast, less attention has been given to those complications of balloon aortic valvuloplasty which more directly threaten life and/or limb. There are at least two reasons why such serious complications may have been underemphasized in these previous studies. First, in none of these previous reports was the issue of complications the principal focus of the investigation. Second, most previous reports typically summarized the experience of a single institution and thereby involved a relatively small number of patients. Availability of the Mansfield Registry data (84) therefore has provided a unique opportunity to investigate this issue systematically in a relatively large cohort of patients. An additional advantage of Registry data for analysis of procedure-related complications is that institutional and investigator anonymity was preserved.

   The results of this Registry analysis indicated that the frequency of catastrophic complications among patients undergoing balloon aortic valvuloplasty was 6.3% of. Furthermore, two findings were common among those patients in whom such complications were recognized: female gender and the use of dual-balloon valvuloplasty. Additional aspects of the individual complication categories merit specific comment.

Ventricular perforation has been previously recognized as a potentially catastrophic complication of percutaneous balloon aortic valvuloplasty (58,85). Analysis of the nine Registry patients in whom this complication occurred in the present study disclosed several important points. First, perforation is not necessarily fatal: Two patients survived following pericardiocentesis alone, while a third improved transiently before successful operative repair. Pericardiocentesis thus appears to be critical in dealing successfully with perforation complicating balloon valvuloplasty; moreover, lack of hemodynamic improvement following balloon valvuloplasty represents an ominous prognostic sign. Second, the high percentage of serial (67%) and dual (78%) balloon inflations suggests that the more maneuvers and instrumentation employed for a particular case, the greater is the likelihood of perforation. While the precise basis for this observation remains to be more fully defined, the relationship may be simply statistical; that is, the more wires and catheters are advanced into the left ventricle, and the more exchangers are required for such instrumentation, the greater is the likelihood that perforation will result. Because the timing of perforation was never precisely identified in any of the nine cases, determination of the instrument responsible for perforation (wire versus diagnostic or dilation catheter) remains uncertain.

Necropsy and operative data from the Registry study does, however, allow conclusions regarding the site of perforation. Although the left ventricular apex, due to the minimal wall thickness typical of that site, generally has been considered to be the most vulnerable site for perforation, perforation during balloon aortic valvuloplasty more commonly involved the base of the left ventricular free wall. In-vitro studies intended to evaluate this point have been carried out in our laboratory in intact hearts obtained fresh at necropsy and have in fact demonstrated that a standard 0.035- or 0.038-in. exchange wire, with and without balloon dilation catheter, introduced retrograde across the aortic valve, have a natural tendency to advance toward the base of the left ventricular free wall; furthermore, both may be easily advanced through even hypertrophied myocardium with no exceptional force (Slovenaki GA, Isner JM, unpublished observations). Age-related angulation of the ventricular septum and diminution in left ventricular chamber size may facilitate this path of catheter/wire advancement. Eccentric malposition of the residual aortic valve orifice due to a congenitally bicuspid valve, documented at necropsy in 1 of the 9 perforations, would be expected to aggravate such catheter/wire misdirection.

While exacerbation of aortic regurgitation has been previously described following balloon aortic valvuloplasty, the magnitude of this complication is typically mild, hemodynamically insignificant, and often resolves spontaneously (58). In contrast, acute severe aortic regurgitation has been rarely observed to complicate percutaneous aortic valvuloplasty. Safian et al. (58) described two patients in whom "important increases in aortic regurgitation" occurred after dilation; one patient died, while the other survived without surgery. Both patients had evidence of leaflet tears. Brady et al. (86) described one patient in whom "a marked increase in aortic regurgitation" developed postvalvuloplasty. Alexopoulous and Sherman (87) described one patient in whom acute onset of severe aortic regurgitation was manifested hemodynamically as transmission of atrial contraction to the aortic pressure tracing. Seifert and Auer (88) successfully repaired an aortic annular disruption in a patient in whom massive, acute aortic regurgitation resulted from dual-balloon aortic valvuloplasty. Among the four patients who developed acute, severe aortic regurgitation in the Registry study, three required aortic valve replacement and a fourth patient died. These four cases were notable for the fact that all were women, and two of four involved the use of dual-balloon inflation. Review of necropsy and operative data suggested four possible bases for the development of acute, severe aortic valvular insufficiency: (1) annular dilation without loss of leaflet integrity; (2) leaflet dehiscence from the site of annular attachment; (3) intraleaflet tear between nodular calcific deposits involving a single leaflet; and (4) intraleaflet tear due to partial fusion of one commissure. The latter three have in common a differential elastic modulus of the calcified versus noncalcified portions of a single leaflet.

The most common catastrophe among the initial 492 patients treated with balloon aortic valvuloplasty in the Mansfield study was a fatal cardiac arrest. This complication has been infrequently documented in previous reports of balloon aortic valvuloplasty (89). Data in the Registry investigation was used to classify patients arbitrarily into three subgroups: (1) the clinical course of 7 patients was consistent with cardiogenic shock; (2) the deaths of 4 patients were caused by recurrent, malignant ventricular tachyarrhythmias; and (3) the basis for abrupt death of 2 additional patients remains uncertain. This classification scheme is compromised by the fact that not all 13 patients underwent necropsy examination; furthermore, most patients did not undergo coronary arteriographic examination. Nevertheless, certain features of this group deserve emphasis. Unlike the sex distribution noted for the other four categories of catastrophic complications, the majority (7/13, 54%) of individuals in whom death was due to a cardiac arrest were male. Six of the 13 patients underwent serial balloon dilation; dual-balloon inflation was employed in 5. A congenitally malformed (bicuspid) aortic valve was documented in 2 patients at necropsy.

Reconstruction of the clinical course of these 13 Registry patients suggests at least three potential mechanisms for fatal cardiac arrest following balloon aortic valvuloplasty. In those patients with a congenitally bicuspid aortic valve, balloon inflation appears to completely occlude the aortic valve orifice (79); in contrast, antegrade blood flow typically persists at each of the three commissural junctions of the congenitally normal, tricuspid aortic valve. A calcified, congenitally bicuspid valve has been previously documented at necropsy in three patients in whom a fatal cardiac arrest occurred as the result of balloon valvuloplasty (79). In at least one of the above 13 patients in whom left main coronary artery stenosis was demonstrated angiographically prevalvuloplasty, fatal cardiac arrest may have resulted from occlusion of the left and/or right coronary ostia during balloon inflation. A similar mechanism may have been responsible for two previously reported cases of nonfatal acute myocardial infarction (58,90). A third potential basis for fatal cardiac arrest in these patients is transient stunning of the left ventricle during the period of balloon inflation. DeLezo et al. (91) have documented a slow, progressive decrease in systolic pressure subsequent to increased left ventricular pressure generated during the first five to six beats of aortic valvular balloon inflation. This decremental pressure pattern was unrelated to balloon deflation and in fact persisted for several beats following balloon deflation, even while aortic pressure was increasing. These hemodynamic changes corresponded to angiographic evidence of dyskinesis and a transient reduction in ejection fraction.

Fatal cerebrovascular accidents occurred in two Registry patients, embolic in one, and possibly hemorrhagic in the other. Interestingly, dual-balloon inflation was utilized in the former. Fatal cerebrovascular accident has been reported in at least one previous patient undergoing balloon valvuloplasty (90). The incidence of nonfatal peripheral embolic phenomena in most published series of balloon aortic valvuloplasty has been less than 2%. Whether such presumed emboli represent calcific emboli from valvular calcific deposits or emboli related to the thrombogenic wires and/or catheters, or even transient hypotension during balloon inflation causing focal ischemia of a watershed or other jeopardized area, remains speculative.

While amputation has not been previously reported as a complication of balloon aortic valvuloplasty, peripheral vascular trauma has consistently been observed as the principal complication of percutaneous aortic valvuloplasty (58,59,74). Two of three Registry patients who required amputation were women. In two of the three, serial balloon inflations were performed with use of a 23-mm-diameter balloon that, because of its bulky size, could not be inserted and removed through conventional introducer sheaths. Previous experience with large-profile balloon-dilating catheters indicated that wire-guided introduction without the use of an introducer sheath was associated with a significant incidence of peripheral vascular trauma unless local surgical cutdown was employed. In one of the three patients requiring amputation, emergency balloon valvuloplasty performed following a cardiac arrest was complicated by rupture of a 23-mm balloon; during catheter withdrawal, the redundant wings of the ruptured balloon became entangled with a previously inserted intraaortic balloon catheter, leading to arterial dissection, and ultimately amputation.

Although most cases of balloon rupture typically involve a longitudinal tear, circumferential tears have been documented as well (92); the latter appear to increase the hazard of vascular trauma during balloon-catheter retrieval. In the absence of data indicating either a favorable effect on acute and/or chronic outcome, these findings raise serious questions regarding the use of intentional balloon rupture as a means of optimizing the results of balloon aortic valvuloplasty.

Two catastrophic complications which have been previously reported by others were not observed among the Registry patients. Lembo et al. (93) described an 86-year-old man in whom serial inflation of 15-mm, 20-mm, 3 × 12-mm (Trefoil), and 23-mm balloons resulted in fatal pericardial tamponade due to a ruptured aorta. In another patient receiving chronic steroid therapy for lupus erythematosus (94), positive blood cultures for staphylococcus epidermis developed 2 weeks postvalvuloplasty. Despite 5 weeks of antibiotic therapy, the patient died. Necropsy findings included a ring abscess around a congenitally bicuspid aortic valve.

h. Conclusion. History has a way of repeating itself, and it is therefore safe to say that the "final chapter" has not been written on the treatment of aortic stenosis. At this stage, however, a few conclusions about *balloon* aortic valvuloplasty are well supported. It appears capable of improving hemodynamics acutely in the majority of patients with calcific stenosis of congenitally normal (three-cuspid) aortic valves. In these patients, even modest amelioration of the aortic valve gradient may be associated with significant clinical improvement. Patients with calcific stenosis of congenitally bicuspid valves may be somewhat immune to any benefit from balloon dilation, and may also be predisposed to significant complications. Restenosis, with the return of critical hemodynamics in most patients, and of symptoms in the majority, is the rule. For this reason, balloon aortic valvuloplasty is restricted to discrete patient populations for whom the more permanent solution of valve replacement is contraindicated.

C. Timing of Surgery

Since mortality is high after the onset of symptoms in patients with severe aortic stenosis, such patients should undergo surgery. Asymptomatic patients should be followed medically (29,40).

Asymptomatic patients with aortic stenosis and left ventricular dysfunction should also be followed medically until the development of symptoms. It has been shown that left ventricular dysfunction is reversible after surgery (41,42).

D. Surgical Treatment

Refer to surgical chapters for detailed discussion.

REFERENCES

1. Roberts WC. The structure of the aortic valve in clinically isolated aortic vascular disease: the case against its being rheumatic etiology. Am J Med 1970; 49:151–9.
2. Roberts WC. The congenitally bicuspid aortic valve: a study of 85 autopsy cases. Am J Cardiol 1970; 26:72–83.
3. Roberts WC. The structure of the aortic valve in clinically isolated aortic stenosis: an autopsy study of 162 patients over 15 years of age. Circulation 1970; 42:91–7.
4. Isner JM, McAllister HA Jr, Fluri-Lundeen J, Ferrans VJ, Khuri S. Gross histologic, and ultrastructural features of cardiac involvement in alkaptonuria (abstr). Lab Invest 1982; 46:40A.
5. Isner JM, Jones AJ, Roberts WC. New risk of an old factor: role of serum cholesterol in calcific disease of the aortic valve (abstr). Circulation 1979; 60:11–47.
6. Isner JM, Chokshi SK, DeFranco A, Braimen J, Slovenkai GA. Contrasting histoarchitecture of calcified leaflets from stenotic bicuspid versus stenotic tricuspid aortic valves. J Am Coll Cardiol 1990; 15:1104–8.
7. Edwards JE. The congenital bicuspid aortic valve. Circulation 1961; 23: 485–8.
8. Nanda NC, Gramiak R, Manning J, Mahoney EB, Lipchik ED, DeWeese JA. Echocardiographic recognition of the congenital bicuspid aortic valve. Circulation 1974; 49:870–5.
9. Brandenburg RO Jr, Tajik AJ, Edwards WD, Reeder GS, Shub C, Seward JB. Accuracy of 2-dimensional echocardiographic diagnosis of congenitally bicuspid aortic valve: echocardiographic-anatomic correlation in 115 patients. Am J Cardiol 1983; 51:1469–73.
10. Whitehead S, Losordo DW, Slovenkai GA, Pandian NG, Isner JM. Transthoracic two-dimensional echocardiography fails to predict native valve morphology in adults with calcific aortic stenosis. Clin Res (in press).
11. Waller BF, Carter JB, Williams HJ Jr, Wang K, Edwards JE. Bicuspid aortic valve: comparison of congenital and acquired types. Circulation 1973; 48: 1140–50.
12. Gussenhoven EJ, vanHerwerden LA, Roelandt J, Bos E, deJong N. Detailed analysis of aortic valve endocarditis: comparison of precordial, esophageal and epicardial two-dimensional echocardiography with surgical findings. JCU 1986; 14:209–11.

13. Fields CD, Isner JM. Balloon valvuloplasty in adults. In: Cleman M, Cabin H, eds. Cardiology Clinics: Interventional Cardiology. Philadelphia: Saundes, 1988:383–419.

14. MacMillan RM, Rees MR, Lumia FJ, Marankao V. Preliminary experience in the use of ultrafast computed tomography to diagnose aortic valve stenosis. Am Heart J 1988; 115:665–71.

15. Fields CD, Isner JM. Ultrafast CT in aortic stenosis (letter). Am Heart J 1988; 116:1647.

16. Isner JM, Losordo DW, Rosenfield K, Ramaswamy K, Kelly S, Pastore JO, Kosowsky BD. Catheter-based intravascular ultrasound discriminates bicuspid from tricuspid valves in adults with calcific aortic stenosis. J Am Coll Cardiol 1990; 15:1310–1317.

17. King RM, Pluth JR, Giuliani ER, Piehler JM. Mechanical decalcification of the aortic valve. Ann Thorac Surg 1986; 42:269–72.

18. Mindich BP, Guarino T, Goldman ME. Aortic valvuloplasty for acquired aortic stenosis. Circulation 1986; 74:I-130-5.

19. Worley SJ, King RM, Edwards WD, Holmes DR. Electrohydraulic shock wave decalcification of stenotic aortic valves: postmortem and intraoperative studies. J Am Coll Cardiol 1988; 12:458–62.

20. Freeman WK, Schaff HV, King RM, Orszulak TA. Ultrasonic aortic valve decalcification: Doppler echocardiographic evaluation (abstr). J Am Coll Cardiol 1988; 11:229A.

21. Isner JM, Braimen J, DeFranco A, Slovenkai GA. Contrasting histoarchitecture of calcific deposits in leaflets from bicuspid versus tricuspid aortic valves. J Am Coll Cardiol 1990; 15:1104–8

22. Chokshi SK, Slovenkai GA, Isner JM. Ultrasonic debridement of aortic valve calcium is effective for three-cuspid, but not congenitally bicuspid, aortic valves (abstr). Clin Res 1989; 37:251A.

23. Kennedy KD, Nishumura RA, Holmes DR, Bailey KR. Natural history of moderate aortic stenosis. J Am Coll Cardiol 1991; 17:313.

24. Wagner W, Selzer A. Patterns of progression of aortic stenosis: a longitudinal hemodynamic study. Circulation 1982; 65:709.

25. Horstkotte D, Loogen F. The natural history of aortic valve disease. Eur Heart J 1988; 9(suppl E):57.

26. Turina J, Hess O, Sepulcri F, Krayenbuehl HP. Spontaneous course of aortic stenosis. Eur Heart J 1987; 8:471.

27. Ross J Jr, Braunwald E. Aortic stenosis. Circulation 1968; 38(suppl V):61.

28. Kelly TA, Rothbart RM. Cooper CM, Kaiser DL, Smucker ML, Gibson RS. Comparison of outcome of asymptomatic to symptomatic patients older than 20 years of age with valvular aortic stenosis. Am J Cardiol 1988; 61:123.

29. Olesen KH, Warburg E. Isolated aortic stenosis—the late prognosis. Acta Med Scand 1957; 160:437.

30. Dineen E, Brent BN. Aortic valve stenosis: comparison of patients with those without chronic congestive heart failure. Am J Cardiol 1986; 57:419.

31. Selzer A. Changing aspects of the natural history of valvular aortic stenosis. N Engl J Med 1987; 317:91.

32. Hakki AH, Kimbiris D, Iskandrian AS, Segal BL, Mintz GS, Bemis CE.

Angina pectoris and coronary artery disease in patients with aortic valvular disease. Am Heart J 1980; 100:441.

33. Ramsdale DR, Bennett DH, Bray CL, Ward C, Beeton DC, Farragher EB. Angina, coronary risk factors and coronary artery disease in patients with valvular disease. A prospective study. Eur Heart J 1984; 5:716.

34. Schaefer A, Jehle J, Loogen F. Indications for coronary angiography in patients with valvular heart disease with respect to risk factors. Z Kardiol 1987; 76:276.

35. Selzer A, Lombard JT. Clinical finding in adult aortic stenosis—then and now. Eur Heart J 1988; 9(suppl E):53.

36. Richards AM, Nicholls MG, Ikram H, Hamilton EJ, Richards RMD. Syncopy in aortic valvular stenosis. Lancet 1984; 327(suppl II):113.

37. Pellikka P, Nishimura RA, Baily KR, Tajik AJ. The natural history of adults with asymptomatic hemodynamically significant aortic stenosis. J Am Coll Cardiol 1990; 15:1012.

38. Chizner MA, Pearle DL, deLeon AC. The natural history of aortic stenosis in adults. Am Heart J 1980; 99:419.

39. Braunwald E. Valvular heart disease. In: Braunwald E, ed. Heart Disease. Philadelphia: Saunders, 1992:1041.

40. Braunwald E. On the natural history of severe aortic stenosis. J Am Coll Cardiol 1990; 15:1018.

41. Croke RP, Pifarre R, Sullivan H, Gunnar R, Loeb H. Reversal of advanced left ventricular dysfunction following aortic valve replacement for aortic stenosis. Ann Thorac Surg 1977; 24:38.

42. Kennedy JW, Doces J, Stewart DK. Left ventricular function before and following aortic valve replacement. Circulation 1977; 56:944.

43. Tuffier T. Etat actuel de la chirugie intrathoracique. Trans Int Cong Med London, 1913:sec. 7, Surg, pt 2, p. 249, 1914.

44. Smithy HG, Parker EF. Experimental aortic valvulotomy. Surg Gynec Obst 1947; 84:625–8.

45. Bailey CP. Surgery of the Heart. Philadelphia: Lea & Febiger, 1955:740–2.

46. Harken DE, Black H, Taylor WJ, Thrower WB, Soroff HS. The surgical correction of calcific aortic stenosis in adults. Results in the first 100 consecutive transaortic valvuloplasties. J Thorac Surg 1958; 36:759–76.

47. MacMillan IKR. Aortic stenosis: a post-mortem cine-photographic study of valve action. Br Heart J 1955; 17:56–62.

48. Kirklin JW, Mankin HT. Open operation in the treatment of calcific aortic stenosis. Circulation 1960; 21:578–86.

49. Hufnagel CA, Conrad PW. Calcific aortic stenosis. N Engl J Med 1962; 266:72–6.

50. Isner JM, Michlewitz H, Clarke RH, Donaldson RF, Konstam MA, Salem DN. Laser-assisted debridement of aortic valve calcium. Am Heart J 1985; 109:448–52.

51. Lock JE, Niemi T, Enzig S, Amplatz K, Burke BA, Bass JL. Transvenous angioplasty of experimental branch pulmonary artery stenosis in newborn lambs. Circulation 1981; 64:886–92.

52. Lababidi Z, Wu JR. Percutaneous balloon pulmonary valvuloplasty. Am J Cardiol 1982; 52:560–3.

53. Jan JS, White RI, Mitchell SE, Gardner TJ. Percutaneous balloon valvuloplasty: a new method for treating congenital pulmonary valve stenosis. N Engl J Med 1982; 307:540–3.

54. Lababidi Z, Wu JR, Walls JT. Percutaneous balloon aortic valvuloplasty: results in 23 patients. Am J Cardiol 1984; 53:194–7.

55. Cribier A, Saoudi N, Berland J, Savin T, Rocha P, Letac B. Percutaneous transluminal valvuloplasty of acquired aortic stenosis in elderly patients: an alternative to valve replacement? Lancet 1986; 1:63–7.

56. McKay RG, Safian RD, Lock JE, Mandell VS, Thurer RL, Schnitt SJ, Grossman W. Balloon dilatation of calcific aortic stenosis in elderly patients: postmortem, intraoperative, and percutaneous valvuloplasty studies. Circulation 1986; 74:119–25.

57. Isner JM, Salem DN, Desnoyers MR, Hougen TJ, Mackey WC, Pandian NG, Eichhorn EJ, Konstam MA, Levine LJ. Treatment of calcific aortic stenosis by balloon valvuloplasty. Am J Cardiol 1987; 59:313–7.

58. Safian RD, Berman AD, Diver DJ, et al. Balloon aortic valvuloplasty in 170 consecutive patients. N Engl J Med 1988; 319:125–30.

59. Cribier A, Savin T, Berland J, Rocha P, Mechmeche R, Saoudi N, Behar P, Letac B. Percutaneous transluminal valvuloplasty of adult aortic stenosis: report of 92 cases. J Am Coll Cardiol 1987; 9:381–6.

60. Kirklin JW, Mankin HT. Open operation in the treatment of calcific aortic stenosis. Circulation 1960; 21:578–86.

61. Desnoyers MR, Isner JM, Salem DN, Wong SS, Pandian NG, Eichhorn EJ, Hougen TJ. Clinical and noninvasive hemodynamic follow-up of patients treated with balloon valvuloplasty for calcific aortic stenosis (abstr). Circulation 1987; 76:IV-303.

62. Block PC, Waldman H, Palacios IF. Follow-up of patients having percutaneous aortic valvuloplasty (abstr). Circulation 1987; 76:IV-1969.

63. Schneider JF, Wilson MA. Restenosis is common six months after balloon valvuloplasty for calcific aortic stenosis in adults (abstr). Circulation 1987; 76:IV-745.

64. Isner JM, Salem DN, Desnoyers MR, Fields CD, Halaburka KR, Slovenkai GA, Hougen TJ, Eichhorn EJ, Rosenfield K. Dual balloon technique for valvuloplasty of calcific aortic stenosis: clinical and necropsy analyses. Am J Cardiol 1988; 61:583–9.

65. Fields CD, Lucas A, Desnoyers MR, Pandian NG, Caldiera M, Salem DN, Isner JM. Follow-up of patients treated with dual balloon valvuloplasty for aortic stenosis: no improvement in restenosis (abstr). Clin Res (in press).

66. Letac B, Cribier A, Koning R, Lefebvre E. Aortic stenosis in elderly patients aged 80 or older: treatment by percutaneous balloon valvuloplasty in a series of 92 cases. Circulation 1989; 80:1514–20.

67. Block PC, Palacios IF. Clinical and hemodynamic follow-up after percutaneous aortic valvuloplasty in the elderly. Am J Cardiol 1988; 62:760–3.

68. Desnoyers MR, Salem DN, Rosenfield K, Mackey W, O'Donnell T, Isner

JM. Successful treatment of cardiogenic shock by emergency aortic balloon valvuloplasty. Ann Intern Med 1988; 108:833–5.

69. Levine MJ, Berman AD, Safian RD, Diver DJ, McKay RG. Palliation of valvular aortic stenosis by balloon valvuloplasty as preoperative preparation for noncardiac surgery. Am J Cardiol 1988; 62:1309–10.

70. Hayes SN, Holmes DR, Nishimura RA, Reeder GS. Palliative percutaneous aortic balloon aortic valvuloplasty before noncardiac operations and invasive diagnostic procedures. Mayo Clin Proc 1989; 64:753–7.

71. Goldman L. Cardiac risks and complications of noncardiac surgery. Ann Intern Med 1983; 98:504–13.

72. Kennedy JW. Complications associated with cardiac catheterization and angiography. Cath Cardiovasc Diag 1982; 8:5–12.

73. Losordo DW, Ramaswamy K, Rosenfield K, Isner JM. Use of emergency balloon dilation to reverse acute hemodynamic decompensation developing during diagnostic catheterization for aortic stenosis ("bailout valvuloplasty"). Am J Cardiol 1989; 63:388–9.

74. McKay RG, Safian RD, Berman AD, Diver DJ, Weinstein JS, Wyman RM, Cunningham MJ, McKay LL, Baim DS, Grossman W. Combined percutaneous aortic valvuloplasty and transluminal coronary angioplasty in adult patients with calcific aortic stenosis and coronary artery disease. Circulation 1987; 76:1298–1306.

75. Hamad N, Pichard A, Lindsay J. Combined coronary angioplasty and aortic valvuloplasty. Am J Cardiol 1987; 60:1184–6.

76. Ports TA, Srebro JP, Manubens SM, White N, Johnson E, Yock PG, Lo E. Simultaneous percutaneous aortic valvuloplasty and coronary artery angioplasty in an elderly patient. Am Heart J 1988; 115:672–5.

77. Isner JM, Fields CD, Halaburka KR, Slovenkai GA, Desnoyers MR, Hougen TJ, Ramaswamy K, Salem DN. Pathologic findings after in vivo aortic and mitral balloon valvuloplasty. J Am Coll Cardiol 1988; 11:229A.

78. Block PC, Palacios IF. Comparison of hemodynamic results of anterograde versus retrograde percutaneous balloon aortic valvuloplasty. Am J Cardiol 1987; 60:659–62.

79. Isner JM. Aortic valvuloplasty: are balloon-dilated valves all they are "cracked" up to be? Mayo Clin Proc 1988; 63:830–4.

80. Safian RD, Mandell VS, Thurer RE, Hutchins GM, Schnitt SJ, Grossman W, McKay RG. Postmortem and intraoperative balloon valvuloplasty of calcific aortic stenosis in elderly patients: mechanisms of successful dilation. J Am Coll Cardiol 1987; 9:655–60.

81. Vahanian A, Guerinon J, Michel PL, Slama M, Grivaux M, Acar J. Experimental balloon valvuloplasty of calcified aortic stenosis in the elderly. Circulation 1986; 74:II-365.

82. Isner JM, Samuels DA, Slovenkai GA, Halaburka KR, Hougen TJ, Desnoyers MR, Fields CD, Salem DN. Mechanism of aortic balloon valvuloplasty: fracture of valvular calcific deposits. Ann Intern Med 1988; 108:377–80.

83. Desnoyers MR, Isner JM, Pandian NG, Wong SS, Hougen T, Fields CD, Lucas AR, Salem DN. Clinical and non-invasive hemodynamic results after

aortic balloon valvuloplasty for aortic stenosis. Am J Cardiol 1988; 62: 1078–84.

84. McKay RG, Safian RD, Lock JE, Diver DJ, Berman AD, Warren SE, Come PC, Baim DS, Mandell VE, Royal HD, Grossman W. Assessment of left ventricular and aortic valve function after aortic valvuloplasty in adult patients with critical aortic stenosis. Circulation 1987; 75:192–203.

85. Kennedy KD, Huack AK, Edwards WD, Holms DR Jr, Reeder GS, Nishimura RA. Mechanism of reduction in aortic valvular stenosis by percutaneous transluminal balloon valvuloplasty: report of five cases and review of literature. Mayo Clin Proc 1988; 63:769–76.

86. Brady ST, Davis CA, Kussmaul WG, Laskey WK, Hirshfield JW, Herrmann HC. Percutaneous aortic balloon valvuloplasty in octogenarians: morbidity and mortality. Ann Intern Med 1989; 110:761–6.

87. Alexopoulos D, Sherman W. Unusual hemodynamic presentation of acute aortic regurgitation following percutaneous balloon valvuloplasty. Am Heart J 1988; 116:1622–3.

88. Seifert PE, Auer JE. Surgical repair of annular disruption following percutaneous balloon aortic valvuloplasty. Ann Thor Surg 1988; 46:242–3.

89. Fields CD, Isner JM. Balloon valvuloplasty in adults. In: Cleman M, Cabin H, eds. Cardiology Clinics: Interventional Cardiology. Vol. 6. Philadelphia: Saunders, 1988:383–419.

90. Voudris V, Drobinski G, Epine YL, Sotirov I, Moussalem N, Canny M. Results of percutaneous valvuloplasty for calcific aortic stenosis with different balloon catheters. Cath Card Diag 1989; 17:80–3.

91. DeLezo JS, Pan M, Romero M, Sancho M, Carrasco JL. Physiopathology of transient ventricular occlusion during balloon valvuloplasty for pulmonic or aortic stenosis. Am J Cardiol 1988; 61:436–40.

92. Weinhaus L, Lababidi Z. Catheter rupture during balloon valvuloplasty. Am Heart J 1987; 113:1035–6.

93. Lembo NJ, King SB, Roubin GS, Hammami A, Niederman AL. Fatal aortic rupture during percutaneous balloon valvuloplasty for valvular aortic stenosis. Am J Cardiol 1987; 60:733–6.

94. Cujic B, McMeekin J, Lopez J. Bacterial endocarditis after percutaneous aortic valvuloplasty. Am Heart J 1988; 115:178.

9

Tricuspid Valve

Paulo A. Ribeiro
Loma Linda University Medical Center
Loma Linda, California

I. INTRODUCTION

The diagnosis and management of tricuspid valve disorders has been hampered by conflicting concepts of the importance of the right heart function. The revolutionary proposals on circulatory physiology introduced by William Harvey included the role of the right ventricle in pumping blood through the lungs (1). This concept gained acceptance over 300 years, until it was challenged by Starr and co-workers (2). These authors demonstrated that venous congestion did not occur after experimentally severely damaging the right ventricular muscle. This elegant experimental work was corroborated by Bakos (3) and Kakan (4). These authors showed that normal right- and left-sided intracardiac pressures were maintained after extensive anatomical damage of the right ventricle. These findings gained clinical support with the demonstration of the feasibility of bypassing the right heart, with the exclusion of both the right atrium and right ventricle, which culminated with the description of the first successful Fontan procedure 20 years ago (5,6).

In contrast, several clinical reports (7,8) have demonstrated the importance of both right ventricular function and the tricuspid valve in maintaining normal cardiovascular physiology, thus supporting William Harvey's concept of the importance of a right-sided heart pump (7). Right ventricular failure may develop in patients with right ventricular infarction (9,10). Tricuspid insufficiency secondary to myocardial ischemia or right ventricular dilatation may increase right atrial pressure and lead to the development of chronic right heart failure in patients with right coronary infarction

(9–11). Experimental animal data from Cohn (12) and associates corroborated these clinical observations and are in contrast with Bakos's (3) and Starr's (2) experimental findings.

The concept of a dispensable tricuspid valve gained support after Arabulu (13) showed the feasibility of tricuspid valvectomy in drug addict patients with tricuspid valve endocarditis. Though many of these patients were still alive after 10 years of follow-up, the majority of them had physical signs of severe tricuspid regurgitation such as a pulsatile liver, and several required insertion of a tricuspid valve prosthesis (13,14). Cardiac output and cardiovascular hemodynamics were not studied in these patients after valvulectomy. The effects of the procedure upon cardiovascular physiology warrants further investigation.

The tricuspid valve and right ventricle may be surgically bypassable in some patients with congenital heart disease with normal pulmonary vascular dynamics, though the role of these structures is unquestionable in patients with increased right ventricular afterload (15–17). For instance, in patients with severe primary pulmonary hypertension with pulmonary valve stenosis, the right ventricle is able to maintain normal cardiac output and the tricuspid valve may be competent (18). The development of tricuspid valve regurgitation in patients with abnormal right ventricular pressures and increased afterload may occur as a result of displacement of papillary muscles, annular dilatation, or papillary muscle ischemia (19–21). Alternatively, the development of tricuspid valve regurgitation may herald primary right ventricular dysfunction (21).

The different etiological factors underlying the development of tricuspid valve regurgitation, whether primary valvular pathology, right ventricular dysfunction, or a combination of these two factors, has not been clarified. The determination of the pathophysiology of tricuspid valve regurgitation is of paramount importance for the clinical management of these patients. The contribution of right ventricular dysfunction in the development of tricuspid regurgitation needs to be defined in each patient. To date, the systematic assessment of right ventricular function has been plagued by methodological problems (22,23).

Despite these controversies, major advances in the conservative surgical treatment of tricuspid valve disease have been made with the introduction of the deVega (24–26) annuloplasty, and more recently with the introduction of the tricuspid valve Duran (27) and Carpentier (28) rings. Tricuspid valvotomy is indicated in the minority of patients who have concomitant severe tricuspid valve stenosis. Several reports of conservative surgical procedures have demonstrated the reduction of the severity of tricuspid valve regurgitation and increase of tricuspid valve area in those patients who have tricuspid valve stenosis (29–31).

The correction in right-sided hemodynamic abnormalities and particularly the increase in cardiac output both at rest and after exercise after tricuspid valve surgery has not been convincingly demonstrated after the surgical procedures (29–31). The effect of surgical intervention on the natural history of patients with tricuspid valve disease warrants a thorough clinical investigation.

The challenge of the tricuspid valve is still very much alive. The characterization of the factors underlying the etiology of tricuspid valve regurgitation and their reaction to right ventricular function are of paramount importance. This goal can be achieved only when clinicians have at their disposal techniques to assess right ventricular function.

II. PATHOLOGY

A. Normal Morphology of the Tricuspid Valve

The normal tricuspid valve has a delicate and complex anatomical structure. The annular circumference of the valve in men is 11.4 ± 1.1 cm and in women is 10.8 ± 1.3 cm (32). The anterior leaflet is the largest of the three leaflets; the posterior leaflet may have between one and four scallops, and the single septal leaflet is the smallest (32). Rarely, small holes are seen near the free margins of the leaflets; these may be secondary to developmental abnormalities (32). The subvalvular tricuspid apparatus is composed of three papillary muscles: The anterior is usually the largest and has a moderator band attached to it; the medial papillary muscles may be rudimentary in adults. On average, 25 chordae insert into the tricuspid valve, 7 to the anterior leaflet, 6 to the posterior leaflet, 9 into the septal leaflet, and 3 into the commissural areas (32). The chordae tendinea may arise from the papillary muscle or from the muscle of the posterior or septal walls of the right ventricle. There are five different types of chordae: fan-shaped, rough chordae, free-edge, deep, and basal chordae. The basal chordae are the shortest and measure an average of 0.6 cm; the deep and rough chordae can be as long as 2.2 cm (32). The fan-shaped chordae form precise landmarks for the commissures and distinguish clefts from the genuine commissures of the leaflets. The deep chordae are not present in the mitral valve, and appear to provide a second arcade for leaflet attachment to the larger tricuspid valve annulus and leaflets (32). The free-edge chordae are also unique to the tricuspid valve; they are single and may originate in the apex of the papillary muscle from its base and insert into the leaflet's free edge. In males the length of the anterior–posterior commissure was an average of 1.1 cm, the posteroseptal 0.8 cm, and the anteroseptal 0.6 cm (32). The histological composition of the tricuspid valve consists of three layers: the atrial surface consisting of collagen and elastin fibers, the middle layer of myxomatous connective tissue, and the ventricular side of collagen fibers (33).

B. Pathological Features of Tricuspid Valve Disease

The incidence of tricuspid valve stenosis is higher at autopsy than in clinical series (34–36). The characteristic pathological features of the different tricuspid valve disorders have been described at autopsy and after surgical excision of the valve (34) (Fig. 1). From 363 diseased tricuspid valves surgically excised at the Mayo Clinic over a 25-year period, the etiology was rheumatic heart disease in 53%, congenital heart disease in 26%, pulmonary venous hypertension in 15%, infective endocarditis in 3%, and carcinoid or trauma in 1% (34). From Hauck (34) series, all patients with rheumatic tricuspid valve disease who had surgical excision of the valve had concomitant pathological evidence of mitral valve involvement. Fifty-one percent of these valves were purely regurgitant; 14 (39%) of 109 valves had chordae fusion.

The pathological features of the purely tricuspid regurgitant valves included fibrosis, leaflet retraction, and chordae fusion; some exhibited commissural fusion (33,34). Pure tricuspid stenosis was rare, and was seen

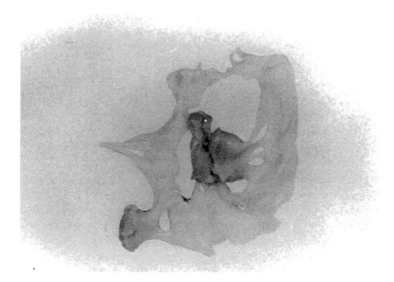

Figure 1 Surgically excised rheumatic tricuspid valve. Note the three papillary muscles and thickened three leaflets with fused commissures.

in 6 of the 194 cases (34): The valves exhibited diffuse leaflet fibrosis and commissural fusion in the closed position.

In our clinical series we observed 43 patients with echocardiographic features of tricuspid stenosis, representing 4% of the total population of patients with rheumatic heart disease (35). A larger series of patients with rheumatic heart disease showed an incidence of 3.1% of severe tricuspid stenosis (31). As mentioned above, the incidence of tricuspid stenosis is higher in autopsy series, ranging between 20% and 40% (31,36,37). Calcification of the tricuspid valve is very rare; the first case was described by Hollman (38), and a further three by Hauck (34). Pathologically, the leaflets are less thickened than the mitral, and the chordae are little affected (34,37,38). Whereas the mitral valve is commonly stenotic in rheumatic heart disease, stenosis occurs less commonly in rheumatic tricuspid valve disease (Fig. 1). In tricuspid stenosis the commissures are fused and are not clearly distinguishable, being covered by a continuous curtain of valve tissue (34) (Fig. 1). In patients with pure tricuspid regurgitation and mitral stenosis, anatomically abnormal tricuspid valves, i.e., with organic disease, have a smaller annular circumference; also, the product of the circumference multiplied by the area is larger than in those patients who exhibit a normal tricuspid valve, i.e., functional tricuspid regurgitation (39).

Congenital malformation of the tricuspid valve accounts for a wide spectrum of valve dysfunction and regurgitation (40,41). Ebstein's anomaly is the most common and may be associated with annulus dysplasia, hypoplasia, or even annulus dilatation (34,41,42). A floppy tricuspid valve (prolapse) exhibits an annulus greater than 14 cm and a larger leaflet area compared to other types of tricuspid pathology (34).

In infective endocarditis the tricuspid leaflet may exhibit vegetations, indentations, or even perforations, and the chordae can be ruptured (13,34). Carcinoid can distort the tricuspid leaflets, and chordae can be thickened and distorted with dense plaques of carcinoid, leading to stenosis, regurgitation, or both (43,44). Endomyocardial fibrosis may involve the tricuspid subvalvular apparatus and cause severe tricuspid regurgitation (45). Rarely, lupus erythematosus involving the tricuspid valve leads to valve stenosis (46). Trauma may rupture the anterior papillary muscle and lead to severe tricuspid regurgitation (47). Coronary disease and myocardial infarction may lead to tricuspid regurgitation (48); pathologically, the papillary muscle of the tricuspid valve may be necrotic or scarred and atrophied (9–11,34).

In many cases of pure tricuspid regurgitation, the only anatomical abnormality is tricuspid valve annulus dilatation (20,21,34,39). The annulus measurement is significantly larger in patients with tricuspid regurgitation secondary to pulmonary hypertension (increased afterload)—the so-called functional tricuspid regurgitation (39).

III. TRICUSPID STENOSIS

A. Pathophysiology

The normal tricuspid valve orifice area at necropsy is at least 7 cm^2. With such a large area, tricuspid stenosis must be severe to be hemodynamically significant. The tricuspid pressure gradient is the hemodynamic marker used routinely to assess the significance of the tricuspid stenosis (48,49). There are inherent limitations in calculating the Gorlin tricuspid valve area (31,50).

A low cardiac output is the major hemodynamic disturbance of this condition. A mean gradient of 2 mm across the tricuspid valve is considered to be indicative of severe tricuspid stenosis (31,48–53) (Fig. 2). With low outputs and slow heart rate, there may be no gradient across the valve despite severe tricuspid stenosis (54). Atropine or fluid challenge may be necessary to expose occult tricuspid valve gradient (54) (Fig. 3). With exercise, the decrease in right ventricular diastolic filling period secondary to tachycardia causes an increase in mean right atrial pressure and tricuspid gradient, with a concomitant decrease in right ventricular diastolic pressure (54). The associated rise in right atrial pressure is presumably due to the reduced time period for right ventricular filling.

Cardiac output can only increase twofold at peak exercise in patients with tricuspid stenosis, accounting for the patients' symptoms of tiredness and shortness of breath with exercise (31,55). The mean right atrial pressure is normal in the majority of patients with severe tricuspid stenosis (31,54) (Fig. 2). The high right atrial pressure observed in patients with tricuspid stenosis usually indicates concomitant severe tricuspid valve regurgitation or a failing right ventricle (31,54). The right atrial pressure tracing exhibits a prominent A wave in the majority of patients with sinus rhythm, and a slow Y descent—indicative of the loss of the rapid filling phase into the right ventricle (31,52–54) (Fig. 2). In a few patients the A wave may be similar to the V wave; this may indicate that the right atrium is failing, and heralds the development of atrial fibrillation (54) (Fig. 2B).

B. History and Clinical Features

The majority of patients with tricuspid stenosis have a history of rheumatic fever (53). The time interval between the episode of rheumatic fever and onset of symptoms varies from a few months to three decades. Tricuspid stenosis is nearly always associated with concomitant mitral stenosis, the latter usually dominating the clinical picture. Exertional dyspnea is present in all cases of isolated tricuspid stenosis, reflecting the low cardiac output in these patients (31,53,56–58). Hemoptysis and right ventricular infarction may occur as a result of emboli from thrombus in the right atrium (53). Hepatomegaly, ascites, and ankle edema may occur in those patients with concomitant severe tricuspid regurgitation who have elevated mean right atrial pressures and right ventricular dysfunction. Orthopnea and paroxysmal nocturnal dyspnea occur in patients with tricuspid stenosis and associated significant mitral valve stenosis.

The clinical diagnosis of tricuspid stenosis may be difficult, since the physical signs can be masked by an associated mitral valve stenosis—for isolated tricuspid valve stenosis is a rare clinical entity (53,55–58). In those patients with sinus rhythm, the A wave in the jugular venous pulse is prominent and increases with inspiration (Fig. 2A). The Y descent is slow, due to the absence of the rapid right ventricular filling phase. The diastolic murmur is mainly presystolic and terminates before the first heart sound (31,53). A diastolic rumble is not diagnostic for tricuspid stenosis, since patients with severe pure tricuspid regurgitation may exhibit diastolic murmurs (59,60). The tricuspid opening snap may be present, and occurs before the mitral opening snap in severe tricuspid stenosis (48,53). The tricuspid rumble usually increases with inspiration and decreases or even disappears with expiration (50,51,53). A diastolic thrill may be palpable, but it is not common (31,55,61). In those patients who are in atrial fibrillation, the tricuspid murmur occurs mainly in the early diastolic period (53,62,63). With long R–R intervals, the murmur may disappear, as there is a longer period for ventricular filling and the tricuspid gradient decreases.

C. Diagnosis of Tricuspid Stenosis

1. Electrocardiogram

The majority of patients with tricuspid valve stenosis are in sinus rhythm (31,54,64). The prominent electrocardiographic features are the dented P waves, usually greater than 3 mm, better seen in leads D2, 3 and AVF, with normal QRS axis and absence of features of right ventricular hypertrophy that may be the clue to the diagnosis. The PR interval may be prolonged in half of the patients with tricuspid valve stenosis. Since the tricuspid stenosis is nearly always associated with concomitant mitral stenosis, the P waves may also exhibit mitral morphology with bi-atrial enlargement.

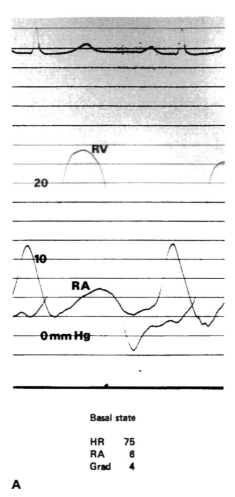

Basal state

HR   75
RA   6
Grad   4

A

Figure 2 (A) Right atrium (RA) and right ventricle (RV) pressure tracings from
a patient with severe tricuspid stenosis. Note the tricuspid diastolic gradient and

2. Radiological Features

Enlargement of the right atrium, with prominence of the right heart border,
is present in the majority of patients. The degree and severity of tricuspid
stenosis has no relation to the size of the right atrium on X-ray. We and
others have seen patients with severe tricuspid stenosis and trivial tricuspid regurgitation who have a normal radiological cardiac silhouette (64).
The dilatation of the right atrium appears to be radiologically more promi-

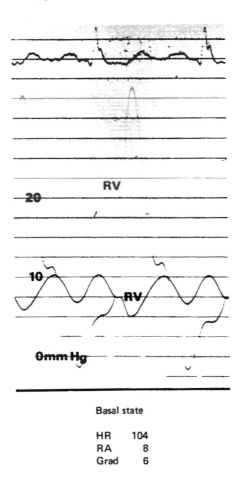

RV

20

RV

10

RV

0mm Hg

Basal state

HR	104
RA	8
Grad	6

B

a large A wave with a slow Y descent. (B) Tricuspid diastolic gradient showing similar A and V waves in a patient with severe rheumatic tricuspid stenosis.

nent in those patients who have concomitant significant tricuspid valve regurgitation (31). Enlargement of the pulmonary artery and left atria is seen in those patients who have associated severe mitral valve disease and pulmonary hypertension.

3. Echocardiography and Doppler Studies

The decrease in the E–F slope was initially described as a useful echo M-mode sign of tricuspid stenosis (65,66). Several other studies showed

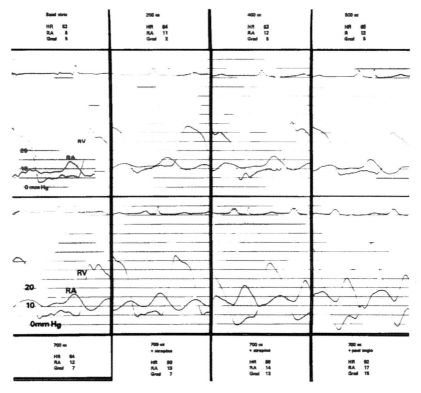

Figure 3 Hemodynamic study from a patient with tricuspid stenosis. Note the small tricuspid diastolic gradient at baseline gradient and the marked increase in tricuspid gradient after fluid challenge and atropine.

that this sign may also be present in patients without tricuspid stenosis (67,68). The echocardiographic features of tricuspid stenosis, i.e., diastolic doming of all three leaflets, and restricted motion, are considered characteristics for tricuspid stenosis (69,70) (Fig. 4). Daniels et al. (71) showed that only 4 of 19 patients studied with the echocardiographic features of tricuspid stenosis had hemodynamically significant tricuspid stenosis. We found that 57% of patients with echo features of tricuspid stenosis had hemodynamically significant tricuspid stenosis (35). The diastolic doming is a sensitive echocardiographic marker of commissural fusion and thickening, but is not a precise indicator of hemodynamically significant tricuspid stenosis (54) (Fig. 4).

The diastolic doming and restricted tricuspid leaflet motion persist after successful tricuspid valvotomy, even after the abolition of the tricuspid

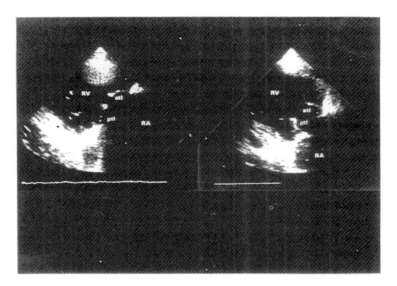

Figure 4 Echocardiographic study in a patient with severe tricuspid stenosis. Right ventricular inflow view. Note the diastolic doming and restrictive motion of the anterior and posterior leaflets (atl and ptl, respectively). Note the marked improvement of leaflet motion after tricuspid valvotomy (right panel).

gradient (55) (Fig. 4). The Doppler tricuspid valve area appeared to correlate fairly well with the Gorlin tricuspid valve area (72–74). Validation studies are warranted to establish this noninvasive technique to quantify the degree of tricuspid stenosis.

4. Hemodynamic Studies

Angiographically, all patients with echocardiographic feature of tricuspid stenosis exhibit tricuspid valve thickening and doming (35,54) (Fig. 5). The right anterior oblique view with 10–15° angulation is the best view for profiling the stenotic tricuspid valve (Fig. 5). Tricuspid regurgitation is noted in nearly all patients with tricuspid stenosis. From 42 consecutive patients with echocardiographic features of tricuspid stenosis, 34 had tricuspid regurgitation grade 1–2/4, 7 had grade 3/4, and one had grade 4/4 according to the Grossman scale (35).

The hemodynamic hallmark of tricuspid stenosis is low cardiac output (31,48). This may increase up to twofold at peak exercise (55). The increase is secondary to the tachycardia, as stroke volume decreases with exercise, together with the pulmonary vascular resistance. Despite the relief of symptoms (29,52), the resting cardiac output may fail to increase

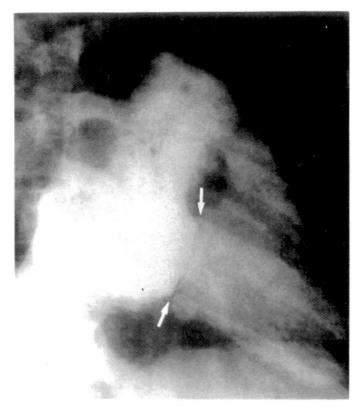

Figure 5 Right atrial angiography is a patient with severe tricuspid stenosis. Note tricuspid thickening and doming (arrows).

after adequate surgical valvotomy. After tricuspid balloon valvotomy the cardiac output has been demonstrated to increase both at rest and with exercise, corroborating the patient's clinical improvement (55,75).

A large A wave may be helpful in the diagnosis of tricuspid stenosis in the absence of pulmonary hypertension (31) (Fig. 2A). An A wave that exceeds the maximum systolic pressure by more than 5 mmHg usually indicates severe tricuspid valve stenosis (31). We have observed a few patients with severe tricuspid stenosis who exhibited similar A and V wave amplitude, indicating that the right atrium is failing or, alternatively, that the tricuspid regurgitation is hemodynamically important (54) (Fig. 2B). Interestingly, the mean right atrial pressure may be normal in many of the patients with severe tricuspid valve stenosis (Figs. 2A and 2B).

The tricuspid diastolic gradient of 2 mmHg is considered to be diagnostic for severe tricuspid valve stenosis (31,48) (Fig. 2). The gradient may be absent in the early stages of tricuspid stenosis, since advanced stenosis is required to be physiologically significant (49). The tricuspid valve gradient increases with volume overload and a rise in heart rate (Fig. 3). The decrease in heart ventricular filling period secondary to tachycardia causes an increase in mean right atrial pressure and tricuspid gradient (54).

There are inherent limitations in calculating the tricuspid valve area using the Gorlin formula (31). The major source of inaccuracy is the concomitant tricuspid regurgitation present in nearly all patients, which results in underestimation of the tricuspid valve area calculation. Two identical right atrium and right ventricle catheters are required to measure the tricuspid gradient simultaneously, since it may be very small as a result of the high degree of compliance of the right atrium and systemic venous system. Not surprisingly, the original study results between anatomical and Gorlin valve area (31,48) had a poor correlation in the absence of a "gold standard" method of calculating the tricuspid valve area; the Doppler-estimated tricuspid valve area appears to correlate moderately well with the Gorlin tricuspid valve area (72–74).

5. Pitfalls in Diagnosis

As the clinical features of tricuspid stenosis may be overshadowed by associated mitral stenosis, the diagnosis should be suspected in all patients with rheumatic valve stenosis, particularly those in atrial fibrillation.

The two-dimensional echocardiographic features of tricuspid stenosis, i.e., leaflet thickening and diastolic doming of all three leaflets, indicates some degree of commissural fusion, but they are not a precise indicator of severe tricuspid stenosis (Fig. 4) (35,69–72). Many patients who exhibit the echo features of tricuspid stenosis have valve areas of 3 cm^2; hemodynamic study is indicated for diagnostic purposes.

The hemodynamic hallmark of tricuspid stenosis is the 2 mm Hg tricuspid gradient measured after careful calibration of two identical catheters placed in the right atrium and right ventricle, respectively (Figs. 2A and 2B). Provocative maneuvers are necessary to expose occult gradients in the minority of patients with severe tricuspid stenosis (Fig. 3) (54).

In patients with concomitant severe tricuspid regurgitation, the mean tricuspid gradient may measure more than 2 mm Hg as a result of the large V waves, in the absence of organic tricuspid stenosis (76,77). In these cases, two-dimensional echocardiographic study is a complementary investigation to the hemodynamic study.

D. Management

From an understanding of the pathophysiology of severe tricuspid stenosis, there appears to be little role for pharmacological treatment. The patient's symptoms are due to the low cardiac output, both at rest and with
exercise. The role of digoxin in increasing cardiac output in patients with
tricuspid stenosis has not been evaluated. The right atrial contraction is
important, and the onset of atrial fibrillation has deleterious hemodynamic
consequences; maintenance of sinus rhythm should therefore be sought.
The tricuspid gradient and right atrium pressure can be reduced with the
use of beta blockade. The decrease of heart rate and increase in right
ventricular diastolic filling period will decrease right atrial pressure and
tricuspid valve gradients (54). The effect of beta blockers would be detri-
mental in the event of further decrease in cardiac output, both at rest and
with exercise, since the cardiac output depends on heart rate.

The majority of patients have normal or slightly raised right atrial pressure and would not benefit from nitrates and diuretic therapy (31,54).
Those who have a failing right atrium, or significant tricuspid regurgitation
with elevated right atrial pressures, will benefit from these drugs, as they
increase venous capacity and decrease intravascular volume.

Tricuspid surgical valvotomy was first recorded by Brofman 40 years
ago (78). The treatment of severe tricuspid stenosis has important clinical
implications for those patients who undergo successful mitral surgery,
since failure to detect and correct severe tricuspid stenosis increases operative mortality and negates patient improvement after mitral valve surgery
(36,79–82). The symptoms are relieved after successful tricuspid valvotomy. Normalization of right atrial pressure and abolition or reduction
in tricuspid gradient may be achieved (31). Severe tricuspid regurgitation
is rare but may develop if commissurotomy is performed too aggressively.
Up to two commissures may be split, and splitting the anteroposterior
commissure should not be attempted (29).

For those patients with concomitant hemodynamically significant tricuspid regurgitation, tricuspid valve repair is indicated in addition to tricuspid valvotomy. The cardiac output may remain low despite the surgical
correction of the tricuspid valve abnormality (31).

A nonsurgical therapeutic alternative to the surgical treatment of severe
tricuspid stenosis was described by Zaibag et al. using valve dilation with
a balloon catheter (Fig. 6) (55,61). An immediate and long-term increase in
tricuspid valve area and a decrease in tricuspid gradient was demonstrated
(61,82). The tricuspid valve areas achieved were similar to those reported
after surgical valvotomy (30); the patient's symptomatic improvement was
corroborated by the increase in cardiac output, both at rest and with exer-

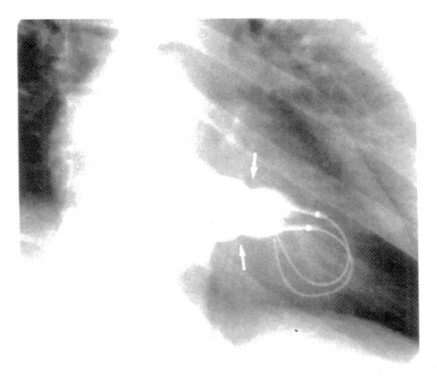

Figure 6 Double-balloon tricuspid valvotomy. Note balloon indentation(arrows) during early inflation.

cise (55,61). Several other authors have confirmed the feasibility of balloon tricuspid valvotomy (83–85). The procedure is indicated for patients with severe tricuspid stenosis and mild to moderate tricuspid regurgitation. The degree of tricuspid regurgitation does not increase in the majority of patients. Since the majority of patients with tricuspid stenosis have concomitant tricuspid regurgitation, few patients will be candidates for this intervention.

IV. TRICUSPID REGURGITATION

A. Pathophysiology

The symptoms of patients with tricuspid valve regurgitation depend on the extent of the cardiovascular hemodynamic disturbances, such as the increase in mean right atrial pressure and decrease in cardiac output (Fig. 7) (60). Conceivably, the decreased renal perfusion leads to sodium and

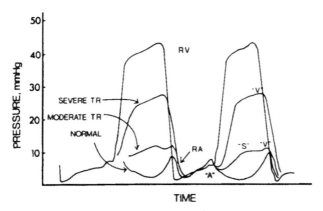

Figure 7   Hemodynamic studies in moderate and severe tricuspid regurgitation. Note the abnormal right atrial pressure wave form compared to normal.

fluid retention and is responsible for the right-sided heart failure symptoms (56,57,76).

The pathophysiology of certain types of organic tricuspid valve regurgitation are well understood: patients with cusp perforation as a result of bacterial endocarditis; tricuspid papillary muscle necrosis following right ventricular infarction; severe tricuspid valve chordae involvement in endomyocardial fibrosis; chordae fusion and failure of the tricuspid coaptation in rheumatic heart disease; marked tricuspid valve prolapse in Marfan's disease.

The mechanism determining the pathophysiology of functional tricuspid valve regurgitation with normal anatomical tricuspid valve leaflets and subvalvular apparatus appears to be annular dilatation (17–21,86). Annular dilatation has been documented in functional tricuspid regurgitation by echocardiographic (17–21,86), angiography (19), and from pathological studies (39). The severity of tricuspid valve regurgitation correlates significantly with the size of the tricuspid valve annulus, in both systole and diastole (17–21). The annulus dilatation is thought to be secondary to right ventricular dilatation in patients with increased right ventricular afterload.

The understanding of the pathophysiological mechanism behind annular dilatation in functional tricuspid regurgitation has important clinical implications. The annular dilatation may reflect anatomical geometrical changes of the right ventricle; in this case, surgical treatment with annular size reduction is indicated. Alternatively, functional tricuspid regurgitation may simply reflect primary right ventricular failure, and surgery will not help these patients.

The high operative and late mortality, and lack of clinical improvement in surgery for tricuspid regurgitation developing late after mitral valve replacement, may indicate that the new tricuspid regurgitation may herald right ventricular dilatation and failure (87). The decrease percentage shortening of the tricuspid annulus size in tricuspid regurgitation compared to normals may indicate impairment of right ventricular systolic function (19,21).

There are inherent limitations in evaluating right ventricular ejection fraction as an index of right ventricular systolic function. Tricuspid regurgitation reduces right ventricular afterload and leads to falsely high right ventricular ejection fraction calculation. Abnormally high levels of pulmonary pressure and resistance may increase the degree of tricuspid valve regurgitation (17). There is an inverse relation between right ventricular ejection fraction and pulmonary artery pressure. Thus the objective evaluation of right ventricular function is complex, particularly in the context of tricuspid valve regurgitation and increased pulmonary vascular resistance. The evaluation of right ventricular ejection fraction is hampered by methodological problems and in normal subjects has a large variability, between 35% and 75% (22,23).

B. Clinical Features

The clinical symptoms and features of patients with tricuspid regurgitation vary according to the severity of the lesion, i.e., magnitude of right atrial pressure and decrease in cardiac output (56,57). All patients complain of dyspnea that is a consequence of decreased cardiac output. Alternatively, it reflects a high pulmonary capillary wedge due to associated mitral valve disease (56). The classical signs of tricuspid regurgitation are present in about one-third of the patients with tricuspid regurgitation (56,57). All patients have a systolic murmur in the tricuspid area (56). This may be difficult to detect in patients with fast atrial fibrillation. The murmur is pansystolic, rough, high-pitched, loudest in the xiphoid area, but can also be heard at the apex. The murmur may not increase with inspiration in some patients (88).

The majority of patients with tricuspid valve regurgitation are in atrial fibrillation, and half of them will exhibit the features of right ventricular failure. The liver is palpable in the majority of them, and ankle edema will be present in 50%. A quarter of the patients will exhibit distended neck veins, ascites, and wasting. A pulsating liver and cyanosis are detected in 10% of patients (56,57). There is wide variability of the character tricuspid valve murmur. According to some authors, the murmur is detected in all patients, but Sepulveda et al. detected the tricuspid systolic murmur in only 18% of their patients (57).

Ninety percent of those patients who have severe tricuspid valve regurgitation will have the Carvallo sign or a pulsatile liver, with prominent V waves (56,57). Rarely, patients may be jaundiced and cyanosed due to the low cardiac output and liver congestion. Splenomegaly is rare and probably related to portal hypertension in those patients who develop liver cirrhosis.

Since solitary, severe tricuspid valve regurgitation is rare (89,90), the clinical features are often masked by those of associated mitral valve disease. In two instances of isolated organic tricuspid valve regurgitation, the patients presented with all the classical features of severe tricuspid valve regurgitation (89,90).

The natural history of severe tricuspid valve regurgitation is difficult to determine, as mitral valve disease nearly always dominates the clinical picture. Patients who underwent tricuspid valvectomy following acute endocarditis may eventually require tricuspid valve replacement due to the development of persistent right-sided heart failure (13).

C. Diagnosis

1. Electrocardiogram

The great majority of patients with tricuspid regurgitation exhibit atrial fibrillation. For the minority who are in sinus rhythm, the P wave is typically broad and notched in standard leads (56), with associated P mitral. The QRS axis is vertical or right, and complete right-bundle bunch block is observed in 51% of patients. Qr or qR complex are seen in lead V1 in 44% of patients. An intrinsic deflection in V1 and V2 is also found in the majority of patients (56,91).

2. Radiography

All patients with tricuspid regurgitation exhibit cardiomegaly. The enlargement of the pulmonary artery shadow is commonly seen and is associated with pulmonary hypertension. The lung fields are oligemic in half of the patients. Hemosiderosis of the lung and pleural effusion may be part of the clinical picture of severe tricuspid regurgitation (56,57).

3. Echocardiography and Doppler Studies

Two-dimensional echocardiographic studies may determine the mechanism of tricuspid regurgitation in organic tricuspid valve disease such as Ebstein's anomaly (41), rheumatic valve disease (35,70), ischemic tricuspid regurgitation (10), carcinoid heart disease (84), endomyocardial fibrosis (92), infective endocarditis, or tricuspid prolapse (68).

In patients with functional tricuspid regurgitation, tricuspid annular dilatation, malalignment coaptation, or anterior displacement of the tricuspid leaflet is observed (20). These abnormalities lead to the separation between leaflet tips, which is the main mechanism responsible for tricuspid valve regurgitation (20,21). The annulus of the tricuspid valve is significantly increased in patients with functional tricuspid regurgitation when compared to normals (19–21). Measurement of the tricuspid valve annulus by two-dimensional echocardiography is a noninvasive method of identifying patients with severe tricuspid regurgitation (18). The percentage shortening of the tricuspid valve annulus is reduced in patients with severe tricuspid regurgitation, and this may indicate primary right ventricular failure (19,21,93).

The echocardiographic features of isolated tricuspid valve regurgitation following tricuspid valvectomy showed progressive right ventricular dilatation and paradoxical intraventricular septal wall motion (89).

The assessment of tricuspid regurgitation by Doppler studies should take into consideration the existence and characteristics of regurgitation patterns observed in normal subjects (94). With continuous-wave Doppler, the prevalence rate of tricuspid regurgitation was 95% according to Yock (95); using color Doppler, the prevalence rate of regurgitation was commonly seen and was age dependent, being more common in younger subjects (94). The mean jet area on color Doppler was 1.5 cm², and the regurgitation flow signals were localized near the site of valve closure. A few studies have attempted to correlate the Doppler severity of tricuspid regurgitation with the angiographic degree of regurgitation (73,74). Color Doppler is being used increasingly for the intraoperative assessment of severe tricuspid regurgitation, and correlative studies with angiography are warranted (96).

The variability of tricuspid valve regurgitation also needs to be considered, the degree of tricuspid regurgitation depending on preload and afterload. The variability of the tricuspid murmurs has been corroborated by hemodynamic studies showing changes in the severity of tricuspid valve regurgitation, and the echocardiographic signal should take this observation into consideration (57,76,97–99).

4. Cardiac Catheterization

The hemodynamic disturbances in tricuspid valve regurgitation are increased right atrial pressure and decreased cardiac output (Fig. 7) (56,57,76). Cardiac output fails to increase with exercise (56). Conceivably, the decrease in renal blood flow may lead to sodium and fluid retention and contribute to right-sided failure (56,100). The mean right atrial pressure is abnormally high, with large V waves (56,57,76). The rapid Y descent appears with inspiration (77). There is a wide hemodynamic spectrum of severity of tricuspid valve regurgitation (Fig. 7).

In mild tricuspid regurgitation, the mean right atrial pressure may be normal, with prominent V waves. The ventricularization of the pattern of right atrial pressure may be total in patients with severe tricuspid regurgitation, and right atrial and right ventricular pressure may be equal (Fig. 7) (77).

Right ventriculography is a valid method for the diagnosis of tricuspid insufficiency using the Ubago technique (101). Using special catheters, tricuspid valve regurgitation is not detected in normal subjects using this technique (101,102).

5. Pitfalls in the Diagnosis of Tricuspid Regurgitation

The clinician should always keep in mind that the classical clinical features of tricuspid regurgitation are present in only a minority of patients who have severe valve regurgitation. The majority may exhibit a systolic murmur that could be confused with mitral regurgitation (103,104). There is a marked variability of tricuspid valve murmur. Contrary to general belief, the failure of the systolic murmur to increase with inspiration does not exclude tricuspid regurgitation (56,57). The presence and severity of tricuspid regurgitation is influenced by preload and afterload, and therefore the character of the murmur may vary (56,99,105). The results of echo and Doppler studies should take this observation into consideration.

The noninvasive cardiologist should also realize that detection of tricuspid valve regurgitation is common in normal subjects (94,95). The characterization of the regurgitation and the Doppler jet signal is important to differentiate between physiological and pathological tricuspid regurgitation (94).

Angiography is the "gold standard" technique for the evaluation of the severity of the tricuspid regurgitation, though it is mandatory to use special techniques (101,102). There may be a discrepancy between the angiographic and hemodynamic degree of severity of tricuspid regurgitation. In our experience, the angiographic degree of tricuspid regurgitation can be severe, while the hemodynamic data may exhibit only mild to moderate hemodynamic disturbance (54). These patients who have been at bed rest before cardiac catheterization may have had a large dose of diuretics with prolonged periods of fasting and may thus be dehydrated.

D. Management

For those patients with moderate and severe tricuspid valve regurgitation, there is a role for medical therapy, in an attempt to avoid the need for tricuspid valve surgery. The therapeutic approach should be aggressive, particularly for those patients who develop tricuspid regurgitation after mitral surgery. Some of these patients have primary right ventricular failure rather than "primary" tricuspid regurgitation. Since the majority of patients are in atrial fibrillation, the ventricular rate should be controlled with digoxin and beta blockade if required. The increase in the diastolic time interval will improve right ventricular diastolic filling and hemodynamics in those patients who are in fast atrial fibrillation. The decrease in right atrial pressure and right heart failure can be achieved with a combination of fluid restriction, low-salt diet, and diuretic therapy. The synergistic effect of a thiazide diuretic such as Metazolone and a loop diuretic may be beneficial in patients with right heart failure that is refractory to medical therapy. Nitrates can increase systemic venous compliance and therefore decrease preload. For those patients who have persistent pulmonary hypertension secondary to mitral valve disease and severe tricuspid regurgitation refractory to medical therapy, surgery should be considered.

The surgical indications will depend on the underlying etiology of the tricuspid regurgitation and on the status of the right ventricular systolic function. A depressed extent of shortening of tricuspid annulus in systole may indicate that primary right ventricular failure may be important in the pathogenesis of tricuspid regurgitation (21,93).

Tricuspid valve replacement with a mechanical prosthesis is not a good therapeutic approach, as the risk of valve thrombosis is very high (106–108). A bioprosthesis inserted in the tricuspid position will probably degenerate. We believe that tricuspid valve repair for both organic and functional tricuspid regurgitation should be attempted in all patients with moderate and severe tricuspid valve regurgitation. Tricuspid regurgitation may be progressive in the course of mitral valve disease (106) and, contrary to early data, does not usually regress after successful mitral valve repair (93).

For patients with functional tricuspid regurgitation, i.e., anatomical normal valve with dilated annulus, the valve can be repaired with a deVega annuloplasty (24,26) or with the insertion of a Duran (27) or Carpentier ring (28). Results of the various techniques are good, though no comparative randomized data are available between the different techniques. The results of tricuspid valve repair for severe tricuspid valve regurgitation are better for functional than for organic valve disease (109).

With the Duran ring, the repair of severe tricuspid valve regurgitation is 100% successful in functional and in organic tricuspid valve disease without tricuspid valve stenosis (109). The success of results persist at 1-year follow-up study. In those patients who have associated organic tricuspid valve disease and also require valvotomy, the success of surgery is maintained in only 60% of patients at 1-year follow-up (109). Randomized surgical studies are indicated to compare the new and existing different techniques for tricuspid valve repair.

Tricuspid valvectomy has been advocated for drug addicts with tricuspid valve endocarditis. Though the patients tolerate the procedure in the absence of the tricuspid valve, many will develop severe tricuspid valve regurgitation and will require tricuspid valve replacement.

ACKNOWLEDGMENTS

We are grateful to Dr. William Sawyer for the detailed revision of the manuscript. We are indebted to Ms. Teresita Datu for her secretarial assistance.

REFERENCES

1. Harvey W. An Anatomical Disguisation on the Motion of the Heart and Blood in Animals, the Works of William Harvey. Translated with a life of the author by R. Willis. New York: Johnson Reprint, 1965:1–86.
2. Starr L, Jeffers WA, Meade RH. The absence of conspicuous increments of venous pressure after severe damage to the right ventricle of the dog, with a discussin of the relation between clinical congestive failure and heart disease. Am Heart J 1943; 26:291–9.
3. Bakos ACP. The question of the function of the right ventricular myocardium: an experimental study. Circulation 1950; 73:724–32.
4. Kagan A. Dynamic response of the right ventricle following extensive damage by cauterization. Circulation 1952; 5:816–23.
5. Sade RM, Castaneda AR. The dispensable right ventricle. Surgery 1975; 77:624–31.
6. Fontan F, Baudet E. Surgical reapir of tricuspid atresia. Thorax 1971; 26: 240–8.
7. Nugent EW, Freedom RM, Nora JJ, Ellison RC, Rowe RD, Nadas A. Clinical course in pulmonary stenosis. Circulation 1977; 56(suppl I):I-138–47.
8. Ribeiro PA, Sivanandan V, Shaikh A, Chalak W, Zaman L, Duran CMG. Decrease in pulmonary artery pressure with slow release nifedipine in Saudi patients with primary pulmonary hypertension. Rev Port Cardiol 1991; 10(5):413–8.
9. Zone DD, Botti RE. Right ventricular infarction with tricuspid insufficiency and chronic heart failure. Am J Cardiol 1976; 37:445–8.
10. Zaus EA, Kearn S. Massive infarction of the right ventricle and atrium. Circulation 1952; 6:593–8.
11. Cohn JN, Guiha NH, Broder MI, Limas CJ. Right ventricular infarction: clinical and hemodynamic features. Am J Cardiol 1974; 33:209–14.
12. Guiha NH, Limas CJ, Cohn JN. Predominant right ventricular dysfunction after right ventricular destruction in the dog. Am J Cardiol 1974; 33:254–8.
13. Arbulu A, Asfaw I. Tricuspid valvulectomy without prosthetic replacement. Ten years of clinical experience. J Thorac Cardiovasc Surg 1981; 82:684–91.

14. Sethia B, Williams BT. Tricuspid valve excision without replacement in a case of endocarditis secondary to drug abuse. Br Heart J 1978; 40:579–80.
15. Ellis JA, Kirch D, Steele PP. Right ventricular ejection fraction in severe chronic airway obstruction. Chest 1977; 77(suppl):281–2.
16. Morrison DA, Goldman S, Henry R, Wright AL, Sorenson S, Caldwell J, Ritchie J. The effect of pulmonary hypertension on right ventricular systolic function. Chest 1983; 84:250–7.
17. Morrison DA, Ouitt T, Hammermeister KE. Functional tricuspid regurgitation and right ventricular dysfunction in pulmonary hypertension. Am J Cardiol 1988; 62:108–12.
18. Fisher EA, Goldman ME. Simple, rapid method for quantification of tricuspid regurgitation by two-dimensional echocardiography. Am J Cardiol 1989; 63:1375–8.
19. Ubago JL, Figueiroa A, Ochoteco A, Colman T, Duran RM, Duran CG. Analysis of the amount of tricuspid valve annular dilatation required to produce functional tricuspid regurgitation. Am J Cardiol 1983; 52:155–8.
20. Mikami T, Kudo T, Sakurai N, Sayamoto S, Tanabe Y, Yasuda H. Mechanisms for development of functional tricuspid regurgitation determined by pulsed doppler and two-dimensional echocardiography. Am J Cardiol 1984; 53:160–4.
21. Tei C, Pilgrim JP, Shah PM, Ormiston JA, Wong M. The tricuspid valve annulus study of size and motion in normal subjects and in patients with tricuspid regurgitation. Circulation 1982; 66:665–71.
22. Ferlinz J, Gorlin R, Cohn PF. Right ventricular performance in patients with coronary disease. Circulation 1975; 52:608–15.
23. Maddahi J, Berman DS, Matsouka DT, Waxman AD, Stankus KE, Forrester JS, Swan HJ. A new technique for assessing right ventricular ejection fraction using rapid multiple gated equilibrium cardiac pool scintigraphy. Circulation 1979; 60:581–9.
24. DeVega NG. La annuloplastia selectiva regulable permanente: una tecnica original para el tratamiento de insuficiencia tricuspide. Rev Esp Cardio 1972; 25:555–60.
25. Chidambaram M, Abdulalili SA, Baliga G, Ionescu M. Long term results of DeVega tricuspid annuloplasty. Ann Thorac Surg 1987; 43:185–8.
26. Grondin P, Meere C, Limet R, Lopez-Bescos L, Delcan JL, Rivera R. Carpentier's annulus and DeVega's annuloplasty: the end of the tricuspid challenge. J Thorac Cardiovasc Surg 1975; 70:852–61.
27. Duran CG, Pomar JL, Colman T, Figueroa A, Revuelta JM, Ubago JL. Is tricuspid valve repair necessary? J Thorac Cardiovasc Surg 1980; 80: 849–60.
28. Carpentier A, Deloche A, Dauptain J, Soyer R, Prigent C, Blondeau P, Piwnica A, Dubost C. A new reconstructive operation for correction of mitral and tricuspid insufficiency. J Thorac Cardiovasc Surg 1971; 61:1–8.
29. Colonna D, Maurat JP, Acar J, Rocache M. Indications et resultats de la commissurotomie tricuspidienne. Coeur et Medicine Intern 1969; 2:209–20. with one year follow-up. Am Heart J 1954; 47:613–7.

30. Trace HD, Bailey CP, Wendhos MH. Tricuspid valve commissurotomy with one year follow-up. Am Heart J 1954; 47:613–7.
31. Kitchen A, Turner R. Diagnosis and treatment of tricuspid stenosis. Br Heart J 1964; 26:354–79.
32. Silver MD, Lam JHC, Rangathan N, Wigle ED. Morphology of the human tricuspid valve. Circulation 1971; 43:333–48.
33. Virmani R. The tricuspid valve. Mayo Clinic Proc 1988; 63:943–6.
34. Hauck AJ, Freeman DP, Ackerman DM, Danielson GK, Edwards WD. Surgical pathology of the tricuspid valve: a study of 363 cases spanning 25 years. Mayo Clinic Proc 1988; 63:851–63.
35. Ribeiro PA, Zaibag MA, Sawyer W. A prospective study comparing the hemodynamic with the cross-sectional echocardiographic diagnosis of rheumatic tricuspid stenosis. Eur Heart J 1989; 10:120–6.
36. Cooke WT, White PD. Tricuspid stenosis with particular reference to diagnosis and prognosis. Br Heart J 1941; 3:147–52.
37. Cabot RC. Facts of the heart. Philadelphia: Saunders, 1926:159–73.
38. Holmann A. Tricuspid valvotomy. Lancet 1956; 1:536–8.
39. Waller BF, Muriarty AT, Eble JN, Davey DM, Hawley DA, Pless JE. Etiology of pure tricuspid regurgitation based on annular circumference and leaflet area: analysis of 45 necropsy patients with clinical and morphological evidence of pure tricuspid regurgitation. J Amer Col Cardiol 1986; 7: 1063–74.
40. Paul MH, Lev M. Tricuspid stenosis with pulmonary atresia; cineangiographic-pathological correlation. Circulation 1960; 22:198–204.
41. Farooki ZQ, Henry JG, Green EW. Echocardiographic spectrum of Ebstein's anomaly of the tricuspid valve. Circulation 1976; 53:63–9.
42. Edwards JE. Pathological features of Ebstein's anomaly of the tricuspid valve. Proc Staff Meet Mayo Clin 1953; 28:89–94.
43. Carpena C, Kay JH, Mendex AM, Redington JV, Zubiate P, Zucker R. Carcinoid heart disease: surgery for tricuspid and pulmonary lesions. Am J Cardiol 1973; 32:229–33.
44. Trell E, Rausing A, Ripa J, Torp A, Waldenstrom J. Carcinoid heart disease. Clinicopathologic finding and follow-up in 11 cases. Am J Med 1973; 54: 433–44.
45. Davies J NP, Ball JD. The pathology of endomyocardial fibrosis in Uganda. Br Heart J 1955; 17:337–42.
46. Gibson R, Wood P. The diagnosis of tricuspid stenosis. Br Heart J 1955; 552–9.
47. Gayet C, Pierre B, Delahaye JP, Champsaurg S, Andrefovet X, Rue FFP. Traumatic tricuspid insufficiency. An underdiagnosed disease. Chest 1987; 92:429–32.
48. Killip T, Lunas DS. Tricuspid stenosis: physiologic criteria for diagnosis and hemodynamic abnormalities. Circulation 1957; 16:3–13.
49. Xavier de Brito AH, Seuff JA, Toledo AN, Zaniolo W, Snitlowsnay R, Costa C, Azevedo AC. Early stages of tricuspid stenosis. Am J Cardiol 1966; 18:57–63.

50. White PD. Heart Disease. 3d ed. New York: Macmillan, 1944:629.
51. Garvin GF. Tricuspid stenosis. Incidence and diagnosis. Arch Intern Med 1943; 72:104–15.
52. Ferrer MI, Harvey RM, Kuschner M, Dickinson WP, Cournand A. Hemodynamic studies in tricuspid stenosis of rheumatic origin. Circ Res 1953; 1: 49–56.
53. Goodwin JF, Rab SM, Sinha AK, Zoob M. Rheumatic tricuspid stenosis. Br Med J 1957; 2:5058–67.
54. Ribeiro PA, Al Zaibag M, Al Kasab S, Idris MT, Halim M, Abdullah M, Shahed M. Percutaneous double balloon valvotomy for rheumatic tricuspid stenosis. Am J Cardiol 1988; 61:660–2.
55. Ribeiro PA, Al Zaibag M, Al Kasab S, Idris MT, Halim M, Abdullah M, Shahed M. Provocation and amplification of the transvalvular pressure gradient of rheumatic tricuspid stenosis. Am J Cardiol 1988; 61:1307–12.
56. Morgan JR, Forker AD, Coates JR, Myers WS. Isolated tricuspid stenosis. Circulation 1971; 44:729–72.
57. Keefe JF, Wolk MJ, Levine HJ. Isolated tricuspid valvular stenosis. Am J Cardiol 1970; 25:252–4.
58. Gueron M, Hirsch M, Borman J, Appelbaum A. Isolated tricuspid valvular stenosis. The pathology and merits of surgical treatment. J Thorac Cardiovasc Surg 1972; 63:760–4.
59. Salazar E, Levine HD. Rheumatic tricuspid regurgitation. The clinical spectrum. Am J Med 1962; 33:111–29.
60. Sepulveda G, Lukas DS. The diagnosis of tricuspid insufficiency. Clinical features in 60 cases with associated mitral valve disease. Circulation 1955; 11:552–63.
61. Al Zaibag M, Ribeiro PA, Al Kasab S. Percutaneous balloon valvotomy for tricuspid stenosis. Br Heart J 1987; 57:51–3.
62. Ockene IS. Tricuspid valve disease. In: DE Dalen, JS Albert, eds. Valvular Heart Disease. Boston: Little, Brown, 1981:281–328.
63. Acar J. Les cardiopathies valvularies acquises. Flammarion Medicine, Sciences, 1985:386–415.
64. Finnegan P, Abrams LD. Isolated tricuspid stenosis. Br Heart J 1973; 35: 1207–10.
65. Shimada R, Takeshita A, Nakamura M, Tokunaga K, Hirata T. Diagnosis of tricuspid stenosis by M-mode and two-dimensional echocardiography. Am J Card 1984; 53:164–8.
66. Joyner CR, Hey EB, Johnson J, Reid JM. Reflected ultrasound in diagnosis of tricuspid stenosis. Am J Cardiol 1967; 19:66–73.
67. Gramiak R, Shah PM. Cardiac ultrasonography: a review of current indications. Radiol Clin N Am 1971; 9:469–90.
68. Feigenbaum H. Echocardiography. 3d ed. Philadelphia: Lea & Febiger, 1981:239–327.
69. Nanna M, Chandrapapna A, Reid C, Nimalasuriya A, Rahimtoola SH. Value of two-dimensional echocardiography in detecting tricuspid stenosis. Circulation 1977; 67:221–4.

70. Guyer DE, Gilliam LD, Foale RA, Clark MC, Dinsmore R, Palacios I, Block P, King ME, Weyman AE. Comparison of the echocardiographic and hemodynamic diagnosis of rheumatic tricuspid stenosis. J Am Coll Cardiol 1984; 3:1135-44.
71. Daniels SJ, Mintz GS, Kotler MN. Rheumatic tricuspid valve disease: two-dimensional echocardiographic, haemodynamic, and angiographic correlations. Am J Cardiol 1983; 51:492-6.
72. Fawzy ME, Mercer EN, Dunn B, Alamri M, Andaya W. Comparison of the echocardiographic and hemodynamic diagnosis of rheumatic tricuspid stenosis. Eur Heart J 1989; 10:985-90.
73. Veyrat C, Kalmanson D, Farjon M, Manin JP, Abitbol G. Non-invasive diagnosis and assessment of tricuspid regurgitation and stenosis using one and two-dimensional echo pulsed Doppler. Br Heart J 1982; 47:596-605.
74. Perez JE, Ludbrook PA, Ahumada GG. Usefulness of Doppler echocardiography in detecting tricuspid valve stenosis. Am J Cardiol 1985; 55:601-3.
75. Ribeiro PA, Al Zaibag M, Sawyer W. Nomenclature for the use of balloon catheters (letter). Am J Cardiol 1989; 63:262.
76. Hansing CE, Rowe GG. Tricuspid insufficiency. A study of hemodynamic and pathogenesis. Circulation 1972; 45:793-9.
77. Cha SD, Desai RS, Gooch AS, Maranhao V, Goldberg H. Diagnosis of severe tricuspid regurgitation. Chest 1982; 82:726-31.
78. Brofman BL. Right auriculoventricular pressure gradients with special reference to tricuspid stenosis. J Lab Clin Med 1953; 42:789-94.
79. Chesterman JT, Whitaker W. Mitral and tricuspid valvotomy from mitral and tricuspid stenosis. Am Heart J 1954; 48:631-6.
80. O'Neill TJE, Janton OH, Glover RP. Surgical treatment of tricuspid stenosis. Circulation 1954; 9:881-5.
81. Pantridge JF, Marshall RJ. Tricuspid stenosis. Lancet 1957; 1:1319-21.
82. Ribeiro PA, Al Zaibag M, Idris MT. Percutaneous double balloon tricuspid valvotomy: three-year follow-up study. Eur Heart J 1990; 11:1109-13.
83. Bourdillon PDV, Hookman LD, Morris SN, Waller BF. Percutaneous balloon valvuloplasty for tricuspid stenosis. Hemodynamic and pathological findings. Am Heart J 1989; 117:492-5.
84. Khalilullah M, Tyagi S, Yagav BS, Jain P, Choudry A, Lochan R. Double balloon valvuloplasty of tricuspid stenosis. Am Heart J 1987; 114:1232-3.
85. Mullins CE, Hill MR, Vick GW, Ludomirsky A, O'Laughlin MP, Bricker JT, Judd VE. Double balloon technique for dilatation of valvular or vessel stenosis in congenital and acquired heart disease. J Am Coll Card 1987; 10:107-14.
86. Miyatake K, Okamoto M, Kinoshita N, Ohta Mitsushige, Kosuka T, Sakakibara H, Nimura Y. Evaluation of tricuspid regurgitation by pulsed Doppler and two-dimensional echocardiography. Circulation 1982; 66:777-84.
87. Michaek-King R, Schaff HV, Danielson GK, Gersh BJ, Orszulak TA, Piehler JM, Puga FJ, Pluth JR. Surgery for tricuspid regurgitation late after mitral valve replacement. Circulation 1984; 70(suppl I)(1):193-7.

88. Muller O, Shillingford J. Tricuspid incompetence. Br Heart J 1954; 16: 195–8.
89. Glancy DL, Marcus FI, Cuadra M, Ewy GA, Roberts WC. Isolated organic tricuspid regurgitation. Am J Med 1969; 46:989–95.
90. Seides SF, De Joseph RL, Brown AE, Damato AN. Echocardiographic findings in isolated surgically created tricuspid insufficiency. Am J Cardiol 1975; 35:679–82.
91. Aceves S, Carral R. The diagnosis of tricuspid valve disease. Am Heart J 1947; 34:114–9.
92. Weyman AE, Rankin R, King H. Locffer's endocarditis presenting as mitral and tricuspid stenosis. Am J Cardiol 1977; 40:438–44.
93. Simon R, Oelert H, Borst HG, Lichlen PR. Influence of mitral valve surgery on tricuspid incompetence concomitant with mitral valve disease. Circulation 1980; 62(suppl I)(1):152–7.
94. Yoshida K, Yoshikawa J, Shakudo M, Akasaka T, Jyo Y, Takao S, Shiratori K, Koizhumi K, Okumachi F, Kato H, Fukaya T. Colour Doppler evaluation of valvular regurgitation in normal subjects. Circulation 1988; 840–7.
95. Yock PG, Naasz C, Schnittger I, Popp RL. Doppler tricuspid regurgitation in normals. Is it real? (abstr). Circulation 1984; 70(suppl II):40.
96. Goldman ME, Fuster V, Guarino T, Mindich BP. Intraoperative echocardiography for the evaluation of valvular regurgitation. Experience in 263 patients. Circulation 1986; 74(suppl I):143–9.
97. Lukas DS, Dotter CT. Modification of the pulmonary circulation in mitral stenosis. Am J Med 1952; 12:639–42.
98. King TW. The valve function on the right ventricle of the human heart. Guy's Hosp. Rep 1837; 2:132.
99. Coelho E. Physiopathologic study (clinical and experimental) of the tricuspid valve. Am J Cardiol 1959; 3:517–23.
100. Strauss MB, Papper S. Sodium and water retention in chronic congestive heart failure. J Chron Dis 1959; 9:536–45.
101. Ubago JL, Figueroa A, Colman T, Ochoteco A, Rodriguez M, Duran CMG. Right ventriculography as a valid method for the diagnosis of tricuspid insufficiency. Cath and Cardiov Diag 1981; 7:443–51.
102. Cha SD, Maranhao V, Lingamneni R, Goldberg H. A new technique: right ventriculography using a preshaped catheter. Cath and Cardiov Diag 1978; 4:311–6.
103. Shilder DP, Harvey WP. Confusion of tricuspid incompetence with mitral insufficiency. A pitfall in the selection of patients for mitral surgery. Am Heart J 1957; 54:353–9.
104. Urrichio JF, Ben Tivoglio L, Gilman R, Likoff W. Tricuspid regurgitation masquerading as mitral regurgitation in patients with pure mitral stenosis. Am Heart J 1958; 25:224–8.
105. McMichael J, Schillinford JP. The role of valvular incompetence in heart failure. Br Med J 1957; 537–40.
106. Jugdutt BI, Fraser RS, Lee SJ, Rossall RE, Callaghan JC. Long term sur-

vival after tricuspid valve replacement. J Thor Cardiovasc Surg 1977; 74: 20–7.

107. Suwansirikul S, Glassman E, Raia F, Spencer FC. Late thrombosis of Stan-Edwards tricuspid ball valve prosthesis. Am J Cardiol 1974; 34:737–9.

108. Daxter RH, Bain WH, Rankin RJ, Turner MA, Escarous AE, Thomson RM, Lorimer AR, Lawrie TDV. Tricuspid valve replacement. A five year appraisal. Thorax 1975; 30:158–65.

109. Ribeiro PA, Mercer EN, Abdan MA, Halees Z, Gometza B, Duran CMG. Tricuspid regurgitation assessed by echo/Doppler after tricuspid repair using the Duran flexible ring: immediate results and 1 year follow-up (abstr). Circulation 1991; 84(II):2551.

Congenital Valvular Heart Disease in Pediatrics

Charles E. Mullins
Baylor College of Medicine
Houston, Texas

Valvular heart disease in children refers primarily to congenital valvular heart disease. There are a few acquired valvular lesions (rheumatic, infectious) which are relatively common in children in the Mideast, Far East, Africa, and in Central and South America. The occurrence of these diseases in children will be covered in separate chapters on those diseases. All four cardiac valves are involved in association with complex congenital lesions—e.g., syndromes of tricuspid, mitral, pulmonary, and aortic valve atresia. These complex and combined lesions each are subjects related to absent or extremely hypoplastic ventricles, with bizarre circulations as a consequence of the underdeveloped ventricle rather than "valvular abnormalities," and will not be covered in detail in this chapter.

I. PULMONARY VALVE

The most common valvular lesion in children and one of the five most common congenital defects is valvular pulmonic stenosis (PS) (1). This occurs in 9–11% of most series of congenital heart disease (1). Except for very severe valve stenosis occurring in the newborn or early infancy, or in the long neglected child, pulmonic stenosis is usually an asymptomatic lesion. It usually presents with a characteristic ejection systolic murmur maximum in the first and second left intercostal spaces at the left sternal border. The duration, intensity, and quality of the murmur varies with the velocity of flow through the stenotic orifice—generally becoming longer, louder, and harsher with increasing degrees of stenosis (2–4). There is usually a prominent ejection click in the pulmonic area, although this may disappear in very severe cases (5). These patients have right ventricular hypertrophy on electrocardiogram usually proportionate to the degree of stenosis (6,7). If right ventricular hypertrophy is not present, the diagnosis is suspect or other significant lesions may exist in conjunction with the pulmonary stenosis (8). The X-ray usually shows a normal heart size with a prominence along the upper left heart border of the main pulmonary artery segment (9–11). The pulmonary vascular markings are normal unless there are associated lesions allowing right-to-left shunting (VSD, ASD/PFO) or, in very severe cases, significant decrease in cardiac output. Valve pulmonary stenosis can be diagnosed and quantitated accurately by careful echo/Doppler studies. There is very accurate correlation between the peak instantaneous calculated gradient and simultaneous hemodynamic peak-to-peak gradients. This allows confident determination of the timing of appropriate and necessary definitive therapy.

Very mild pulmonic valve stenosis (10 to 20 mm peak systolic gradient) usually remains mild or nonprogressive (12), while more severe stenosis tends to progress proportionate to the growth of the patient (12,13). Older patients with unrecognized or unattended significant pulmonic valve stenosis can present like the infant with very severe stenosis, with signs of right heart failure (14), syncope, or cyanosis in the presence of a PFO/ASD. On X-ray they will have a large dilated heart secondary to right ventricular and right atrial dilation.

The differential diagnosis of valve pulmonary stenosis includes supravalve pulmonary stenosis, branch pulmonary stenosis, and pulmonary stenosis associated with other lesions, particularly atrial septal defect, branch pulmonary stenosis, ventricular septal defect, and/or hypoplastic right ventricle (15). If the associated defect is small or minor, the differentiation from pure pulmonary stenosis is possible only by echo and/or cardiac catheterization. The dysplastic pulmonary valve with pulmonary stenosis which accounts for 5–10% of isolated valve PS also may be determined only at the time of attempted catheter therapy or surgery. Certain somatic syndromes (Noonan's) (16) and/or the detection of an unusually small pulmonary valve annulus by echo may suggest, but are not unequivocal for, the diagnosis of a dysplastic pulmonary valve.

The definitive diagnosis of valve pulmonary stenosis can be made by echo. The determination of the valve anatomy and the gradient across the valve is quite specific by echo/Doppler studies, with excellent correlation between peak instantaneous echo and peak-to-peak hemodynamic gradients (17,18). Cardiac catheterization with quality cardiac angiography may still be necessary diagnostically to verify hemodynamics, determine precise anatomy, and rule out a dysplastic valve or other associated lesions.

The treatment of valvular pulmonary stenosis now is balloon dilation of the stenotic valve (19–21). In the past, when surgery was the treatment for valvular pulmonic stenosis, it was usually reserved for patients with a resting (sedated at catheterization) gradient of 50 mmHg across the valve. This took into account the significant morbidity and risks of the surgery in combination with what was known about the natural history of the disease. Most centers now agree that a resting valve gradient of 40 mmHg or even less in the presence of right ventricular hypertrophy warrants therapeutic intervention by balloon dilation. A single balloon with a diameter of 1.4 to 1.5 times the diameter of the valve annulus (22), or two balloons side by side with combined balloon diameters of 1.6 to 1.8 times the diameter of the annulus, are used (23,24). In experienced hands, with accurate valve and annulus measurements and strict attention to technique, the gradient across the valve should be reduced to less than 10 to 15 mmHg with minimal risk to the patient by balloon dilation. Although there have been cases where the right ventricular pressure has actually increased due to infundibular reaction following the dilation of a very severe stenosis, the phenomenon of the "suicide right ventricle" with deterioration of the patient as seen following surgical valvotomy for very severe stenosis has not been reported following valve dilation. The truly dysplastic valve, documented most conclusively by failed balloon valvuloplasty, requires surgical correction (16,25–27). Usually, valvular excision and annular patching are necessary for good relief of obstruction from the dysplastic valve.

Severe valvular pulmonic stenosis in the newborn or young infant presents with heart failure, cyanosis from shunting at the foramen ovale, often a short nondescript murmur, and massive cardiomegaly on X-ray. These infants are very fragile (28,29). They can be treated with pulmonary balloon valvuloplasty but require very careful control of their ventilation, because of frequent acidosis and bradyarrhythmias. The procedure must be performed dexterously, with only very brief excursions across the stenotic valve, and often graduated valvuloplasty starting with small coronary balloons to initiate any opening in the valve (30,31).

Severe pulmonary valve stenosis with hypoplastic right ventricle (32,33) is a problem with the underdeveloped ventricle identical to pulmonary valve atresia with intact ventricular septum and is not within the scope of this chapter. Similarly, pulmonary stenosis with ventricular septal defect, tetralogy of Fallot, and absent pulmonary valve syndrome all involve the pulmonary valve or annular stenosis but represent far more than the problem with the pulmonary valve and will not be considered in this discussion of valvular lesions.

II. AORTIC VALVE

Like the pulmonary valve, the predominant congenital lesion of the aortic valve is congenital aortic stenosis. Also like pulmonary stenosis, congenital aortic valve stenosis usually presents in childhood as an incidental ejection murmur (34,35). Like the pulmonary stenosis patients, these children, even with quite significant stenosis, recognize no symptoms (34,36). After successful relief of a stenotic aortic valve, however, many patients will retrospectively recognize that their exercise tolerance was decreased prior to the successful therapy. Chest pain and fatigue are reported symptoms of moderate to severe aortic stenosis, but the first symptom of severe valve aortic stenosis may be syncope or even sudden death, presumably due to ventricular fibrillation. The intensity, quality, and duration of the ejection murmur varies approximately with the severity of the stenosis. The more severe lesions have a long, harsh (angry!) ejection systolic murmur associated with a systolic thrill (34). The murmur is usually maximal in the first and second right intercostal spaces with radiation across the sternum to the lower left sternal border to an area of secondary intensity at the apex (37). In very severe cases there can be radiation of the murmur through bone conduction to boney prominences—e.g., the shoulder, elbow, and even the wrist. There usually is a prominent ejection click over the apex and occasionally even in the aortic area (38,39). Along with the systolic murmur, many of these patients will have a decrescendo diastolic murmur of associated aortic regurgitation (38).

The electrocardiogram tends to show dominance of left ventricular forces. Eventually with severe stenosis, there will be frank left ventricular hypertrophy with strain (35,40). This finding, unfortunately, does not always vary in direct proportion to the degree of severity and cannot be used as a reliable means of determining severity (41,42), Likewise, even with severe stenosis, the heart size is usually normal on X-ray (38). Dilation of the ascending aorta with prominence of the upper right mediastinal shadow and aortic nob may be present and suggest the diagnosis, but again is no help in determining severity (38,42).

The echo/Doppler is helpful in establishing the diagnosis (43). The severity of the aortic valve stenosis can be estimated by echo/Doppler but not as accurately as in pulmonic stenosis (44–46). The Doppler peak instantaneous gradient usually significantly overestimates the hemodynamic peak-to-peak gradient (47). Unfortunately, this is not always the case, and the magnitude of the overestimation is not consistent. Unless the estimated Doppler gradient is extremely high (5 m/s or more when the diagnosis is unequivocal) or, at the other extreme, very low, these patients will usually require cardiac catheterization to determine the exact severity of the obstruction and particularly to make thoughtful decisions about appropriate therapy.

Cardiac catheterization is performed when a definitive diagnosis or precise hemodynamics are required or when it is suspected that there is significant enough stenosis to require therapeutic intervention. Catheterization of these patients requires entrance into the left ventricle. This can be accomplished by either the retrograde arterial or transseptal atrial puncture technique (48). The transseptal technique has the advantage of being a reliable approach to the ventricle no matter what the anatomy of the valve nor the degree of stenosis and with no compromise of an artery regardless of how large a catheter is placed in the ventricle for quality angiocardiograms. Simultaneous left ventricular and aortic root pressures or a continuous withdrawal pressure across the valve are required to measure the valvular gradient (36). In equivocal cases, an accurate and nearly simultaneous cardiac output determination should be made for precise valve area determinations (49,50). Biplane angiocardiograms with injection into the left ventricle and the heart in simultaneous left anterior oblique-cranial and a right anterior oblique-caudal angulation will usually cut the left ventricular outflow tract and the aortic valve on edge in each plane (51,52). These angiocardiograms should clearly define the anatomy and establish the diagnosis.

The differential diagnosis of aortic valve stenosis in childhood includes sub- and supravalve aortic stenoses, both of which may have similar murmurs although no ejection click (37). In the infant with severe aortic stenosis, the differential includes sepsis, cardiomyopathy, and even arrhythmias (53). Significant aortic valve stenosis usually is not associated with other congenital cardiac lesions but rarely can be seen with coarctation or ventricular septal defects. An anatomic bicuspid aortic valve is frequently associated with coarctation of the aorta, but this rarely results in aortic valve stenosis of any hemodynamic significance, at least in childhood. The overall natural history of aortic stenosis is somber, with 60% of these patients dying by the age of 40 years and half of these dying with sudden, unexpected death (54,55).

Because of the natural history of this lesion, a peak-to-peak resting (sedated) systolic gradient of 60 mmHg or greater in an active child or teenager, even without symptoms or other signs of deterioration, is considered an indication for therapeutic intervention. The preferred therapy in childhood for significant valvular aortic stenosis now is balloon dilation of the aortic valve (56). The results and complications (57,58) of balloon dilation appear comparable to surgery and the risks considerably less than surgical therapy (56). There are, however, still many centers where this technique is not available or where balloon dilation has not been accepted as appropriate therapy, and in these centers surgical valvotomy is still the standard treatment. For dilation of the aortic valve, the valve is crossed retrograde and one or preferably two balloons are positioned across the valve and inflated. A single balloon with a diameter equal to, or slightly smaller than, the valve annulus diameter (57), or two balloons with a combined diameter 10–20% greater than the aortic valve annulus diameter, are used for the dilation (23). When balloon dilation is unsuccessful at relieving the stenosis, a surgical valvotomy is indicated. Occasionally, valve replacement will be necessary as the initial therapy for severely deformed and stenotic valves which cannot be opened by balloon or surgical valvotomy or valves which after either balloon or surgical valvotomy become severely incompetent (59,60).

Very severe aortic stenosis in the newborn or young infant, like severe pulmonary valve stenosis, presents as an acute emergency. These infants present with low cardiac output, shock, acidosis, and marked cardiomegaly on X-ray. Even more so than infants with severe pulmonary stenosis, these infants are very fragile and even more difficult to treat (53,61,62). Balloon dilation of the aortic valve is more difficult, not only because of the necessary retrograde arterial approach, but because of the different developmental and physiological responses of the left ventricle to the severe stenosis. This response can vary from a small contracted, truly hypoplastic left ventricle (61) through an entire spectrum to the other extreme of a massively dilated, poorly contracting left ventricle. Patients with very small or hypoplastic ventricles with severe aortic stenosis die, almost regardless of the type of therapy (63). Infants with dilated ventricles also have a high early mortality but do better with valve dilation or surgery.

Isolated congenital aortic valve regurgitation does occur very rarely. However, aortic regurgitation usually is in conjunction with either aortic stenosis, a ventricular septal defect, or as a result of endocarditis or rheumatic carditis (acute or chronic). These associated lesions or illnesses should be ruled out before the diagnosis of isolated congenital aortic valve insufficiency is made. Aortic regurgitation presents with a decrescendo diastolic murmur along the left sternal border. The intensity and duration of this murmur usually varies with the severity of the valvular leak. More significant degrees of regurgitation will be associated with a diastolic rumble over the apex, the so-called Austin-Flint murmur caused by encroachment on the mitral valve by the regurgitant jet in the left ventricular outflow tract. An additional important physical finding with aortic regurgitation is the presence of very prominent and collapsing pulses, which are frequently visible even in the suprasternal notch and carotids. In more severe cases the pulses will be visible in the axillary, brachial, and femoral areas, particularly in infants.

The patients with even moderately significant aortic regurgitation usually have left ventricular hypertrophy on ECG and some cardiac enlargement on X-ray as a consequence of the left ventricular volume overload and left ventricular dilation. The echo/Doppler will document, but not accurately quantitate, the degree of aortic regurgitation. The echo should diagnose the presence of any associated lesion, especially a high ventricular septal defect, a subarotic membrane, or even a vegetation of endocarditis as the cause of the regurgitation. The M-mode and 2-D echos are extremely valuable for following the effect of the regurgitant volume overload on the left ventricular function—especially the left ventricular dimensions and left ventricular shortening fraction. These patients should have regular and repeated echos for determination of left ventricular size and function. In the presence of aortic regurgitation, to compensate for the ejection of the regurgitant fraction as well as normal stroke volume, the ventricular function by echo should be supernormal. In order to medically follow these patients safely, the patient should have a left ventricular shortening fraction of greater than 35% and no sequential decreases in this shortening fraction at follow-up visits. Any valid and significant decrease in the shortening fraction on serial echocardiographic studies is an indication for more aggressive therapy.

The initial treatment of aortic regurgitation in children should be conservative for several reasons. First, the patients and their left ventricles usually tolerate all but the most severe regurgitation very well with no symptoms, and of most importance, good preservation of left ventricular function. Second, the "definitive" therapy, when required, is valve replacement. In small children this creates additional problems, with the need for some type of chronic anticoagulation as well as no chance for valve growth. This prosthetic valve will require repeat surgery because of the patient's growth as well as the wear of the valve (60,64).

Both acute rheumatic fever and bacterial endocarditis, when they involve the aortic valve in children, usually result in acute aortic regurgitation. Because this regurgitation usually occurs with a previously nonhypertrophied ventricle, acute-onset regurgitation often is not well tolerated. The underlying illness must be treated while carefully watching the effect of the regurgitation on the ventricular function. With the occasional resultant acute and massive aortic regurgitation with either of these conditions, an emergency valve replacement will be necessary to salvage the patient from acute left ventricular failure and pulmonary edema. Otherwise the regurgitation associated with the acute disease should be managed medically with digoxin, diuretics, and afterload reducers as long as ventricular function can be preserved.

As with the atretic pulmonary valve and hypoplastic right ventricle, the atretic or severely hypoplastic aortic valve is associated with a hypoplastic left ventricle and represents a separate disease entity from aortic valve disease, which will not be covered in this chapter.

III. TRICUSPID VALVE

Isolated congenital involvement of either atrioventricular valve is rare in childhood. Extremely rare cases of tricuspid stenosis are encountered—usually with some hypoplasia of the right ventricle and an interatrial communication (32). These patients may have very subtle signs and recognize few symptoms. The more severely involved patients with tricuspid stenosis present with cyanosis and/or hepatovenous congestion and the signs of other associated intracardiac defects. The diagnosis requires a high degree of suspicion and then very accurate echocardiographic interrogation and specific angiocardiographic visualization at the time of catheterization. Therapeutically, if the ventricle is only minimally hypoplastic, the valve can be opened with expectations of resultant reasonable cardiac function. With more severe degrees of ventricle hypoplasia, the ventricle is the primary problem and an entity which will not be covered under congenital valve diseases in children.

At the opposite extreme of tricuspid stenosis, Ebstein's malformation of the tricuspid valve is more common, produces varying degrees of tricuspid valve regurgitation, and rarely is associated with some stenosis. Pathologically, Ebstein's malformation of the tricuspid valve also includes abnormalities of the right ventricle, sometimes to an extreme degree (65). The degree of involvement of the ventricle in general determines the clinical presentation. Ebstein's malformation usually is associated with an atrial septal defect/open patent foramen ovale. The presence of this defect or, in particular, its absence affect the signs and symptoms as well as the outcome of these patients. The pathological abnormality consists of varying degrees of displacement of the attachment of the tricuspid valve into the body of the right ventricle away from the normal atrioventricular annulus. The leaflets are deformed and plastered against the wall of the right ventricle. This impairs the function of the valve and reduces the effective functional size of the right ventricle. The combination causes significant (frequently massive) tricuspid valve regurgitation. Occasionally, there is separate true valve pulmonary stenosis (65) or, more commonly, a tricuspid valve leaflet is displaced so far into the ventricle that the right ventricular outflow tract is obstructed by the tricuspid leaflet, causing functional pulmonary stenosis. Either of these right ventricular outflow obstructive abnormalities markedly aggravates the tricuspid regurgitation. Although mild cases do occur with very little displacement of the valve and very little functional abnormality, the vast majority of patients with Ebstein's malformation have a severe degree of involvement.

As a consequence, most patients with Ebstein's malformation present in the newborn period with marked cyanosis and "right heart" failure (66). In the absence of any, or with only a small inter atrial communication, the consequence of this tricuspid regurgitation is massive right atrial dilation and resultant massive cardiomegaly (the largest cardiac silhouettes that are seen), severe right heart failure, and low cardiac output. With or without any right ventricular outflow obstruction, these symptoms are aggravated by the normally high pulmonary resistance in the newborn. In the usual infant, there will be some interatrial communication with resultant shunting of varying degrees of systemic venous blood from right to left atrium, and in turn, systemically. The resultant cyanosis often is severe. While these infants will be severely hypoxic, they tend to have a better cardiac output than the infant with an intact atrial septum. The classic patient, in addition to the cyanosis, will have a systolic murmur of tricuspid regurgitation, and even more characteristically, a quadruple cadence to the heart sounds with a prominent S-3 and S-4 in addition to the first and second heart sounds. The electrocardiogram shows right atrial enlargement and an atypical right bundle branch block with a paucity of "right ventricular" or anterior forces (67). Many of these patient will have a pattern of aberrant atrioventricular conduction (e.g., WPW-type complexes) on their electrocardiogram, and some even present with supraventricular tachycardia (68,69).

The diagnosis in the child or older patient should be quite obvious from the clinical findings. The differential diagnosis in the child includes any cause of massive cardiac enlargement with signs of right heart failure and cyanosis. This would include atrial septal defect with pulmonary vascular disease, primary pulmonary hypertension, or end-stage severe pulmonary stenosis with right heart failure. The diagnosis can be confirmed with a good 2-D echocardiogram, which will show the displacement of the tricuspid valve (70–72). Cardiac catheterization is seldom necessary just to confirm the diagnosis, but may be necessary to sort out the hemodynamics. These patients are very prone to arrhythmias and tolerate them very poorly; however, when they have been anticipated and prepared for, these can be rapidly controlled or converted with electrical cardioversion or overdrive pacing in the catheterization laboratory.

The differential diagnosis in the newborn also includes any lesion which causes cyanosis, failure, and cardiomegaly. This must be differentiated from persistent fetal circulation with secondary tricuspid regurgitation, very severe pulmonary stenosis with a dilated failing right ventricle, pulmonary atresia with an intact septum, or tricuspid atresia. In the newborn, the diagnosis also usually can be made from the clinical findings including exam, electrocardiogram, X-ray, and echocardiogram, but occasionally catheterization is necessary to determine the correct course of therapy.

Therapy depends on the age of presentation and the clinical presentation. The best therapy in the newborn is support for symptoms and an attempt to avoid intervention at that time. Oxygen and even ventilation may be needed until the pulmonary resistance decreases. If there is no atrial communication and a severe degree of Ebstein's malformation, the infant may need a balloon or blade septostomy to allow some right-to-left shunting to increase effective systemic output. If there is severe cyanosis with hypoxemia in spite of oxygen and ventilation or as a result of the septostomy, then a systemic-to-pulmonary shunt will be necessary. Once past the newborn period, many of these patients do remarkably well in spite of their cyanosis and massive cardiomegaly (73). When they reach mid-childhood or older, they can be considered for a tricuspid valve repair with plication of the right atrium (74,75) or a caval-pulmonary ("Fontan")-type repair (76). If they have aberrant conduction on their electrocardiogram and certainly if they have had recurrent arrhythmias, their aberrant tracts should be divided at the surgery.

Tricuspid valve atresia, like tricuspid stenosis with a hypoplastic right ventricle, is a problem of a functionally missing ventricle and not a "valve" problem. The presentation, resultant bizarre hemodynamic abnormalities, and the therapy, like many other congenital lesions, depend on the associated abnormalities and will not be addressed here.

IV. MITRAL VALVE

Congenital mitral valve disease usually is in combination with other defects, particularly other left heart lesions. In rare instances it can be involved as an isolated defect or, more commonly, when in combination with other lesions, it is the dominant or persistent remaining lesion when the others have been corrected. Congenital mitral valve stenosis is a rare lesion which usually involves the entire valve apparatus, unlike aortic, pulmonic, or even tricuspid stenosis, mitral stenosis usually results in a bizarre malformation of the valve (77). The valve often has a single leaflet with a single papillary muscle—the so-called parachute mitral valve. The chordae are fused and shortened, the annulus is small, and there often is a membrane above the annulus. Any of these abnormalities can exist alone, but usually several or at least some degree of each lesion occur together to make up the bizarre valves. The degree of stenosis has little or no correlation with the appearance of the valve. Any one of the areas of narrowing is capable of creating severe stenosis. The clinical findings relating to the mitral valve vary with the degree of functional mitral stenosis, not with the anatomy of the valve. Isolated congenital mitral stenosis (not atresia) may but seldom does present in the newborn period. With significant stenosis, older children will have some fatigue, exercise intolerance, and in particular shortness of breath with exertion. Characteristically, they will have a low-frequency presystolic crescendo diastolic murmur maximal over the apex. They may or may not have a pansystolic murmur of associated mitral regurgitation. If the stenosis is very severe, the patients will also have signs of pulmonary hypertension with a very loud single second heart sound and a right ventricular lift. Since there are commonly associated other left heart lesions (subaortic or valvular aortic stenosis, or coarctation of the aorta), the findings from these lesions may be coexistent or overshadow the mitral findings.

The diagnosis should be fairly straightforward from the clinical findings unless overshadowed by other defects. With significant stenosis, the X-ray will show a normal or slightly enlarged heart size, left atrial enlargement, increased pulmonary venous markings, and in severe cases, Curley-B lines. The electrocardiogram will show varying degrees of left atrial enlargement and/or right ventricular hypertrophy. The diagnosis should be confirmed and the type and severity of the stenosis determined by the echocardiogram/Doppler. Cardiac catheterization will be necessary to determine the hemodynamics absolutely, particularly when there is a significant cardiac defect in addition to the mitral stenosis.

The therapy of congenital mitral stenosis is medical until one is forced into some interventional therapy because of uncontrollable symptoms due to the mitral obstruction or signs of severe pulmonary hypertension. Unfortunately, since the valve is so complex and bizarre in its anatomy, a "simple" surgical commissurotomy or valve repair is seldom satisfactory for relief of symptoms. Frequently, when surgery is required, valve replacement is necessary, with the resultant necessity of chronic anticoagulation therapy (78) and unequivocal repeat valve replacement. In spite of the need for anticoagulation, mechanical prosthetic valves are used in children because of the rapid deterioration (calcification) of tissue valves in children (79). More recently, surprisingly favorable results have been obtained by balloon dilation of these congenitally stenotic mitral valves regardless of their underlying anatomy (80). A double-transseptal, double-balloon technique has been used with the best results and the least complications (80). Because of the unfavorable anatomy, the complexity and risks of the procedure, and the theoretical strong likelihood of destroying the valve and creating significant mitral regurgitation, balloon dilation of the congenital mitral valve has been reserved for the very symptomatic patient or the patient with severe secondary pulmonary hypertension, either of which conditions would require surgery as an alternate therapy.

Isolated congenital mitral valve regurgitation exists, but is an even rarer lesion than congenital mitral stenosis (81). Although it may be the dominant lesion, it also more frequently exists with other defects, particularly coarctation of the aorta or endocardial cushion defects, which will be discussed later. Unless it is aggravated by significant elevation of afterload (systemic hypertension, coarctation, aortic stenosis), congenital mitral regurgitation is quite well tolerated for years. The patients will have chronic fatigue and some shortness of breath, but usually no acute symptoms until very late in the course of the disease (81,82). They usually will preserve left ventricular function quite well. The first significant symptomatic deterioration often occurs with the onset of atrial arrhythmias. Clinically they present with a pansystolic murmur, maximum over the apex. This is frequently associated with a mid-diastolic rumble, also over the apex. Chest X-ray shows significant cardiomegaly, especially left atrial enlargement with increased pulmonary (venous) markings. The electrocardiogram will show left atrial enlargement and left ventricular hypertrophy. Echocardiogram will demonstrate but not accurately quantitate the mitral regurgitation and will rule out other abnormalities of the mitral valve or other associated defects.

Therapy for congenital mitral regurgitation is first medical, with diuretics, digoxin, and afterload reducers. Surgical removal of structural causes of increased afterload will improve the congenital mitral regurgitation. When medical management fails and the valve must be addressed surgically, mitral annuloplasty or valve repair should be attempted. However, when surgery is required, mitral valve replacement is usually required, if not initially, almost invariably later, at subsequent surgery. The same type of valve is used and the same problems exist whether the valve is replaced for regurgitation or stenosis (83).

REFERENCES

1. Nadas AS, Fyler DC. Pediatric Cardiology. 34th ed. Philadelphia: Saunders, 1972.
2. Vogelpool L, Schrire V. Auscultatory and phoncardiographic assessment of pulmonary stenosis with intact ventricular septum. Circulation 1960; 22:55.
3. Dimond EG, Lin TK. The clinical picture of pulmonary stenosis (without ventricular septal defect). Ann Intern Med 1954; 40:1108.
4. Mannheimer E, Jonsson B. Heart sounds and murmurs in congenital pulmonary stenosis with normal aortic root. Acta Paediatr 1954; 43(suppl 100):167.

5. Hultgren HN, Reeve R, Cohn K, McLeod R. The ejection click of valvular pulmonic stenosis. Circulation 1969; 40:631.

6. Bassingthwaighte JB, et al. The electrocardiographic and hemodynamic findings in pulmonary stenosis with intact ventricular septum. Circulation 1963; 28:893.

7. Ellison RC, et al. Indirect assessment of severity in pulmonic stenosis. Circulation 1977; 56(suppl I):114.

8. Emmanouilides GC, Baylen BG. Pulmonary stenosis. In: Adams FH, Emmanouilides GC, eds. Heart Disease in Infants, Children, and Adolescents. 3d ed. Baltimore: Williams & Wilkins, 1983.

9. Blount SG Jr, McCord MC, Komesu S, Lanier RR. Roentgenological aspects of isolated valvular pulmonic stenosis. Radiology 1954; 62:337.

10. Dow JW, et al. Studies of congenital heart disease. IV: Uncomplicated pulmonic stenosis. Circulation 1950; 1:267.

11. Greene DG, et al. Pure congenital pulmonary stenosis and idiopathic congenital dilatation of the pulmonary artery. Am J Med 1949; 6:24.

12. Levine RO, Blumenthal S. Pulmonic stenosis in five congenital cardiac defects. Circulation 1965; 31–32(suppl III):33.

13. Lange PE, Onnasch DGW, Heintzen PH. Valvular pulmonary stenosis: natural history and right ventricular function. In: Doyle EF et al., eds. Pediatric Cardiology. New York: Springer-Verlag, 1986.

14. Krabill KA, Wang Y, Einzig S, Moller JH. Rest and exercise hemodynamics in pulmonary stenosis: comparison of children and adults. Am J Cardiol 1985; 56:360.

15. Cheatham JP. Pulmonary stenosis. In: Garson A, Bricker JT, McNamara DG, eds. Science and Practice of Pediatric Cardiology. Vol. II. Philadelphia: Lea & Febiger, 1990.

16. Noonan JA. Hypertelorism with Turner phenotype: a new syndrome with associated congenital heart disease. Am J Dis Child 1968; 116:373.

17. Oliveira TC, et al. Noninvasive prediction of transvalvular pressure gradients in patients with pulmonary stenosis by quantitative two-dimensional echocardiographic Doppler studies. Circulation 1983; 67:866.

18. Ishizawa A, et al. Noninvasive and quantitative evaluation of the severity of isolated pulmonary valvular stenosis by two-dimensional pulsed Doppler echocardiography. In: Doyle EF, et al., eds. Pediatric Cardiology. New York: Springer-Verlag, 1986.

19. Lababidi Z, Wu J. Percutaneous balloon pulmonary valvuloplasty. Am J Cardiol 1983; 52:560.

20. Kan JS, et al. Percutaneous transluminal balloon valvuloplasty for pulmonary valve stenosis. Circulation 1984; 69:554.

21. Stanger P, Cassidy SC, Girod DA, Kan JS, Lababidi Z, Shapiro S. Balloon pulmonary valvuloplasty: results of the Valvuloplasty and Angioplasty of Congenital Anomalies Registry. Am J Cardiol 1990;65:775–783.

22. Radtke W, et al. Percutaneous balloon valvotomy of congenital pulmonary stenosis using oversized balloons. J Am Coll Cardiol 1986; 8:909.

23. Mullins CE, Nihill MR, Vick III GW, Ludomirsky A, O'Laughlin MP, Bricker JT, Judd VE. Double balloon technique for dilation of valvular or vessel stenosis in congenital and acquired heart disease. J Am Coll Cardiol 1987; 10(1):107.

24. Ali Khan MA, Al Yousef S, Mullins CE. Percutaneous transluminal balloon pulmonary valvuloplasty for the relief of pulmonary valve stenosis with special reference to double-balloon technique. Am Heart J 1986; 112:158.

25. Edwards JE: Congenital malformation of the heart and great vessels. In: Gould SE, ed. Pathology of the Heart and Blood Vessels. 34th ed. Springfield, IL: Charles C. Thomas, 1968.

26. Kortezky ED, et al. Congenital pulmonary stenosis resulting from dysplasia of valve. Circulation 1969; 40:43.

27. Musewe NN, Robertson MA, Benson LN, Smallhorn JF, Burrows PE, Freedom RM, Moes CAF, Rowe RD. The dysplastic pulmonary valve: echocardiographic features and results of balloon dilatation. Br Heart J 1987; 57: 364.

28. Gersony WM, Bernhard WF, Nadas AS, Gross RE. Diagnosis and surgical treatment of infants with critical pulmonary outflow obstruction. Circulation 1967; 35:765.

29. Coles JG, Freedom RM, Olley PM, Coceani F, Williams WG, Trusler GA. Surgical management of critical pulmonary stenosis in the neonate. Ann Thorac Surg 1984; 358:458.

30. Ali Khan MA, Al Yousef S, Sawyer W. Graduated sequential balloon dilatation as a treatment for severe pulmonary valve stenosis in infants and children. Pediatr Cardiol 1987; 8:212.

31. Zeevi B, Keane JF, Fellows K, Lock JE. Balloon dilation of critical pulmonic stenosis in the first week of life. J Am Coll Cardiol 1988; 11:821.

32. Williams JCP, Barratt-Boyles BG, Lowe JB. Underdeveloped right ventricle and pulmonary stenosis. Am J Cardiol 1963; 11:458.

33. Freed MD, et al. Critical pulmonary stenosis with dimuntive right ventricle in neonates. Circulation 1973; 48:875.

34. Ellison RC, Wagner HR, Weidman WH, Miettinen OS. Congenital valvular aortic stenosis: clinical detection of small pressure gradient. Prepared for the Joint Study on the Natural History of Congenital Heart Defects. Am J Cardiol 1976; 37:757.

35. Wagner HR, Weidman WH, Ellison RC, Miettinen OS. Indirect assessment of severity in aortic stenosis. Circulation 1977; 56(suppl I):I-20.

36. Alpert BS, et al. Hemodynamic responses to ergometer exercise in children and young adults with left ventricular pressure on volume overload. Am J Cardiol 1983; 52:563.

37. Latson LA. Aortic stenosis: valvular, supravalvular, and fibromuscular subvalvular. In: Garsen A, Bricker JT, McNamara DG, eds. Science and Practice of Pediatric Cardiology. Vol. II. Philadelphia: Lea & Febiger, 1990.

38. Braunwald E, et al. Congenital aortic stenosis. I: Clinical and hemodynamic findings in 100 patients; and Marrow AG, et al. II: Surgical treatment and results of operation. Circulation 1963; 27:426.

39. Cohen LS, Friedman WF, Braunwald E. Natural history of mild congenital aortic stenosis elucidated by serial hemodynamic studies. Am J Cardiol 1972; 30:1.

40. Fowler RS, et al. The ECG in aortid stenosis. Value of TAVF and QV_6. Pediatr Cardiol 1982; 3:213.

41. Reynolds JL, Nadas AS, Rudolph AM, Gross RE. Critical congenital aortic stenosis with minimal electrocardiographic changes. N Engl J Med 1960; 262:276.

42. Mody MR, Mody GT. Serial hemodynamic observations in congenital valvular and subvalvular aortic stenosis. Am Heart J 1975; 89:137.

43. Seitz WS, et al. Echocardiographic application of the Gorlin formula for assessment of aortic stenosis. Correlation with cardiac catheterization in pediatric patients. Am Heart J 1986; 111:1118.

44. Glanz S, Hellenbrand WE, Berman MA, Talner NS. Echocardiographic assessment of the severity of aortic stenosis in children and adolescents. Am J Cardiol 1976; 38:620.

45. DeMaria AN, et al. Value and limitations of cross-sectional echocardiography of the aortic valve in the diagnosis and quantification of valvular aortic stenosis. Circulation 1980; 62:304.

46. Huhta JC, et al. Surgery without catheterization for congenital heart defects: management of 100 patients. J Am Coll Cardiol 1987; 9:823.

47. Peller OG, Wallerson DG, Devereux RB. Role of Doppler and imaging echocardiography in selection of patients for cardiac valvular surgery. Am Heart J 1987; 114:1445.

48. Duff DF, Mullins CE. Transseptal left catheterization in infants and children. Cath Cardiovasc Diagn 1978; 4:213.

49. Gorlin R, et al. Dynamics of the circulation in aortic valvular disease. Am J Med 1955; 18:855.

50. Bache RJ, Jorgenson CR, Yang Y. Simplified estimation of aortic valve area. Br Heart J 1972; 34:408.

51. Fellows KE, Keane JF, Freed MD. Angled views in cineangiocardiography of congenital heart disease. Circulation 1977; 56:485.

52. Ceballos R, Soto B, Bargeron LM. Angiographic anatomy of the normal heart through axial angiography. Circulation 1981; 64:351.

53. Harstreiter AR, et al. Congenital aortic stenosis syndrome in infancy. Circulation 1963; 28:1084.

54. Campbell M. The natural history of congenital aortic stenosis. Br Heart J 1968; 30:514.

55. Frank S, Johnson A, Ross J Jr. Natural history of valvular aortic stenosis. Br Heart J 1973; 35:41.

56. Rocchini AP, Beekman RH, Shachar GB, Benson L, Schwartz D, Kan JS. Balloon aortic valvuloplasty: results of the Valvuloplasty and Angioplasty of Congenital Anomalies Registry. Am J Cardiol 1990; 65:784.

57. Lababidi Z, Wu JR, Walls TJ. Percutaneous balloon aortic valvuloplasty: results in 23 patients. Am J Cardiol 1984; 53:194.

58. Choy M, et al. Percutaneous balloon valvuloplasty for aortic stenosis in infants and children. Am J Cardiol 1987; 59:1010.

59. Milano A, et al. Late results after left-sided cardiac valve replacement in children. J Thorac Cardiovasc Surg 1986; 92:218.

60. Makhlouf A, et al. Prosthetic heart valve replacement in children. Results and follow-up of 273 patients. J Thorac Cardivasc Surg 1987; 93:80.

61. Nadas AS, Mody MR. Preductal coarctation and hypoplastic left heart complexes, with comments on the premature closure of the foramen ovale. In: Cassels ED, ed. Heart and Circulation in the Newborn and Infant. New York: Gruen & Stratton, 1966:225.

62. Keane JF, Bernhard WF, Nadas AS. Aortic stenosis surgery in infancy. Circulation 1975: 52:1138.

63. Mocelin R, et al. Reduced left ventricular size and endocardial fibroelastosis as correlates of mortality in newborns and young infants with severe aortic valve stenosis. Ped Cardiol 1983; 4:265.

64. Borkon AM, et al. Five year follow-up after valve replacement with the St. Jude Medical valve in infants and children. Circulation 1986; 74(suppl I):I-110.

65. Anderson KR, et al. Morphologic spectrum of Ebstein's anomaly of the heart: a review. Mayo Clin Proc 1979; 54:174.

66. Schiebler GL, et al. Clinical study of twenty-three cases of Ebstein's anomaly of the tricuspid valve. Circulation 1959; 19:165.

67. Follath F, Hallidie-Smith KA. Unusual electrocardiographic changes in Ebstein's anomaly. Br Heart J 1972; 34:513.

68. Lev ML, Gibson S, Miller RA. Ebstein's disease with Wolff-Parkinson-White syndrome: report of a case with a histopathologic study of possible conduction pathways. Am Heart J 1955; 49:724.

69. Schiebler GL, Adams P Jr, Anderson RC. The Wolff-Parkinson-White syndrome in infants and children: a review and a report of 28 cases. Pediatrics 1959; 24:585.

70. Hirschklau MJ, et al. Cross-sectional echocardiographic features of Ebstein's anomaly of the tricuspid valve. Am J Cardiol 1977; 40:400.

71. Gussenhoven EJ, et al. "Offsetting" of the septal tricuspid leaflet in normal hearts and in hearts with Ebstein's anomaly: anatomic and echographic correlation. Am J Cardiol 1984; 54:172.

72. Gussenhoven WJ, et al. The role of echocardiography in assessing the functional class of the patient with Ebstein's anomaly. Eur Heart 1984; 5:490.

73. Watson H. Natural history of Ebstein's anomaly of tricuspid valve in childhood and adolescence: an international co-operative study of 505 cases. Br Heart J 1974; 36:417.

74. Mair DD, Seward JB, Driscoll DJ, Danielson GK. Surgical repair of Ebstein's anomaly: selection of patients and early and late operative results. Circulation 1985; 72(suppl 2):II-70.

75. Danielson GK, Maloney JD, Devloo RAE. Surgical repair of Ebstein's anomaly. Mayo Clin Proc 1979; 54:185.

76. Glenn WWL, Browne M, Whittemore R. Circulatory bypass of the right side of the heart cavapulmonary artery shunt—indications and results (report of a collected series of 537 cases). In: Cassels DE, ed. The Heart and Circulation in the Newborn and Infant. New York: Grune & Stratton, 1966:345.
77. Grenadier E, et al. Two-dimensional echo Doppler study of congenital disorders of the mitral valve. Am Heart J 1984; 107:319.
78. Bradley LM, et al. Anticoagulant therapy in children with mechanical prosthetic cardiac valves. Am J Cardiol 1985; 56:533.
79. Wada J, et al. Long-term follow-up of artificial valves in patients under 15 years old. Ann Thorac Surg 1980;29:519.
80. Grifka RG, Nihill MR, Mullins CE. Percutaneous transseptal double balloon valvuloplasty for congenital mitral stenosis (abstr). Presented at American Academy of Pediatrics, Boston, MA, Oct 5–7, 1990.
81. Braunwald E, Ross RS, Morrow AG, Roberts WC. Differential diagnosis of mitral regurgitation in childhood: clinical pathological conference at the National Institutes of Health. Ann Intern Med 1961; 54:1223.
82. Braunwald E. Heart Disease: A Textbook of Cardiovascular Medicine. Philadelphia: Saunders, 1984.
83. Chadha SK, et al. Mitral valve disease in young: review of surgical treatment. Ind J Thorac Cardiovasc Surg 1983;2:29.

11

Acute Mitral and Aortic Valve Regurgitation

Kenneth R. Jutzy
Loma Linda University Medical School, Loma Linda, California

Muayed Al Zaibag
Armed Forces Hospital, Riyadh, Saudi Arabia, and Loma Linda University Medical Center, Loma Linda, California

I. ACUTE MITRAL REGURGITATION

A. Introduction

Acute mitral regurgitation (MR) differs significantly from chronic MR. These differences are not only in pathophysiology and clinical features, but more important, in prognosis and treatment. Hence it is imperative that these differences be kept in mind so that early diagnosis and prompt management of this acute condition can be accomplished.

Acute MR varies in degree of severity, but in clinical practice we are concerned with moderately severe to severe forms of regurgitation. These conditions are associated with high mortality and morbidity if diagnosis and treatment are delayed or missed.

B. Etiology

Acute regurgitation of the mitral valve results from rupture of chordae tendineae, dysfunction or rupture of a papillary muscle, or disruption of a valve leaflet. Table 1 summarizes the various etiologies of acute MR. Spontaneous idiopathic chordal rupture, acute coronary ischemia, infective endocarditis, myxomatous degeneration, and degeneration of bioprosthetic valves are the most common underlying etiologies (1–3).

Table 1 Causes of Acute Mitral Regurgitation

1. Mitral annulus disorders
   a. Infective endocarditis, e.g., abscess formation
   b. Trauma e.g., valvular heart surgery
   c. Paravalvular leak due to suture interruption, e.g., surgical technical problems or infective endocarditis
2. Mitral leaflet disorders
   a. Infective endocarditis, e.g., perforation or interfering with valve closure by vegetation
   b. Trauma, e.g., tear during percutaneous mitral balloon valvotomy or penetrating chest injury
   c. Tumors, e.g., atrial myxoma
   d. Myxomatous degeneration
   e. Systemic lupus erythematosus, e.g., Libman-Sacks lesion
3. Rupture of chordae tendineae
   a. Idiopathic, e.g., spontaneous
   b. Myxomatous degeneration, e.g., mitral valve prolapse, Marfan's syndrome, and Ehlers-Danlos syndrome
   c. Infective endocarditis
   d. Acute rheumatic fever
   e. Trauma, e.g., percutaneous balloon valvotomy, blunt chest trauma
4. Papillary muscle disorders
   a. Coronary artery disease, e.g., causing dysfunction and rarely rupture
   b. Acute global left ventricular dysfunction
   c. Infiltrative diseases, e.g., amyloidosis, sarcoidosis
   d. Trauma
5. Primary mitral valve prosthetic disorders
   a. Porcine cusp perforation, e.g., endocarditis
   b. Porcine cusp degeneration
   c. Mechanical failure, e.g., strut fracture
   d. Immobilized disc or ball of the mechanical prosthesis

Coronary artery disease is the most common cause of acute MR (2). This is not surprising since the incidence of acute myocardial infarction is high; in the United States it is 1.5 million cases annually (4). The incidence of angiographic MR after infarction is 13–18% (5,6). Idiopathic rupture of chordae tendineae, however, is the most common pathological condition that produces severe acute MR (1), whereas acute myocardial infarction and infective endocarditis are the principal etiologies in fatal acute severe MR (3).

1. Rupture of Chordae Tendineae

It is widely popularized that spontaneous rupture of chordae tendineae is often of unknown etiology. In 1972, 65 patients with spontaneous rupture of chordae were studied: two-thirds of these patients had no apparent previous cardiac disease, while 32% had ischemic, rheumatic, or infective heart disease (7). Mitral valve prolapse (MVP) most likely was underdiagnosed, and currently there is a consensus that MVP is often associated with spontaneous chordal rupture. In a study of 60 patients who underwent surgery because of pure severe MR associated with MVP, chordal rupture was found in 22% (8). At necropsy, the overall incidence of MVP was reported to be 1% in 1969, but in 1982 had risen to 7.4% (9,10). This difference is probably due to increased awareness of this pathological entity and the availability of more sensitive diagnostic tests, namely echocardiography.

In a more recent study, ultrastructural examination of the mitral valve apparatus in patients with spontaneous chordal rupture revealed changes consistent with myxomatous degeneration of the leaflets, causing their dilatation and subsequent regurgitation from severe prolapse or chordal rupture (11). This suggests that there is a close relationship between spontaneous chordal rupture, MVP, and myxomatous degeneration of the mitral valve.

2. Coronary Artery Disease

During or following acute coronary ischemic episodes, various degrees of acute MR can occur due to papillary muscle disorders (2,5,6,12–16). The latter may range from mild dysfunction to partial or even complete rupture.

The posteromedial papillary muscle is most vulnerable to ischemia because of the pattern of its blood supply. Generally, this muscle has blood supply only from the posterior descending branch of the dominant right or circumflex coronary artery, while the anterolateral papillary muscle has dual supply from the left anterior descending and circumflex coronary arteries (17). Thus, acute inferoposterior infarction is most likely to result in papillary muscle rupture, which can occur even in patients with small or nontransmural infarctions and well-preserved global left ventricular function (1,6,18). Nevertheless, since anterior myocardial infarction is generally more frequent than inferior infarction, the overall observed incidence of papillary muscle rupture causing acute severe MR is approximately equal after anterior and inferior myocardial infarctions (1,5).

Although catastrophic complete rupture of the papillary muscle is rare, dysfunction of this muscle is fairly common after acute myocardial infarction (2,5,6,14–16). The size of infarction does not reliably predict the occurrence or the severity of acute MR. For example, severe acute MR may result from an occlusion of a small obtuse marginal or diagonal branch of the circumflex and left anterior descending arteries, respectively.

It is noteworthy that the reported incidence of acute MR following acute myocardial infarction varies widely; this is partly because of the different methods of detecting MR. For example, by physical examination, a new apical murmur has been found in about 50% of patients with acute infarction (14,15). The level of detection of such a murmur following an infarction may vary with the severity of regurgitation; in two separate studies, only a few (7% and 13%) patients—with angiographically confirmed mild to moderate MR—had audible murmurs following infarction, while 50% of those with severe degree of regurgitation had murmurs (5,6). Murmurs in acute MR may not be detectable because of posteriorly directed regurgitant jets, abnormal chest wall anatomy, or interference by ambient noise, especially in patients with severe pulmonary edema or on artificial ventilators.

Using left ventriculography within hours after the onset of acute myocardial infarction, MR was detected in 13–18% of cases; moderately severe to severe regurgitation, however, was seen in only 2–3% (5,6). By contrast, using a more sensitive technique, pulsed-wave Doppler echocardiography, MR was diagnosed in 50% of patients with acute anterior infarctions and 27% of those with acute inferior infarctions. Three months later, using the same method, regurgitation was found in 83% of anterior and 43% of inferior infarct patients (16). This increase in incidence of MR over time could be due to left ventricular dilatation with consequent incomplete mitral leaflet closure (IMLC). Other causes may include papillary muscle misalignment from fibrosis of the head of the papillary muscle or adjacent myocardium during healing of the infarcted area, and finally the increased incidence of MR may be due to technically superior Doppler images obtained in a cooperative, stable patient.

Episodic acute coronary ischemia in unstable angina or postinfarction angina may cause intermittent papillary muscle dysfunction. This can result in sudden-onset, severe MR (12,18,19), precipitating "flashing" pulmonary edema. This recently recognized condition can be of clinical importance since urgent medical treatment or revascularization may result in a drastic improvement in the severity of acute MR (20), thus avoiding mitral valve replacement.

Animal studies suggest that the cause of acute ischemic MR may not be limited to papillary muscle dysfunction (21–23). Kaul's elegant study showed that acute ischemic MR is the result of global left ventricular dysfunction that occurs during global or even regional myocardial ischemia (21). The mechanism of the regurgitation in that situation is incomplete mitral leaflet closure (IMLC).

3. Infective Endocarditis

Active infective endocarditis may cause acute severe MR by destruction of valve leaflets or, less often, rupture of chordae tendineae (24).

4. Prosthetic Valve Dysfunction

With mechanical prosthesis, acute regurgitation may result from strut fracture with embolization of disc or leaflet, immobilization of mechanical leaflets by vegetation or thrombus, or prosthetic paravalvular regurgitation from infective endocarditis.

Bioprosthetic valvular degeneration usually develops gradually with rapidly increasing congestive heart failure (Fig. 1). However, acute severe MR may occur in such valves. Infective endocarditis can result in acute severe MR by leaflet destruction or paravalvular regurgitation and valve dehiscence.

5. Trauma

Blunt chest trauma can cause acute MR by damaging the valve leaflets, papillary muscles, or chordae tendineae (25). Penetrating chest trauma,

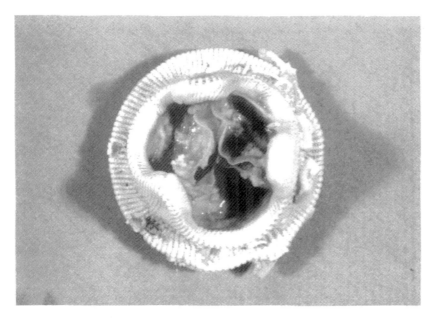

Figure 1 Bioprosthetic (Hancock) valve showing marked pathological degenerative changes in its leaflets.

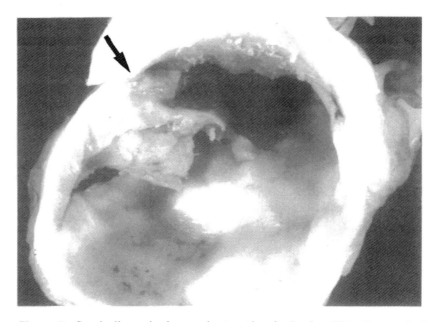

Figure 2   Surgically excised severely stenotic mitral valve. Note the tear in the large anterior leaflet (arrow) resulting in acute severe mitral regurgitation. This is a rare complication of percutaneous mitral balloon valvotomy.

on the other hand, rarely damages the mitral apparatus, but is usually fatal due to concomitant injuries (26).

Iatrogenic trauma to the mitral apparatus can occur from cardiac surgery or percutaneous balloon valvotomy. The latter procedure has been recognized as treatment of choice for suitable patients with severe mitral stenosis. The mechanism underlying acute MR in balloon mitral valvotomy can be oversplitting of fused leaflet commissures, leaflet tears (Fig. 2), or tearing of chordae. Acute severe iatrogenic MR following balloon valvotomy results in unique pathophysiological changes that are secondary to the abrupt transition from severe mitral stenosis to severe MR. In our laboratories 4–5% of patients developed acute severe MR with this procedure, though only one-third (1.5% of the total series) of them required urgent surgery (27). Table 1 lists other uncommon conditions that may rarely cause acute MR.

C. Pathophysiology

In all forms of MR, defective closure of the mitral valve allows reflux of blood retrogradely from the left ventricle into the left atrium during ventricular systole. The hemodynamic consequences of such regurgitation depend on the pressure gradient between the left ventricle and atrium during systole and the size of the regurgitant volume. The systolic gradient, however, is influenced by many factors, including left ventricular function, systolic pressure, left atrial compliance, and systemic vascular resistance (afterload).

In chronic MR, gradual development of the condition allows the left atrium to dilate and become compliant. In turn, this allows the atrium to accommodate increased volume without an increase in pulmonary venous pressure. In addition, the left ventricle dilates (Fig. 3) and hypertrophies, enabling it to deliver an increased stroke volume and to maintain adequate forward cardiac output. [Total stroke volume (TSV) = forward stroke volume (FSV) + regurgitation volume.] In more advanced cases of chronic MR, left atrial pressure increases and the pulmonary artery will

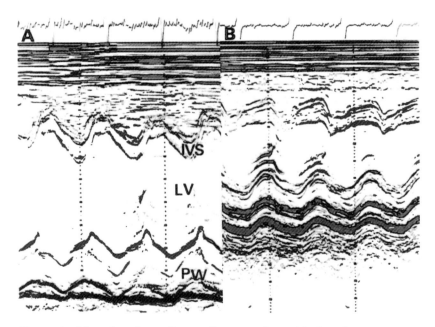

Figure 3 M-mode echocardiogram from a patient with chronic severe compensated mitral regurgitation (MR). Note the dilated left ventricle with preservation of function (A) developed as part of the compensatory mechanisms to accommodate the increased left ventricular stroke volume. (B) Return of left ventricular size to normal after correction of the severe MR by mitral valve replacement. IVS = interventricular septum; LV = left ventricle; PW = posterior wall.

then adjust to this increase by vasoconstriction and arterial wall hypertrophy.

In acute severe MR, on the other hand, the normal-sized left atrium is suddenly presented with pressure and volume overload from the regurgitant valve. Because the atrium is poorly compliant, the massive systolic regurgitant flow will result in a large pressure peak in systole, manifested by a giant "V" wave in the left atrial pressure tracing. This sudden increase in left atrial pressure is transmitted retrogradely, resulting in increased pulmonary venous pressure and often increased pulmonary arterial pressure as well. The "V" wave may reach 70–80 mmHg or more and is usually clearly seen in pulmonary capillary wedge, and at times in the pulmonary artery pressure tracing (Fig. 4). If pulmonary venous pressure exceeds plasma oncotic pressure, *interstitial* pulmonary edema will occur. If the rate of accumulation of fluid in the pulmonary interstitium exceeds the ability of lymphatics to remove the fluid, *alveolar* pulmonary edema will result.

In the presence of MR, much of the stroke volume is directed retrogradely into the left atrium. Forward cardiac output will depend on left ventricular end-diastolic volume, ejection fraction, left atrial compliance, and systemic vascular resistance *(see Chapter 16)*. In mild to moderate cases of acute MR, forward cardiac output may still be maintained by increased left ventricular contractility and heart rate; this is true even in the presence of a normal left ventricular size. In the presence of acute severe MR, however, the increase in total stroke volume produced by various compensatory mechanisms will not be sufficient to maintain adequate forward cardiac output; this is because of the sudden onset of severe MR. Any preexisting left ventricular systolic dysfunction will exacerbate this process.

Acute severe MR may complicate percutaneous balloon mitral valvotomy in 4–5% of patients (27). These patients usually have chronic severe mitral stenosis with resultant high left atrial pressure and significant pulmonary venous and arterial hypertension. We have noticed that such patients can tolerate acute severe MR relatively well with medical therapy of vasodilators and diuretics. Patients with preexisting increased pulmonary vascular resistance may be somewhat protected from the pulmonary edema of acute MR.

D. Natural History

With large regurgitant volumes, the sudden increase in left atrial pressure will result in acute pulmonary edema. As discussed above, forward cardiac output also acutely decreases. Left ventricular dysfunction, resulting from acute myocardial ischemia or other factors, will further reduce car-

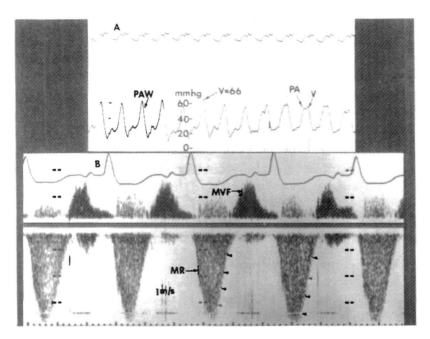

Figure 4 Pressure recordings from right heart catheterization (upper panel A) and continuous-wave Doppler recording from the apical position (lower panel B) in a patient with acute severe mitral regurgitation (MR) due to infective endocarditis. The pressure tracing from pulmonary artery wedge (PAW) position shows a gigantic "V" wave of 66 mmHg. The systolic pulmonary artery (PA) pressure tracing appears bifid; the first peak represents the PA systolic pressure (arrow) and the second peak is due to an overlapping "V" wave (arrow). The continuous-wave Doppler recording (B) shows an intense signal during systole due to severe MR. The deceleration slope of this MR signal is very steep and rapid (four small arrowheads) consistent with a prominent "V" wave. The forward diastolic mitral valve flow (MVF) is also increased due to severe MR. Calibration marks are at an interval of 1 m/sec.

diac output. If left untreated, the combination of acute pulmonary edema and low cardiac output generally leads to early systemic hypoxemia, poor peripheral tissue oxygenation, and often death. This natural history can be influenced strongly by the underlying cause of the regurgitation, for example myocardial ischemia, concomitant infected structures in infective endocarditis, and other valvular lesions in rheumatic heart disease.

On the other hand, if the regurgitant volume is small and left ventricular function is preserved, acute regurgitation may be tolerated with medical therapy.

E. Clinical Manifestation

The signs and symptoms of acute MR differ somewhat depending on etiology, severity of regurgitation, and underlying ventricular function. In mild acute mitral regurgitation, the condition may be clinically silent, with no symptoms due to regurgitation. In such cases, the predominant cardiac symptoms are that of the underlying condition that caused the regurgitation, such as myocardial infarction, unstable angina, or infection.

The clinical presentation of acute severe MR is that of acute pulmonary edema, quiet different from chronic severe MR (Table 2). The patient generally complains of a sudden onset of severe dyspnea, orthopnea, paroxysmal nocturnal dyspnea, and cough. These dramatic symptoms can be overshadowed by those associated with the underlying etiology causing the acute severe MR. This is especially true in patients with acute myocardial infarction, presenting usually with severe chest pain.

Physical examination usually reveals a patient who appears ill, often in respiratory distress. Sinus tachycardia is common in an attempt to maintain cardiac output, and in severe cases, systemic hypotension or pulsus alternans can be present. Systemic venous pressure can be elevated due to elevated right ventricular end-diastolic pressure (EDP) from the acute onset of pulmonary arterial hypertension. Cardiac examination generally does not reveal a left ventricular heave. A systolic thrill may rarely be present at the lower left sternal border or apex. On auscultation, the first heart sound is generally diminished. A third heart sound is common, but may be difficult to appreciate because of tachycardia and pulmonary crackles. The murmur of MR can vary in intensity from loud enough to create a palpable thrill to a murmur barely heard. The intensity of the murmur depends on the systolic pressure gradient between the left ventricle and left atrium and, to some degree, on the direction of flow of the regurgitant jet. Jets directed posteriorly into the left atrial cavity will be more difficult to detect when listening anteriorly on the chest. On the other hand, with posterior chordal rupture the anteriorly directed jet will cause a precordial basal murmur that may be mistaken for an aortic murmur.

Other aspects of the examination may give clues to the etiology of the regurgitation. In patients with infective endocarditis, there may be signs of vasculitis, septic emboli, fever, or other systemic features of this disease.

F. Investigations

1. Electrocardiogram

The electrocardiogram is generally of little help in the diagnosis or management of acute MR. The most common abnormality is sinus tachycardia. Occasionally, atrial fibrillation may be present, but this is less common

Table 2 Differential Diagnosis of Acute Versus Chronic Severe Mitral Regurgitation

	Chronic severe	Acute severe
Clinical		
Onset	Chronic and gradual dyspnea	Acute
Appearance	Normal/mildly dyspneic	Severely ill
Blood pressure	Variable	Variable
Tachycardia	Variable/not striking	Almost always
Apical impulse	Displaced and forcible (large heart)	Not displaced
Apical systolic thrill	Common	No
S1	Normal or soft	Usually normal or mildly increased
S2	Wide splitting	Usually normal
S3	Common	Common
S4	Rare	Common
Apical mitral murmur	Harsh parasystolic	Soft or absent early systolic and decrescendo
-radiation of murmur	Axilla	Axilla, spine, or base
Basal ejection systolic murmur	No	With posterior leaflet chordal rupture (not aortic in origin)
Apical rumbling diastolic murmur	Infrequent	Common and short
ECG/LVH	Almost always	No
Chest X-ray	Severe cardiomegaly	No cardiomegaly
Lung fields	Pulmonary venous congestion	Pulmonary edema
Echocardiography		
LV size	Dilated	Normal
LV function	Variable	Hyperactive
LA size	Dilated	Normal
Look for clues of underlying etiology		
Myocardial infaction	History, ECG, and echo	
Endocarditis	Peripheral signs, echo (vegetation)	
Leaking mitral prosthesis	Transesophageal echo and Fluoroscopy (clots, vegetation)	

than in patients with chronic MR. If the regurgitation is due to acute myocardial infarction or other acute ischemic events, the electrocardiogram can provides clues to the location and extent of the infarction or ischemia. Acute myocardial ischemic events involving the left circumflex coronary artery and its branches can alter anterolateral papillary muscle

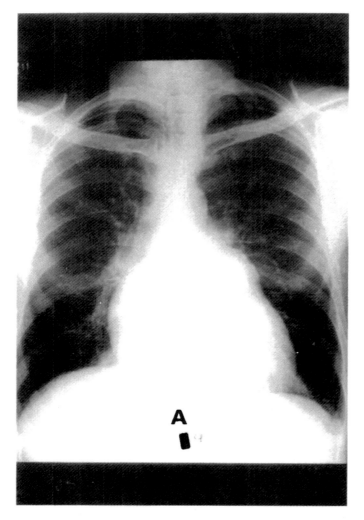

Figure 5 (A) Chest X-ray of patient with severe chronic mitral regurgitation. Note the marked cardiomegaly and minimal pulmonary vascular changes.

function, even with relatively small areas of ischemia. Such episodes may show little or no electrocardiographic evidence of the underlying ischemia.

2. Chest X-Ray

In contrast to chronic severe MR (Fig. 5A), the most common chest X-ray finding in patients with acute severe MR is pulmonary edema without cardiomegaly (Fig. 5B). If acute MR is superimposed on chronic MR,

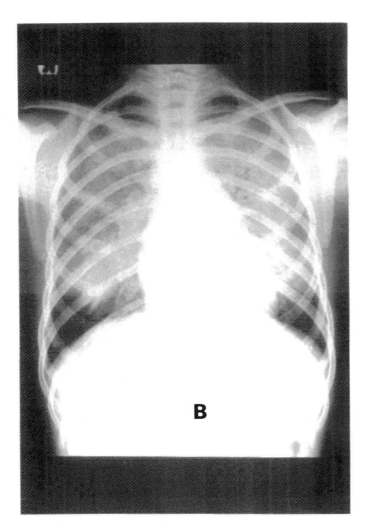

Figure 5 (B) In contrast, the chest X-ray of patient with severe acute mitral regurgitation shows pulmonary edema with no cardiomegaly.

there may be signs of left atrial enlargement on X-ray, but the heart size is often enlarged.

3. Echocardiography

Two-dimensional echocardiography (2D-echo) is useful in assessing ventricular function and valvular morphology. Left ventricular and atrial sizes are usually normal in acute MR unless the acute phase is superimposed

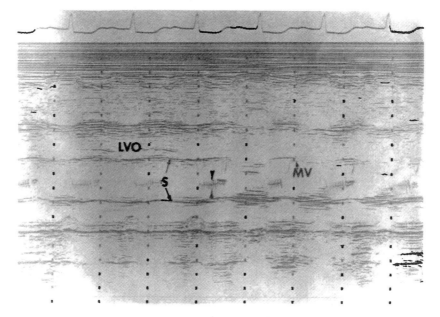

Figure 6   M-mode echocardiogram from a patient with 10-year-old bioprosthetic mitral valve who presented with acute pulmonary edema. The opening of the mitral valve (MV) in diastole is normal. However, during systole, high-frequency vibrations are noted (between arrowheads) consistent with a ruptured and flail leaflet. LVO = left ventricular outflow tract; S = stents.

on chronic regurgitation. Left ventricular ejection fraction is usually normal and hyperdynamic. This is true unless the underlying etiology is acute myocardial ischemia, when left ventricular function may then be impaired, with segmental left ventricular wall abnormalities.

Mitral valve morphology can be assessed with 2D-echo, demonstrating abnormalities such as vegetations, redundant or myxomatous valve tissue, papillary muscle dysfunction, chordae tendineae rupture, and valve leaflet defect *(see Chapter 3)*. Degeneration of bioprosthetic valve can result in leaflet rupture, and echocardiography may reveal evidence of flail leaflet (Fig. 6).

Pulsed-wave Doppler is helpful in assessing left ventricular compliance and degree of regurgitation. Color flow Doppler can further increase the ability to assess degree and spacial pattern of regurgitation. *Continuous-wave* Doppler across the tricuspid valve can be used to estimate right ventricular systolic pressure. When the mitral valve or subvalvular structure is difficult to assess with conventional transthoracic echocardiography, the transesophageal technique has been demonstrated to be a helpful adjunct. When the regurgitant jet is eccentric, severe MR may be missed by conventional transthoracic studies; this is particularly true when evaluating mitral valve prostheses. In these circumstances, and if significant regurgitation is clinically suspected, transesophageal studies are mandatory. Refer to *Chapter 3* for detailed discussion on echocardiographic examination.

4. Cardiac Catheterization

With adequate echocardiography, cardiac catheterization is rarely needed to confirm the diagnosis of acute MR, but it is useful in assessing concomitant problems. Intracardiac pressures can be accurately measured, including left ventricular end-diastolic pressure (EDP) and pulmonary artery pressure. As mentioned above, measurement of pulmonary capillary wedge pressure (PCW) is useful in determining the hemodynamic consequences of regurgitation. Left ventriculography can be performed to assess left ventricular function and degree of MR; however, these parameters can be evaluated with less morbidity by Doppler/echocardiography.

Coronary arteriography is indicated when regurgitation is a result of coronary disease or when surgery is contemplated in patients at risk for coronary artery disease. Fluoroscopy can be used to evaluate the mobility of mechanical leaflets of prosthetic valves (Figs. 7 and 8).

G. Pitfalls in Diagnosis

The prognosis and management of acute severe MR differ from those of chronic regurgitation. A high index of suspicion must be maintained to avoid missing the diagnosis; the diagnosis should be entertained in any patient with sudden-onset pulmonary edema. This is true even when the typical murmur of MR is not heard, since this murmur, as described previously, can be atypical or even absent in acute regurgitation. In patients with acute severe MR, the pattern of acute pulmonary edema on chest X-ray may be misinterpreted as an infectious process. In experienced hands, Doppler/echocardiography, especially with color flow mapping, should be diagnostic for acute MR.

The characteristic "V" waves seen in pulmonary wedge (PCW) tracing during cardiac catheterization can be very tall and confuse the interpretation of the pulmonary artery tracing, unless careful attention is paid to the timing of the wave (Fig. 4).

H. Management

Management of acute severe MR involves urgent attempts at compensating for the hemodynamic abnormalities and thereafter correcting the underlying cause; the latter is usually a surgical procedure.

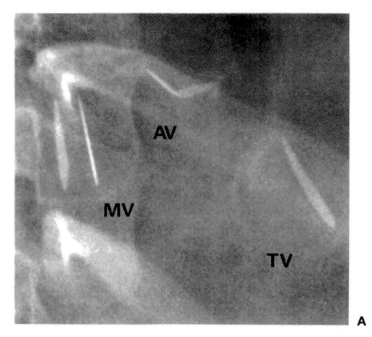

Figure 7 Fluoroscopic images in a patient with bileaflet mechanical valves (St. Jude) in the aortic, mitral, and tricuspid positions. (A) In diastole, shows normal closed aortic valve (AV) and normal open mitral valve (MV).

In mild cases with low regurgitant volume, no specific therapy may be needed apart from treating the underlying disease. Patients with moderate to severe degrees of acute regurgitation generally need prompt intervention, starting with traditional therapy for congestive heart failure such as diuretics. More specifically, arterial vasodilator therapy is beneficial by decreasing systemic vascular resistance, reducing regurgitant volume, and allowing more forward flow. Thus, treatment with a vasodilator, such as intravenous nitroprusside or oral angiotensin-converting-enzyme inhibitor, will lower pulmonary venous pressure (Fig. 9, A and B), improve pulmonary edema, and increase systemic cardiac output.

If systemic blood pressure is not high enough for the patient to tolerate aggressive arterial vasodilators, this treatment can be combined with inotropic support, such as intravenous dopamine and/or intra-aortic balloon pump therapy (IABP). The balloon is located in the descending aorta, immediately distal to the left brachial artery. During ventricular diastole,

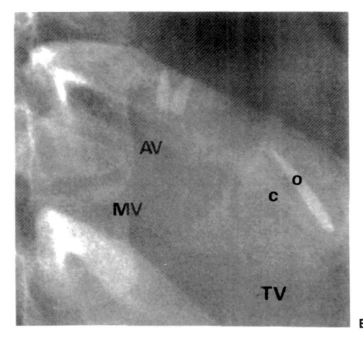

Figure 7 (B) In systole, shows normal open aortic (AV) and normal closed mitral valve (MV). The tricuspid valve (TV) leaflets, however, remain immobile through-out the cardiac cycle, with one leaflet fixed in the closed (c) and the other in the open (o) position. This is due to mechanical impingement of the leaflet by thrombus formation.

the inflated balloon augments the diastolic ascending aortic pressure and coronary blood flow. During ventricular systole, on the other hand, the balloon is deflated, potentiating a negative pressure in the aorta and reduc-ing systemic resistance (afterload), thus augmenting systemic forward blood flow and reducing regurgitant flow. Properly timed, the balloon counterpulsation is very useful in patients with acute MR (Fig. 9D). How-ever, arterial vasodilator therapy appears to be more efficient in reducing pulmonary wedge pressure than IABP (Fig. 9, A–D). On the other hand, IABP is more useful in patients with acute coronary ischemic disease because it augments diastolic coronary artery perfusion.

Treatment designed to compensate for the hemodynamic compromise of acute MR is often only temporarily successful. Attention should be directed toward treating the underlying regurgitant lesion by surgical

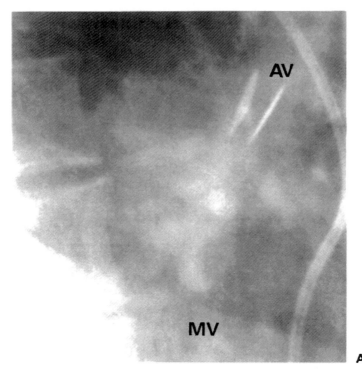

A

Figure 8 Fluoroscopic images in patient with bileaflet mechanical valves (St. Jude) in the aortic and mitral positions. (A) In systole, shows opened aortic (AV) and closed mitral valve (MV).

means. If valve anatomy allows repair, this is preferable, but otherwise valve replacement is necessary. This is done with highest success when the patient is stabilized before surgery.

In acute coronary ischemic events, emergency coronary arteriography will identify the coronary artery narrowing or occlusion. Urgent revascularization of ischemic myocardium by percutaneous angioplasty may relieve ischemia and prevent necrosis, thus reducing or even abolishing the regurgitation (20). Hence, successful revascularization would alleviate the need for mitral valve surgery, which carries a high mortality in such an acute condition.

The timing of surgical mitral repair or replacement in acute severe MR due to acute myocardial infarction has long been debated. Optimally, surgery should be delayed for several weeks following infarction. This allows the infarct to heal, which makes working with necrotic myocardial tissue

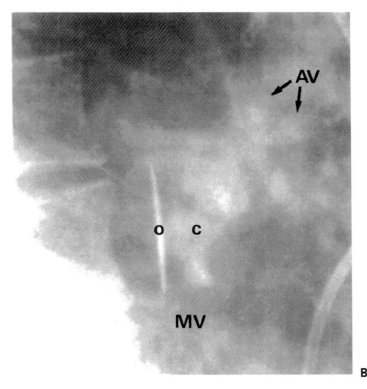

Figure 8 (B) In diastole, shows closed aortic valve (AV); however, the mitral valve (MV) has one leaflet in the normal open position (o) while the other is in closed (c) position. This patient presented with clinical picture of mitral stenosis. This is due to mechanical impingement of the leaflet caused by pannus and thrombus formation.

technically easier. However, many patients cannot wait several weeks because of hemodynamic instability and may not survive if corrective measures are delayed. Others can initially be stabilized, but deteriorate hemodynamically over time. At present, the consensus of a reasonable approach would be aggressive stabilization of patients using medical and/ or mechanical therapies; once stabilized, most patients should undergo early surgical valve repair or replacement, together with indicated coronary bypass surgery. A subset of patients with a favorable prognosis may be expected to be more stable over time, as judged by degree of regurgitation, left ventricular function, pulmonary artery pressure, and coronary artery anatomy. These patients can be watched carefully and undergo

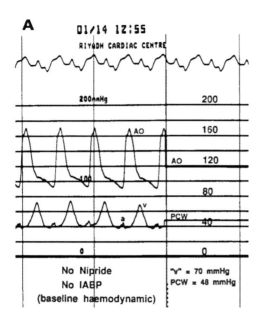

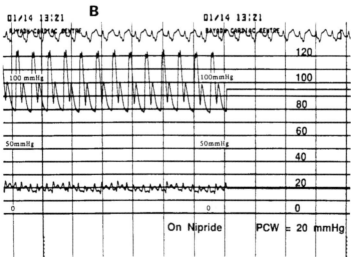

Figure 9 Pressure recordings from pulmonary artery/capillary wedge (PCW) and femoral artery positions in a patient with acute mitral regurgitation due to acute myocardial infarction. (A) Baseline hemodynamic parameters, before the use of any therapeutic maneuver; note the gigantic "V" wave and markedly elevated PCW pressure. (B) Marked reduction of PCW pressure and disappearance of the gigantic "V" wave after administration of intravenous nitroprusside.

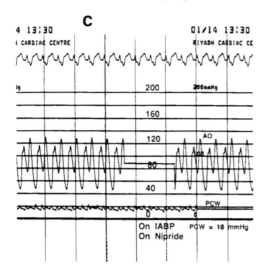

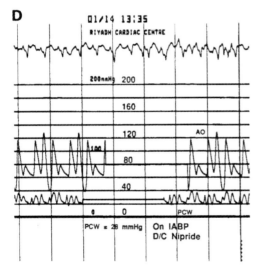

Figure 9 (C) Minimal additional benefit of IABP therapy to nitroprusside. (D) Rapid rise of PCW pressure from 18 to 28 mmHg, shortly after discontinuing nitroprusside while the patient is still on IABP. This signifies the superior benefit of nitroprusside therapy to IABP in this case.

surgery electively several weeks after infarction, or continue to be managed medically.

II. ACUTE AORTIC REGURGITATION

A. Introduction

Acute aortic regurgitation (AR) differs from chronic AR. These differences include etiology, clinical presentation, diagnosis, treatment, and prognosis. Recognizing these differences is of utmost importance in managing patients with these disorders.

B. Etiology

Acute AR can result from the following: defects in aortic valve cusps, disruption of support of the aortic cusps, and diseases of the ascending aorta.

In the United States, the most common cause of aortic valve cusp defects resulting in acute AR is infective endocarditis (24). Acute AR in patients with endocarditis results from perforation or destruction of the cusps by infection, interference with leaflet closure by large vegetations, or erosion of the aortic ring with consequent lack of support to the leaflets. The aortic valve was the principal cardiac valve affected in 70% of patients with infective endocarditis (24). The bicuspid aortic valve is more prone to infection; however, this is an uncommon congenital anomaly, found in only 1–2% of autopsies (28). Tricuspid aortic valve was identified in 50% of patients with infective endocarditis of the aortic valve (24,29). In fatal cases of aortic valve endocarditis, a tricuspid aortic valve was frequently noticed (24,29). These observations have led investigators to suggest that the "normal-looking" tricuspid aortic valves are often infected with more virulent organisms, causing early and rapid valve destruction with high incidence of intramyocardial and annular (ring) abscesses (Fig. 10). The use of a sensitive diagnostic method, transesophageal echocardiography, has highlighted the frequent involvement of subaortic structures in patients with aortic valve infective endocarditis (30); it was demonstrated in 44% of such patients.

Although acute AR was found to be the most common valvular injury in survivors of patients with major closed-chest trauma (31), it is a rare cause of acute AR (25,26). Valvular traumatic injury due to percutaneous aortic balloon valvuloplasty is rare, but it is often a fatal complication of this procedure (32–34). Acquired rheumatic aortic valve disease, congenital aortic valve disease, and degenerative aortic valve disease may cause chronic AR, but rarely cause acute AR.

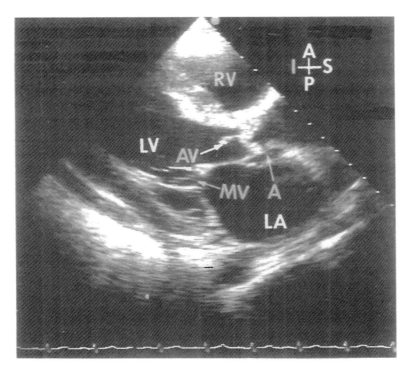

Figure 10 Parasternal long-axis view of 2D-echocardiogram, from a patient with an aortic valve endocarditis, showing a large vegetation (AV) attached to the ventricular surface of the aortic valve cusp. An echo-free space is noted in the posterior aortic root (A) due to annular abscess. LA = left atrium; LV = left ventricle; MV = mitral valve; RV = right ventricle.

Bioprosthetic valve leaflets tend to degenerate over time with calcification, fibrosis, and eventual disruption of the bioprosthetic leaflets (Fig. 1). This leads to aortic stenosis, chronic regurgitation, or occasionally acute AR. Mechanical aortic valve prosthesis may become acutely regurgitant if the leaflet function is suddenly impaired, keeping the leaflet in an "open position"; this is due to mechanical impingement of leaflet closure by thrombus, endothelial tissue overgrowth, or vegetation. Acute AR, however, is rarely caused by mechanical failure of the prosthesis; it is usually due to strut fracture resulting in leaflet dislodgment or embolization and often death. Paraprosthetic leak of the mechanical valve, causing acute or subacute AR, is more common and results from infective endocarditis or failure of the suture line soon after surgery.

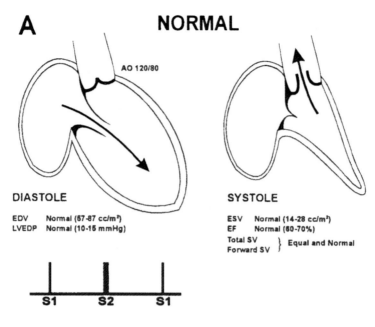

A   NORMAL

AO 120/80

DIASTOLE

EDV   Normal (57-87 cc/m²)
LVEDP   Normal (10-15 mmHg)

SYSTOLE

ESV   Normal (14-28 cc/m²)
EF   Normal (60-70%)
Total SV   } Equal and Normal
Forward SV }

S1   S2   S1

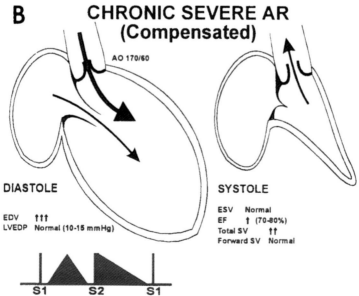

B   CHRONIC SEVERE AR
(Compensated)

AO 170/60

DIASTOLE

EDV   ↑↑↑
LVEDP   Normal (10-15 mmHg)

SYSTOLE

ESV   Normal
EF   ↑ (70-80%)
Total SV   ↑↑
Forward SV Normal

S1   S2   S1

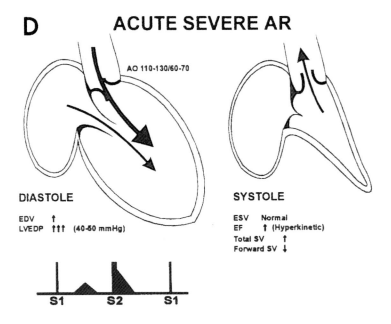

D ACUTE SEVERE AR

AO 110-130/60-70

DIASTOLE

EDV ↑
LVEDP ↑↑↑ (40-50 mmHg)

SYSTOLE

ESV Normal
EF ↑ (Hyperkinetic)
Total SV ↑
Forward SV ↓

S1 S2 S1

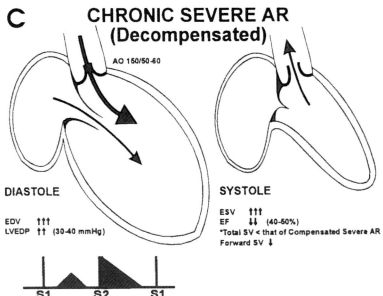

C CHRONIC SEVERE AR (Decompensated)

AO 150/50-60

DIASTOLE

EDV ↑↑↑
LVEDP ↑↑ (30-40 mmHg)

SYSTOLE

ESV ↑↑↑
EF ↓↓ (40-50%)
*Total SV < that of Compensated Severe AR
Forward SV ↓

S1 S2 S1

Figure 11 Hemodynamic (upper panel of each diagram) and auscultatory (lower panel) changes occurring in patient with severe compensated (B) and decompensated (C) chronic aortic regurgitation (AR), acute severe AR (D), and in normal subject (A). Shaded areas in the auscultatory panels represent the type and severity of the murmurs. EDV = end-diastolic volume; LVEDP = left end-diastolic pressure; ESV = end-systolic volume; EF = ejection fraction; SV = stroke volume; AO = aortic pressure; S1 = first heart sound; S2 = second heart sound.

Diseases of the aorta that can cause acute AR include acute aortic dissection, sudden aortic root dilatation in patients with annular aortic ectasia, or, more rarely, infective aortitis. Acute dissection of the ascending aorta with involvement of the aortic annulus occurs most commonly in patients with systemic hypertension, Marfan's syndrome, and rarely pregnancy (35–37).

C. Pathophysiology

The presence of aortic valvular cusp perforation, or failure of adequate diastolic closure of the aortic cusps, results in reflux of blood from the aortic root into the left ventricle during diastole; this results in an increase in left ventricular end-diastolic volume (LVEDV). The hemodynamic consequences of such regurgitation will depend on the ability of the left ventricle to compensate for this increase in diastolic volume.

In chronic AR, the primary mechanism of compensation is left ventricular dilatation and eccentric hypertrophy *(see Chapter 16)*. This can be accomplished when the onset of the regurgitation is gradual and, therefore, no significant changes in the left ventricular end-diastolic pressure (LVEDP) can be detected. In these circumstances the increased left ventricular contractility, together with marked increase in LVEDV and relatively normal end-systolic size (LVESV), leads to greatly increased left ventricular stroke volume (SV) that maintains adequate forward cardiac output despite severe AR (Fig. 11B). These compensatory changes explain the normal peripheral systemic resistance, absent sinus tachycardia, and wide pulse pressure in patients with chronic severe AR.

In advanced cases of severe chronic AR, the left ventricular end-systolic volume (ESV) increases, resulting in a gradual decrease in forward stroke volume (FSV)/cardiac output and ejection fraction while still maintaining a relatively high total stroke volume (TSV) (Fig. 11C). These final pathophysiological changes occur as a result of left ventricular impairment and dramatically exacerbate the natural history of this condition *(see Chapter 7)*.

In contrast to chronic AR, the left ventricle in acute AR is suddenly presented with a volume overload and high systemic resistance. These pathophysiological changes occur before compensatory adjustments in the left ventricle, namely increased left ventricular diastolic volume and increased wall thickness. The principal compensatory mechanism in acute AR is merely sinus tachycardia and increased left ventricular contractility, resulting in the early and marked increase in LVEDP (Fig. 11D) and reduction in forward SV/cardiac output (38,39). The elevated LVEDP will then be transmitted retrogradely, causing a marked increase in left atrial and

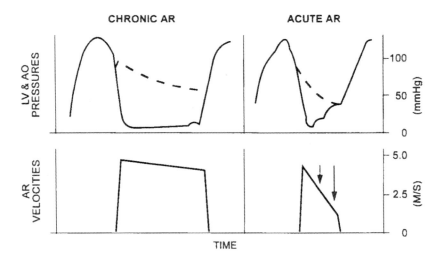

Figure 12   Simultaneous left ventricular (continuous line) and aortic (dotted line) pressure tracings (upper panels) and continuous-wave Doppler recordings (lower panels) from patients with chronic and acute aortic regurgitation (AR). The shaded areas in the upper panels and the continuous-wave Doppler recordings in the lower panels reflect the aortic diastolic pressure gradients. In patient with acute AR, the slope of continuous-wave Doppler recording is rapid (arrows); this is due to rapid drop in pressure gradient in mid-late diastole, as also seen in the upper panels (shaded area). AR = aortic regurgitation; AO = aorta; LV = left ventricle.

pulmonary venous pressures, resulting in acute pulmonary edema. Since there is no significant increase in stroke volume, systolic aortic pressure will not change and the wide pulse pressure observed in chronic AR will not occur. The dramatic increase in LVEDP will result in its rapid equalization with aortic diastolic pressure (Figs. 12 and 13D). These pathophysiological hemodynamic abnormalities explain the short decrescendo diastolic aortic murmur (Fig. 11D) and the premature mitral valve closure in patients with acute AR (Fig. 14A). The latter explains the presence of a soft S1 and shortening of the Austin Flint murmur (40). In contrast to patients with chronic AR, patients with acute AR have increased peripheral systemic resistance due to low forward cardiac output.

D. Natural History

In patients with acute AR, the combination of acute pulmonary edema and low cardiac output leads to a severe decrease in organ perfusion,

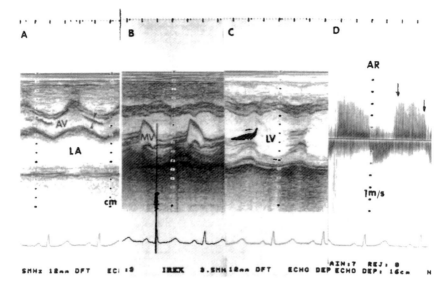

Figure 13 M-mode and Doppler recordings from a patient with aortic valve endocarditis due to *Staphylococcus aureus* resulting in acute severe aortic regurgitation (AR) (A) Normal opening of the aortic valve cusps (AV). During systole, there is mild thickening of the aortic valve echo signals, and high-frequency vibrations (arrowheads) are noted indicating flail leaflet. (B) Normal M-mode echo recording of the mitral valve (MV). A vertical line marking end-diastole shows no evidence of premature closure of MV, which is frequently noted in patients with acute AR. (C) M-mode recording of the left ventricle (LV), which is minimally dilated and has normal systolic function. Trivial pericardial effusion is noted posteriorly. (D) Continuous-wave Doppler recording from the apical position, showing severe AR with rapid deceleration rate and low end-diastolic velocity (arrows). Calibration marks are 1 m/sec apart in the Doppler recording and 1 cm apart in the M-mode recording. LA = left atrium.

systemic hypoxemia, and eventual death from a combination of these factors. The natural history of acute AR, as with acute MR, is influenced by the etiology. The above hemodynamic consequences are further complicated by the presence of infection, aortic dissection, or other injuries in the multiple-trauma patient. For example, aortic valve infective endocarditis, resulting in acute AR, carries a poor prognosis. It is usually caused by virulent organisms, such as *Staphylococcus*, that are associated with a high incidence of aortic ring and intramyocardial abscesses. Therefore, prompt diagnosis and early treatment are essential.

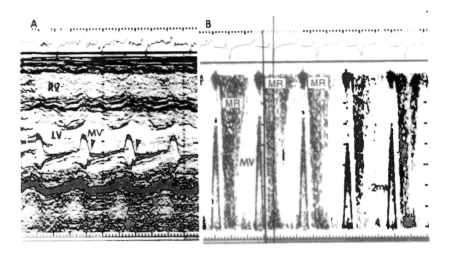

Figure 14 M-mode (A) and pulsed Doppler (B) recordings of the mitral valve from a patient with acute aortic regurgitation (AR) due to infective endocarditis. (A) Premature closure of the mitral valve (arrowheads). This is characteristic of acute AR and high left ventricular end-diastolic pressure (LVEDP). (B) Diastolic (presystolic) mitral regurgitation (MR) due to high LVEDP. The MR begins during late diastole (i.e., before the peak of the QRS on the ECG) and continues throughout systole. The calibration markers in M-mode recording are 1 cm apart and in Doppler recording at 0.2 m/sec. LV = left ventricle; MR = mitral regurgitation; MV = mitral valve; RV = right ventricle.

E. Clinical Manifestations

The clinical features of patients with acute AR differ markedly from those with chronic severe AR (Table 3). Patients with acute severe AR present with a combination of acute pulmonary edema and low forward cardiac output. Thus the symptoms consist of acute or relatively rapid onset of dyspnea, often with severe orthopnea. Patients may also complain of severe fatigue, listlessness, or lethargy.

Physical examination usually shows a very ill-looking patient with orthopnea who may be lethargic or mentally confused. Examination of the peripheral arterial pulses reveals a diminished pulse volume without the collapsing (water hammer) character often found in patients with severe chronic AR. The lung field examination reveals diffuse bilateral crackles, consistent with pulmonary edema. Cardiac examination demonstrates sinus tachycardia with no displacement of the cardiac impulse. The first

Table 3 Differential Diagnosis of Acute Versus Chronic Severe Aortic Regurgitation

	Chronic severe	Acute severe
Clinical		
Onset	Chronic and gradual dyspnea	Acute
Appearance	Normal/mildly dyspneic	Severely ill
Blood pressure	Wide pulse pressure (very low diastolic and high systolic BP)	Not striking, normal, or even low
Tachycardia	Variable/not striking	Always
Peripheral arterial signs (Table 2)	Obvious	No
Apical impulse	Displaced and forcible (very large heart)	No
Basal diastolic thrill	Rare	More common (perforation)
Basal systolic thrill	Common	No
S1	Usually normal	Soft
S2	Usually normal (soft calcific valve)	Soft
S3	Common with LV failure	Common
Basal ejection systolic murmur	Common and harsh	Common and soft
Basal early diastolic murmur	Long, blowing and decresendo	Short, soft, or loud and musical with perforation
Apical rumbling diastolic murmur	Common	Common but with no presystolic accentuation
ECG/LVH	Almost always	No
Chest X-ray		
Cardiomegaly	Severe	No
Lung fields	Usually normal	Pulmonary edema
Echocardiograph		
LV size	Severely dilated	Normal
LV function (EF)	Variable	Hyperactive
Premature closure of mitral valve	No	Common
Diastolic mitral regurgitation	No	Common
Late mitral valve opening	No	Common
Look for clues of underlying etiology		
Marfan's syndrome	General appearance and other associated features	
Aortic dissection	Peripheral pulses	
Prosthetic aortic valve dysfuction	ECG of acute myocardial infarction or pericarditis	
Infective endocarditis	Transesophageal echo or CT scan	
	Clots or vegetations (echo and fluoroscopy)	
	Peripheral signs, vegetation (echo)	

heart sound (S1) may be soft or absent due to early closure of the mitral valve. The second heart sound (S2) is usually normal, but the aortic component (A2) may be diminished if there is disruption of the aortic valve leaflets. In mechanical aortic valve prosthesis with failure of leaflet mobility due to thrombus or vegetation, the click of mechanical leaflet closure will be greatly diminished or absent. Because of the rapid increase in LVEDP during the late phase of ventricular diastole, the early diastolic decrescendo murmur classically heard in chronic regurgitation will be markedly shortened (Fig. 11D), or even inaudible with the presence of ambient noise. Basal systolic low murmur and a rather short Austin Flint murmur are a common finding (Fig. 11D).

Thorough physical examination may provide clues to the underlying diseases causing the acute AR. This would include stigmata of infective endocarditis, such as systemic emboli, or signs of acute aortic dissection, such as blood pressure differential in the extremities.

F. Investigations

1. Electrocardiogram

The resting electrocardiogram (ECG) is usually of little help in making the diagnosis of acute AR. It usually shows sinus tachycardia and there may be nonspecific ST-segment and T-wave changes. This is in contrast to patients with chronic severe AR, in whom ECG changes of left ventricular hypertrophy and strain are common (Fig. 15). In patients suspected to have acute AR, the ECG findings of acute myocardial infarction would suggest the diagnosis of acute aortic dissection. Conduction abnormalities such as heart block on ECG almost always indicate ring abscesses.

2. Chest X-ray

The chest X-ray generally shows a pattern of pulmonary edema, with no signs of left ventricular enlargement. Enlargement of the ascending aorta would raise the suspicion of aortic dissection as a cause of acute regurgitation. Rocking movement of the prosthetic aortic valve or immobile leaflet, on fluoroscopy, may be detected in patients with prosthetic valve dysfunction.

3. Echocardiography

M-mode, 2D-echo, and Doppler examination are the most important diagnostic tests in patients with acute AR. The M-mode study will show normal left ventricular end-diastolic dimension (Fig. 13C) with normal to slightly enhanced fractional shortening and early closure of mitral valve (Fig. 14A).

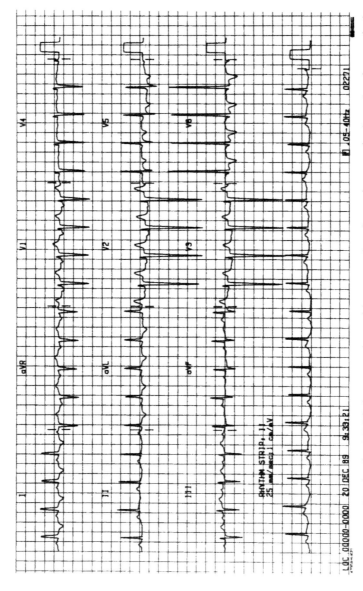

Figure 15 Twelve lead ECG from a patient with severe chronic aortic regurgitation, showing marked left ventricular hypertrophy and strain pattern.

2D-echo imaging of the aortic valve may show valve leaflet disruption and prolapse, accompanying vegetations (Fig. 10), or rarely leaflet fenestrations. The presence of an aortic ring abscess (Fig. 10) and intramyocardial abscesses may also be detected. 2D-echo examination, particularly using the transesophageal approach, may visualize dilatation or dissection of the ascending aorta. This approach is probably superior to aortography and computed-tomography (CT) scan in the diagnosis of aortic dissection (41). The detection of pericardial effusion in patients with acute AR suggests a possible underlying diagnosis of aortic root dissection.

A combination of pulsed, continuous, and color flow Doppler recordings can accurately outline the location and severity of the regurgitation. The continuous-wave Doppler signal across the aortic valve is distinctly different in acute and in chronic AR. In acute AR, diastolic regurgitant flow rapidly diminishes because of the rapid increase in LVEDP; thus, the shape of the resulting Doppler envelope is distinctly different from that seen in chronic regurgitation (Figs. 12, 13D, 16).

A pressure half-time of less than 200 msec indicates a severe form of AR. The more acute the slope of the continuous-wave Doppler, the more severe is the AR (Fig. 16) *(see Chapter 3)*.

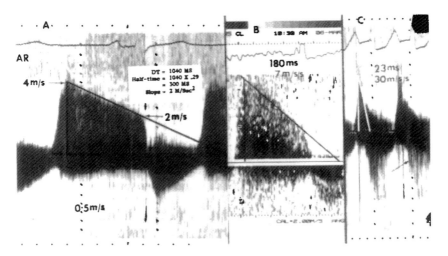

Figure 16 Continuous-wave Doppler recordings from three patients with various degrees of severity of aortic regurgitation (AR). (A) Pressure half-time of 300 msec indicating mild AR. (B and C) Pressure half-time of 180 msec and 23 msec signifying chronic severe AR and acute severe AR respectively. A pressure half-time of less than 200 msec is inconsistent with severe AR.

Although transthoracic 2D-echo is usually the best method to view the aortic valve leaflets, the transesophageal approach is superior in looking at the ascending aorta for signs of enlargement and/or dissection and for detecting subaortic structural involvement in infective endocarditis.

4. Cardiac Catheterization

With adequate transthoracic and transesophageal Doppler/echocardiography, cardiac catheterization is usually not necessary to establish the diagnosis of acute AR. It may be essential, however, to assess the presence of coronary artery disease in patients in whom cardiac surgery is contemplated and who may be at risk for such a disease.

Ascending aortography and CT scan of the chest may be useful to assess the integrity of the aortic root when other examinations are inconclusive. Fluoroscopy may be used to evaluate the mobility of mechanical leaflets of prosthetic valves (Figs. 7 and 8).

G. Pitfalls in Diagnosis

It is difficult to diagnose AR of acute form because the classical physical signs that are the hallmark of chronic AR are generally absent; in addition, the signs of acute AR are subtle and easily missed in the acute form. Thus, to make the diagnosis, a very high index of suspicion must be maintained in a patient presenting with acute pulmonary edema and low cardiac output. Important clues as to etiologies that can lead to this acute condition can be gleaned from the history, general physical examination, and laboratory investigations. If the disorder is suspected, a prompt Doppler/echocardiographic examination performed by an experienced physician is generally diagnostic. Other lesions, such as rupture of the sinus valsalva, may occasionally mimic this disorder.

H. Management

The only effective management for acute AR is prompt surgical repair. In most cases, this will require aortic valve replacement (AVR) and correction of any associated defects such as aortic annulus involvement with infection or dissection, aortic root destruction with dissection, and intramyocardial abscesses. Therefore, in addition to AVR, other complicated surgical procedures carrying a high risk may also be required.

If the etiology of the AR is infective endocarditis, careful preoperative evaluation of the annular and subvalvular cardiac structures, including anterior mitral valve leaflet and the fibrous area between aortic and mitral valves, must be accomplished to prevent the risk of leaving infected tissue after successful valve replacement (30); this can best be accomplished by transesophageal echocardiography.

The timing of cardiac surgery depends on the degree of hemodynamic compromise the patient exhibits, the etiology of the regurgitation, and concomitant medical problems. It is preferable to stabilize an acutely ill patient with intensive medical therapy before major surgery; this allows for full investigation and treatment of concomitant medical problems. In patients with infective endocarditis, for instance, intravenous administration of appropriate antibiotics for 1 week before valve replacement is strongly advisable in an attempt to prevent recurrence of infection postoperatively. However, this may not be possible in patients with severe hemodynamic compromise due to acute AR.

Some have suggested that bioprosthetic valves are more resistant to early postoperative infection than mechanical prosthesis, and that aortic homograft may be the most suitable valve for acute infective endocarditis (42–44). The mortality rate, however, remains high for patients presenting with severe congestive heart failure and severe AR, particularly if it is associated with infective endocarditis (45).

If aortic dissection is the cause of acute AR, surgical correction should not be delayed because of the known high risk of mortality in delaying such treatment (45). If the patient does not have Marfan syndrome and valve replacement can be avoided, aortic valve resuspension and reconstruction with repair of the aortic wall dissection can be contemplated. Otherwise, the use of composite valve graft conduit and reimplantation of the coronary arteries into the graft is the treatment of choice (45).

As with acute MR, successful management of the patient with acute AR depends primarily on a high index of suspicion and rapid diagnosis. A decision can then be made, with both cardiologists and cardiac surgeons participating, as to the optimal time of surgical intervention, weighing such factors as immediate hemodynamic stability, concomitant medical problems, and need for other therapy.

REFERENCES

1. Depace NL, Nestico PF, Morganroth J. Acute severe mitral regurgitation: pathophysiology, clinical recognition and management. Am J Med 1985; 78: 293.
2. Roberts WC. Morphological features of the normal and abnormal mitral valve. Am J Cardiol 1983; 51:1005.
3. Roberts WC, Danjel JC, Buckley BH. Nonrheumatic valvular cardiac disease: a clinicopathological survey of 27 different conditions causing valvular dysfunction. Cardiovasc Clin 1973; 5(2):334.
4. American Heart Association, National Center for Health Statistics, 1991.

5. Lehmann KG, Francis CK, Dodge HT, and the TIMI Study Group. Mitral regurgitation in early myocardial infarction: incidence, clinical detection and prognostic implications. Ann Intern Med 1992; 177:10.
6. Tcheng JE, Jackman JD Jr, Nelson CL, Gardner LH, Smith LR, Rankin JC, Califf RM, Stack RS. Outcome of patients sustaining acute ischemic mitral regurgitation during myocardial infarction. Ann Intern Med 1992; 117:18.
7. Selzer A, Katayama F. Mitral regurgitation: clinical pattern, pathophysiology and natural history. Medicine 1972; 51:343.
8. Waller BF, Morrow AG, Maron BJ, Del Negro AA, Kent KM, McGrath FJ, Wallace RB, McIntosh CL, Roberts WC. Etiology of clinically isolated severe chronic pure mitral regurgitation, analysis of 97 patients over 30 years of age having MVR. Am Heart J 1982; 104:276.
9. Pomerance A. Ballooning deformity (mucoid degeneration) of atrioventricular valves. Br Heart J 1969; 31:343.
10. Lucas RV Jr, Edwards JE. The floppy mitral valve. Curr Prob Cardiol 1982; 7:148.
11. Scott-Jupp W, Barnett LN, Gallagher PJ, Monro JL, Ross JK. Ultrastructural changes in spontaneous rupture of mitral chordae tendineae. J Pathol 1981; 133:462.
12. Burch GE, DePasquale NP, Philips JH. The syndrome of papillary muscle dysfunction. Am Heart J 1968; 75:399.
13. Cederquist L, Sodestrom J. Papillary muscular rupture in myocardial infarctions, a study based upon an autopsy material. Acta Med Scand 1964; 176: 287.
14. Heikkila J. Mitral incompetence as a complication of acute myocardial infarction. Acta Med Scand 1967; 475(Suppl):1–149.
15. Gahl K, Sutton R, Pearson M, Gaspari P, Lairet A, McDonald L. Mitral regurgitation in coronary heart disease. Br Heart J 1977; 39:13.
16. Loperfido F, Biascucci LM, Pennestri F, Laurenzi F, Gimigliano F, Vigna C, Rossi E, Favuzzi A, Santavelli P, Manzoli U. Pulsed-waved Doppler echocardiographic analysis of mitral regurgitation after myocardial infarction. Am J Cardiol 1986; 58:692.
17. Estes EH, Dalton FM, Entman ML, Dixon HB, Hackel DB. The anatomy and blood supply of the papillary muscle of the left ventricle. Am Heart J 1966; 7:356.
18. Hickey MSt, Smith LR, Muhlbaier LH, Harrel F Jr, Reves JG, Hinohaara T, Califf RM, Pryor DB, Rankin JS. Current prognosis of ischemic mitral regurgitation: implications for future management. Circulation 1988; 78(Suppl I):1–51.
19. Feuvre CL, Metzger JP, Lachurie ML, Georges JL, Baubion N, Vacheron A. Treatment of severe mitral regurgitation caused by ischemic papillary muscle dysfunction: Indications for coronary angioplasty. Am Heart J 1992; 123:860.
20. Shawl FA, Forman MB, Punja S, Goldbaum TS. Emergency coronary angioplasty in the treatment of acute ischemic mitral regurgitation: long-term results in five cases. J Am Coll Cardiol 1989; 14:986.

21. Kaul S, Spotnitz WD, Glasheen WP, Touchstone DA. Mechanism of ischemic mitral regurgitation: an experimental evaluation. Circulation 1991; 84:2167.
22. Tsakiris AG, Rastelli GC, Amorium DD, Titus JL, Wood EH. Effect of experimental papillary muscle damage on mitral valve closure in intact anaesthetized dogs. Mayo Clin Proc 1970; 45:275.
23. Mittal AK, Langston M, Cohn KE, Selzer A, Keith WJ. Combined papillary muscle and left ventricular wall dysfunction as a cause of mitral regurgitation: an experimental study. Circulation 1971: 44:174.
24. Arnett EN, Roberts WC. Active infective endocarditis: a clinicopathological analysis of 137 necropsy patients. Curr Probl Cardiol 1976; 1:2.
25. Parmely LF, Manion WC, Mattingly GW. Non-penetrating traumatic injury of the heart. Circulation 1958; 18:371.
26. Parmely LF, Mattingly GW, Manion WC. Penetrating wounds of the heart and aorta. Circulation 1958; 17:953.
27. Al Zaibag MA, Ribeiro P. The future of balloon valvotomy. In: Topol EJ, ed. Textbook of Interventional Cardiology. Philadelphia: WB Saunders, 1990:912.
28. Roberts WC. The congenitally bicuspid aortic valve, a study of 85 autopsy patients. Am J Cardiol 1970; 26:72.
29. Davies MJ. In: Pathology of Cardiac Valve. London: Butterworths, 1980.
30. Karalis DG, Bansal RC, Hauck AJ, Ross JJ Jr, Applegate PA, Jutzy KR, Mintz GS, Chandrasekaran K. Transesophageal echocardiography recognition of subaortic complications in aortic valve endocarditis; clinical and surgical implications. Circulation 1992; 86:353.
31. Levine RJ, Roberts WC, Morrow AG. Traumatic aortic regurgitation. Am J Cardiol 1962; 10:752.
32. Lembo NJ, King SB, Roubin GS. Fatal aortic rupture during percutaneous balloon valvuloplasty for valvular aortic stenosis. Am J Cardiol 1987; 60: 733.
33. Lewin RF, Dorros G, King JF, Seifert PE, Schamal TM, Aner JE. Aortic annular tear after valvoplasty; the role of aortic annulus echocardiographic measurement. Cathet Cardiovasc Diagn 1989; 16:123.
34. Cribier A, Gerber L, Letac B. The future of balloon valvotomy. In: Topol EJ, ed. Textbook of Interventional Cardiology. Philadelphia: WB Saunders, 1990:849.
35. Eagle AK, Desanctis RW. Aortic dissection. Curr Probl Cardiol 1989;14: 231.
36. Ergin MA, Galla JD, Lansman S. Acute dissection of the aorta. Current surgical treatment. Surg Clin North Am 1985;65:721.
37. Katz NM, Collea JV, Morant JV. Aortic dissection durign pregnancy: treatment of emergency cesarian section immediately followed by operative repair of aortic dissection. Am J Cardiol 1984; 54:699.
38. Parker JO, Case RB. Normal LV function. Circulation 1979; 60:4.
39. Welch GH Jr, Braunwald E, Sarnoff SJ. Hemodynamic effects of quantitatively varied experimental aortic regurgitation. Circ Res 1957: 5:546.

40. Fortuin NJ, Craige E. On the mechanism of the Austin Flint murmur. Circulation 1972; 45:558.
41. Erbel R, Engberding R, Daniel C, Roelandt J, Visser C, Rennollet H, and the European Cooperation Study Group for Echocardiography. Echocardiography in the diagnosis of aortic dissection. Lancet 1989; 457.
42. Kirklin JW, Barratt-Boyes BG. Aortic valve disease. In: Cardiac Surgery. New York: Wiley, 1986:373.
43. Miller C. Predictions of outcome in patients with prosthetic valve endocardidis (PVE) and potential advantage of homograft aortic root replacement for prosthetic ascending aortic valve—graft injection. J Cardiac Surg 1990; 5:53.
44. Ross D. Allagraft root replacement for prosthetic endocardidis. J Cardiac Surg 1990; 5:68.
45. Cohn LH, Birjinink V. Therapy of acute aortic regurgitation. In: Carabello B, ed. Cardiology Clinic. Philadelphia: WB Saunders, 1991:341.

12

Mitral and Tricuspid Valve Prolapse

Pravin M. Shah
Loma Linda University Medical Center
Loma Linda, California

I. DEFINITIONS

Mitral valve prolapse (MVP) is one of the few entities which may mean different things to different specialists. A great deal of confusion and misunderstanding has arisen from lack of universal definition of MVP. It truly is an example of the ancient tale of seven blind men feeling different anatomic parts of an elephant and each having a different definition of the animal. To a clinical cardiologist, MVP conjures a picture of a patient with numerous ill-defined but protracted symptoms, inconstant systolic click(s), and late systolic murmur, which are typically influenced by bedside maneuvers such as the Valsalva maneuver. An angiographer views MVP as predominantly a posterior leaflet pathology with frequent association of posterobasal asynergy. A surgeon views prolapse on the anatomical basis of valve incompetence, such as leaflet coaptation, chordal integrity, and annular dilation. A gross pathologist looks for annular dilation, increased leaflet volume, and redundancy. The histologist confirms by detection of "myxoid degeneration" of the leaflet(s). An echocardiographer

---

This chapter, not withstanding the title, will deal in detail with mitral valve prolapse, leaving tricuspid valve prolapse as a single section for specific comments. There is voluminous literature on mitral valve prolapse, and tricuspid valve prolapse is only rarely seen in the absence of mitral prolapse. The two coexist in nearly half the patients diagnosed with mitral valve prolapse.

is able to provide significant anatomical, functional, and physiological information in advanced cases, but struggles to differentiate mild cases of MVP from normal superior systolic displacement.

A great deal of the apparent controversy and confusion can be avoided by acknowledging that MVP represents a broad spectrum. A normal-appearing valve with intermittent and possibly focal pathology is strikingly different from a grossly pathological valve with advanced mitral regurgitation. Although both of these carry the designation of MVP, they are as dissimilar as the trunk is from the tail of an elephant.

MVP thus constitutes a cluster of clinical entities with a common finding of prolapse of one or both leaflets. The identification of prolapse is aided by a combination of clinical and echocardiographic clues. The only true hemodynamic consequence of MVP is mitral regurgitation with associated clinical presentation which is related to its severity and rate of progression. The rate of progression of mitral regurgitation is adversely influenced by chordal rupture or infective endocarditis. The nonhemodynamic correlates of MVP include neuropsychiatric syndromes, neuroendocrine or autonomic dysfunction, cardiac arrhythmias with a rare potential for sudden death, and embolic events with neurological deficits. Many of these clinical entities have apparently little to do with the mitral valve prolapse except for its association.

In the era of increasing attempts at surgical reconstruction of myxomatous floppy valves to correct mitral regurgitation, it is imperative to develop commonly agreed-upon definitions and terminologies among cardiologists, cardiac surgeons, and cardiac pathologists.

II. HISTORICAL BACKGROUND

MVP, although thought to be a malady of the second half of the twentieth century, has clearly been around for a much longer time. Pocock, who, in 1846, edited the American edition of James Hope's classical treatise on heart disease, wrote:

> Regurgitation through the mitral valve during the systole of the heart often takes place without any striking organic lesion in persons of irritable temperament, upon the occurrence of any mental agitation or upon sudden exertion. Under such circumstances, the systole of the heart is accompanied by a slight blowing sound, heard near the apex, not perceptible over the aorta, and ceasing when the disturbing cause has passed by (C. W. Pocock, *Hope on the Heart*, 1846).

This description may best be explained on the basis of MVP.

In addition, Wooley has conducted a scholarly search on the historical aspects of MVP and makes a persuasive argument that designations often used in the past, such as DaCosta's syndrome, soldier's heart, and neurocirculatory asthenia may indeed refer predominantly to those that at present would carry a diagnosis of MVP (1). Gallavardin reported in 1913 an association between late systolic click and pleuropericardial adhesions. It became a part of standard teaching that mid or late systolic clicks were extracardiac in origin. Paul Dudley White considered these clicks to be caused, at least in some cases, by chordal mechanism. It is of interest to note that master clinical Paul Wood, who dominated much of the thinking on bedside cardiac diagnosis in the 1950s, failed to associate these sounds with the mitral apparatus and did not appreciate mitral valve prolapse as an entity.

The modern resurgence in defining and diagnosing mitral valve prolapse is credited to Barlow and colleagues (2), who confirmed prolapse by ventriculography and associated it with mid-systolic click. Criley, who pointed Barlow to a correct interpretation of the angiogram, reported a series with angiographic documentation and coined the term, "prolapse of the mitral valve" (3). The first report of the diagnosis by M-mode echocardiography was by Shah and Gramiak, who emphasized different patterns based on orientation of the M-mode beam relative to the prolapsing segment of the valve (4). The advent of two-dimensional echocardiography with its superior anatomical orientation has resulted in redefining the diagnosis of MVP based on systolic position of the leaflets relative to the annular plane. Kisslo and associates utilized the parasternal long-axis views (5), and Morganroth and associates emphasized the appearance using the apical cross sections (6). Although the apical views seemed to provide a better assessment of the annular plane, some normal subjects were observed to show systolic displacement of the anterior mitral leaflet beyond the annular plane in the apical four-chamber view. Ormiston and colleagues described an echocardiographic method to assess the mitral annular size in humans and reported mitral annular dilatation in a subset of patients with diagnosis of MVP (7,8). Shah proposed that the echocardiographic diagnosis of MVP be based not solely on the leaflet displacement beyond the annular plane, but also include "myxomatous" thickening of the valve leaflets, annular dilatation, involvement of the tricuspid valve, and less often the semilunar valves (9). It was suggested that a combination of findings be used to diagnose true or pathological mitral valve prolapse (also termed mitral valve prolapse syndrome). More recently, Levine et al. have suggested that the mitral annuls is nonplanar, with a saddle-shaped outline such that the annular segments seen in apical four-chamber view are more apically displaced (10,11). This nonplanarity of the annulus served to explain a common perplexing appearance of echocardiographic prolapse, using this cross section, in otherwise normal valves. They recommended that only the parasternal long axis be used to diagnose mitral valve prolapse. A recently completed study in the author's laboratory suggests that the mitral annulus, while being nonplanar, is not truly a saddle-shaped configuration. This study demonstrated the annulus at the point of anterior leaflet attachment to be apically displaced (or lower), but not at the point of attachment of the posterior leaflet as visualized in the apical four-chamber view. This served to explain why posterior leaflet prolapse, even in apical four-chamber view, is almost never encountered in normal subjects.

Since our concepts on mitral valve prolapse are in evolution, a final chapter in the history of the disease has yet to be written.

III. ETIOLOGICAL CLASSIFICATION

True mitral valve prolapse, i.e., abnormal displacement of mitral leaflet(s) into the left atrium, may be primary and idiopathic, or secondary to other pathology.

Primary or idiopathic prolapse is associated with "myxomatous" change and is the most common form of mitral valve prolapse encountered. The term mitral valve prolapse generally refers to this type. It may also be termed mitral valve prolapse syndrome, when associated with autonomic or neuroendocrine dysfunction.

Secondary prolapse may be caused by a number of disorders, including the following:

1. Rheumatic: Rheumatic valvulitis, especially acute rheumatic fever, may result in annular dilatation and mitral valve prolapse, which is almost indistinguishable from the idiopathic variety except by pathological examination.
2. Infective endocarditis: Infective endocarditis may complicate idiopathic mitral valve prolapse with chordal rupture (flail mitral valve) when the infection develops on a normal valve.
3. Trauma: Nonpenetrating trauma may result in chordal rupture in a previously healthy valve or in a myxomatous valve. Typically, a steering-wheel injury in an automobile accident could result in a flail mitral valve.
4. Acute myocardial infarction: Necrosis and rupture of head of a papillary muscle results in acute severe mitral regurgitation, with flail valve with papillary muscle and attached chordae prolapsing into the left atrium.
5. Acute myocardial ischemia: It is postulated, with some experimental support, that acute papillary muscle ischemia results in its failure to shorten during systole (or its actual elongation) and subsequent valve prolapse.

6. Marfan's syndrome: Marfan's syndrome, as a disorder of generalized connective tissues, commonly involves the mitral valve leaflets and the annulus, resulting in valve prolapse.
7. Ehlers-Danlos syndrome: Types 1, 3, and 4 are known to be associated with mitral valve prolapse. In a family of a proband with classic type 4 disease, only those with abnormal production of a specific collagen had mitral valve prolapse as an associated finding (13).
8. Distortion of left ventricular geometry: Since the length of the chordal apparatus is relatively fixed, major reduction or distortion in the left ventricular cavity may be associated with prolapse. Typical examples of such geometric distortions are (a) atrial septal defect with right ventricular volume overload, (b) massive pericardial effusion with compression and underfilling of the left ventricle, and (c) severe pulmonary hypertension without left heart disease. It is not clear if prolapse can occur with acute intravascular volume depletion with tachycardia and hypotension, and resulting reduction in LV volumes.

This chapter will deal primarily with idiopathic mitral valve prolapse, and the term mitral valve prolapse will be used to imply the idiopathic or primary or myxomatous variety.

IV. PATHOLOGY (See Chapter 1)

In the severe forms of mitral valve prolapse, pathological findings are characteristic, but in the more subtle forms, recognition may depend on careful morphometric methods. Lucas and Edwards have proposed interchordal leaflet hooding as a major criterion of morphological diagnosis. Waller and associates proposed a morphometric approach to measure annular circumference (in centimeters) and leaflet area (in square centimeters) and calculate a circumference area product (in cubic centimeters (12). A basis for this approach rests on the characteristic leaflet redundancy and annular dilation, both of which are generally present to varying degrees. Associated morphological features include elongated chordae tendineae, fibrotic thickening of leaflet surfaces, and ventricular endocardial friction lesions.

Histological features include an increase in the spongiosa component (the portion containing mucopolysaccharide material). The increased spongiosa has been inappropriately termed myxoid degeneration. More correctly, there is encroachment of the spongiosa on the fibrosa, resulting in focal disruption of the fibrosa.

The posterior mitral leaflet has three well-defined scallops: medial, middle, and lateral. Prolapse of any one or more of these scallops may be observed. Although the anterior leaflet does not have any well-defined scallops, they may form with redundancy and elongation of the leaflet.

V. PREVALENCE

The familial occurrence of mitral valve prolapse has been found in members of both sexes in two or three generations in several families. The genetic studies suggest that the propensity for the development of mitral valve prolapse is inherited as an autosomal dominant trait with variable expression (14). The expression of the mitral valve prolapse gene appears to be affected by box sex and age. Women predominate in most population surveys and familiar studies, and it is suggested that echocardiographic prolapse is penetrant in 90% to 100% of women but in only about 50% of men with the gene. The influence of age is somewhat complex and less well defined. The prevalence of mitral valve prolapse is low in childhood and adolescence but increases after age 20 years. Another complicating epidemiological observation is that prevalence in women but not in men appears to decrease with age.

There is also a predilection of mitral valve prolapse for certain types of body habitus. The subjects with prolapse are leaner, with narrower anteroposterior chest dimensions, longer arms spans, and a high incidence of thoracic skeletal deformities. This has led to a suggestion that a significant portion of patients with mitral valve prolapse have autosomally dominant, inherited body habitus, suggesting that mitral valve prolapse is only one component of a generalized developmental syndrome.

VI. CLINICAL ASPECTS

A. Symptoms

Patients often seek medical attention for various ill-defined symptoms that seem to have strong underlying features of anxiety neurosis. In most epidemiological studies, a large number of patients are symptom free. One study suggests that the incidence of these vague symptoms is no different in patients with mitral valve prolapse than in those without. Nonetheless, the symptoms often thought to be associated with mitral valve prolapse include the following:

1. Fatigue and lassitude.
2. Chest pain. The pain is generally atypical, unrelated to exertion, and often localized without a typical radiation pattern. However,

in a few patients, some of the features may be suggestive of angina,
and a diagnosis of atypical angina is often entertained.
3. Dyspnea. Patients often complain of difficulty in breathing, either
on exertion or at rest. A careful history once again shows the sensation to be one of breath "sticking," inability to move air, feeling
of a need for more oxygen, and so on, and not true dyspnea.
4. Palpitation is a frequent symptom and consists of awareness of
heartbeat and frequently localized pain and tenderness over the
apical impulse. Other forms of palpitations include skipped beats,
a fluttering sensation, and rapid heart action.
5. Dizziness/syncope. Patients often complain of dizziness, although
frank syncope is less common. These symptoms are at times aggravated on upright posture and are associated with low blood
pressure.
6. Agoraphobia. Some patients complain of extreme anxiety and
unexplained fear and panic. These may come on as panic attacks,
characterized by the frightening occurrence of simultaneous severe
anxiety and multiple cardiovascular and autonomic symptoms including palpitations, dyspnea, chest pain, and dizziness.

Thus, a combination of multiple ill-defined symptoms in a patient with
little in the way of objective evidence of organic cardiac disease leads to
a suspicion of underlying mitral valve prolapse. However, a number of
recent epidemiological studies question the association of these symptoms
and mitral valve prolapse. Thus, earlier reports of a high incidence of
prolapse in panic attacks (agoraphobia) is not confirmed in more recent
studies. The Framingham Study of the general population examined 2931
subjects (age range 20 to 2 years) and concluded that cardiovascular symptoms were no more common in persons with than in those without echocardiographic mitral valve prolapse.

B. Physical Signs

The characteristic physical signs that provide important clues to the bedside diagnosis of mitral valve prolapse include the following.

1. Mid-systolic to late systolic click. A high-pitched mid-systolic
to late systolic click heard over the apex is most commonly due to mitral
valve prolapse. Careful timing with selective angiocardiography and with
echocardiography has shown the click to coincide with the apex of the
prolapsing motion of the valve leaflet. A sudden tensing of the chordal
leaflet structure at the height of prolapse is considered to be a mechanism

of production of this sound. At times, multiple clicks are present. The click or clicks may typically be noted to shift in timing to an earlier or later portion of systole based on changes in left ventricular volume and geometry. Thus, maneuvers that reduce left ventricular volume result in an earlier timing of prolapse and hence the click, and vice versa. The Valsalva maneuver is well suited to demonstrate variation in timing of the systolic click. It moves progressively earlier in systole during phases 2 and 3 and may indeed coincide with the first heart sound. Following release of Valsalva strain during phase 4, as filling of the left ventricle increases progressively, the click moves later in systole and may be heard just before the aortic component of the second heart sound.

2. Systolic murmur. A high-pitched, blowing, systolic murmur commonly accompanies the click and is heard over the apex. The murmur may start before the click but typically follows it. In some patients, a holosystolic murmur is present, although late systolic accentuation is common.

A characteristic apical "whoop" or honk is audible in some patients, especially related to body position. It is often loud and may be heard or felt by the patient. A change in posture from sitting to supine often eliminates the honking nature of the murmur.

3. First heart sound (S_1). Intensity of the mitral component of the first heart sound may vary depending on the timing and type of prolapse. Tei and associates reported that early or pansystolic prolapse is generally associated with a loud S_1 over the apex, whereas mid-systolic to late systolic occurrence of prolapse is associated with normal S_1 (15). Patients with flail mitral valve secondary to rupture of chordae tendineae generally have a soft or absent S_1. This bedside clue may be helpful in characterizing the timing and mechanism of prolapse. The loud S_1 observed with pansystolic prolapse may merely represent coincident timing of the systolic click and S_1, whereas the attenuated S_1 in flail mitral valve is secondary to failure of leaflet coaptation at the time of valve closure.

4. Diastolic sounds. An early diastolic sound coincident with full opening of the valve leaflet may be observed in phonocardiographic recordings and may sometimes be audible. This occurs at the time of the mitral opening snap but is generally of low intensity.

5. Jugular venous pulse and the carotid arterial pulse are normal in contour.

6. Apical impulse has often shown midsystolic retraction by apexcardiography, and this may be appreciated during careful inspection and palpation of the apex beat.

The underlying mechanisms of physical signs are more clearly defined and can be related to the timing and occurrence of valve prolapse. Thus the systolic click coincides with the apex of leaflet prolapse, and multiple clicks may represent different scallops of the valve prolapsing at slightly different times. The systolic murmur is one of mitral regurgitation.

As many as 50% of patients with mitral valve prolapse may demonstrate tricuspid valve prolapse, and the physical findings may be indistinguishable except for a more defined localization of a click or murmur along the lower left sternal edge. If clicks are heard along the lower right sternal edge, associated tricuspid valve prolapse is likely to be present. Tricuspid valve prolapse may occasionally occur as an isolated finding. Thus a careful evaluation of the tricuspid valve should also be undertaken by echocardiography in patients with typical auscultatory findings indicative of valve prolapse but without abnormalities of the mitral valve.

C. Bedside Maneuvers

As pointed out earlier in this section, several bedside maneuvers may assist in providing diagnostic confirmation, especially when the auscultatory signs are not typical or prominent.

1. Posture

Assumption of the upright posture, by reducing venous return and cardiac filing, results in earlier occurrence of the click and murmur, although their intensities may be softer. Opposite behavior in these physical signs is noted with squatting. As described earlier, some patients demonstrate a loud whooping or honking murmur in certain positions in a reproducible manner.

2. Valsalva Maneuver

A sustained forced expiration against a closed glottis held over 15–20 s before release results in typical changes in ventricular filling, stroke volume, blood pressure, and heart rate. An early occurrence of the click, at times coincident with S_1, and earlier initiation of the systolic murmur are noted during phases 2 and 3, when left ventricular volume is reduced and tachycardia is present. The opposite occurs during phase 4, when the left ventricular volume is increased and bradycardia is present.

3. Amyl Nitrite Inhalation

A decrease in arterial pressure and ensuing tachycardia are associated with reduced left ventricular volume and associated with earlier occurrence of the click and an earlier but softer systolic murmur.

4. Postectopic Potentiation

After an ectopic beat, left ventricular volume increases because of the compensatory pause; thus, late occurrence of the clicks in relation to the first heart sound is expected. However, because of a marked increase in inotropy due to postectopic potentiation, the clicks occur earlier and the interval between the first heart sound and clicks decreases. It has been suggested that in individual patients the left ventricular systolic dimension at which mitral valve prolapse occurs is relatively fixed; thus the first heart sound-click interval may shorten during the postectopic beat because the click dimension is reached earlier during ejection as a result of marked increase in contractility.

D. Intermittency of Physical Signs

The characteristic auscultatory features may be intermittently present in a patient, at times without obvious explanation. The typical click or murmur may be absent at examination and quite evident at a subsequent time. This well-known clinical finding makes the use of auscultatory signs as "gold standard" for diagnosis somewhat unreliable. Although the presence of typical auscultatory findings strongly supports a diagnosis of mitral valve prolapse, their absence cannot be used to exclude the diagnosis. Placing excessive value on clinical findings to determine the presence or absence of mitral valve prolapse, as proposed by some investigators, cannot be considered accurate (16).

1. Prolapse Without Auscultatory Signs

It is well recognized that an obvious mitral valve prolapse, noted by either angiocardiography or echocardiography, may be observed in the absence of any physical signs, even with bedside maneuvers. However, the prevalence of prolapse without auscultatory signs in population studies has not been well defined. The Framingham Study of 2931 subjects, which defined mitral valve prolapse based on M-mode echocardiography criteria, reported that less than 15% of patients with prolapse had a click or murmur on both heard on auscultation. This question will need to be readdressed with the use of more rigid echocardiographic criteria of diagnosis, requiring both morphological as well as functional aspects of prolapse.

2. Auscultatory Signs of Prolapse Without Echocardiographic Confirmation

It is generally held that when typical auscultatory findings are present, it is not necessary to obtain confirmation by echocardiography, because negative results do not rule out the clinical diagnosis. However, other, less common causes of mid-systolic to late systolic clicks include interatrial septal aneurysm, intracardiac tumors, and rarely pleuropericardial disease. In instances when auscultatory findings are typical of prolapse but the results of echocardiography are negative, it is advisable to document the presence of a typical click and murmur, in resting condition as well as with bedside maneuvers (e.g., Valsalva maneuver) by phonocardiography. It is certainly possible for prolapse to be localized to a small portion of a leaflet (e.g., a scallop of a posterior leaflet), which may not have been visualized by echocardiographic technic. Such a likelihood is minimized by obtaining multiple cross sections from several transducer orientations and not excluding the apical views. A click may rarely be caused by prolapse of the tricuspid valve in the absence of the mitral valve prolapse.

E. Signs of Autonomic Dysfunction

Autonomic dysfunction has been reported in patients with mitral valve prolapse syndrome (17,18). The clinical observations include a sudden unexplained sinus tachycardia or unusual increase in heart rate following upright posture, and unexplained changes in blood pressures, especially hypotension. The various reported abnormalities of neuroendocrine and autonomic function may be summarized as follows [as suggested by Boudoulas and colleagues (19)]:

1. Evidence of high adrenergic activity. The 24-hour urinary catecholamines were higher in symptomatic patients than in normal controls. Plasma catecholamine values at rest were higher in symptomatic patients, in both supine and upright positions. A repeat measurement in the same patients after 6 years showed persistent elevations of plasma catecholamines (20).
2. Evidence of abnormal catecholamine regulation. Acute volume expansion with 2.5–3 L of isotonic saline given intravenously over 10 hours failed to result in a decrease in plasma catecholamine values in patients with mitral valve prolapse syndrome, in contrast to normal subjects.
3. Evidence of abnormal symptomatic response to adrenergic stimulation. Isoproterenol infusions reproduced symptoms including chest pain, fatigue, dyspnea, dizziness, and panic attacks only in patients with mitral valve prolapse syndrome. The increase in heart rate was significantly greater.
4. Evidence for decreased intravascular volume. Several studies have demonstrated reduced intravascular volumes. There is also an inverse relationship between plasma volume and peripheral vascular resistance on standing.
5. Evidence for abnormal renin-aldosterone regulation. Volume depletion with intravenous furosemide resulted in a greater increase

in plasma norepinephrine, a lesser increase in plasma renin activity, and a greater decrease in plasma aldosterone in patients with mitral valve prolapse syndrome than in control subjects.

6. Evidence for abnormal parasympathetic activity. Studies examining heart rate response to the Valsalva maneuver showed higher rates during strain period and inappropriate bradycardia during recovery, suggesting excessive vagal tone in some patients. Evidence for abnormal baroreflex modulation was a different heart rate response to phenylephrine infusion than in normal controls.

7. Atrial natriuretic factor. Some patients show an increase in atrial natriuretic factor, and this is associated with a lower blood volume. A second group had normal values. The meaning of differences between the groups is not known.

Although these studies emphasize abnormal autonomic and neuroendocrine function, the basic mechanisms involved and their precise correlations with symptoms or with associated MVP have yet to be elucidated

VII. LABORATORY INVESTIGATIONS

A. Routine 12-Lead Electrocardiogram

Approximately 10–15% of patients with mitral valve prolapse demonstrate abnormal ST- and T-wave changes in the inferior and lateral leads. The basis for this abnormality is not understood. A combination of ECG changes along with auscultatory findings was referred to as an auscultatory-echocardiographic subset of the mitral valve prolapse syndrome. Supraventricular or ventricular dysrhythmias may be observed on routine ECG.

B. Chest X-Ray Film

The cardiac silhouette is most often normal, although narrowed anteroposterior dimensions, pectus excavatum, loss of dorsal spine curvature ("straight back"), and various degrees of kyphoscoliosis may be observed. The thoracic skeletal abnormalities occur in approximately 60–70% of patients, although they are often not pronounced.

VIII. ECHOCARDIOGRAPHIC DIAGNOSIS

A. M-Mode Echocardiography

Although M-mode parameters for mitral prolapse were developed before the advent of two-dimensional echocardiography, the limitations of M-mode include uncertain or "blind" beam direction and lack of spatial display with a limited window.

B. Two-Dimensional Echocardiography

As a result of better spatial orientation and ease of determining the mitral annular plane, two-dimensional echocardiography has become the imaging modality with which the diagnosis of functional mitral valve prolapse is made. In some patients, the main limitation of the method is a technical inadequacy in obtaining the multiple anatomical cross sections needed to image all major segments of both valve leaflets. All cross sections providing separation between the left ventricle and the left atrium and a view of the mitral annular plane may be used to diagnose mitral valve prolapse. In all views, the point of coaptation of the leaflets is an important observation. Pronounced mitral valve prolapse without chordal rupture consists of billowing of the leaflets, with posterosuperior displacement of the body of the leaflet(s) being greater than the free margins of coaptation. The resulting appearance is one of convexity of the leaflet body as it protrudes into the left atrium. The tip coaptation is preserved normal in mild cases and may be displaced in more severe cases, with a separation between leaflets rendering them incompetent.

The more important two-dimensional characteristics of primary mitral valve prolapse include the following:

1. Functional prolapse of a localized portion of one or both leaflets may be observed. It is viewed as a systolic displacement of the prolapsing segment of the valve into the left atrium posterosuperior to the mitral annular plane. The two-dimensional cross section that permits its visualization depends on the segment of the leaflet involved in prolapse. The parasternal or apical long-axis view transects the medial aspect of the anterior leaflet and the middle scallop of the posterior leaflet. Prolapse of these components is best diagnosed using the long-axis views. The apical four-chamber view visualizes the medical aspect of the anterior leaflet and generally the lateral scallop of the posterior leaflet or lateral aspect of the middle scallop. The apical two-chamber view permits visualization of the lateral aspect of the anterior leaflet and the medial scallop of the posterior leaflet. Thus the two-dimensional view with the most diagnostic information will depend on the segment or segments of the leaflet involved. Two cautionary notes are important. First, the body of the anterior leaflet may appear to prolapse in the apical four-chamber view in some normal subjects. This is due to the mitral annulus being nonplanar such that at its anterior leaflet attachment it is more apically positioned. How-

ever, even in this view, posterosuperior displacement of the coaptation point or of the posterior leaflet is not a normal finding. Second, the apical two-chamber view is a posteriorly oriented cross section. Because the entire heart moves anteriorly during systole, this cross section may transsect the leaflets in diastole and the posterior annulus in systole. This cross section may provide an erroneous suggestion of prolapse because the annulus is normally curved posteriorly. Nevertheless, a major point that should be emphasized is that all available two-dimensional views should be used in order to diagnose mitral valve prolapse, which in some patients may be a focal abnormality. A recent suggestion that only long-axis views be used to make the diagnosis is inappropriate, because a distinct prolapse of the posterior leaflet may easily be missed. Evidence is not sound to support the contention that apical views are not relevant.

2.   Thickened mitral valve leaflets with redundant tissue of one or both leaflets are generally assessed visually, although comparisons with a structure such as the posterior aortic wall may compensate for differences in gain settings. The thickening may also be focal and may require to be examined in multiple views.

3.   Dilation of the mitral annulus is best evaluated by using the apical views to reconstruct the annulus and measure its circumference and the area. As a general guide, the maximum diameter of the annulus in the apical four-chamber is generally less than 3.5 cm in an adult. An annular diameter in excess of 4.0 cm is nearly always indicative of its dilation, and in excess of 3.5 cms is suggestive of its being dilated. Since the annular dilation occurs in more advanced cases, its presence should be carefully sought.

4.   Coexistence of prolapse of other cardiac valves most commonly involves the tricuspid valve, which is best observed in the views from the right ventricular apex with visualization of the right ventricle, the right atrium, and the tricuspid annular plane. Idiopathic prolapse of the aortic valve cusp is less common and may be observed in the parasternal or the apical long-axis views. Redundancy and prolapse of the pulmonary valve may be present occasionally.

Flail mitral valve is diagnosed using the following two-dimensional echocardiographic criteria:

1.   Absence of leaflet coaptation at the tips or free margins may be noted in one or more apical or parasternal cross sections, depending on the size of the flail leaflet. The flail leaflet protrudes into the left atrium such that its free margin is more posteriosuperiorly

displaced than its body. This results in an appearance that contrasts from the severe billowing of the valve.

2. Sudden whipping motion of a leaflet from the left ventricle to the left atrium may be observed when a large portion of a leaflet is flailing.

3. A leaflet or a portion of one of the leaflets may prolapse into the left atrium, beginning in presystole after the end of the P wave and continuing into ventricular systole. A frame-by-frame evaluation showing presystolic prolapse is characteristic of a flail leaflet, which is generally not observed in the other forms of mitral valve prolapse. Flail mitral valve is most often indicative of ruptured chordae tendineae leaving unsupported leaflet time.

4. Remnants of ruptured chordae tendineae may be seen in the left atrium attached to its prolapsing free margin. This is generally better appreciated with transesophageal than with transthoracic echocardiography.

C. Doppler Echocardiography

Pulsed Doppler technique provides additional evidence of valve regurgitation. The sample volume is located in the mitral apparatus or immediately proximal to the mitral valve in the left atrium. A late-systolic flow velocity turbulence is always abnormal and is indicative of mitral regurgitation. This is typically seen in patients with late-systolic click and murmur of mitral valve prolapse. The abnormal velocity signal may be observed even in the absence of a systolic murmur. Early systolic regurgitation lasting less than 100 ms of systole is less likely to be pathological. On the other hand, pansystolic regurgitation and with aliased signal is nearly always pathological.

Although presence or absence of mitral regurgitation is useful in evaluation of a patient with mitral valve prolapse, its presence cannot be used to diagnose or its absence to exclude valve prolapse.

Color flow imaging, besides providing visualization of the regurgitation jet, may also give insight into its origin and mechanism. Significant mitral regurgitation secondary to prolapse is nearly always eccentric, and its direction provides a clue to its origin. Anterior leaflet prolapse results in a regurgitation jet directed posterolaterally, seen best in the long-axis views. Posterior-leaflet middle scallop pathology is associated with a jet directed medially and anteriorly behind the aortic root, which is also well seen in the long-axis views. Posterior-leaflet lateral scallop pathology results in a medially directed jet toward the interatrial septum and is visualized best in the four-chamber view. Pathology of the medial scallop (least common) results in laterally and somewhat anteriorly directed jet, seen best in the short-axis views. Extensive pathology of several segments of the leaflet would naturally produce a more diffuse or less localizing regurgitation jet.

When does prolapse visualized on echocardiography constitute a pathological syndrome of mitral valve prolapse? As stated earlier, the echocardiographic evidence of mitral valve prolapse may represent a nonpathological functional state resulting from changes in left ventricular geometry and size. The question arises as the significance of echocardiographic mitral valve prolapse. When should an echocardiographic diagnosis of "definite," and "probable," mitral valve prolapse be made? Given the present knowledge about prolapse, the following guidelines may be useful in the clinical setting.

1. Definite mitral valve prolapse syndrome with clinical-pathological significance may be diagnosed when two or more of the following echocardiographic signs are present: leaflet prolapse into the left atrium; thickened, redundant valve leaflets; dilated mitral annulus; associated tricuspid valve prolapse with dilation of the tricuspid annulus; associated aortic valve prolapse. The emphasis in making a diagnosis of definite mitral valve prolapse is on the combination of functional as well as structural changes. This subset of patients generally exhibits the typical physical signs.
2. Probable mitral valve prolapse may be diagnosed when the following is present: functional mitral valve prolapse on two-dimensional echocardiography with clinical signs to support the diagnosis but without structural changes (i.e., thickened leaflets or dilated annulus).
3. No mitral valve prolapse. An echocardiographic diagnosis of mitral valve prolapse cannot be supported under the following circumstances:
    a. Superior displacement of body of anterior mitral leaflet without displacement of the coaptation point or of the posterior leaflet in the apical four-chamber view may be viewed a normal superior systolic motion (especially if the maximum displacement is less than 1.0 cm from the annular plane).
    b. Geometric distortion of the left ventricle may be associated with functional prolapse which, in the absence of structural abnormalities, does not indicate true mitral valve prolapse.

IX. COMPLICATIONS

The complications of mitral valve prolapse include the following: progressive mitral regurgitation and heart failure, chordal rupture with flail mitral valve, cardiac arrhythmias, sudden death, infective endocarditis, and systemic embolism. Although the incidence of these complications appears to be low and the subset of patients susceptible to a given complication is not defined accurately, the serious nature of many of these complications cannot be ignored.

A. Progressive Mitral Regurgitation and Heart Failure

In affluent parts of the world, where the incidence of rheumatic fever is sharply reduced, a common cause of mitral regurgitation is the mitral valve prolapse syndrome. The mechanisms for a progressive increase in mitral regurgitation in the absence of chordal rupture include increasing degrees of prolapse resulting from more extensive leaflet "degeneration" and redundancy or elongation of chordal tendineae, and progressive dilation of the mitral annulus, which in the initial stages is primary (i.e., unrelated to the size of the left ventricle or left atrium). In later stages, secondary annular dilation is superadded from increased mitral regurgitation and chamber enlargement. Thus, chronic mitral regurgitation begets more mitral regurgitation.

The incidence of progressive mitral regurgitation in a population of patients with mitral valve prolapse is not known. It generally reaches the symptomatic stage after the fifth decade of life. For some unknown reason, it appears that men are more prone to develop this complication. This is in striking contrast to the greater prevalence of prolapse among women in the second and third decades of life. Increased physical exertion, higher systemic arterial blood pressure, or some yet unknown factors may be responsible for this disparity.

Presenting symptoms are often those of pulmonary congestion with effort dyspnea, orthopnea, and paroxysmal nocturnal dyspnea. The physical signs are those of severe mitral regurgitation with signs of left ventricular enlargement, a holosystolic mitral regurgitation murmur, and S_3 gallop with or without middiastolic flow murmur. In many patients, the first heart sound (S_1) over the apex is accentuated and is associated with early systolic or pansystolic prolapse.

Progressive pulmonary hypertension, right heart chamber dilation, and chronic congestive heart failure are late developments. Ideally, surgical correction should be undertaken before this stage of advancement.

B. Flail Mitral Valve Syndrome

Rupture of the chordae tendineae, which results in flail mitral valve syndrome, is most commonly secondary to the "degenerative" mitral valve prolapse syndrome, although other causes include infective endocarditis and blunt chest trauma. The chordal rupture in patients with mitral valve prolapse is commonly spontaneous. Rupture of primary chords attached to or near the free margins of the leaflets results in increased mitral regurgitation. The severity of regurgitation is related to the extent of unsupported leaflet tissue based on the size and number of ruptured chordae. The degree of annular dilation and of leaflet redundancy is variable.

Presenting symptoms are similar to those described earlier, although acute onset may be heralded by rupture of a chord, resulting in prolapse of a larger volume of unsupported valve tissue. A subacute course with symptoms progressing over weeks or a more chronic course is more common. The physical signs are as described earlier for more chronic cases, except for an attenuated or absent S_1. The signs of acute mitral regurgitation are rather characteristic and consist of a short early systolic murmur, prominent S_4, early signs of pulmonary hypertension, and right ventricular decompensation. In more acute cases, the cardiac chambers are only slightly dilated.

Management of a flail mitral valve syndrome is surgical, although timing of surgery may be guided by the severity and progression of symptoms and of left ventricular function.

C. Cardiac Dysrhythmias

Early reports have emphasized a high incidence of ventricular and supraventricular arrhythmias in patients with mitral valve prolapse (21). In some patients the arrhythmias are serious enough to be life threatening, and sudden death has generally been associated with malignant ventricular dysrhythmias. The early ambulatory ECG monitoring studies revealed between 50% and 80% incidence of ventricular premature contractions (VPCs), and complex or frequent VPCs were noted in 30% to 50% of patients. The ventricular arrhythmias are typically reduced in frequency of occurrence at night and exaggerated after exercise. The incidence of nonsustained or sustained ventricular tachycardia in patients seen at tertiary referral centers has varied between 10% and 25%. Spontaneous brief episodes of ventricular fibrillation may occur, and torsades de pointes has been reported. Mechanisms of ventricular dysrhythmias are not clarified. Focal cardiomyopathy has been offered as an explanation. Vectorcardiographic evidence that the majority of VPCs originate in the posterobasal left ventricular myocardium may lend support to this theory. The dysrhythmias have not correlated with prolapse of one or both leaflets; however, the severity of mitral leaflet thickening as judged by echocardiogram has correlated with a higher incidence of arrhythmias. Prolongation of the QT interval has also been implicated. There is also a high incidence of repolarization abnormalities in the resting ECG.

Supraventricular arrhythmias are also common in patients with mitral valve prolapse. Paroxysmal supraventricular tachycardia is probably the most common sustained tachyrhythmia in patients with the mitral valve prolapse syndrome. Electrophysiological studies have implicated atrioventricular nodal reentry as the mechanism in some, and a high incidence of bypass tracts precipitating the tachycardia has been reported. Although earlier reports emphasized a preponderance of left-sided accessory pathways in cases of mitral valve prolapse, a recent study found no pattern of association with the location of the accessory pathway.

Conduction abnormalities have also been reported and associated with mitral valve prolapse. Sinus node dysfunction and various grades of atrioventricular block as well as bundle branch block may be noted. Electrophysiological studies have revealed abnormal sinus node function, prolongation of the atrioventricular interval, and intrahisian block, as well as functional bundle branch block.

D. Sudden Death

A number of reports as well as clinical experience indicate that sudden death may occur in persons with mitral valve prolapse as the only pathological cardiac finding. In most such instances, antecedent serious recurrent ventricular dysrhythmias have been observed. In some cases, complete atrioventricular block or sinoatrial arrest is an underlying factor responsible for sudden death. A role of antiarrhythmic agents in preventing sudden death remains to be established.

E. Infective Endocarditis

The occurrence of infective endocarditis in patients with mitral valve prolapse has been recognized, although it is not certain if this represents a coincidental association or is indicative of an increased risk offered by valvular pathology. A controlled study confirmed an increase in risk for endocarditis associated with mitral valve prolapse (22). It has been suggested that persons with mitral valve prolapse are five to eight times more likely to have infective endocarditis than normal persons. Although clinical reports have demonstrated the occurrence of endocarditis regardless of the presence or absence of an associated murmur, a murmur of mitral regurgitation is thought to provide additional risk. It also appears that thickened redundant valves and severe prolapse are more frequently associated with infection.

It has been recommended that prophylaxis for infective endocarditis be instituted only for patients with a heart murmur. This seems somewhat illogical, because patients with clicks alone are known to have suffered from endocarditis, and murmurs may be intermittent. Some patients with a distinct mitral regurgitation jet of mild or even moderate severity may have no discernible heart murmur. The author subscribes to a view that patients who fulfill stringent criteria for diagnosis based on structural and functional evidence of mitral valve prolapse should receive prophylaxis for endocarditis, regardless of the physical findings of valvular regurgitation.

F. Systemic Embolism

A large body of clinical evidence implicates mitral valve prolapse as a cause of transient ischemic attacks (TIA) or stroke, especially in younger patients. The neurological literature is replete with association of TIA, stroke, and mitral valve prolapse. Patients are also reported to develop retinal emboli. A study of 141 patients over 45 years of age (mean, 64.7 years) and 40 patients under 45 years old (mean, 33.9 years) demonstrated an incidence of valve prolapse in the older group to be 5–7% and in younger patients to be 40% (23). Some patients also had other potential causes of cerebral ischemia, suggesting that detection of mitral valve prolapse does not confirm a causative role and other potential causes should be sought. A precise mechanism for systemic embolism has not been defined, although platelet aggregates over a redundant and thickened valve may provide an explanation. A study of platelets in patients with mitral valve prolapse has reported increased platelet coagulant activities, and patients with thromboembolism also demonstrated an increased proportion of circulating platelet aggregates. This study appears to support a potential role of platelets in the purported association of thromboembolism and mitral valve prolapse.

X. NATURAL HISTORY

It is difficult to define with accuracy the natural history of so common and varied a disorder as mitral valve prolapse (24,25). Most long-term follow-up studies originate from tertiary referral centers and have for a large part included retrospective data analysis. Although this approach defines the likely complications that may develop during the lifetime of a patient with this disorder, current evidence points to a specific subset of patients being more at risk for some of the complications, as discussed earlier.

Most long-term follow-up studies demonstrate that the vast majority of patients remain stable and without progression of mitral regurgitation. The incidence of infective endocarditis appears to be low and may be largely preventable. Progression of mitral regurgitation appears to develop more frequently in older men with redundant, thickened valves and often with associated chordal rupture. Sudden death is a rare complication and is almost always associated with malignant ventricular dysrhythmias. Patients with an abnormal resting ECG may be at increased risk. Systemic embolism is a rare complication, and younger patients (<45 years) with thickened redundant valve leaflets appear to be at greater risk.

XI. MEDICAL TREATMENT

Because mitral valve prolapse is generally a benign condition with a low incidence of complications, which may yet be quite devastating, a physician often faces a real dilemma about the wisdom of informing a patient of the presence of this condition and educating him or her about the possibility of serious complications. The basic principles of management are as follows.

A. Patient Education and Reassurance

Patient education and reassurance constitute a most important therapeutic intervention once a diagnosis of definite or highly probable mitral valve prolapse is established. This is especially necessary in symptomatic patients who suffer from high-level anxiety.

B. Symptomatic Treatment

Because many of the symptoms have no well-defined organic basis, there is little place for cardioactive drugs to treat symptoms such as chest pain, palpitations, dizziness, and so on. Beta-adrenergic blocking agents have been used, with relief of various vague symptoms, including anxiety attacks. In more persistent cases, use of tranquilizers may be indicated. However, it is much more important to listen to patients' descriptions of symptoms and give reinforcing assurance of the excellent long-term prognosis from one visit to the next.

In occasional patients, when coronary artery spasm can be documented, treatment with calcium channel blockers or with nitrates may be indicated. Similarly, specific treatment aimed at arrhythmias or hypotension may relieve associated symptoms.

C. Prevention of Complication

Even though they are infrequent, the complications do tend to have serious consequences, and hence a prophylactic approach is advisable.

D. Treatment of Complications

1. Infective Endocarditis

It is controversial whether all patients in whom a diagnosis of mitral valve prolapse is made by clinical or echocardiographic criteria should receive prophylaxis against endocarditis. Clemens and Ransohoff (26) have estimated the early risk of endocarditis for a person with mitral valve prolapse to be approximately 5:100,000. This low risk of endocarditis for an individual, despite increased overall risk compared with a normal person, can be explained by the high prevalence of mitral valve prolapse in the general population and the relative rarity of endocarditis (1.1:100,000 per year). It has been suggested that routine prophylaxis with parenteral penicillin is not cost-effective and also may cause a net loss of life, because the risk of endocarditis after dental procedures would be outweighed by the risks of anaphylaxis. Thus, for routine prophylaxis, oral antibiotics are recommended.

The following groups are at increased risk of infective endocarditis:

1. Patients with thickened redundant valve leaflets determined by echocardiography
2. Patients with associated mitral regurgitation jet
3. Patients with frequent bacteremia (e.g., drug addicts)

Those with structurally normal-appearing valve leaflets with a suggestion of probable prolapse and without a regurgitation jet should not receive routine prophylaxis.

2. Sudden Death

The most frequent underlying cause of sudden death is cardiac dysrhythmias. Hence the prevention consists of proper recognition and effective treatment of arrhythmias. Because mitral valve prolapse is such a common condition, it would not appear practical to carry out ambulatory ECG monitoring on all patients with this diagnosis. The following situations are offered as practical guidelines for undertaking 24-hour Holter monitoring:

1. Presence of cardiac arrhythmias on routine 12-lead ECG
2. Presence of repolarization abnormalities (ST and T changes) on 12-lead ECG
3. Symptomatic patients with palpitations, dizziness, or syncope
4. Prolonged QT interval or preexcitation syndrome on ECG
5. Special work-related categories (e.g., pilots)

Although class 1 antiarrhythmics (i.e., quinidine, procainamide) are commonly used, neither effectiveness nor safety is established. In many patients, propranolol appears to be effective. Similarly, phenytoin sodium has been used with some success. In more recalcitrant cases with malignant forms of ventricular dysrhythmia, it would be appropriate to use more potent drugs such as amiodarone, despite a risk of side effects. In some patients, the use of mechanical devices such as an implanted defibrillator may have to be considered.

Occasional success in terms of reduction of serious life-threatening ventricular dysrhythmias has been reported following replacement of the mitral valve. However, this radical form of therapy is generally not indicated for arrhythmias and should be reserved for patients with severe mitral valve regurgitation and hemodynamic compromise.

3. Systemic Embolism

It has been proposed that patients with a history of systemic embolism should receive antiplatelet agents to prevent recurrences. Although this approach is a reasonable one, no definitive evidence of efficacy exists at present. The use of anticoagulants may be reserved or patients with recurrent embolism despite antiplatelet therapy.

4. Congestive Heart Failure

Because congestive heart failure may develop from either a progressive increase in mitral valve regurgitation or rupture of chordae tendineae, there is no adequate known prophylactic measure.

XII. SURGICAL TREATMENT

Role of surgery in mitral valve prolapse is limited to correction of severe mitral regurgitation, although rare cases of surgical intervention for recurrent sudden death episodes, refractory to drug therapy, have been reported with mixed results.

A. Timing of Surgery

Timing of surgery for correction of mitral regurgitation can be one of the most vexing problems in decision making. Since an ideal valve prosthesis does not exist and success of valve repair cannot be assured with complete confidence, it is preferable to seek a time for surgery when in the natural history of the disease, risk–benefit ratio favors such course. The natural history of chronic severe mitral regurgitation is one of clinical and functional stability along with progressively increasing regurgitation and dilation of the left ventricle. No single parameter, noninvasive or invasive, exists which is capable of defining a precise time for surgery. Left ventricular ejection fraction, a commonly used index of left ventricular function, is unreliable in the setting of mitral regurgitation, since a major portion of left ventricular emptying occurs in the low-resistance, low-pressure left atrium. Indeed, mitral valve surgery for regurgitation is nearly always followed by a drop in ejection fraction. A clinically useful way to follow asymptomatic patients with chronic mitral regurgitation is with serial echocardiographic measures of left ventricular dimensions, volumes, and ejection fractions. When the left ventricular end diastolic dimension exceeds 7.0 cm, the end diastolic volume exceeds 200 ml/M^2, and ejection fraction drops to 50% or less, surgical option even for an asymptomatic patient should be seriously entertained. A major risk to the patient is in waiting until the left ventricular function has deteriorated to a value of ejection fraction below 35%, when irreversible myocardial damage is likely to have occurred and long term results of surgery are of marginal benefit. End systolic stress has been offered as a more accurate endpoint for timing of surgery, but other studies have not confirmed this. A recent observation in our laboratory suggested usefulness of left ventricular *dp/dt* evaluated by continuous-wave Doppler signal of mitral regurgitation jet (27). A value of left ventricular of *dp/dt* below 1000 mmHg/s/s was associated with poor postoperative recovery.

Among other factors which play a role in timing of surgery are feasibility of valve repair versus replacement and associated conditions. Availability of a surgical team experienced in and willing to undertake reconstructive surgery in suitable patients tends to favor one toward earlier surgery in those with valve pathology that is more suitable for repair. Similarly, coexistence of other conditions, such as aortic valve surgery or coronary artery disease, may influence the timing of mitral valve surgery.

B. Role of Echocardiography in Detection of Valve Pathology More Suitable for Valve Repair

Although a final decision for mitral valve repair or replacement is made by the operating surgeon after careful examination of the valve pathology, a number of echocardiographic clues can provide accurate prediction of the valve pathology. An echocardiographer must utilize multiple cross sections to assess the extent and location of valve pathology, and clues from color flow imaging to assess the exact site of origin of the regurgitant jet. The following echocardiographic guidelines favor valve repair:

1. Predominant posterior leaflet pathology with normally preserved anterior leaflet function

2. Dilation of the annulus
3. Anterior leaflet billowing without chordae rupture and associated with chordal elongation
4. Anterior leaflet flail localized to less than a third of the leaflet tissue and associated with primary or free margin chordae rupture
5. Localized perforation in a leaflet secondary to prior infective endocarditis
6. Cleft mitral valve pathology

C. Intraoperative Role of Echocardiography in Mitral Valve Surgery

Availability of transesophageal echocardiography has had a major impact on valvular surgery, especially for mitral regurgitation. The crisp and high-resolution images of valve apparatus can be obtained prior to thoracotomy, and additional quantitation of pathology including the size of the mitral annulus can be assessed. Success of an attempted surgical repair can be assessed accurately after the patient comes off cardiopulmonary bypass with the chest open. Evaluation of residual regurgitation, if any, of systolic anterior motion and dynamic outflow obstruction, if present, of mitral diastolic gradients, and of left ventricular function can be made by using transesophageal echocardiography.

It is necessary for the cardiovascular surgeon and echocardiographer to work closely and communicate effectively for successful management of patients in need of surgical correction in order to maximize immediate and long-term results of surgery.

XIII. TRICUSPID VALVE PROLAPSE

A. Prevalence

Proper echocardiographic technics have demonstrated that tricuspid valve prolapse (TVP) is present in approximately 50% of patients with definite or probable evidence of MVP. No detailed epidemiological studies exist with regard to age and sex distribution or natural history of TVP. It must be remembered that, on occasion, TVP may exist without MVP.

B. Clinical Aspects

Clinical signs: It is difficult, if not impossible to differentiate the systolic click of MVP from that of TVP. A murmur is soft, low pitched, and localized to the lower sternal edge.

C. Echocardiographic Diagnosis

Two-dimensional echocardiography is generally required for assessment of TVP. The right ventricular inflow view obtained with the transducer over the right ventricular apex is most useful. At times, TVP may be obvious in the apical four-chamber view or in the low-parasternal short-axis view. The septal and anterior cusps of the tricuspid valve are more readily visualized. The general criterion of prolapse is one used for MVP, i.e., displacement of the tricuspid valve tissue behind the tricuspid annular plane into the right atrium. A caution must be used in diagnosis of TVP when the septal cusp above shows this displacement. For reasons possibly of nonplanarity of the tricuspid valve, the diagnosis should not be based solely on septal cusp "prolapse," unless it is marked (>1.0 cm) and associated with atypical jet of tricuspid regurgitation. Redundancy and prolapse of the anterior cusp can be diagnosed in the right ventricular inflow view or the apical four-chamber view. A visualization of the posterior cusp requires a cross section nearly orthogonal to the right ventricular inflow view such that aortic root is present. In this plane, the anterior and posterior cusps can be observed.

The tricuspid annulus, being nearly circular, can be examined in any one view showing its maximal diameter. In an adult, the tricuspid annulus is normally less than 4.0 cm in diameter. Patients with TVP often shown dilation of the annulus, which may be further increased with progressive tricuspid regurgitation and dilatations of the right ventricle and atrium.

The Doppler methods are used to detect and assess severity of tricuspid regurgitation.

D. Complications

Although no systemic studies of complications are available, they are likely to be associated with similar complications, except for systemic embolism. Infective endocarditis, especially in intravenous drug users, is a likely complication. Progressive tricuspid regurgitation may occur but is uncommon, possibly owing to low pressures in the right heart cavities.

E. Treatment

No specific management guidelines exist other than a need to replace or repair the valve in the presence of severe symptomatic tricuspid regurgitation. Tricuspid anuloplasty is generally successful.

REFERENCES

1. Wooley CF. Where are the diseases of yesteryear? DaCosta's syndrome, soldiers heart, the effort syndrome, neurocirculatory asthenia—and the mitral valve prolapse syndrome. Circulation 1976; 53:749.

2. Barlow JB, Bosman CK, Pocock WA, et al. Late systolic murmur and none-jection (mid-late) systolic clicks. Br Heart J 1968; 30:203.

3. Criley JM, Lewis KB, Humphries JO, et al. Prolapse of the mitral valve: clinical and cineangiocardiographic findings. Br Heart J 1966; 28:488.

4. Shah PM, Gramiak R. Echocardiographic recognition of mitral valve prolapse (abstr). Circulation 1970: 42(suppl 3):45.

5. Kisslo J, vonRamm OT, Thurstone FL. Cardiac imaging using a phased-array ultrasound system. II. Clinical technique and application. Circulation 1976; 50:262.

6. Morganroth J, Mardelli TJ, Naito M, et al. Apical cross-sectional echocardiography: standard for the diagnosis of idiopathic mitral valve prolapse syndrome. Chest 1981; 79(1):23.

7. Ormiston JA, Shah PM, Tei C, Wong M. Size and motion of the mitral valve annulus in man. I: A two-dimensional echocardiographic method and findings in normal subjects. Circulation 1981; 64:113.

8. Ormiston JA, Shah PM, Tei C, Wong M. Size and motion of the mitral valve annulus in man. II. Abnormalities in mitral valve prolapse. Circulation 1982; 65:713.

9. Shah PM. Update of mitral valve prolapse syndrome: when is echo prolapse a pathological prolapse? In: Echocardiography: A Review of Cardiovascular Ultrasound. Vol. 1. Futura Publishing Co., Mount Kisco, NY. 1984:87.

10. Levine RA, Triulzi MO, Harrigan P, Weyman AE. The relationship of mitral annular shape to the diagnosis of mitral valve prolapse. Circulation 1987; 75:756.

11. Levine RA, Stathogiannis E, Newell JB, Harrigan P, Weyman AE. Reconsideration of echocardiographic standards for mitral valve prolapse: lack of association between leaflet displacement isolated to the apical four chamber view and independent echocardiographic evidence of abnormality. J Am Coll Cardiol 1988; 11:1010.

12. Waller BF, Morrow AG, Maron BJ, et al. Etiology of clinically isolated, severe, chronic, pure, mitral regurgitation: analysis of 97 patients over 30 years of age having mitral valve replacement. Am Heart J 1982; 104:288.

13. Jaffe AS, Geltman EM, Rodney GE, Utto J. Mitral valve prolapse: a consistent manifestation of type IV Ehlers-Danlos syndrome: the pathogenic role of the abnormal production of type III collagen. Circulation 1981; 64:121.

14. Devereux RB, Brown T, Kramer-Fix R, Sachs I. Inheritance of mitral valve prolapse: effect of age and sex on gene expression. Ann Intern Med 1982; 97:826.

15. Tei C, Shah PM, Cherian G, et al. The correlates of abnormal first heart sound in mitral valve prolapse syndromes. N Engl J Med 1982; 307:334.

16. Perloff JK, Child JS, Edwards JE. New guidelines for the clinical diagnosis of mitral valve prolapse. Am J Cardiol 1986; 57:1124.

17. Gaffney FA, Bastian BC, Lane LB, et al. Abnormal cardiovascular regulation in the mitral valve prolapse syndrome. Am J Cardiol 1983; 52:316.

18. Coghlan HC, Phares P, Cowley M, et al. Dysautonomia in mitral valve prolapse. Am J Med 1979; 67:236.

19. Boudoulas H, Reynolds JC, Mazzaferri E, Wooley CF. Metabolic studies in mitral valve prolapse syndrome. Circulation 1980; 61:1200.

20. Boudoulas H, Reynolds JC Mazzaferri E, Wooley CF. Mitral valve prolapse syndrome: the effect of adrenergic stimulation. J Am Coll Cardiol 1983; 2: 638.

21. Winkle RA, Lopes MG, Popp RL, Hancock EW. Life threatening arrhythmias in mitral valve prolapse syndrome. Am J Med 1976; 60:961.

22. Clemens JD, Horwitz RI, Jaffee CC, et al. A controlled evaluation of the risk of bacterial endocarditis in persons with mitral valve prolapse. N Engl J Med 1982; 307:776.

23. Barnett HJM, Bongliner DR, Taylor W, et al. Further evidence relating to mitral valve prolapse to cerebral ischemic events. N Engl J Med 1980; 302: 139.

24. Bisset GS, Schwartz DC, Meyer RA, et al. Clinical spectrum and long-term follow up of isolated mitral valve prolapse in 119 children. Circulation 1980; 52:423.

25. Oakley CM. Mitral valve prolapse: harbinger of death or variant of normal. Br Med J 1984; 288:1853.

26. Clemens JD, Ransohoff DF. A quantitative assessment of predental antibiotic prophylaxis of patients with mitral valve prolapse. J Chronic Dis 1984; 37:531.

27. Pai RG, Bansal R, Shah PM. Doppler derived rate of left ventricular pressure rise: its correlation with postoperative left ventricular function in mitral regurgitation. Circulation 1990; 82:514.

13

Infective Endocarditis

Anilkumar Mehra and Shahbudin H. Rahimtoola
University of Southern California, Los Angeles, California

Infective endocarditis refers to bacterial, fungal, rickettsial, and possibly viral infections of heart valves or mural endocardium as well as infections of vascular endothelium (enarteritis) (1a). It remains an important cause of cardiovascular morbidity and mortality despite an increased clinical awareness of the need for early diagnosis and treatment and advances in its medical and surgical treatment (1). Bacterial endocarditis is the most common form of infective endocarditis and is often classified as acute or subacute on the basis of the clinical course of the patient, which is dependent on the invasiveness of the infecting organism.

I. PATHOGENESIS

A. Predisposing Factors

Subacute bacterial endocarditis usually develops in the setting of an underlying structural abnormality; the bacteria are most frequently of low virulence, such as viridans streptococci. Cardiovascular abnormalities with significant pressure gradient between two cardiac chambers generates turbulent blood flow which damages the surface of the abnormal valve or adjacent endocardium within the lower pressure chamber (2). Formation of sterile platelet-thrombi on the damaged endothelium becomes nidus for bacterial adhesion in the course of bacteremia and multiplication of the bacterial organisms in the platelet-fibrin mesh forms vegetations. Cardiac lesions which do not generate turbulent blood flow, such as isolated atrial septal defect, usually do not predispose to bacterial endocarditis (1a).

In acute bacterial endocarditis, there is usually no apparent underlying heart disease or stimulus for formation of sterile thrombi and the infection results from a more virulent organism such as *Staphylococcus aureus (Staph. aureus)* or from inadequate host defenses (3). Systemic disease, such as diabetes mellitus or collagen vascular disease, may suppress host responses. In addition, intravenous drug usage with infected syringes and/ or needles leads to infective endocarditis in patients with normal valves.

The majority of patients with bacterial endocarditis have underlying heart disease. Approximately 50% have rheumatic valve disease, and 10–15% have congenital heart disease such as tetralogy of Fallot, ventricular septal defect, patent ductus arteriosus, coarctation of aorta, and bicuspid aortic valves (1a,4). Forty percent or more of patients with infective endocarditis have no prior history of heart disease and includes patients with subclinical rheumatic or congenital heart disease, mitral valve prolapse with mitral regurgitation, hypertrophic cardiomyopathy, and patients with no identifiable underlying heart disease (1a).

B. Pathology

The hydrodynamics of flow through an orifice from a high- to a low-pressure chamber allows preferential deposition of bacteria on the low-pressure side of the orifice or at the site where the jet stream impacts on the endothelial surface (2). Therefore, typically the site of vegetations in mitral regurgitation is on the atrial surface of the mitral valve or the wall of the left atrium and in aortic regurgitation, the ventricular surface of the aortic valve. Similarly, in ventricular septal defect, the right ventricular surface of the defect and the right ventricular wall opposite to it are commonly involved (1a).

Infective endocarditis involves the left heart valves more frequently than the right; the aortic, mitral, both valves, tricuspid, and pulmonic valves, in that order of frequency (5). In intravenous drug abusers, the left heart valves are involved in approximately 50% of cases. In prosthetic valve endocarditis, the aortic valve is more frequently affected than the mitral valve. The incidence of endocarditis is similar in mechanical and bioprosthetic valves.

Fresh vegetations in infective endocarditis are pink, red, large, friable and may easily embolize. The largest vegetations develop in fungal and in some cases of *Staph. aureus* endocarditis. In some cases, vegetations may grow large enough to obstruct the valvular orifice; and if they embolize, they may occlude major systemic arteries (6a).

If infection remains uncontrolled, necrosis of the affected valve leaflets may lead to perforation of the cusps and/or formation of aneurysms. Extension of the infectious process into the adjacent structures may lead to rupture of chordae tendinae, root abscesses, paravalvular leak, perforation of ventricular or atrial septa, myocardial abscess, and suppurative pericarditis (6a).

C. Port of Entry

Although a number of procedures and instrumentations lead to transient bacteremias, only a limited number of bacterial species and transient bacteremias lead to infective endocarditis (6). Dental procedures are a common predisposing event. Surgery and diagnostic procedures, particularly those involving the genitourinary and gastrointestinal tract, may result in significant transient bacteremia.

The incidence of transient bacteremia associated with dental extraction has been reported to range from 18% to 85%; streptococci being the commonest organism. The dental and oral procedures associated with transient bacteremia are scaling of teeth, peridontal operations, brushing of teeth, chewing hard candy, tonsilloadenoidectomy, bronchoscopy, orotracheal intubation, and nasal operations (6a).

Transient bacteremia with barium enema, sigmoidoscopy, or upper gastrointestinal endoscopy is reported in about 10% of patients, viridans streptococci being the most common organism. The incidence is lower with upper endoscopy than colonoscopy. A large number of urological procedures including cytoscopy, urethral catheterization, and urethral dilatation result in transient bacteremias; gram-negative bacilli are the most common organisms (6a).

Obstetrical and gynecological procedures have been reported to account for 26% of the cases of infective endocarditis in females (7). Bacteremia and infective endocarditis may occur following, vaginal delivery with manual removal of the placenta, dilatation and curretage, and infected intrauterine contraceptive devices. Although infective endocarditis has been reported to occur following a normal vaginal delivery, it is rare (7).

Prolonged use of intravenous catheters, such as central venous lines, pulmonary artery catheters, and hyperalimentation lines, is associated with increased risk of endocarditis due to colonization of the tip of the catheter. The site of entry of organisms is at the location of skin insertion. Other nosocomial endocarditis occur with postoperative wound infections, hemodialysis shunts, and transvenous pacemaker insertions. Staphylococci are the most common organisms in procedures that involve interruption of skin integrity (1a).

Intravenous drug usage has become an increasingly frequent risk factor for the development of acute infective endocarditis in recent years (8).

D. Microbiology

Many bacterial organisms have been implicated in infective endocarditis (Table 1) (11). Streptococci and staphylococci account for more than 80% of the infections; gram-negative bacilli 7%; and fungal, rickettsial, or chlamydial infections 5% of cases. "Culture-negative" endocarditis is seen in 5–15% of patients with endocarditis (9–11).

The organisms that cause subacute bacterial endocarditis, are usually found within the body's normal flora, are of low virulence and establish infection in the presence of previous cardiac abnormalities. Streptococci

Table 1   Incidence of Endocarditis Due to Various Infectious Agents

Organism	Percentage with natural valve	Percentage with prosthetic valve
Streptococci	60–80	10–35
Viridans streptococci	30–40	3–23
S. sanguis		
S. mutans		
S. mitior		
Enterococci	5–18	5–9
Other streptococci	15–25	1–4
Staphylococci	20–35	40–50
S. aureus	10–30	15–20
S. epidermidis	1–3	20–30
Gram-negative aerobic bacilli	1.5–13	10–20
(*Pseudomonas,*		
Enterobacteriaceae)		
Diphtheroids	<10	4–10
Fungi (*Aspergillus, Candida,*	2–4	5–15
Histoplasma)		
Miscellaneous	<5	<1
Gonococci		
Borrella		
Listeria		
Meningococci		
Bacteroides		
Hemophilus		
Rickettsiae (*Coxiella burnetii*)		
Chlamydia psittaci		
Cell-defective bacteria		

Source: From Ref. 11, with the permission of Little, Brown & Co.

and *Staphylococcus epidermidis* are usually of low virulence. In streptococcal endocarditis of the native valve, viridans streptococci account for approximately 70% of the cases; enterococci (group D streptococci) for 10%; and nonhemolytic, microaerophilic, anaerobic, or nonenterococcal group D streptococci for 20% of the cases (1,1a,4,9).

   More virulent organisms, such as *Staph. aureus, Streptococcus pneumoniae, Neisseria meningitis, Neisseria gonorrhae, Streptococcus pyogenes*, and hemophilus influenzae, often result in fulminant acute bacterial endocarditis (6a,8). These agents commonly affect hospitalized patients and intravenous drug abusers.

   In contrast to native valve endocarditis, staphylococcus is the most common organisms for early prosthetic valve endocarditis, *Staph. epidermidis* being the most common organism (11). Gram-negative bacilli, fungi, and to a lesser extent *Staph. aureus* are more common in early than late prosthetic valve endocarditis. In late prosthetic valve endocarditis, both streptococci (*Strep. viridans*) and staphylococci occur with equal frequency; however, *Staph. epidermidis* is more common than *Staph. aureus* (1a).

   A number of gram-negative bacilli, such as *Serratia, Acinetobacter, Pseudomonas cepacia, Pseudomonas aeruginosa*, Bacteroides, as well as gram-positive organisms such as group B, D, and L streptococci, lactobacilli, *Legionella*, and mycobacteria affect prosthetic heart valves more frequently than native valves (6a,12). Endocarditis caused by atypical mycobacteria— *Mycobacterium chelonei, Mycobacterium gordonae*, and *Mycobacterium fortuitum*—usually occurs only with porcine valve endocarditis (6a). The recent increase in the incidence of fungal endocarditis may be because of increased use of prosthetic valves, hyperalimentation, intravenous catheters, long-term antibiotic therapies, and intravenous drug abuse (1a).

E. Immunology

Immunological phenomena are more common in subacute that in acute bacterial endocarditis and are related to the duration of the infection. In subacute bacterial endocarditis, high titers of rheumatoid factor are detected in up to 50% of patients (13). Specific agglutinating, complement-fixing antibodies, and cryoglobulins with specific affinities for the renal glomerular membrane, vascular walls, and myocardium are increased in the serum of patients with infective endocarditis, especially the subacute form. Other immunological abnormalities detected in some patients are increase in antinuclear antibody, depression in total hemolytic complement, C3, and C4, and increase in circulating immune complexes. Circulating immune complexes are demonstrated in up to 97% of patients with subacute and 45% of patients with culture-negative endocarditis (6a).

Clinical manifestations of the immunological phenomena are glomerulonephritis, Roth spots, Janeway lesions, Osler nodes, and arthritis.

II. CLINICAL FEATURES

Infective endocarditis presents with a number of clinical manifestations that mimic many other disease states (Table 2). The clinical features are related to the disease state itself, and the noncardiac or cardiovascular complications. It may be useful to classify infective endocarditis into acute, with signs/symptoms present for few days; or subacute, with clinical features present for few weeks to months before diagnosis; as this may have practical implications with regard to probable bacterial etiology and urgency of therapy (1a). The "classic" triad of fever of more than several days' duration without apparent cause, significant heart murmur, and anemia should raise the possibility of infective endocarditis (7,14). Fever is present in almost 100% of patients who have not received previous antibiotic therapy or antipyretics or antiinflammatory agents (1). A

Table 2 Clinical Presentations of Endocarditis

Fever and heart murmur
Sepsis
Fever of unknown origin
Transient ischemic attacks or stroke
Meningitis
Subarachnoid hemorrhage
Peripheral arterial embolization
Myocardial infarction
Unexplained congestive heart failure
Pulmonary infarction, necrotizing pneumonia
Constitutional symptoms suggestive of
　neoplasm
　collagen vascular disease
Musculoskeletal complaints suggestive of
　polymyalgia rheumatica
　acute rheumatic fever
　rheumatoid arthritis
Anemia
Renal failure

Source: From Ref. 11, with the permission of Little, Brown & Co.

normal temperature pattern under reliable observation makes the diagnosis unlikely. Occasional exceptions to this rule may be seen in patients with uremia, congestive heart failure, and debilitating illnesses (4). In the subacute form, the fever is generally low-grade remittent; whereas in the acute form, it may exceed 103°F (39.5°C) and be accompanied by rigors (7).

The development of a new cardiac murmur or a change in character or intensity of a preexisting murmur is an important feature of the disease (7). However, the finding of the presence or a change in character of a murmur is the exception rather than the rule in patients with infective endocarditis (1,4,15). It is common to observe some change in the intensity of the murmur due to tachycardia, anemia, and/or fever. Infective endocarditis without a significant murmur may be seen early in the course of endocarditis or with infections involving mural rather than valvular endothelium. New murmurs or significant changes in intensity of murmurs usually result from regurgitant valvular lesions (1a).

The incidence of "peripheral signs" of endocarditis, such as splenomegaly, petechiae (often conjunctival), Osler nodes, Janeway lesions, clubbing, and subungual or retinal hemorrhages increases with the duration and chronicity of the illness; therefore the frequency of these peripheral manifestations has decreased in the antibiotic era (4,7). These manifestations are helpful in supporting the diagnosis, but their absence is not helpful in excluding the diagnosis of infective endocarditis. Splenomegaly is still a particularly important sign of subacute infective endocarditis (7).

A. Cutaneous Manifestations

Cutaneous manifestations classically described for infective endocarditis are petechiae, subungual hemorrhages, Osler nodes, and Janeway lesions. Petechiae (most commonly involving the conjunctional or oral mucosa) are observed in 26% of patients (1). Subungual splinter hemorrhages are most often due to trauma, so they have less diagnostic value. Osler nodes are tender erythematous lesions on the palms and terminal phalanges of the hand or soles of the feet, whereas Janeway lesions are nontender, maculonodular hemorrhagic areas present on palms and soles (7).

B. Renal Manifestations

Renal involvement is relatively common in both the acute and subacute forms. Renal infarction due to embolic occlusions of renal artery occur in approximately 60% of patients with left-sided endocarditis; they are frequently sterile and silent, or sometimes may cause pain and hematuria, but usually do not result in renal failure (1,16). Septic infarctions with subsequent abscesses are rare. Both focal and diffuse glomerulonephritis are immunologically mediated by renal deposition of circulating immune complexes (16). Focal glomerulonephritis is more common and results in proteinuria and hematuria but rarely in renal failure (1a). Diffuse glomerulonephritis may result in significant renal failure. The incidence of diffuse glomerulonephritis is related to duration of the disease and is less common now than in the preantibiotic era. Renal insufficiency due to diffuse glomerulonephritis frequently reverses with appropriate therapy of the infection (1a). Differentiation between renal failure due to immune complex injury from drug therapy-related nephrotoxicity or interstitial nephritis may be very difficult and is an important clinical problem. Discontinuation of antibiotic therapy usually reverses the renal insufficiency that is related to drugs. If renal insufficiency persists after temporary discontinuation of antimicrobial therapy and the infection is not controlled, then it may be related to the infective endocarditis. It may be necessary to differentiate immune complex-mediated nephrotoxicity from injury due to antibiotics by renal biopsy.

C. Neurological Manifestations

Approximately one-third of patients with infective endocarditis develop neurological or psychiatric signs and symptoms as part of the initial presenting symptom complex or as a late complication of bacterial endocarditis (17,18). Stroke due to nonhemorrhagic or hemorrhagic infarct and toxic encephalopathy presenting as mental status disturbances with focal neurological deficits are common presenting symptoms (1a). Strokes manifesting as aphasia, ataxia, cortical sensory loss, hemiplegia, or homonymows hemianopsia may be due to emboli or rupture of a mycotic aneurysm. Embolic cerebral infarction is the most common neurological complication; it occurs in approximately 20% of patients with infective endocarditis (19). Meningitis, meningoencephalitis, brain abscess, mononeuritis, mycotic aneurysm, or intracerebral bleeds may sometimes be seen as neurological complications. In patients with meningitis, the cerebrospinal fluid is more often normal or "aseptic," with lymphocytic or mixed lymphocytic polymorphonuclear pleocytosis, and indicates infection with less virulent organisms such as viridans streptococci (17). Purulent fluid usually suggests endocarditis with virulent organisms, such as staphylococci or pneumococci. Suspicion of infective endocarditis should be raised in any patient of any age who presents with fever and/or murmur and neurological signs and symptoms (1a).

III. COMPLICATIONS OF INFECTIVE ENDOCARDITIS

A. Recurrent or Persistent Fever

When appropriate antibiotic therapy is initiated, there is usually a prompt decline in fever and an improvement in the symptomatic status. With sensitive organisms, this may occur in 24–48 hours; but with resistant organisms such as *Staph. aureus*, it may take several days to 2–3 weeks before the patient is afebrile (1a). The most common problem seen during the therapy of infective endocarditis is the persistence or recurrence of fever. Bacteriological failure is unlikely if the infecting organism is known to be sensitive and appropriate antibiotics are used; in this instance, it suggests the presence of a "loculated" infection, such as an abscess. If the infecting organism is known to have a fairly significant degree of antibiotic resistance, recurrence or persistence of fever indicates the need for valve replacement (1a). Other causes of persistent or recurrent fever have to be considered and excluded, including septic or sterile phlebitis, especially with use of indwelling catheters; metastatic abscesses, especially with staphylococcal endocarditis; recurrent embolization from vegetations; deep-vein thrombosis; and superimposed infections, particularly of the urinary and respiratory tracts. Drug fever is a common cause of recurrent fever, and this diagnosis should be considered especially when the infecting organism is known to be sensitive to the antibiotics administered. If fever persists, antibiotic therapy may be stopped temporarily after a careful reevaluation for other causes of fever. Drug fevers usually clear in 24–48 hours but may persist for 72–96 hours. If the fever clears and it was the sole manifestation of an adverse drug reaction and further antibiotic therapy is necessary, one can reinstitute the same antimicrobial therapy or alternative non-cross-reacting drugs to which the organism is sensitive. If the fever does not clear, antibiotic therapy should be restarted and other causes of the fever diligently sought for (1a).

B. Cardiac Vascular Complications

Infective endocarditis is a highly destructive process which may result in a number of potentially lethal cardiovascular complications (Table 3) (15).

Congestive heart failure is the most common serious cardiac complication of infective endocarditis; it is the major cause of mortality, accounting for approximately 60% of the deaths (1). Heart failure is almost always due to valve regurgitation. Valvular destruction by highly virulent organisms such as *Staph. aureus*, rupture of chordae tendinae, erosion of annulus by root abscesses, or perforation or prolapse of valve leaflets may

Table 3 Cardiovascular Complications of Infective Endocarditis

---

Congestive heart failure, usually due to valve destruction leading to valve regurgitation
Localized suppuration
  Perivalvular or myocardial abscesses
  Creation of left-to-right shunts (sinus of Valsalva rupture, ventricular septal defects, aortopulmonary fistula, ventriculoatrial fistula)
Emboli
  Systemic
  Coronary artery
Mycotic aneurysms
Conduction abnormalities; rhythm disturbances
Suppurative pericarditis
Myocarditis

Source: From Ref. 15, with the permission of Mosby Year Book Medical Publishers.

result in acute valvular or paravalvular regurgitation and congestive heart failure (20). Acute myocarditis or coronary embolization with myocardial infarction which may be silent may on occasion contribute to congestive heart failure. Chronic congestive heart failure may result from scarring of the valve or supporting structures, even when the infection has cleared. Aortic valve regurgitation is the most common cause of congestive heart failure; up to 80% of patients with aortic valve endocarditis and 50% of patients with mitral valve endocarditis develop congestive heart failure (21).

Valvular obstruction is occasionally seen with large vegetations, such as with fungal or rarely staphylococcal endocarditis, especially in mitral prosthetic valve endocarditis. Extension of the infectious process into the myocardium can lead to myocardial abscesses and is seen in 20% of patients with infective endocarditis at autopsy (1). Myocardial abscesses may be suspected when conduction abnormalities, arrhythmias, antibiotic failure, intracardiac fistula with left-to-right shunt, and congestive heart failure is seen. The most common causes of left-to-right shunt are rupture of an aneurysm of the sinus of Valsalva, septal perforation with the development of a ventricular septal defect, aortopulmonary fistula, or ventriculoatrial fistula.

New conduction abnormalities in the absence of other known causes occur, especially with aortic valve involvement, and should raise the possibility of myocardial abscesses. Temporary pacing is indicated if Mobitz II or a higher-grade heart block is present. Extension of the infectious process into the pericardial space may result in suppurative pericarditis. Pericarditis with pericardial effusions may also result from immunological reaction, congestive heart failure, or uremia. Pericardial effusions are seen with two-dimensional echocardiography in 54% of patients with infective endocarditis and are generally associated with a benign clinical course (22).

Mycotic aneurysms may develop in up to 15% of patients. They result most commonly from embolic occlusion of the vascular vasa vasorum but may also occur from intracranial involvement due to direct invasion of bacteria into the vessel wall or from deposition of immune complexes into arterial wall with subsequent arteritis (23). The most common sites of mycotic aneurysms are the brain, peripheral vessels, abdominal aorta, superior mesenteric, or splenic arteries. Although cerebral mycotic aneurysms are usually thought to be clinically silent, intracranial or subarachnoid hemorrhage is preceded by premonitory sudden severe headache or focal neurological deficits in up to 50% of cases (23). Cerebral angiography is indicated in patients presenting with sudden severe headache or focal neurological deficits, especially if valve replacement is indicated. The question of medical versus surgical management of asymptomatic mycotic aneurysms is controversial. Since rupture and hemorrhage can occur during or after therapy and are associated with high morbidity and mortality, elective surgery may be recommended if the aneurysm is recognized, is in a surgically accessible site, and can be corrected at low risk.

C. Emboli

Clinically recognized systemic embolic occur in one-third of cases of infective endocarditis, cerebral embolism being the most common (19). Clinical manifestations result from vascular occlusions; acute neurological symptoms including hemiplegia, aphasia, and sensory loss result from cerebrovascular involvement, hematuria from renal artery occlusions, acute abdominal pain from mesenteric or splenic artery emboli, chest pain from coronary or pulmonary emboli, or limb involvement from peripheral vascular emboli. Myocardial infarction due to coronary embolism is not common; it is usually seen in aortic valve endocarditis, is frequently not seen electrocardiographically, and occasionally may contribute to the development of congestive heart failure. The majority of systemic emboli (90%) occur before the initiation or within 48 hours of starting antibiotic therapy and in patients with uncontrolled infections (19). Systemic embolization may rarely occur up to months after successful antimicrobial therapy. Risk of embolization is higher in patients with left-sided endocarditis and large vegetations (>10 mm) (24–26). Presence of systemic emboli is a predictor of in-hospital mortality in patients with infective endocarditis (24). The incidence of systemic embolization is not related to the type of infecting organisms.

IV. DIAGNOSIS

The greatest difficulty in diagnosing infective endocarditis is not thinking of it; therefore, a high index of suspicion is needed (27). The most useful clinical findings are fever, cardiac murmur, or presence of preexisting cardiac disease that is known to be at risk for development of infective endocarditis and positive blood cultures. In this circumstance, the diagnostic difficulty arises in a patient with preexisting heart disease who has fever and another clinical condition that may be the cause of the positive blood cultures. With the exception of positive blood cultures, other laboratory findings are variable, and often of little definitive diagnostic value (Table 4).

A. Nonspecific Findings

Erythrocyte sedimentation rate is elevated in almost 90–100% patients who are not in congestive heart failure. Mild to moderate normocytic-

Table 4 Laboratory Manifestations of Endocarditis

Laboratory finding	Incidence (%)
Hematological	
Anemia	70–90
Thrombocytopenia	5–15
Leukocytosis[a]	20–30
Leukopenia	5–15
Histiocytosis	25
Elevated ESR	90–100
Serological	
Hypergammaglobulinemia	20–30
Rheumatoid factor	40–50
Hypocomplementemia	5–15
Immune complexes	90–100
Mixed cryoglobulins	80–95
Urine	
Proteinuria	50–65
Microscopic hematuria	30–50
RBC casts	10–12
Bacteremia	
Positive blood cultures	95
Intraleukocytic bacteria	50

[a] Primarily in acute endocarditis.
Source: From Ref. 11, with the permission of Little, Brown & Co.

normochromic anemia is common; its severity being related to the duration of the illness. Peripheral leukocyte counts are usually moderately elevated or may be normal, although marked leukocytosis may be seen in acute infections. Thrombocytopenia may be seen in patients with acute infections and occasionally in patients with splenomegaly. Rheumatoid factor is present in 40–50% of patients with subacute bacterial endocarditis. Microscopic hematuria and proteinuria are frequent, whereas red cell casts may be seen with glomerulonephritis (1a). Presence of *Strep. bovis* bacteremia should prompt workup for gastrointestinal malignancies. In the appropriate clinical circumstances, presence of circulating immune complexes and mixed cryoglobulins is a very helpful finding.

B. Blood Cultures

In endocarditis, bacteremia is persistent in the majority of cases and is usually not intermittent. Therefore, large numbers of blood cultures are not necessary, and their timing during the 24 hours is not critical (28). The majority of cases of infective endocarditis can be diagnosed by three paired blood cultures (six bottles: three vented, three unvented, drawn over a 2-h period); however, at least six paired blood cultures are necessary for testing before diagnosis of culture negative can be made. Blood cultures are usually positive in 85–95% of cases (1a,7). When acute endocarditis is suspected, three or four blood cultures taken from separate venipuncture sites at 15-min intervals are adequate for identifying more than 90–95% of patients with acute bacterial endocarditis before initiating empiric antibiotic therapy. When the presentation is subacute, six separate cultures over a 1- to 2-day period should be done before initiating therapy (1a).

If blood cultures remain negative after a few days and endocarditis is clinically suspected, the laboratory should be asked to hold blood cultures for at least 3 weeks, as some organisms grow very slowly (29). In approximately 10–20% of patients with infective endocarditis, blood cultures will be negative. The blood cultures are most likely to be negative in patients who have received previous antibiotic therapy, or if the causative agents require special culture techniques. In patients who are treated with antibiotics in the previous 2 weeks, the antibiotics should be discontinued if clinically possible; and blood should be done after 24–48 hours. The other important cause of culture-negative endocarditis is the presence of anerobic and nonbacterial infections such as fungal endocarditis. If the initial blood cultures are negative after a few days, the patients should have blood cultures repeated twice during a 7-day interval; and if the cultures remain negative, then a diagnosis of culture-negative endocarditis can be made; however, alternative diagnoses, such as collagen vascular disease, atrial myxoma, or marantic endocarditis should also be considered (7).

C. Echocardiography

Two-dimensional transthoracic echocardiography will reveal vegetations in approximately 70–80% of patients with endocarditis (30). The availability of transesophageal echocardiography has increased the sensitivity and specificity of detection of vegetations, especially in patients with prosthetic valve endocarditis (Figs. 1 and 2) (25,26,31,32) . Absence of vegetation is not useful in excluding infective endocarditis. Its presence in a patient with positive blood cultures who is clinically suspected of having endocarditis is of some prognostic value (7). Echocardiography is helpful in the diagnosis of endocarditis in patients with low clinical suspicion who have positive blood cultures or in patients with high clinical suspicion who have negative blood cultures (33).

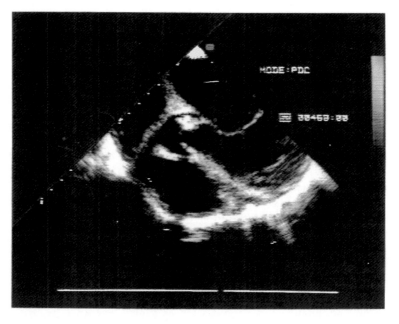

Figure 1 Transesophageal echocardiogram in a patient with St. Jude aortic prosthetic valve endocarditis. A large vegetation is seen on the aortic valve. Courtesy of P.A.N. Chandraratna, M.D.

Echocardiography is also very useful in the assessment of complications of endocarditis (34). Doppler echocardiography and color Doppler echocardiography is of value in the noninvasive assessment of the presence and severity of valvular regurgitation (35). Contrast echocardiography can be used to detect intracardiac shunts. Transesophageal echocardiography is superior to transthoracic echocardiography in the detection of many complications of infective endocarditis, such as paravalvular leak, aortic root abscesses, aneurysm of sinus of Valsalva, and assessment of patients with suspected prosthetic valve endocarditis (25,26,31,32). The presence of vegetations as well as their size has been reported to correlate with the development of future embolic events or progressive congestive heart failure (24,25,34). Tissue characterization of vegetations may be of help in differentiating new from old vegetations and thus in diagnosing recurrences of endocarditis (34a).

V. TREATMENT

A. General Guidelines

Bacteria within the vegetations are very high in density, have reduced rates of metabolism, and are surrounded by fibrin, so they are somewhat protected from normal host defences. Therefore, to achieve a bacteriological cure with sterilization of lesions, high doses of an appropriate intravenous bactericidal antibiotic usually needs to be administered for at least 4 weeks, and preferably for 6 weeks (35).

Urgency of initiation of antibiotic therapy on a presumptive diagnosis of infective endocarditis before blood cultures results are available depends on the clinical presentation: In patients in whom acute infective endocarditis is suspected, it is imperative to initiate appropriate antibiotic therapy promptly after obtaining four to six sets of blood cultures over a 1-h period. In some patients, a gram stain of the peripheral blood buffy coat smear, or the clinical settings, e.g., infected sternal wounds, intravenous catheters, intravenous drug abuse, may help to identify the causative organism. In patients with a nonspecific clinical picture with possible subacute infective endocarditis and very stable cardiac hemodynamic status with no hemodynamic impairment, it may be best to await blood culture results before initiating antibiotics; this may require 1–3 days.

The choice of antibiotics, their combination, dosage, and duration of therapy depends on the identification of the causative organism and the minimal inhibitory concentration (MIC) as well as minimal bactericidal concentration (MBC) of appropriate antibiotics against the infecting organism by tube dilution and standard disk susceptibility testings.

Assessment of adequacy of antibiotic therapy is usually not necessary in patients receiving high doses of intravenous penicillin for endocarditis with highly susceptible organisms such as viridans streptococci. However, in patients with endocarditis due to more resistant organisms, and those receiving combination therapy determination of serum bactericidal levels is very useful. Ideally, the patient's serum should achieve peak minimal bactericidal concentration (MBC) of at least 1:8 and preferably 1:16 or greater (1a).

B. Antibiotic Therapy for Specific Types of Endocarditis

In patients with normal renal function, Tables 5–10 summarize antibiotic therapy and dosages for most common forms of endocarditis in adult patients (37,38); these are the recommendations of the American Heart Association.

Most streptococci except enterococci and some viridians streptococci are very sensitive to penicillin alone. The dividing line between "sensitive" or susceptible and relatively resistant streptococci is an MIC level of 0.1 μg/mL; the sensitive streptococci have MIC ≤0.1 μg/mL. Addition of aminoglycoside to penicillin therapy results in synergistic bactericidal action; the combination of aminoglycoside with penicillin may be used for the first 2 weeks, followed by penicillin alone for 2 weeks, for the treatment of *Strep. viridans* endocarditis. The additional therapy for the first 2 weeks with aminoglycoside should be avoided in elderly patients, patients with renal insufficiency, and those with auditory or vestibular disorders (1a).

Enterococci require penicillin plus aminoglycocide for the full course of antibiotic therapy. The majority of enterococci are susceptible to gentamicin, and in-vitro synergism with penicillin for enterococci is always demonstrable as opposed to synergism with streptomycin, which is rare. It is preferable to use 4–6 weeks of combination therapy, and more than 3 months in patients with a complicated course.

Patients with suspected or proven *Staph. aureus* endocarditis should be treated with penicillinase-resistant semisynthetic penicillin prior to determination of susceptibilities. Nafcillin or oxacillin is preferred because of the high incidence of methicillin-induced interstitial nephritis. In patients with endocarditis due to "tolerant" strains of *Staph. aureus*, it may be reasonable to combine gentamicin therapy with penicillin. The 6-week course is recommended for patients with an initial delayed clinical response or complicated clinical course (1a). For methicillin-resistant *Staph. aureus* endocarditis, vancomycin is the drug of choice. As *Staph. aureus*

Table 5 Suggested Regimens for Therapy for Endocarditis Due to Penicillin-Susceptible *Viridans* Streptococci and *Streptococcus bovis* (Minimum Inhibitory Concentration, ≤0.1 μg/mL)[a]

Antibiotic	Adult dose and route[b]	Pediatric dose and route	Duration, wk
1. Aqueous crystalline penicillin G[c]	10–20 million U/24 h IV either continuously or in 6 equally divided doses	150,000–200,000 U/kg per 24 h IV (not to exceed 20 million U/24 h) either continuously or in 6 equally divided doses	4
2. Aqueous crystalline penicillin G[d]	10–20 million U/24 h IV either continuously or in 6 equally divided doses	150,000–200,000 U/kg per 24 h IV (not to exceed 20 million U/25 h) either continuously or in 6 equally divided doses	2
With streptomycin[e]	7.5 mg/kg IM (not to exceed 500 mg) every 12 h	15 mg/kg IM (not to exceed 500 mg) every 12 h	2
or with gentamicin[e]	1 mg/kg IM or IV (not to exceed 80 mg) every 8 h	2.0–2.5 mg/kg IV (not to exceed 80 mg) every 8 h	2
3. Aqueous crystalline penicillin G[d]	10–20 million U/24 h IV either continuously or in 6 equally divided doses	150,000–200,000 U/kg per 24 h IV (not to exceed 20 million U/24 h) either continuously or in 6 equally divided doses	4
With streptomycin[e]	7.5 mg/kg IM (not to exceed 500 mg) every 12 h	15 mg/kg IM (not to exceed 500 mg) every 12 h	2
or with gentamicin[e]	1 mg/kg IM or IV (not to exceed 80 mg) every 6 h	2.0 to 2.5 mg/kg IV (not to exceed 80 mg) every 8 h	2

[a] Therapy for penicillin-allergic patients; antibiotic doses for patients with impaired renal function should be modified appropriately.
[b] IV indicates intravenously and IM, intramuscularly.
[c] Preferred in most patients older than 65 years of age and in those with impairment of the eighth nerve or of renal function.
[d] Or procaine penicillin G, 1.2 million U IM every six hours. Procaine penicillin G is not recommended for treatment of endocarditis due to viridans streptococci in children.
[e] Should be given in addition to penicillin, II regimen 3 is selected, streptomycin or gentamicin should be given for the first two weeks. Peak steptomycin levels of approximately 20 μg/mL and peak gentamicin levels of approximately 3 μg/mL are desirable. Dosing of aminoglycosides on a milligrams per kilogram basis will produce higher serum concentrations in obese than in lean patients. Relative contraindications to use of aminoglycosides are age greater than 65 years or renal or eighth nerve impairment.
Source: From Ref. 38, with permission of the American Medical Association and the American Heart Association.

Table 6   Therapy for Endocarditis Due to Penicillin-Susceptible *Viridans* Streptococci and *Streptococcus bovis* (Minimum Inhibitory Concentration, ≤0.1 μg/mL) in Patients Allergic to Penicillin[a]

Antibiotic	Adult dose and route[b]	Pediatric dose and route	Duration, wk
1. Cephalothin[c,d]	2 g IV every 4 h	100–150 mg/kg per 24 h IV (not to exceed 12 g/24 h) in equally divided doses every 4 to 6 h	4
or Cefazolin[d]	1 g IM or IV every 8 h	80–100 mg/kg per 24 h IM or IV (not to exceed 3.0 g/24 h) in equally divided doses every 8 h	4
2. Vancomycin[e]	30 mg/kg per 24 h IV in 2 or 4 equally divided doses, not to exceed 2 g/24 h unless serum levels are monitored	40 mg/kg per 24 h IV in 2 or 4 equally divided doses, not to exceed 2 g/24 h unless serum levels are monitored	4

[a] Vancomycin dose should be reduced in patients with renal dysfunction; cephalosporin dose may need to be reduced in patients with moderate to severe renal dysfunction.
[b] IV indicates intravenously and IM, intramuscularly.
[c] Streptomycin or gentamicin may be added to cephalothin or cefazolin for first two weeks in doses recommended in Table 1.
[d] There is potential cross-allergenicity between pencillins and cephalosporins. Cephalosporins should be avoided in patients with immediate-type-hypersensitivity to penicillin.
[e] Peak serum concentrations of vancomycin should be obtained one hour after infusion and should be in the range of 30 to 45 μg/mL, for twice daily dosing and 20 to 35 μg/mL for four times daily dosing. Vancomycin or aminoglycosides given on a milligram per kilogram basis will produce higher serum concentrations in obese than in lean patients. Each dose of vancomycin should be infused over one hour.
Source: From Ref. 38, with permission of the American Medical Association and the American Heart Association.

is the most common organism in patients with acute infective endocarditis, an empiric antibiotic regimen of IV ampicillin, Nafcillin, and gentamicin is recommended as the initial treatment (1a). In patients who are allergic to penicillin, vancomycin and gentamicin is used.

Pneumomococcal, gonococcal, and meningococcal endocarditis should be treated with IV penicillin G for 4 weeks. Haemophilius endocarditis should be treated with ampicillin plus gentamicin for 6–8 weeks. Enteric gram-negative rods are relatively drug resistant and are difficult to treat;

Table 7   Therapy for Endocarditis Due to Strains of *Viridans* Streptococci and *Streptococcus bovis* Relatively Resistant to Penicillin G (Minimum Inhibitory Concentration, >0.1 μg/mL and <0.5 μg/mL)[a]

Antibiotic	Adult dose and route[b]	Pediatric dose and route	Duration, wk
Aqueous crystalline penicillin G	20 million U/24 h IV either continuously or in 6 equally divided doses	200,000 to 300,000 U/kg per 24 h IV (not to exceed 20 million U/24 h) given continuously or in 6 equally divided doses	4
With streptomycin[c]	7.5 mg/kg IM (not to exceed 500 mg) every 12 h	15 mg/kg IM (not to exceed 500 mg) every 12 h	2
or with gentamicin[c]	1 mg/kg IM or IV (not to exceed 80 mg) every 8 h	2.0 to 2.5 mg/kg IM or IV (not to exceed 80 mg) every 8 h	2

Cephalothin or cefazolin (with an aminoglycoside for the first two weeks) or vancomycin alone can be used in patients whose penicillin hypersensitivity is not of the immediate type. Vancomycin also can be used in patients with immediate penicillin allergy. Antibiotic doses should be modified appropriately for patients with impaired renal function.
IV indicates intravenously and IM, intramuscularly.
Streptomycin or gentamicin should be given in addition to penicillin for the first two weeks. Peak streptomycin levels of approximately 20 μg/mL and peak gentamicin levels of about 3 μg/mL are desirable. For the rare viridans streptococcus with minimum inhibitory concentration greater than or equal to 0.5 μg/mL of penicillin G, aminoglycoside therapy should be continued for four weeks with appropriate monitoring of serum levels of streptomycin or gentamicin. Aminoglycosides given on a milligram per kilogram basis will produce higher serum concentrations in obese than in lean patients.
Source: From Ref. 38, with permission of the American Medical Association and the American Heart Association.

Table 8   Therapy for Endocarditis Due to Enterococci (or to *Viridans* Streptococci with a Minimum Inhibitory Concentration, ≥0.5 μg/mL)[a]

Antibiotic	Adult dose and route[b]	Pediatric dose and route	Duration, wk
	Regimen for Non-Pencillin-Allergic Patients		
1. Aqueous crystalline penicillin G	20 to 30 million U/24 h IV given continuously or in 6 equally divided doses	200,000 to 300,000 U/kg per 24 h IV (not to exceed 30 million U/24 h) given continuously or in 6 equally divided doses	4–6

Table 8 (*Continued*)

Antibiotic	Adult dose and route[b]	Pediatric dose and route	Duration, wk
With gentamicin[c,d,e]	1 mg/kg IM or IV (not to exceed 80 mg) every 8 h	2.0 to 2.5 mg/kg IM or IV (not to exceed 80 mg) every 6 h	4–6
or with streptomycin[c,d,e]	7.5 mg/kg IM (not to exceed 500 mg) every 12 h	15 mg/kg IM (not to exceed 500 mg) every 12 h	4–5
2. Ampicillin	12 g/24 h IV given continuously or in 6 equally divided doses	300 mg/kg per 24 hr IV (not to exceed 12 g/24 h) in 4 to 6 equally divided doses	4–6
With gentamicin[c,d,e]	1 mg/kg IM or IV (not to exceed 80 mg) every 8 h	2.0 to 2.5 mg/kg IM or IV (not to exceed 80 mg) every 8 h	4–6
or with streptomycin[c,e,f]	7.5 mg/kg IM (not to exceed 500 mg) every 12 h	15 mg/kg IM (not to exceed 500 mg) every 12 h	4–6
Regimen for Penicillin-Allergic Patients (Desensitization Should Be Considered; Cephalosporins Are Not Satisfactory Alternatives)			
Vancomycin[g]	30 mg/kg per 24 h IV in 2 or 4 equally divided doses, not to exceed 2 g/24 h unless serum levels are monitored	40 mg/kg per 24 h IV in 2 or 4 equally divided doses, not to exceed 2 g/24 h unless serum levels are monitored	4–6
With gentamicin[c,d,e]	1 mg/kg IM or IV (not to exceed 80 mg) every 8 h	2.0 to 2.5 mg/kg IM or IV (not to exceed 80 mg) every 8 h	4–6
or with streptomycin[c,e,f]	7.5 mg/kg IM (not to exceed 500 mg) every 12 h	15 mg/kg IM (not to exceed 500 mg) every 12 h	4–6

[a] Antibiotic doses should be modified appropriately in patients with impaired renal function.

[b] IV indicates intravenously and IM, intramuscularly.

[c] Choice of aminoglycoside depends on resistance level of infecting strain (see text). Enterococci should be tested for high-level resistance (minimum inhibitory conentration, $\geq$ 2000 μg/mL).

[d] Serum concentration of gentamicin should be monitored and dose adjusted to obtain a peak level of approximately 3 μg/mL.

[e] Dosing of aminoglycosides and vancomycin on a milligram per kilogram basis will give higher serum concentrations in obese than in lean patients.

[f] Serum concentration of streptomycin should be monitored if possible and dose adjusted to obtain a peak level of approximately 20 μg/mL.

[g] Peak serum concentrations of vancomycin should be obtained one hour after infusion and should be in the range of 30 to 45 μg/mL for twice daily dosing and 20 to 35 μg/mL for four times daily dosing. Each dose should be infused over one hour.

Source: From Ref. 38, with permission of the American Medical Association and the Heart Association.

Table 9 Therapy for Endocarditis Due to *Staphylococcus* in the Absence of Prosthetic Material[a]

Antibiotic	Adult dose and route[b]	Pediatric dose and route	Duration
Methicillin-Susceptible Staphylococci			
Regimen for non-penicillin-allergic patients			
Nafcillin	2 g IV every 4 h	150–200 mg/kg per 24 h IV (not to exceed 12 g/24 h) in 4 to 6 equally divided doses	4–6 wk
or oxacillin	2 g IV every 4 h	150–200 mg/kg per 24 h IV (not to exceed 12 g/24 h) in 4 to 6 equally divided doses	4–6 wk
With optional addition of gentamicin[c,d]	1 mg/kg IM or IV (not to exceed 80 mg) every 8 h	2.0–2.5 mg/kg IV (not to exceed 80 mg) every 8 h	3–5 d
Regimen for penicillin-allergic patients			
1. Cephalothin[e]	2 g IV every 4 h	100–150 mg/kg per 24 h IV (not to exceed 12 g/24 h) in equally divided doses every 4 to 6 h	4–6 wk
or Cefazolin	2 g IV every 8 h	80–100 mg/kg per 24 h IV (not to exceed 6 g/24 h) in equally divided doses every 8 h	4–6 wk
With optional addition of gentamicin[c]	Same as for non-penicillin-allergic patient	Same as for non-penicillin-allergic patient	

therefore, therapy is usually selected according to the most active agents determined by tube dilution susceptibility tests. *Pseudomonas* endocarditis is usually seen in drug addicts and is treated with ticarcillin plus an aminoglycoside for 6 weeks. Treatment with piperacillin results is rapid development of resistance to the drug (1a). For anerobic infections except *B. fragilis* endocarditis, penicillin is the drug of choice. For *B. fragilis*

Table 9 (*Continued*)

Antibiotic	Adult dose and route[b]	Pediatric dose and route	Duration
2. Vancomycin[f]	30 mg/kg per 24 h IV in 2 or 4 equally divided doses, not to exceed 2 g/24 h unless serum levels are monitored	40 mg/kg per 24 h IV in 2 or 4 equally divided doses, not to exceed 2 g/24 h unless serum levels are monitored	4–6 wk
	Methicillin-Resistent Staphylococci		
Vancomycin[c,d]	30 mg/kg per 24 h IV in 2 or 4 equally divided doses, not to exceed 2 g/24 h unless serum levels are monitored	40 mg/kg per 24 h IV in 2 or 4 equally divided doses, not to exceed 2 g/24 h unless serum levels are monitored	4–6 wk

[a] Antibiotic doses should be modified appropriately for patients with impaired renal function. For treatment of endocarditis due to penicillin-susceptible staphylococci (minimum inhibitory concentration, ≤0.1 μg/mL), aqueous crystalline penicillin G (Table 1, first regimen) should be used for four to six weeks instead of nalcillin or oxacillin. Shorter antibiotic courses have been effective in some drug addicts with right-sided endocarditis due to *Staphylococcus aureus*. See text for comments on use of rifampin.

[b] IV indicates intravenously and IM, intramuscularly.

[c] Dosing of aminoglycosides and vancomycin on a milligram per kilogram basis will give higher serum concentrations in obese than in lean patients.

[d] Benefit of additional aminoglycoside has not been established. Risk of toxic reactions due to these agents is increased in patients who are older than age 65 years or who have renal or eighth nerve impairment.

[e] There is potential cross-allergenicity between penicillins and cephalosporins. Cephalosporins should be avoided in patients with immediate-type hypersensitivity to penicillin.

[f] Peak serum concentration of vancomycin should be obtained one hour after infusion and should be in the range of 30 to 45 μg/mL for twice daily and 20 to 35 μg/mL for four times daily dosing. Each dose of vancomycin should be infused over one hour. See text for consideration of optional addition of gentamicin.

Source: From Ref. 38, with permission of the American Medical Association and the American Heart Association.

endocarditis, metronidazole is superior to clindamycin or chloramphenicol, as both of them are primarily bacteriostatic.

In patients with high clinical suspicion of endocarditis with negative blood cultures, a combination of penicillin plus an aminoglycoside is used initially. If the patient becomes afebrile within a week of initiation of therapy, then this combination is continued for 4–6 weeks. If response to therapy is poor and the clinical diagnosis of endocarditis is highly sus-

Table 10 Treatment of Staphylococcal Endocarditis in the Presence of a Prosthetic Valve or Other Prosthetic Material[a]

Antibiotic	Adult dose and route[b]	Pediatric dose and route	Duration wk
Regimen for Methicillin-Resistant Staphylococci			
Vancomycin[c,d]	30 mg/kg per 24 h IV in 2 or 4 equally divided doses, not to exceed 2 g/24 h unless serum levels are monitored	40 mg/kg per 24 h IV in 2 or 4 equally divided doses, not to exceed 2 g/24 h unless serum levels are monitored	4
With rifampin[e]	300 mg PO every 8 h	20 mg/kg per 24 h PO (not to exceed 900 mg/24 h) in 2 equally divided doses	
and with gentamicin[d,f,g]	1.0 mg/kg IM or IV (not to exceed 80 mg) every 8 h	2.01–2.5 mg/kg per 24 h IV (not to exceed 80 mg) every 8 h	
Regiman for Methicillin-Susceptible Staphylococci			
Nalcillin or oxacillin[b]	2 g IV every 4 h	150–200 mg/kg per 24 h IV (not to exceed 12 g/24 h) in 4 to 5 equally divided doses	
With rifampin[e]	300 mg PO every 8 h	20 mg/kg per 24 h PO (not to exceed 900 mg/24 h) in 2 equally divided doses	6
and with gentamicin[d,g]	1.0 mg/kg IM or IV (not to exceed 80 mg) every 8 h	2.0–2.5 mg/kg IV (not to exceed 80 mg) every 8 h	

[a] Vancomycin and gentamicin doses must be modified appropriately in patients with renal failure.

[b] IV indicates intravenously; PO, orally; and IM, intramuscularly.

[c] Peak serum concentrations of vancomycin should be obtained one hour after infusion and should be in the range of 30 to 45 μg/mL for twice daily dosing and 20 to 35 μg/mL for four times daily dosing. Each dose should be infused over one hour.

[d] Aminoglycosides or vancomycin given on a milligram per kilogram basis will produce higher serum concentrations in obese than in lean patients.

[e] Rifampin is recommended for therapy of infection due to coagulase-negative staphylococci. Its use in coagulase-positive staphylocooccal intects is controversial. 6 Rifampin increases the amount of warfarin sodium required for antihrombolic therapy.

[f] Serum concentration of gentamicin should be moritored and dose should be adjusted to obtain a peak level of approximately 3 μg/mL.

[g] Use during initial two weeks. See text on alternative aminoglycoside therapy for organisms resistant to gentamicin.

[h] First-generation cephalosporins or vancomycin should be used in penicillin-allergic patients. Cephalosporins should be avoided in patients with immediate-type hypersensitivity to penicillin and in patients infected with methicillin-resistant staphylococci.

Source: From Ref. 38, with permission of the American Medical Association and the American Heart Association.

pected, other combination(s) of antibiotics may be considered before surgery is recommended.

Fungal endocarditis requires a combined chemotherapeutic and surgical therapy, as complete bacteriological cure is highly unlikely with bulky
vegetations, especially in prosthetic valve endocarditis. Amphotericin-B
is the most potent bactericidal agent available, but it has a high incidence
of renal and bone marrow toxicity. Potentiation of Amphotericin-B activity against *Candida* species may be achieved by addition of oral fungistatic
drugs, 5-Flucytosine, or rifampin. The best therapy for fungal endocarditis
is early surgical intervention and prolonged postoperative amphotericin-
B therapy.

C. Patients with Allergy to Antibiotics

In patients with possible penicillin allergy, it is preferable to skin-test for
penicillin allergy and to give penicillin G if the results are negative. If the
patient has a history of severe allergic reactions to penicillin and/or if the
skin tests are positive with penicillin but negative for cephalosporins, a
first-generation cephalosporin can be used. Still, the initial doses should
be given very cautiously, under a physician's close observation. If skin
tests for cephalosporins are also positive or if one is awaiting skin tests
to be performed, vancomycin, is the treatment of choice. Because of the
high incidence of resistance, cephalosporins are not useful alternative
drugs in the treatment of enterococcal endocarditis (1a). The second- and
third-generation cephalosporins offer no advantage over first-generation
cephalosporins.

D. Anticoagulation

Patients with systemic emboli and native or bioprosthetic valve endocarditis in normal sinus rhythm do not require anticoagulation therapy. The
indications for anticoagulation therapy in this situation are based on comorbid factors, such as atrial fibrillation or evidence of left atrial thrombus
(39). However, anticoagulation therapy should be continued in patients
with mechanical prosthetic valve endocarditis unless there are specific
contraindications.

E. Surgical Therapy

The indications for surgery and valve replacement in infective endocarditis are summarized in Table 11 (40–42).

The mortality in infective endocarditis is high; and in 80% of them, the
cause of death is congestive heart failure which is usually secondary to

Table 11 Indications for Surgery in the Treatment of Infective Endocarditis

Congestive heart failure
Infections
    Uncontrolled by antibiotic therapy
    Fungal, usually with staphylococcal infections, aortic and mitral valves, and
        gram-negative bacillary infections
Recurrent systemic emboli
New heart block or conduction defects
Other
    Suppurative pericarditis
    Mycotic aneurysm of sinus of valsalva
    Rupture of sinus or valsalva, rupture of ventricular or atrial septa, or others
        (e.g., development of arteriovenous and ventriculoatrial shunts)
    "Very large" mobile vegetations

Source: From Ref. 15, with the permission of Mosby Year Book Medical Publishers.

valvular regurgitation. Early recognition, and prompt medical as well as surgical therapy has dramatically reduced mortality in patients with infective endocarditis (43,44). Medical therapy guided by hemodynamic monitoring should be promptly initiated and consists of digoxin, diuretics, and veno- as well as arterial vasodilators. In mild congestive heart failure controlled well with medical therapy, antibiotics should be continued for 4–6 weeks, with reassessment for the need for surgical intervention at the end of antibiotic therapy. In moderate congestive heart failure, especially if the heart failure is not easily controlled by medical therapy, urgent valve replacement is recommended. In severe heart failure, urgent valve replacement is usually needed. Valve replacement, by alleviating the hemodynamic burden of valvular regurgitation, has been shown to reduce the mortality from 66% to 15% in patients with infective endocarditis with moderate to severe congestive heart failure (40).

Incidence of antibiotic failure in patients with native valve endocarditis is about 7% (45). Antibiotic failure usually occurs when (1) the organisms are highly virulent, such as with gram-negative organisms or *Staph. aureus*; and (2) the organisms are inaccessible to antibiotics and natural defense mechanisms, which is seen in patients with large vegetations, fungal infections, and local extension of infectious process into surrounding tissues, for example, with development of myocardial abscesses, mycotic aneurysms, or purulent pericarditis. Antibiotic failure is suspected when the patient remains symptomatic and the blood cultures remain positive after 72–96 hours of appropriate optimal antimicrobial therapy. Persistent fever and positive blood cultures may result from infection elsewhere in the body; therefore, noncardiac sources of persistent infection must be investigated before considering valve replacement.

Presence of myocardial abscess(es) is suggested by the development of new conduction abnormalities or arrhythmias in the absence of other identifiable causes; if confirmed or very strongly suspected, then surgical intervention should be considered.

Rupture of myocardial abscesses or mycotic aneurysms in the sinus of Valsalva, interatrial, and/or interventricular septa may result in development of acute intracardiac shunts and congestive heart failure and usually is an indication for surgery. Suppurative pericarditis is relatively uncommon but usually requires surgical therapy.

Staph. aureus endocarditis is a highly destructive process and is associated with high mortality, ranging from 45% to 73% with medical therapy alone (40). Therefore, early urgent valve replacement is indicated in patients with *Staph. aureus* endocarditis of the aortic or mitral valves who fail to respond to aggressive medical therapy. Tricuspid or pulmonic valve *Staph. aureus* endocarditis usually responds well to aggressive medical treatment alone (46); however, therapeutic failures due to drug resistance, progressive hemodynamic deterioration, or embolization may require valvectomy or valvuloplasty with debridement of the infected tissue, followed, if necessary, by valve replacement (40,46).

Fungal endocarditis is associated with morality rates of 80–100% with medical therapy alone; therefore, early valve replacement and prolonged postoperative amphotericin-B therapy is indicated in almost all cases (47). Gram-negative endocarditis is frequently resistant to antimicrobial therapy; therefore, surgical therapy is frequently indicated. Culture-negative endocarditis that does not respond well to antibiotic therapy is also an indication for surgical intervention.

Most of the systemic embolic in patients with infective endocarditis occur on initial clinical presentation or shortly thereafter, that is, before the infection is controlled (19). The risk of recurrent embolism is low when the infection is controlled. Recurrent systemic emboli despite optimal antibiotic therapy usually indicates failure of control of infection. There is evidence that echocardiographic visualization of vegetations is associated with higher risk for major complications, such as heart failure, death, and embolism, and also a need for surgery (24–26,34). Although this is statistically the case, not all patients with vegetations have these complications, and vegetations have not been shown to be an important independent predictor of the need for surgery. Furthermore, it is not clear whether large (>10 mm) as opposed to small (<10 mm) vegetations and left-sided vegetations indicate an additional risk for any of these complications. Therefore, a reasonable guideline is that, in the absence of other indications of surgery (for example, heart failure, uncontrolled infection, recurrent emboli, fungal infection, intramyocardial abscess), the presence of large vegetations alone, or early emboli before control of infection per se, do not appear to clinically warrant valve replacement. However, if systemic emboli recurs despite 48–72 hours of appropriate optimal antibiotic therapy, especially in association with echocardiographic evidence of large vegetations, surgical intervention should be considered. Prior to recommending surgical treatment for recurrent systemic emboli, one should determine the nature of emboli, as comorbid factors such as atrial fibrillation or the presence of left atrial thrombus also increase the incidence of nonseptic emboli in patients with infective endocarditis. As opposed to left-sided endocarditis, recurrent pulmonary embolization from right-sided endocarditis alone is not necessarily an indication for surgery.

Infective endocarditis in intravenous drug abusers is a special surgical problem because of complicating issues of possible persistent drug abuse and recurrent infection after valve replacement. However, therapeutic failures due to drug resistance, progressive hemodynamic deterioration, or recurrent pulmonary emboli leading to the possibility of respiratory insufficiency due to tricuspid valve infection indicate a need for surgery (46).

Prosthetic valve endocarditis requires special urgent consideration. Early surgical intervention in prosthetic valve endocarditis has reduced the mortality rate from 61% with medical therapy alone to 38% overall (40). The indications for surgery include: (1) heart failure due to prosthetic valve dysfunction; (2) other indications as for native valve endocarditis (Table 11); (3) unstable prosthesis on fluoroscopy, indicative of significant valve dehiscence; (4) extension of the infection beyond the valve annulus; (5) valve obstruction; (6) persistent infection, e.g., positive blood cultures after several days of antibiotic therapy; (7) early prosthetic valve endocarditis with or without evidence of valve dysfunction or failure; and (8) relapse of infection (40,48,49). Relapse of infection is a relative indication for surgery; one can attempt another course of antibiotic therapy depending on the clinical condition and antibiotic sensitivity of the organism. More than one relapse indicates a need for valve re-replacement. If the patient is not a surgical candidate, a prolonged course of parenteral antibiotics followed by long-term oral suppressive therapy may be advisable.

Timing of valve replacement in both native and prosthetic valve endocarditis should be dictated by the hemodynamic state and other clinical aspects of the patient and not by the duration of antibiotic therapy. Contrary to earlier concerns of performing valve implantation during active infective endocarditis, the risk of early reinfection of the prosthetic valve implanted during uncontrolled active infection is low (6%) (50,51). Other serious potential postoperative complications after valve re-replacement in infective endocarditis are valve dehiscence and instability of the valve prosthesis with paravalvular leak. Use of homograft valves has reduced the risk of early postoperative prosthetic valve infection.

VI. ANTIBIOTIC PROPHYLAXIS

The substantial morbidity and mortality in patients who develop infective endocarditis emphasize the importance of chemoprophylaxis in patients with increased susceptibility to the development of infective endocarditis. The recommendations of the American Heart Association for the cardiac conditions more commonly associated with endocarditis and the dental and surgical procedures that are more likely to cause endocarditis are listed in Tables 12 and 13 (52).

Antibiotic prophylaxis should be directed against the most common organisms causing bacteremia and endocarditis from these procedures. Standard recommendations outlined by the American Heart Association for prophylactic antibiotics and their dosages are shown in Tables 14, 15, and 16 (52).

Table 12   Cardiac Conditions[a]

Endocarditis prophylaxis recommended
Prosthetic cardiac valves, including bioprosthetic and homograft valves
Previous bacterial endocarditis, even in the absence of heart disease
Most congenital cardiac malformations
Rheumatic and other acquired valvular dysfunction surgery
Hypertrophic cardiomyopathy
Mitral valve prolapse with valvular regurgitation
Endocarditis prophylaxis not recommended
Isolated secundum atrial septal defect
Surgical repair without residua beyond 6 mo of secundum atrial septal defect,
    ventricular septal defect, or patent ductus arteriosus
Previous coronary artery bypass graft surgery
Mitral valve prolapse without valvular regurgitation[b]
Physiologic, functional, or innocent heart murmurs
Previous Kawasaki disease without valvular dysfunction
Previous rheumatic fever without valvular dysfunction
Cardiac pacemakers and implanted defibrillators

---

[a] This table lists selected conditions but is not meant to be all-inclusive.
[b] Individuals who have a mitral valve prolapse associated with thickening and/or redundancy of the valve leaflets may be at increased risk for bacterial endocarditis, particularly men who are 45 years of age or older.
Source: From Dajani AS et al, JAMA 264:2919, 1990, with permission of the American Medical Association and the American Heart Association,

Table 13   Dental or Surgical Procedures[a]

Endocarditis prophylaxis recommended
Dental procedures known to induce gingival or mucosal bleeding, including professional cleaning
Tonsillectomy and/or adenoidectomy
Surgical operations that involve intestinal or respiratory mucosa
Bronchoscopy with a rigid bronchoscope
Sclerotherapy for esophageal varices
Esophageal dilatation
Gallbladder surgery
Cystoscopy
Urethral dilatation
Urethral catheterization if urinary tract infection is present
Urinary tract surgery if urinary tract infection is present[b]
Prostatic surgery
Incision and drainage of infected tissue[b]
Vaginal hysterectomy
Vaginal delivery in the presence of infection[b]
Endocarditis prophylaxis not recommended[c]
Dental procedures not likely to induce gingival bleeding, such as simple adjustment of orthodontic appliances or fillings above the gum line
Injection of local intraoral anesthetic (except intraligamentary injections)
Shedding of primary teeth
Tympanostomy tube insertion
Endotracheal intubation
Bronchoscopy with a flexible bronchoscope, with or without biopsy
Cardiac catheterization
Endoscopy with or without gastrointestinal biopsy
Casarean section
In the absence of infection for urethral catheterization, dilatation and curettage, uncomplicated vaginal delivery, therapeutic abortion, sterilization procedures, or insertion or removal of intrauterine devices

---

[a] This table lists selected procedures but is not meant to be all-inclusive.
[b] In addition to prophylactic regimen for genitourinary procedures, antibiotic therapy should be directed against the most likely bacterial pathogen.
[c] In patients who have prosthetic heart valves, a previous history of endocarditis, or surgically constructed systemic-pulmonary shunts or conduits, physicians may choose to administer prophylactic antibiotics even for low-risk procedures that involve the lower respiratory, genitourinary, or gastrointestinal tracts.
Source: From Dajani AS et al, JAMA 264:2919, 1990, with permission of the American Medical Association and the American Heart Association.

Table 14 Recommended Standard Prophylactic Regimen for Dental, Oral, or Upper Respiratory Tract Procedures in Patients Who Are at Risk[a]

Drug	Dosing regiment
	Standard Regimen
Amoxicillin	3.0 orally 1 h before procedure: then 1.6 g 6 h after initial dose
	Amoxicillin/penicillin-allergic patients
Erythromycin or	Erythromycin ethylsuccinate, 800 mg, or erythromycin stearate, 1.0 g orally 2 h before procedure; then half the dose 6 h after initial dose
Cindamycin	300 mg orally 1 h before procedure and 150 mg 6 h after initial dose

[a] Includes those with prosthetic heart valves and other high-risk patients.

[b] Initial pediatric doses are as follows: amoxicillin, 50 mg/kg; erythromycin ethylsuccinate or erythromycin stearate, 20 mg/kg; and cindamycin, 10 mg/kg. Follow-up doses should be one half the initial dose. Total pediatric dose should not exceed total adult dose. The following weight ranges may also be used for the initial pediatric dose of amoxicillin: <15 kg, 750 mg; 15 to 30 kg, 1500 mg; and >30 kg, 3000 mg (full adult dose).

Source: From Dajani AS et al, JAMA 264:2919, 1990, with permission of the American Medical Association and the American Heart Association.

VII. SPECIAL CLINICAL CIRCUMSTANCES

A. Infective Endocarditis in Intravenous Drug Abusers

At many medical centers, infective endocarditis due to intravenous drug abuse has become one of the most common forms of endocarditis. Symptoms are usually acute, and fever is almost always observed. It frequently develops on previously normal cardiac valves. *Staph. aureus* is the responsible organism in 50% of cases (46). Streptococci, including enterococci, account for 20%, gram-negative bacilli, including *Pseudomonas*, 15–20%, and fungi, mainly the *Candida* species, about 10% of cases (1a,42).

The incidence of tricuspid valve involvement with and without left-heart involvement is approximately 50%. Its clinical manifestations include abrupt onset of fever, chills, rigors, and pulmonary symptoms including dyspnea, cough, pleuritic chest pain, and occasionally hemoptysis. With isolated tricuspid involvement, there is usually absence of neurological and other peripheral signs of endocarditis, and a murmur of tricuspid insufficiency is present in only one-third of patients at the time of initial presentations. Chest X-ray findings of multiple septic emboli are present in up to 70% of patients at initial presentation (53).

Table 15 Alternate Prophylactic Regimens for Dental, Oral, or Upper
Respiratory Tract Procedures in Patients Who Are at Risk

Drug	Dosing regimen[a]
Patients unable to take oral medications	
Ampicillin	Intravenous or intramuscular administration of ampicillin, 2.0 g, 30 min before procedure; then intravenous or intramuscular administration of ampicillin, 1.0 g, or oral administration of amoxicillin, 1.5 g, 6 h after initial dose
Ampicillin/amoxicillin/penicillin-allergic patients unable to take oral medications	
Cindamycin	Intravenous administration of 300 mg 30 min before procedure and an intravenous or oral administration of 150 mg 6 h after initial dose
Patients considered high risk and not candidates for standard regimen	
Ampicillin, gentamicin, and amoxicillin	Intravenous or intramuscular administration of ampicillin, 2.0 g, plus gentamicin, 1.5 mg/kg (not to exceed 80 mg), 30 min before procedure; followed by amoxicillin, 1.5 g, orally 6 h after initial dose; alternatively, the parenteral regimen may be repeated 6 h after initial dose
Ampicillin/amoxicillin/penicillin-allergic patients considered high risk	
Vancomycin	Intravenous administration of 1.0 g over 1 h, starting 1 h before procedure; no repeated dose necessary

[a] Initial pediatric doses are as follows: ampicillin, 50 mg/kg; clindamycin, 10 mg/kg; gentamicin, 2.0 mg/kg; and vancomycin, 20 mg/kg. Follow-up doses should be one half the initial dose. Total pediatric dose should not exceed total adult dose. No initial dose is recommended in this table for amoxicillin (25 mg/kg is the follow-up dose).
Source: From Danjani AS et al, JAMA 264:2919, 1990, with permission of the American Medical Association and the American Heart Association.

Left-sided endocarditis alone occurs in 48% of patients and tricuspid valve involvement alone in 42–47% of patients with endocarditis associated with IV drug abuse (46). The remaining 5–10% of patients have both left-heart and tricuspid valve involvement. Aortic valve alone is involved in 23% of cases, and mitral valve alone in 10%. With left-sided endocarditis, the clinical symptomatology is similar to that in nonaddicts (53).

The antimicrobial therapy of endocarditis in intravenous drug abusers follow the same principles as in nonaddict patients, and the indications for surgery for left-sided endocarditis are also similar to non-addict pa-

Table 16   Regimens for Genitourianry/Gastrointestinal Procedures

Drug	Dosage regimen[a]
	Standard regimen
Ampicillin, gentamicin, and amoxicillin	Intravenous or intramuscular administration of ampicillin 2.0 g, plus gentamicin, 1.5 mg/kg (not to exceed 80 mg), 30 min before procedure; followed by amoxicillin, 1.5 g orally 6 h after initial dose; alternatively, the parenteral regimen may be repeated once 8 h after initial dose
	Ampicillin/amoxicillin/penicillin-allergic patient regimen
Vancomycin and gentamicin	Intravenous administration of vancomycin, 1.0 g over 1 h plus intravenous or intramuscular administration of gentamicin, 1.5 mg/kg (not to exceed 80 mg), 1 h before procedure; may be repeated once 8 h after initial dose
	Alternate low-risk patient regimen
Amoxicillin	3.0 g orally 1 h before procedure; then 1.5 g 6 h after initial dose

[a] Initial pediatric doses are as follows: ampicillin, 50 mg/kg; amoxicillin, 50 mg/kg; gentamicin, 2.0 mg/kg; and vancomycin, 20 mg/kg. Follow-up doses should be half the initial dose. Total pediatric dose should not exceed total adult dose.
Source: From Dajani AS et al, JAMA 264:2919, 1990, with permission of the American Medical Association and the American Heart Association.

tients. For isolated tricuspid valve endocarditis with resistant organisms or recurrent pulmonary emboli with respiratory insufficiency, valvectomy without valve replacement is indicated and well tolerated in the absence of high right ventricular pressures. Valve replacement may be indicated at later date if significant right heart failure develops.

B. Prosthetic Valve Endocarditis

The incidence of prosthetic valve endocarditis (PVE) in recent years is approximately 3% in the first postoperative year and 0.5% per year thereafter. Endocarditis occurs in equal frequency in both bioprosthetic and mechanical valves. PVE is divided into early- and late-onset types, early PVE occurring within 2 months after surgery. More recently, it has been suggested that early PVE should include infections occurring in the first postoperative year. The infection in early PVE is presumed to have been acquired at the time of surgery or early postoperative period (48), potential sources of infections being intraopertive contamination of the heart-lung machine, intravenous and urinary catheters, blood transfusions, or bacterial seeding from postoperative infections such as pneumonia, sternal wound infections, urinary tract infections. In most cases, a definite source of infection is usually not identified (1a). Mortality is higher in early PVE than late PVE.

Staph. epidermidis and *Staph. aureus* account for almost 50% of the cases of prosthetic valve endocarditis (11). The incidence of culture-negative endocarditis may be higher in PVE (10). In early PVE, the most common organism is *S. epidermidis*, and resistant organisms such as gram-negative rods, diphtheroids, fungi, and *Staph. aureus* are more common than in late PVE. Microbiology of late PVE is similar to native valve endocarditis; streptococcal viridans being the most common organism, except that *Staph. epidermidis* is common, accounting for more than 20% of the infections. In contrast to native valve endocarditis, the aortic valve is more commonly involved than the mitral valve in PVE, and infection frequently extends into adjacent tissues, causing ring abscesses, paravalvular leak, and congestive heart failure. With bioprosthetic valves, especially in the mitral position, stenosis and obstruction by the vegetative material is more frequent than with mechanical valves.

An unexplained persistent fever, refractory heart failure or new regurgitant murmurs may serve as important clues to the diagnosis of PVE (48). The diagnosis of infective endocarditis in patients with sustained bacteremia without cardiac or peripheral manifestations of endocarditis may be difficult, especially in the early postoperative period. However, in the absence of an apparent extracardiac source of bacteremia, patients should be treated for endocarditis.

Transesophageal echocardiography is more sensitive and specific than transthoracic echocardiography especially in mitral position, in detecting vegetations, transvalvular or paravalvular regurgitation, and ring abscesses or aneurysms in prosthetic valve endocarditis (Figs. 1 and 2). Both transthoracic and transesophageal echocardiography should be used in patients with suspected prosthetic valve endocarditis (25,26,31,32).

Initial therapy with vancomycin and gentamicin should be started in patients with suspected PVE while blood culture results are pending (Table 10). Amikacin may be substituted for gentamicin in hospitals with a high prevalence of gentamicin resistance. Every effort should be made to achieve maximum bactericidal levels. Treatment is readjusted after blood culture and sensitivity results are known, and therapy is continued for 6 weeks for sensitive organisms and for 8 weeks for more resistant organisms. In order to monitor response to therapy, blood cultures should be done every other day early in the course of treatment, at least weekly

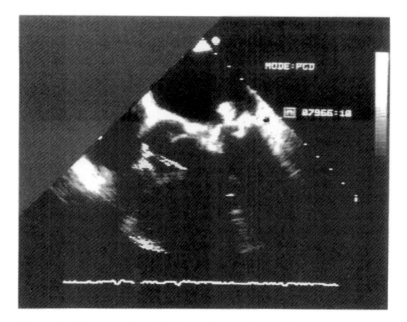

Figure 2 Transesophageal echocardiogram in a patient with mitral bioprosthesis showing a large vegetation on the atrial side of the mitral valve. Patient also had 4+ mitral regurgitation and congestive heart failure. Courtesy of P.A.N. Chandraratna, M.D.

thereafter, and on several occasions for 1–2 months after therapy is discontinued. Indications for surgical intervention in PVE were discussed earlier.

REFERENCES

1. Weinstein L, Rubin RH. Infective endocarditis—1973. Prog Cardiovasc Dis 1973; 16:239,–74.
1a. Brandriss MW. Cardiac Infections. In: Reese RE, Douglas, Jr., RG, eds. 2nd ed. Boston: Little Brown and Company. 1986:258–283.
2. Gonzalez-Lavin L. Lise M, Ross D. The importance of the "jet lesion" in bacterial endocarditis involving the left heart. J Thorac Cardiovasc Surg 1970; 59:185–92.
3. Buchbinder NA, Roberts WC. Left-sided valvular active infective endocarditis: a study of forty-five necropsy patients. Am J Med 1972; 53:20–35.
4. Lerner PI, Weinstein L. Infective endocarditis in the antibiotic era. N Engl J Med 1966; 274:199–206, 259–66, 323–31, 388–93.

5. Roberts WC. Characteristics and consequences of infective endocarditis (active and healed or both) learned from morphologic studies. In: Rahimtoola SH, ed. Infective Endocarditis. New York: Grune & Stratton, 1978:55–123.
6. Everett ED, Hirschmann JV. Transient bacteremia and endocarditis: a review. Medicine 1977; 56:61–77.
6a. Weinstein L: Infective endocarditis. In: Braunwald E, ed. Heart disease. 3rd ed. W.B. Saunders Company. 1988, 1093–1134.
7. Reid CL, Elkayam U, Rahimtoola SH. Infective endocarditis in pregnancy. In: Elkayam U, Gleicher N, eds. Cardiac Problems in Pregnancy, 2d ed. New York: Alan R. Liss, 1990:119–211.
8. Reisberg BE. Infective endocarditis in the narcotic addict. Prog Cardiovasc Dis 1979; 22:193–204.
9. Pelletier LL, Petersdorf RG. Infective endocarditis: a review of 125 cases from the University of Washington Hospitals, 1963–72. Medicine 1977; 56: 287–313.
10. Van Scoy RE. Culture-negative endocarditis. Mayo Clin Proc 1982; 57: 149–54.
11. Sande MA, Small PM. Infective Endocarditis. In: Stein JH, ed. Internal Medicine, 3d ed. Boston: Little Brown, 1990:140–9.
12. Geraci JE, Wilson WR. Endocarditis due to gram-negative bacteria: report of 56 cases. Mayo Clin Proc 1982; 57:145–48.
13. Phair JP, Clarke J. Immunology of infective endocarditis. Prog Cardiovasc Dis 1979; 22:137–44.
14. McAnulty JH, Rahimtoola SH, DeMots H, Griswold HE. Clinical features of infective endocarditis. In: Rahimtoola SH, ed. Infective Endocarditis. New York: Grune & Stratton, 1978:125–48.
15. Reid Cl, Chandraratna PAN, Rahimtoola SH. Infective endocarditis: improved diagnosis and treatment. Current Probl Cardiol 1985; 10:1–51.
16. Wilson JW, Houghton DC, Bennett WM, Porter GA. The kidney and infective endocarditis. In: Rahimtoola SH, ed. Infective Endocarditis. New York: Grune & Stratton, 1978:179–94.
17. Pruit AA, Rubin RH, Karchmer AW, Duncan GW. Neurologic complications of bacterial endocarditis. Medicine 1978; 57:329–43.
18. Zimet I. Nervous system complications in bacterial endocarditis. Am J Med 1969; 47:593–607.
19. Hart RG, Foster JW, Luther MF, Kanter MC. Stroke in infective endocarditis. Stroke 1990; 21:695–700.
20. Roberts WC, Buchbinder NA. Healed left-sided infective endocarditis: a clinicopathologic study of 59 patients. Am J Cardiol 1977; 40:876–88.
21. Mills J, Utley J, Abbott J. Heart failure in infective endocarditis: predisposing factors, course, and treatment. Chest 1974; 66:151–7.
22. Nimalasuriya A, Chandraratna PAN, Wong E, Wong R, Rahimtoola SH. Incidence and clinical correlates of pericardial effusions detected by 2-D echocardiography in infective endocarditis (abstr). Circulation 1983; 68: 111–205.

23. Wilson WR, Giuliani ER, Danielson GK, Geraci JE. Management of complications of infective endocarditis. Mayo Clin Proc 1982; 57:162–70.

24. Jaffe WM, Morgan DE, Perlman AS, Otto CM. Infective endocarditis. 1983–1988: echocardiographic findings and factors influencing morbidity and mortality. J Am Coll Cardiol 1990; 15:1227–33.

25. Mugge A, Daniel WG, Frank G, Lichtlen PR. Echocardiography in infective endocarditis: reassessment of prognostic implications of vegetations size determined by the transthoracic and transesophageal approach. J Am Coll Cardiol 1989; 14:631–8.

26. Erbel R, Rohmann S, Drexler M, Mohr-Kahaly S, Gerharz DC, Iversen S. Improved diagnostic value of echocardiography in patients with infective endocarditis by transesophageal approach. Eur Heart J 1988; 9:43–53.

27. McAnulty JH, Rahimtoola SH. Surgery for infective endocarditis. JAMA 1979; 242:77–9.

28. Belli J, Waisbren BA. The number of blood cultures necessary to diagnose most cases of bacterial endocarditis. Am J Med Sci 1956; 232:284–8.

29. Washington JA. The role of the microbiology laboratory in the diagnosis and antimicrobial treatment of infective endocarditis. Mayo Clin Proc 1982; 57: 22–32.

30. Martin RP, Meltzer RS, Chia BL, Stinson EB, Rakowski H, Popp RL. Clinical utility of two-dimensional echocardiography in infective endocarditis. Am J Cardiol 1980; 46:379–85.

31. Pederson WR, Walker M, Olson JD, Gobel F, Lange HW, Daniel JA, Rogers J, Longe T, Kane M, Mooney MR, Goldenberg IF. Value of transesophageal echocardiography as an adjunct to thrasthoracic echocardiography in evaluation of native and prosthetic valve endocarditis. Chest 1991; 100:351–6.

32. Shivley BK, Gurule FT, Rodlan CA, Leggett JH, Schiller NB. Diagnostic value of transesophageal compared with transthoracic echocardiography in infective endocarditis. J Am Coll Cardiol 1991; 18:391–7.

33. Rubenson DS, Tucker CR, Stinson EB, London EJ, Oyer P, Moreno-Cabral R, Popp RL. The use of echocardiography in diagnosing culture-negative endocarditis. Circulation 1981; 64:641–6.

34. Wong DH, Chandraratna PAN, Wishnow R, Dusitnanond V, Nimalasuriya A. Clinical implications of large vegetations in infectious endocarditis. Arch Intern Med 1983; 143:1874–7.

34a. Tak T, Rahimtoola SH, Kumar A, Gamage N, Chandraratna PAN. Value of digital image processing of two-dimensional echocardiograms in differentiating acute from chronic vegetations of infective endocarditis. Circulation 1988; 78:116–23.

35. Reid CL, Kawanishi DT, McKay CR, Elkayam U, Rahimtoola SH, Chandraratna PAN. Accuracy of evaluation of presence and severity of aortic and mitral regurgitation by contrast two-dimensional echocardiographic technique. Am J Cardiol 1983; 52:519–24.

36. Wilson WR, Guiliani ER, Danielson GK, Geraci JE. General considerations in the diagnosis and treatment of infective endocarditis. Mayo Clin Proc 1982; 57:81–5.

37. Sande MA, Scheld WM. Combination antibiotic therapy of bacterial endocarditis. Ann Intern Med 1980; 92:390–5.

38. Bisno AL, Disumkes WE, Durack DT, et al. Antimicrobial treatment of infective endocarditis due to viridans streptococci, enterococci, and staphylococci. JAMA 1989; 261:1471–7.

39. Levine HJ, Pauker SG, Salzman EW. Antithrombotic therapy in valvular heart disease. Chest 1989; 95:985–1065.

40. Richardson JV, Karp RB, Kirklin JW, Dismukes WE. Treatment of infective endocarditis: a 10 year comparative analysis. Circulation 1978; 58:589–97.

41. Brandenburg RO, Guiliani ER, Wilson WR, Geraci JE. Infective endocarditis: a 25 year overview of diagnosis and treatment. J Am Coll Cardiol 1983; 1:280–91.

42. Stinson EB. Surgical treatment of infective endocarditis. Prog Cardiovasc Dis 1979; 22:145–68.

43. Rahimtoola SH. Valvular heart disease: a perspective. J Am Coll Cardiol 1983; 1:199–215.

44. Craft CH, Woodward W, Elliott A, Commerford PJ, Barnard CN, Beck W. Analysis of surgical versus medical therapy in active complicated native valve infective endocarditis. Am J Cardiol 1983; 51:1650–5.

45. Black S, O'Rourke RA, Karliner JS. Role of surgery in the treatment of primary infective endocarditis. Am J Med 1974; 56:357–68.

46. Stimmel B, Dack S. Infective endocarditis in narcotic addicts. In: Rahimtoola SH, ed. Infective Endocarditis. New York: Grune & Stratton, 1978:195–209.

47. McLeod R, Remington JS. Fungal endocarditis. In: Rahimtoola SH, ed. Infective Endocarditis. New York: Grune & Stratton, 1978:211–90.

48. Mayer KH, Schoenbaum SC. Evaluation and management of prosthetic valve endocarditis. Prog Cardiovasc Dis 1982; 25:43–54.

49. Karchmer AW, Dismukes WE, Buckley MJ, Austen WG. Late prosthetic valve endocarditis: clinical features influencing therapy. Am J Med 1978; 64: 199–206.

50. Cukingman RA, Carey JS, Wittig JH, Cimochowski GE. Early valve replacement in active infective endocarditis: results and late survival. J Thorac Cardiovasc Surg 1983; 85:163–73.

51. Wilson WR, Danielson GK, Guiliani ER, Washington JA, Jaumin PM, Geraci JE. Valve replacement in patients with active infective endocarditis. Circulation 1978; 58:585–8.

52. Dajani As, Bisno AL, Chang KJ, et al. Prevention of bacterial endocarditis. Clin Cardiol 1990; 264:2919–22.

53. Chanbers HF, Korzeniowski OM, Sande MA, National Collaborative Endocarditis Study Group. *Staphylococcus aureus* endocarditis: clinical manifestations in addicts and nonaddicts. Medicine 1983; 63:170–7.

14

Electrocardiographic Changes and Complicating Arrhythmias in Valvular Heart Disease

Moh'd Ali Habbab
Armed Forces Hospital, Riyadh, Saudi Arabia

Nabil El-Sherif
State University of New York—Health Science Center, Brooklyn, New York

I. INTRODUCTION

Valvular heart disease may cause pressure-volume overload leading to altered myocardial function and various chamber abnormalities (enlargement or hypertrophy). When they are significant enough, these changes will produce characteristic electrocardiographic changes in the 12-lead electrocardiogram and may lead to various cardiac arrhythmias. Cardiac arrhythmias also can be produced and aggravated by the direct involvement of the various myocardial tissues by the underlying valvular disease as in rheumatic heart disease. Various hemodynamic changes, as well as other serious complications such as embolization and sudden death, may be caused by these cardiac arrhythmias during the course of the valvular heart disease. Also, some arrhythmias, either preexisting or newly occurring, may complicate the pre- or postsurgical period.

II. MITRAL STENOSIS

A. Electrocardiographic Changes (Fig. 1)

1. Left Atrial Enlargement

Left atrial enlargement is a principal electrocardiographic feature of mitral stenosis and is found in 90% of patients with significant mitral stenosis and

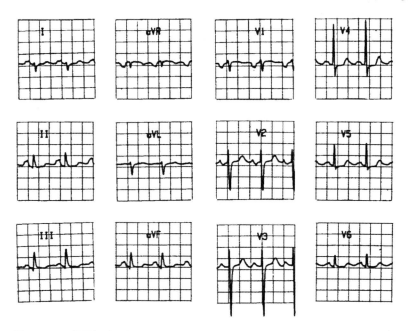

Figure 1 ECG obtained from a 22-year-old patient in sinus rhythm with rheumatic mitral stenosis. The clear evidence of left atrial enlargement is shown by the increased duration of the notched P wave (P mitrale) in leads I and II, and the deep negative P force in V1.

sinus rhythm (1). The characteristic ECG signs of left atrial enlargement include P-wave duration in lead II of more than 0.12 s (P mitrale, which may be notched, bifid, or have a flat top), terminal negative P force in lead V1 of more than 0.03 mV/s, P-wave axis between $+45°$ and $-30°$. These signs correlate more closely with left atrial volume than with left atrial pressure (2) and often regress following successful valvotomy (3). The development of atrial fibrillation correlates with the preexistent ECG diagnosis of left atrial enlargement and is related to the size and extent of fibrosis of the left atrial myocardium (4). Contrary to prior belief (5), coarse atrial fibrillation, which has large fibullatory waves greater than 0.1 mV in V1, does not correlate well with the presence or absence of mitral valve disease or with the size of the left atrium as detected by the electrocardiogram (6,7).

2. Right Ventricular Hypertrophy

The level of right ventricular systolic pressure will determine the ECG evidence of right ventricular hypertrophy, which is infrequent in patients with right ventricular systolic pressure less than 70 mmHg (1).

About half of all patients with right ventricular systolic pressure between 70 and 100 mmHg manifest the electrocardiographic criteria of right ventricular hypertrophy, including both a mean QRS axis greater than 80° in the frontal plane and an R:S ratio greater than 1.0 in V1 (8). When right ventricular systolic pressure exceeds 100 mmHg, ECG evidence of right ventricular hypertrophy is found quite consistently. The mean QRS axis averages plus + 150°, and there is a Q-R morphology in the right precordial leads with inverted or biphasic T waves (9). In pure mitral stenosis, the QRS axis in the frontal plane often correlates with the severity of valvular obstruction and the level of pulmonary vascular resistance. A mean frontal axis between 0 and + 60° suggests that the mitral valve area exceeds 1.3 cm², and an axis greater than 60° generally indicates that the valvular area is less than 1.3 cm². Also, in patients with pulmonary vascular resistance of more than 650 dynes-s-cm⁻⁵, the mean axis usually exceeds plus 110° (8).

B. Complicating Arrhythmias

1. Atrial Fibrillation

Atrial fibrillation is one of the most common complications of mitral stenosis. It may occur as a transient episode or as a sustained arrhythmia. The combination of mitral valve disease and atrial inflammation secondary to rheumatic carditis causes left atrial dilatation, fibrosis of the atrial wall, and disorganization of the atrial muscle bundles; the latter leads to disparate conduction velocities and inhomogeneous refactory periods. Premature atrial activation, due either to an automatic focus or to reentry, may stimulate the left atrium during the vulnerable period and may thus precipitate a bout of atrial fibrillation. Coronary atrial fibrillation results in turn in diffuse atrophy of the muscle, which causes further inhomogenouity of refractoriness, and conduction leads to irreversible atrial fibrillation (4).

The occurrence of atrial fibrillation seems to be related to the degree of left atrial dilatation (10), the extent of fibrosis in the left atrium (4), the duration of atriomegaly, and the age of the patient (10,11). Henry et al. have shown a close correlation between echocardiographic left atrial size and atrial fibrillation (10). When the left atrium was smaller than 4 cm, only 3 of 117 patients had atrial fibrillation; however, when the left atrium was more than 4 cm, 80 of 148 patients had atrial fibrillation. According to Deverall et al. (12), the incidence of atrial fibrillation in patients with mitral stenosis was clearly related to age when the patient was first seen [11–20 years (0%), 21–30 years (17%), 31–40 years (45%), 41–50 years (60%), and over 51 years (80%)].

Atrial contraction augments the presystolic transmitral valvular gradient by approximately 30% in patients with mitral stenosis (13). When atrial fibrillation occurs, it is frequently accompanied by a sudden hemodynamic and symptomatic degeneration and a decrease of about 20% in cardiac output (14). Chronic mitral stenosis results in elevated left atrial pressure, which in turn leads to the enlargement of the left atrium and raises pulmonary venous and capillary pressures. The more rapid ventricular rate that is common in atrial fibrillation raises the transvalvular pressure gradient. Tachycardia shortens diastole more than systole and diminishes the time available for flow across the mitral valve. Therefore it augments the transmitral valvular pressure gradient and elevates the left atrial pressure and the pulmonary venous pressure further (15,16). According to the hydraulic (Gorlin) formula, doubling the flow rate will quadruple the pressure gradient (17), so that stress such as exercise in patients with moderate to severe mitral stenosis will cause marked elevation in left atrial pressure (18). This explains the sudden development of dyspnea and pulmonary edema in previously asymptomatic patients with mitral stenosis who experience atrial fibrillation with rapid ventricular rate (14) and the equally rapid improvement in patients when the ventricular rate is slowed by means of digitalis or propranolol and other beta-blocking agents (19–21).

Treatment of atrial fibrillation should be directed toward reducing the ventricular rate and, if possible, reestablishing sinus rhythm by a combination of pharmacological treatment and cardioversion. Digitalis, with or without propranolol or other beta-blocking agents, should be used to slow the ventricular rate (19–21). Digitalis may also be used in preventing paroxismal atrial fibrillation. Quinidine or quinidinelike antiarrhythmics can be used to revert the rhythm pharmacologically to normal sinus rhythm or to maintain sinus rhythm after electrical cardioversion. Cardioversion is more successful in young patients with mild mitral stenosis without marked left atrial enlargement who have been in atrial fibrillation less than 6 months, and who have been treated with adequate doses of quinidine (22). Repeated cardioversion is not indicated if the patient has not sustained sinus rhythm while on adequate doses of quinidine. The immediate success rate with quinidine is about 50–55% in patients with mitral stenosis versus 20–25% in patients with mitral regurgitation (23). With chronic atrial fibrillation, elective anticoagulation should be instituted 2–3 weeks before cardioversion—either pharmacological or electrical. This treatment reduces, but does not eliminate, the embolic risk, both at the time of the procedure and within the first week after conversion, as atrial function recovers and a thrombus may be dislodged (24). Systemic embolization occurs in 1–2% of patients with mitral stenosis following electrical or pharmacological cardioversion. Paroxysmal atrial fibrillation and repeated conversions, spontaneous or induced, carry the risk of embolization (25). Following conversion, the risk of reversion to atrial fibrillation is high in the first days and weeks after cardioversion. If conversion or maintenance of sinus rhythm cannot be achieved, the ventricular rate at rest should be maintained at approximately 60–65 beats/min with digitalis with or without beta-blockers (21).

2. Atrial Fibrillation and Systemic Embolization

Embolization is most common in patients with advanced disease, atrial fibrillation, and a large left atrial appendage. The overall incidence of systemic embolization in patients with rheumatic mitral valve disease is approximately 1.5% per patient-year (26). The risk of embolization is increased sevenfold by the presence of atrial fibrillation, and there is a temporary relationship between the onset of fibrillation and the occurrence of embolic, since 33% of emboli occur in the first month after the onset of atrial fibrillation, and 66% occur within the first year (26). Atrial fibrillation is of the two factors most closely associated with systemic embolization in patients with mitral stenosis, in addition to age.

The size of the left atrium is relevant in that as it enlarges it increases the probability of atrial fibrillation (27). Coulshed et al. (28) showed that the overall incidence of embolization in patients with mitral stenosis was 9%. The incidence varied with age and rhythm: In patients who were 35 years old and under, the incidence was 5% with normal sinus rhythm and 27% with atrial fibrillation; and in patients who were more than 35 years old, the incidence was 11% with normal sinus rhythm and 32% with atrial fibrillation (28). Bannister (29) followed 105 patients with mild mitral stenosis for an average of 4.5 years. Systemic embolization occurred in 21% of all patients and in more than 50% of those patients who were over 40 years and had atrial fibrillation. Thus it is clear that patients with mitral stenosis who are older than 35 years or who are in atrial fibrillation should be treated with long-term anticoagulation.

III. MITRAL REGURGITATION

A. Electrocardiographic Changes (Fig. 2)

1. Left Atrial Enlargement

In chronic mitral regurgitation, left atrial enlargement is as common as in mitral stenosis and can alter the P wave in the same way (30,31). If atrial fibrillation has developed, atrial enlargement is suggested by the coarse fibrillatory pattern (32). In acute mitral regurgitation the ECG is usually

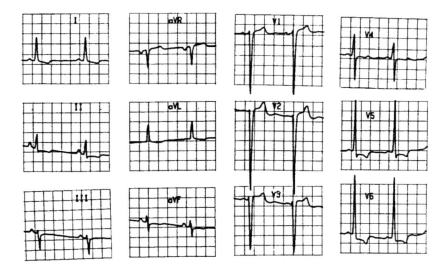

Figure 2 ECG obtained from a 35-year-old patient in sinus rhythm and severe mitral regurgitation showing evidence of left atrial enlargement and left ventricular diastolic volume overload (see text for details).

normal, although ECG evidence of left atrial enlargement can occur early, particularly in lead V1, and probably reflects elevated left atrial pressure rather than true hypertrophy (33).

2. Left Ventricular Hypertrophy

A left ventricular diastolic volume overload pattern of increased voltage amplitude occurs in about 40–50% of patients with severe mitral regurgitation (30). The ECG pattern is one of left ventricular hypertrophy but with a prominent Q wave in the leads facing the left side of the septum, namely, leads I, aV1, V5, and V6, and a prominent R wave in the leads facing the right side of the septum, namely, V1 and V2. The Q wave is narrow, measuring 0.025 s or less, and its depth is 0.2 mV or greater (34).

3. Right Ventricular Hypertrophy

In mitral regurgitation, the pulmonary vascular resistance is generally not elevated to the same extent as in mitral stenosis. Thus the ECG evidence of right ventricular hypertrophy and right axis deviation is much less frequent and is seen in only about 15% of patients (30). Also, moderate right ventricular hypertrophy rarely produces any characteristic ECG changes, both because of the insensitivity of the ECG to RVH and because left ventricular hypertrophy due to left ventricular volume overload balances the electrical impulses (35).

4. Other Changes

When ischaemic heart disease is the mechanism for mitral regurgitation, ECG changes of recent or old myocardial infarction (usually inferior or posterior) (35,35a) or definite ischemic changes are often present. Although S-T changes have been attributed to papillary muscle dysfunction, these are nonspecific and can occur due to left ventricular hypertrophy, conduction defects, and digitalis (36).

B. Complicating Arrhythmias

1. Atrial Fibrillation

Incompetence of the mitral valve during systolic ejection permits regurgitation into the left atrium and pulmonary veins, and massive enlargement of the left atrium occurs with severe and long-standing regurgitation. Atrial fibrillation eventually accompanies this left atrial enlargement and becomes a common finding in chronic regurgitation. As in the case of mitral stenosis, the occurrence of atrial fibrillation seems to be related to the extent of left atrial dilatation, and its incidence increases with age (10). Rheumatic involvement of the left atrial wall may also play a role in the redevelopment of atrial fibrillation (37). Although deterioration may occur when atrial fibrillation occurs, this is usually much less dramatic than that seen in mitral stenosis. The large, distensible left atrium prevents a rapid rise of left atrial pressure when fibrillation beings, and hence protects the lungs. The left ventricular filling is not so dependent on the length of diastole as in mitral stenosis, and therefore is not reduced to the same extent by the rapid heart rate that usually accompanies uncontrolled atrial fibrillation (38). The control of atrial fibrillation rate produces a dramatic improvement, which is why digitalis plays a major role in the management of mitral regurgitation.

Quinidine or procainamide may be helpful in suppressing frequent atrial premature contractions as well as maintaining sinus rhythm following electrical or pharmacological conversion from atrial fibrillation. Because of larger left atrial dimensions in mitral regurgitation than in mitral stenosis, the immediate success rate of cardioversion is less than 20–25% for mitral regurgitation and 50–55% for mitral stenosis (23), and that rate is likely to be even less if the rhythm is long-standing (more than 1 year) (24). It is rarely worthwhile trying to convert atrial fibrillation to sinus rhythm without correcting the mitral regurgitation, since fibrillation soon recurs.

IV. MITRAL VALVE PROLAPSE

A. Electrocardiographic Changes (Fig. 3)

1. ST-T Changes

The most common ECG abnormality in mitral valve prolapse is flattened, inverted, or biphasic T-wave and nonspecific ST changes in leads II, III, and AVF and occasionally in the anterolateral leads as well (39). These changes may be related to ischemia of papillary muscles, or of the left ventricle at the basis, resulting from increased tension on these structures or possibly even stimulating local coronary spasm produced by the prolapsing valve (40,41), or they may reflect an underlying cardiomyopathy (42).

Also, some studies suggest that these changes may be due to an autonomic inbalance resulting in sympathetic overactivity (43,44). These ECG changes are commonly seen in symptomatic patients and have been reported in about 30% of patients in hospital-based series (45) and approximately 15% of patients detected in screening studies (46,47). Amylnitrate and exercise may exaggerate these ST-T changes, thus exercise stress test reduces a high incidence of more than 53% positive tests (more than 1 mm ST depression) in patients with mitral valve prolapse and normal coronary arteries (48).

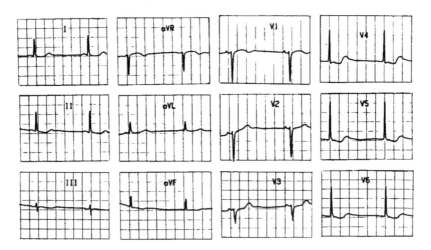

Figure 3 Nonspecific ST changes and T-wave flattening as well as biphasic T waves in the inferior lateral leads obtained from a 38-year-old female with echocardiographically documented mitral valve prolapse.

2. Left Atrial and Left Ventricular Hypertrophy

When significant mitral regurgitation occurs, the expected ECG changes of left atrial and left ventricular hypertrophy may become apparent.

B. Complicating Arrhythmias

1. Ventricular Arrhythmias

The cause of arrhythmias in patients with mitral valve prolapse is multifactorial and appears to be related to the anatomic subtrade and the modulating role of the autonomic nervous system (49). Ventricular arrhythmias are slightly more common than supraventricular arrhythmias in patients with mitral valve prolapse (50).

The incidence of PVCs found by ambulatory electrocardiographic monitoring has been reported to range from 49% to 85% (51,52), compared to about 50% in the general population (53,54). In symptomatic patients, Winkle et al. (50) described 75% with PVCs, 42% with multiform PVCs, 50% with cuplets, and 21% with ventricular tachycardia. The prevelance of complex ventricular arrhythmias was reported to vary between 43% and 56% (55). In patients without hemodynamically significant mitral regurgitation, Kramer et al. (56) found 63% to have PVCs, with multiform PVCs in 43%, PVC cuplets in 6%, and VT in 5%. Only 40% of this group of patients were symptomatic. Exercise testing appears to increase the incidence of arrhythmias in mitral valve prolapse patients (from 50% at rest to 75% with treadmill exercise testing) (57).

Many mechanisms have been proposed for the genesis of these ventricular arrhythmias. The most common clinical pathological features of mitral valve prolapse appear to result from hypermobility of the mitral apparatus that is produced by dysfunction of the annulus fibrosis (58,59). This altered position of the valve apparatus permits the chordae to erupt against the ventricular endocardium. This endocardial friction by the chordae (60) or the leaflet (61), and the effects of intramyocardial extension of surface fibrosis produced by this friction (61), may cause the arrhythmias.

Excessive traction of the papillary muscle by the prolapsed leaflets (62), which tend to cause an earlier local ventricular activation in the area of traction and relative prolongation of the ventricular functional refractory period in the area of traction, may lead to the induction or exhibitation of ventricular ectopic activity (63). Ventricular fibrosis, which appears to be present in a high percentage of symptomatic patients (70% with abnormal endocardial and interstitial fibrosis on right ventricular biopsy) (64) and patients who have died suddenly (65), is another possible mechanism of ventricular ectopy. Wellens (66) has demonstrated reentry as the mechanism of ventricular arrhythmias in a few patients with mitral valve prolapse. The anatomic substrate of the entrant circuit could involve a contact lesion, an area of localized myocardial ischemia, or cardiomyopathy (67). Platelet aggregation, hemorrhage, and fibrin deposits have been observed in the angle between the left atrium and the posterior mitral leaflet, and microembolism from these deposits may involve the coronary circulation with subsequent myocardial ischemia and ventricular arrhythmias, as these deposits have been suggested to be the source of fatal coronary emboli (68).

The presence of mitral regurgitation and left ventricular enlargement is likely to be associated with an increased incidence of significant arrhythmia ectopy (69). There is also an increased association between mitral valve prolapse and prolongation of the QT interval, and this association may play a role in the genesis of ventricular arrhythmias (70,71). Autonomic dysfunction, in the form of increased sympathetic activity, may initiate, precipitate, or contribute to ventricular arrhythmia in patients with mitral valve prolapse. Autonomic studies showed that patients with mitral valve prolapse have higher resting and standing plasma catecholamine levels than controls, and the highest plasma values were seen in patients with QTc prolongation (70). Also, patients with mitral valve prolapse have a greater increase in heart rate and more marked QT interval prolongation than controls during isoproterenol infusion, and there is parallel response of the 24-hour urine catecholamine secretion to the frequency of ventricular ectopic beats (72). The results of these and other studies (73,74) demonstrate the increased sympathetic activity which may initiate, precipitate, or contribute to the ventricular activity in patients with mitral valve prolapse. For these reasons, the use of beta-blockers is the treatment of choice for ventricular arrhythmias in mitral valve prolapse (75,76). They strikingly reduce ventricular ectopic frequency, possibly because they have both an antiarrhythmic effect and reduce the degree of prolapse by depressing contractility and increasing left ventricular volume (77). Special attention should be paid to mitral valve prolapse patients with ventricular arrhythmias and prolonged QT interval. These patients should be treated with beta-blockers. Maintenance of normal serum potassium is extremely important (mitral valve prolapse patients may be prone to be hypokalemia because of the hyperadrenergic state) (72), and other antiarrhythmics that prolong the QT interval should be avoided.

If therapy with beta-blockers proves ineffective, moricizine may be used effectively, while class 1A antiarrhythmics are usually not effective (78) and should be avoided because they prolong QT interval.

2. Supraventricular Arrhythmias

The incidence of PACs in symptomatic patients with mitral valve prolapse ranges from 35% to 63% (50,79). Pooled data from recent studies (51,56) showed a trend toward a high prevalence of supraventricular tachycardia in mitral valve prolapse (28%) versus controls (17%). The most common sustained tachyarrhythmia in patients with mitral valve prolapse is paroxysmal supraventricular tachycardia, the mechanism of which is related to the increased incidence of a dual AV node pathway (80) and accessory atrioventricular pathways (81) in these patients. These pathways were found in 58% of patients with mitral valve prolapse, versus 20% in the control group; they were concealed in 57% and left-sided in all patients (81). Conversely, patients with Wolff-Parkinson-White syndrome have a high incidence of mitral valve prolapse (82).

As in the case of ventricular arrhythmias, numerous mechanisms have been proposed for the genesis of supraventricular arrhythmias.

The experimental studies of Wit et al. (83,84) demonstrated spontaneous phase 4 (diastolic) depolarization from the atriumlike muscle fibers of the anterior mitral leaflet after stretching or exposure to catecholamines. Also, the pathological findings of dense laminated collagen-containing elastic issue in the atrial endocardium and fibrous nodules in the left atrial wall (68), and the fatty infiltration in the approaches to both sinoatrial and atrioventricular nodes (65), may partially explain the striking incidence of spontaneous and inducive atrial flutter and fibrillation in patients with mitral valve prolapse. Alternation in atrial refractoriness between the high and low right atrium (possibly autonomic mediated) was described in patients with mitral valve prolapse, and producible atrial flutter compared with normal (85). Similar to its effect on ventricular arrhythmias, the autonomic dysfunction of increased sympathetic acticity may initiate, precipitate, or contribute to supraventricular arrhythmias. Mitral regurgitation producing left atrial enlargement has an increased incidence of atrial fibrillation and flutter, described in mitral regurgitation with left atrial enlargement, due to other pathological entities.

While PACs usually do not require therapy, proprenolol is effective in a high percentage of patients (75). Treatment of supraventricular tachycardia requires the identification of the specific tachycardia. AV nodal reentrant tachycardia usually is treated with beta-blocking agents, digitalis, or calcium channel blockers.

Specific therapy for accessory pathway reentrant tachycardia requires assessment by means of electrophysiological study. Atrial flutter and fibrillation are treated effectively with class 1A or 1C antiarrhythmics plus digitalis or beta-blockers. Caution is required with regard to QT interval prolongation.

3. Bradyarrhythmias

Bradycardiac rhythms, notably sinus bradycardia, sinus exit block, and atrial ventricular conduction defects including high-grade blocks, have usually been described in symptomatic patients, most noticeably those with syncopy (79,86–88). Bundle-branch block appears to be common in patients with mitral valve prolapse (88,89), its incidence reaching 22.5% in one study (90).

The mechanism for these bradyarrhythmias can be explained on a pathological basis (65,88,91)—marked fatty infiltration in the approaches to the sino-atrial and atrio-ventricular nodes in the region of the atrial preferential pathway—or on autonomic reflexes (92,93). Patients with severe bradyarrhythmias have occasionally required pacemaker therapy.

4. Sudden Death and Mitral Valve Prolapse

The relationship between the mitral valve prolapse syndrome and sudden death is not clear (94) because of the heterogeneity of reported cases, differences in case selection, and the absence of adequate controlled data (68). Sudden death occurs in a small portion of patients, and the immediate cause is probably a tachyarrhythmia (68), although complete heart block with prolonged asystole has also been reported in mitral valve prolapse syndrome and cannot be excluded (86). The risk is extremely low in patients with only a click, or no abnormal auscultatory findings (77). High risk for sudden death may be expected in patients with clinical evidence of mitral regurgitation and a history of syncopy episode, a family history of sudden death, complex arrhythmias on 24-hour ECG or induced by exercise, or by abnormal resting ECG (77).

V. AORTIC STENOSIS

A. Electrocardiographic Changes (Fig. 4)

1. Left Ventricular Hypertrophy

The characteristic electrocardiographic changes in severe aortic stenosis are those of ventricular hypertrophy (95). They are the classical systolic or pressure-overload changes, which are usually characterized by tall R waves in the left precordial leads and deep S waves in the right precordial leads, and ST segment depression with P-wave inversion in leads 1, AVL, V5, and V6. This may be accompanied by left-axis deviation. Although the features of left ventricular hypertrophy are seen in the majority (about 85%) of cases with severe aortic stenosis, the full left ventricular hypertro-

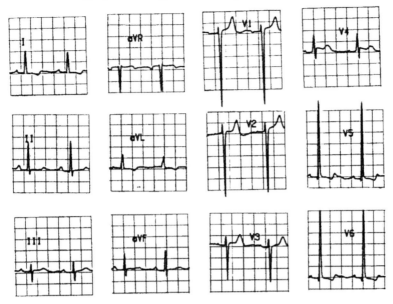

Figure 4   Classical systolic or pressure-overload ECG changes (see text for details) obtained from a 60-year-old male with aortic stenosis.

phy with strain pattern is seen in only 50% of cases (96). The higher the gradient across the aortic valve, the more likely is the strain or systolic overload pattern (97,98).

Also, ST-segment depressions greater than 0.3 mV in patients with aortic stenosis suggests the presence of severe left ventricular hypertrophy. In aortic stenosis with no evidence of mitral, coronary, or myocardial disease, the total 12-lead QRS amplitude in millivolts correlates well with the height of the left ventricular systolic pressure in millimeters Hg (99). Although the features of left ventricular hypertrophy become more marked as the stenosis increases, in a few cases the ECG may be normal or show only minor T-wave abnormalities (100,101), and 9% of patients who die suddenly have a normal ECG (102,103).

Occasionally, loss of R waves in the right precordial leads, simulating anterior septal infarction (pseudo-infarction pattern), is present when there is left-axis deviation. It has been reported that 10% of all cases of left anterior hemiblock are due to aortic valve disease (104).

2. Left Atrial Hypertrophy

Electrocardiographic evidence of left atrial hypertrophy is seen in 80% of patients with severe isolated aortic stenosis (105). The principal manifestation is prominent late negativity of the P wave in V1 rather than an increased duration in lead 2, suggesting that hypertrophy rather than dilatation is present. This reflects a significant and sustained elevation of left ventricular diastolic pressure seen with marked ventricular hypertrophy and in decompensated lesion. Although left atrial hypertrophy in patients with aortic stenosis should raise the suspicion of an associated mitral lesion, it may be seen without accompanying mitral valve disease in severe aortic stenosis (106).

B. Complicating Arrhythmias

1. Ventricular Arrhythmias

Ambulatory electrocardiography frequently shows high-grade ventricular ectopy in patients with isolated aortic stenosis (107,108). Sixty-four percent of these patients were found to have multiform PVCs, cuplets, or nonsustained ventricular tachycardia. The occurrence of ventricular arrhythmia is unrelated to the severity of the stenosis, or the presence or absence of coronary artery disease (107), but it correlates significantly with deficits in myocardial function reflected by low ejection fraction and high wall stress (108).

The pathophysiological mechanisms underlying ventricular arrhythmias in patients with aortic stenosis are unclear. Myocardial ischemia resulting solely from impaired coronary blood flow is not the primary mechanism for arrhythmias (107). The interrelation of increased myocardial mass, the degree of ventricular dilatation, and ventricular wall stress could be the most important factor (109,110).

Patients with chronic pressure overload and hypertrophy of the left ventricle have increased ventricular wall stress (111), reduced blood flow per unit mass of myocardium (112), subendocardial ischemia despite normal coronary arteries (113,114), and reduced density per myocardial mass (115,116). Greater increases in left ventricular volumes relative to ventricular mass might result in inadequate hypertrophy, and this high-stress hypertrophy state is associated with elevations in wall stress and increased myocardial oxygen requirements (117), as well as decreased myocardial contractility (26). Echocardiographic findings in patients with aortic stenosis and normal coronary arteries demonstrated that differences in wall hypertrophy relative to ventricular cavity size might contribute to arrhythmogenesis. Patients demonstrating complex ventricular arrhythmias had a significantly higher ratio of left ventricular chamber radius to wall thickness, as well as a higher left ventricular volume-to-mass ratio, than patients without complex arrhythmias—suggesting that complex arrhythmias may be associated with greater intramyocardium wall stress (109,118).

2. Conduction Defects

Varying degrees of atrioventricular and intraventricular block may be seen in patients with calcific aortic stenosis (119–121). These conduction defects may result from septal trauma incidental to high intramyocardial tensions, from hypoxic damage to the conduction fibers, or from extension of valvular calcification into the fibrosis septum. Atrio-ventricular block is usually a late manifestation and associated with the spread of calcification into the conduction tissue. The prevelance of conduction defects (atrioventricular block, sino-atrial disease, bundle branch block, left anterior hemiblock, or intraventricular conduction defect) is higher in aortic stenosis patients older than 60 years with mitral annular calcium (58%) than those without (25%) (121). This is most likely due to the close proximity of the aortic route and mitral annulus to the AV node and bundle of His.

3. Sudden Cardiac Death

Sudden death occurs in 10–20% of patients with aortic stenosis (122). This is particularly likely when there has been preceding syncope or angina or there has been heart failure. However, it can occur in asymptomatic individuals. The cause remains unclear: It has been attributed to various mechanisms, including inability to increase cardiac output in the presence of dilatation (97,123) transient tachyarrhythmias (123), ventricular asystole (97,124), and complete atrioventricular block due to calcific disease of the His conduction system (125).

Before the use of surgery for valvular heart disease, 73% of deaths in patients with aortic stenosis were sudden (126). Although the safe and effective replacement of the aortic valve has reduced the incidence of sudden death in patients with aortic stenosis (127), patients with valve replacement remain at some risk for sudden death due to arrhythmias, prosthetic valve dysfunction, or coexistent coronary heart disease (128).

Sudden death accounts for 21% of total deaths following valve replacement surgery (129); the incidence increases 3 weeks after operation and levels off after 8 months. A high incidence of ventricular arrhythmias has been observed during follow-up of patients with valve replacement, especially in those who had aortic stenosis, multiple valve surgery, or cardiomegaly (130). Sudden death during follow-up was associated with ventricular arrhythmias and thromboembolism.

VI. AORTIC REGURGITATION

A. Electrocardiographic Changes (Fig. 5)

1. Left Ventricular Hypertrophy

The ECG usually demonstrates left ventricular preponderance in patients with aortic regurgitation. Left-axis deviation and increased left ventricular

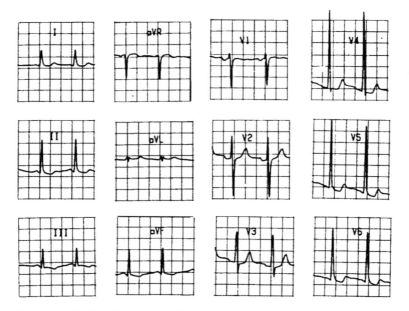

Figure 5 ECG evidence of left ventricular hypertrophy with diastolic overload pattern (see text for details) obtained from a patient with severe aortic regurgitation.

voltage are common. In moderate aortic regurgitation, the diastolic overload pattern of the left ventricle is seen in the lateral leads (I, aV1, V_3-V_6), which often demonstrates a small Q wave, a tall R wave, an isoelectric S-T segment, and an upright T wave. With more severe degrees of aortic regurgitation, the S-T segment may be depressed, down-sloping or both, and the T waves are inverted in the lateral leads (131).

In acute aortic regurgitation, the ECG may or may not show left ventricular hypertrophy, despite the presence of left ventricular failure, depending on the severity and duration of regurgitation (22). However, nonspecific S-T segment and T-wave changes are common.

B. Complicating Arrhythmias

1. Conduction Defects

Intraventricular conduction defects occur late in aortic regurgitation and are usually associated with left ventricular dysfunction. Prolonged PR intervals, Mobitz type I, AV block, or bundle branch blocks may be seen in patients with aortic regurgitation secondary to inflammatory processes and most frequently when secondary to rheumatoid arthritis, ankylosing spondylitis, or lupus erythymatosus (132). Also, conduction defects may be seen with aortic regurgitation secondary to severe calcific aortic valve disease.

2. Ventricular Arrhythmias

Ventricular arrhythmias do not usually occur with aortic regurgitation unless congestive heart failure is present.

VII. TRICUSPID STENOSIS

A. Electrocardiographic Abnormalities (Fig. 6)

1. Right Atrial Enlargement

The most characteristic ECG feature is pulmunale with tall, peaked P waves which exceed 0.3 mV in leads II, III, aVF, and V1 (133,134). Prolongation of the PR interval may coexist, and depression of the PR segment—resulting from increased magnitude of the atrial T wave—may also be seen. Since most patients with tricuspid stenosis have mitral valve disease, the ECG findings of biatrial enlargement with abnormally tall, broad P waves in leads II, III, and aVF and common positive and negative deflection in V1 are commonly found. Right atrial dilatation may rotate the ventricular septum and affect QRS morphology in such a manner that the large volume of the right atrium between the exploring electrode and

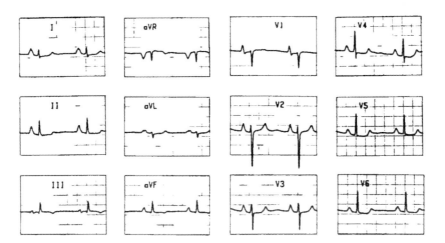

Figure 6 P pulmonale in a patient with severe tricuspid stenosis. Note the tall, peaked P waves in the inferior and anterior leads.

the ventricles reduces the amplitude of the QRS complex in V1 (which often has a Q wave), whereas the QRS complex is much taller in V2 (22).

B. Complicating Arrhythmias

1. Atrial Fibrillation

Atrial fibrillation is seen in less than one-third of patients with tricuspid stenosis, and such patients have a high incidence of sinus rhythm, seen in at least two-thirds of patients—which is somewhat remarkable considering the advanced degree of rheumatic involvement usually present with tricuspid stenosis.

VIII. TRICUSPID REGURGITATION

A. Electrocardiographic Findings

1. Biatrial Enlargement (Fig. 7)

The ECG findings of tricuspid regurgitation are usually masked by the changes caused by associated mitral or aortic valvular involvement and attendent pulmonary hypertension. Usually less than 20% of patients with tricuspid regurgitation present with sinus rhythm. Almost all patients who are in sinus rhythm demonstrate ECG findings of bi-atrial enlargement, which include broad and notched P waves in the limb leads and a large negative component of biphasic P wave in the right precordial leads (135).

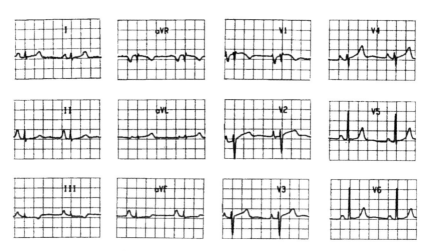

Figure 7 ECG evidence of bi-atrial enlargement commonly seen in patients with tricuspid regurgitation and normal sinus rhythm (see text for details).

ECG evidence of right atrial enlargement is relatively uncommon, but definite Q waves in lead V1 are seen in about 44% of patients, felt to be related to right atrial enlargement (136).

2. Right Ventricular Hypertrophy

Voltage criteria for right ventricular hypertrophy are usually seen in about one-third of patients with tricuspid regurgitation; 65% of them show some form of right bundle branch block. Although incomplete right bundle branch block was seen in about half of patients with tricuspid regurgitation, complete right bundle branch block is relatively uncommon and is seen in only about 4% of cases (135).

B. Complicating Arrhythmias

1. Atrial Fibrillation

Chronic atrial fibrillation is common and is seen in more than 80% of patients with tricuspid regurgitation (135).

2. Ebstein's Anomaly and Tricuspid Regurgitation

Wolf-Parkinson-White pattern with right-sided accessory pathways is seen in 5–10% of these patients. Evidence of right atrial dilatation is often seen, with peaked P waves and a deep Q wave in V1 (136). Complete or incomplete right bundle branch block is usually present. The PR interval is prolonged in about one-third of patients. Supraventricular arrhythmias, generally paroxysmal, are common; and ventricular arrhythmias are also seen and may be a significant cause of morbidity and mortality.

C. Traumatic Tricuspid Regurgitation

Conduction disturbances are specially common in this group: 92% of these patients have complete or incomplete right bundle branch block, and 41% have an additional component of left anterior (23%) or left posterior (18%) hemi block. Supraventricular arrhythmias are usually seen in 41%, which is significantly less than tricuspid regurgitation secondary to pulmonary hypertension and left heart disease (137).

IX. PULMONARY STENOSIS

A. Electrocardiographic Findings (Fig. 8)

1. Right Ventricular Hypertrophy

The ECG may be normal in mild pulmonary stenosis; however, in moderate to severe disease, a right ventricular hypertrophy pattern is generally

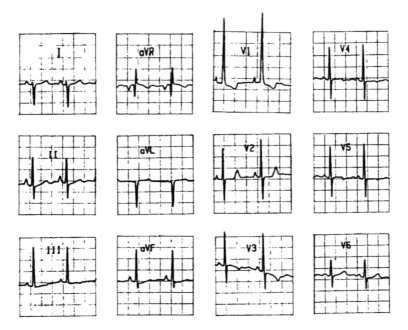

Figure 8 ECG obtained from an 18-year-old male with severe congenital pulmonary stenosis. Note the ECG evidence of right ventricular and right atrial enlargement (see text for details).

evident (138). In mild pulmonary stenosis the ECG may be normal or show anterior axis rotation in the precordial leads, with R/S in V1 equal to or greater than 1.0. In severe pulmonary stenosis the R is generally dominant in V1 (typically 10 mm in children), with a deep S wave in V6. T-wave inversion may or may not appear in V1 to V4. The presence of these changes usually indicates a right ventricular systolic pressure greater than 100 mmHg (139,140); however, there absence does not exclude this degree of right ventricular hypertension.

2. Right Atrial Enlargement
If it is present, P pulmonale indicates severe pulmonic stenosis, though it is an insensitive sign.

B. Complicating Arrhythmias

1. Tachyarrhythmias
Although arrhythmias are very uncommon in isolated pulmonary stenosis, they occasionally pose a problem in the immediate postoperative period

(141). Tachyarrhythmias, both supraventricular as well as ventricular, can occur and are possibly due to ischemia of the hypertrophied right ventricle.

X. PULMONARY REGURGITATION

A. Electrocardiographic Changes

1. Right Ventricular Hypertrophy

The ECG is usually normal. The presence of right ventricular hypertrophies suggests superimposed pulmonary hypertension (142).

REFERENCES

1. Cooksey JD, Dunn M, Massie E. Clinical Vectocardiography and Electrocardiography. 2d ed. Chicago: Year Book Medical Publishers, 1977:272.
2. Kasser I, Kennedy JW. The relationship of increased left atrial volume and pressure to abnormal P waves on the electrocardiogram. Circulation 1969; 39:339.
3. Wood P. An appreciation of mitral stenosis. Br Med J 1954; 1:1051, 1113.
4. Unverferth DV, Fertel RH, Unverferth BJ, Leier CV. Arterial fibrillation in mitral stenosis: histologic, hemodynamic and metabolic factors. Int J Cardiol 1984; 5:143.
5. Mounsey P. The atrial electrocardiogram as a guide to prognosis after mitral valvulotomy. Br Heart J 1961; 21:617.
6. Morganroth J, et al. Relationship of atrial fibrallatory wave amplitude to left atrial size and etiology of heart disease. Am Hear J 1979; 97:184.
7. Garber EB, Morgan MG, Glasser SP. Left atrial size in patients with atrial fibrillation. An echo-cardiographic study. Am J Med Sci 1976; 272:57.
8. Cueto J, Toshima J, Armyo G, Tuna N, Lillehei CW. Vectorcardiographic studies in acquired valvular disease with reference to the diagnosis of right ventricular hypertrophy. Circulation 1967; 33:588.
9. Taymor RC, Hoffman I, Henry E. The Frank vectorcardiogram in mitral stenosis. Circulation 1964; 30:865.
10. Henry WL, Morganroth J, Pearman AS, Clark CE, Redwood DR, Itscoitz SB, Epstein SE. Relationship between echocardiographically determined left atrial size and atrial fibrillation. Circulation 1976; 53:273.
11. Probst P, Goldschlager N, Selzer A. Left atrial size and atrial fibrillation in mitral stenosis: factors influencing their relationship. Circulation 1973; 48:1281.
12. Deverall PB, et al. Incidence of systemic embolism before and after mitral valvotomy. Thorax, 1968; 23:530.
13. Lorell BH, Grossman W. dynamic and isometric exercises during cardiac catheterisation. In: Grossman W, ed. Cardiac Catheterisation and Angiography. 3d ed. Philadelphia: Lea & Febiger, 1986:P251.

14. Selzer A. Effects of atrial fibrillation upon the circulation in patients with mitral stenosis. Am Heart J 1960; 59:518.
15. Arandi DT, Carleton RA. The deleterious role of tachycardia in mitral stenosis. Circulation 1967; 36:511.
16. Dalen JE. Mitral stenosis. In: Dalen JE, Alpert JS, eds. Valvular Heart Disease. 2d ed. Boston: Little, Brown, 1987:49.
17. Gorlin R, Gorlin SG. Hydraulic formula for calculation of the area of stenotic mitral valve, other cardiac valves and central circulatory shunts. Am Heart J 1951; 41:1.
18. Nakhjavan FK, Katz MR, Maranhao V, Goldberg H. Analysis of influence of catecholamine and tachycardia during supine exercise in patients with mitral stenosis and sinus rhythm. Br Heart J 1969; 31:753.
19. Bhatia ML, Shrivastava S, Roy SB. Immediate hemodynamic effects of beta adrenergic blocking agent, propanolol in mitral stenosis at fixed heart rates. Br Heart J 1972; 34:638.
20. Meister SG, Engel TR, Feitosa GS, et al. Propranolol in mitral stenosis during stress rhythm. Am Heart J 1977; 94:685.
21. Giuffrida G, Bonzani G, Betocchi S, et al. Hemodynamic response to exercise after propranolol in patients with mitral stenosis. Am J Cardiol 1979; 44:1076.
22. Braunwald E. Valvular heart disease. In: Braunwald E, ed. Heart Disease: A Text Book of Cardiovascular Medicine. 3d ed. Philadelphia: Saunders, 1988:1023.
23. Goldman MJ. The management of chronic atrial fibrillation, indications for and method of conversion to sinus rhythmn. Prog Cardiovasc Dis 1960; 2: 465.
24. Mancini GBJ, Goldberger AL. Cardioversion of atrial fibrillation: consideration of embolisation anticoagulation, prophylactic pacemaker and long term success. Am Heart J 1982; 104:617.
25. Levine HJ. Which atrial fibrillation patients should be on chronic anticoagulation? J Cardiovasc Med 1981; 6:843.
26. Szekely P. Systemic embolistiobn and anticoagulant prophylaxis in rheumatic heart disease. Br Med J 1964; 1:1209.
27. Sherrid MV, Clark RD, Cohn K. Echocardiographic analysis of left atrial size before and after operation in mitral valve disease. Am J Cardiol 1979; 43:171.
28. Coulshed N, et al. Systemic embolism in mitral valve disease. Br Heart J 1970; 32:26.
29. Bannister RG. The risks of deferring valvotomy in patients with moderate mitral stenosis. Lancet 1960; 2:329.
30. Bentoviglio LG, Uricchio JF, Waldow A, Likoff W, Goldberg H. An electrocardiographic analysis of mitral regurgitation. Circulation 1956; 18: 572.
31. Morris JJ, Estes E II, Whalen RE, et al. P wave analysis in valvular heart disease. Circulation 1964; 29:242.

32. Peter RH, Morris JJ Jr, McIntosh HD. Relationship of fibrillatory waves and P waves in the electrocardiogram. Circulation 1966; 33:599.

33. Josephson ME, Kastor JA, Morganroth J. Electrocardio-graphic left atrial enlargement. Electrophysiologic, echocardiographic and haemodynamic correlates. Am J Cardiology 1977; 39:967.

34. Fisch C. Electrocardiography and vectorcardiography. In: Braunwald E, ed. Heart Disease: A Text Book of Cardiovascular Medicine. 3d ed. Philadelphia: Saunders, 1988:180.

35. Diagnosis and investigation of rheumatic and nonrheumatic mitral valve disease. In: Hall RJ, Julian DG, eds. Diseases of the Cardiac Valves. New York: Churchill Livingstone 1989:176.

35a. Neikkila J. Mitral incompetence complicating acute myocardial infarction. Br Heart J 1967; 29:162.

36. Burch GE, DePasquale NP, Phillips JH. The syndrome of papillary muscle dysfunction. Am Heart J 1968; 75:399.

37. Bailey GWH, Braniff BA, Hancock EW, Cohn KE. Relation of left atrial pathology to atrial fibrillation in mitral valvular disease. Ann Intern Med 1968; 69:13.

38. Rheumatic mitral valve disease. In: Hall RJ, Julian DG, eds. Diseases of the Cardiac Valves. New York: Churchill Livingstone, 1989:176.

39. Pocock WA. Mitral leaflet billowing and prolapse. In: Barlow JB, ed. Perspectives on the Mitral Valve. Philadelphia: Davis, 1987:45.

40. Pocock WA, Barlow JB. Etiology and electrocardio-graphic features of the billowing posterior mitral leaflet syndrome: analysis of a further 130 patients with a late systolic murmur or non ejection systolic click. Am J Med 1971; 51:731.

41. Cobbs BW. Clinical recognition and medical management of rheumatic heart disease and other acquired valvular heart disease. In: Hurst JW, Logna RB, Schlant RC, Wenger NK, eds. The Heart. 3d ed. New York: McGraw-Hill, 1974:883.

42. Newman H, et al. Relation of left ventricular function and prognosis in hypertrophic cardiomyopathy: an angiographic study. J Am Coll Cardiol 1985; 5:1064.

43. Abinader EG. Adrenergic beta blockade and ECG changes in the systolic click murmur syndrome. Am Heart J 1976; 91:297.

44. Sloman G, Stannard M, Hare WSG, Goble AH, Hunt D. Prolapse of the posterior leaflet of the mitral valve. Israel J Med Sci 1969; 5:727.

45. Barlow JB, Pocock WA. The problem of non ejection systolic clicks and associated mitral systolic murmurs: emphasis on the billowing mitral leaflet syndrome. Am Heart J 1975; 90:636.

46. Procacci PM, Saravan SV, Schreiter SL, et al. Prevalence of clinical mitral valve prolapse in 1169 young women. N Engl J Med 1976; 294:1086.

47. Markiewicz W, Stoner J, London E, et al. Mitral valve prolapse in one hundred presumably healthy young females. Circulation 1976; 53:64.

48. Massie B, Botvinick EH, Shames D, et al. Myocardial perfusion scinitgraphy in patients with mitral valve prolapse. Circulation 1978; 57:19.

49. Wooley CF. Where are the diseases of yesteryear? Da Costa's syndrome, soldier's heart, the effort syndrome, neurocirculatory asthenia—and the mitral valve prolapse syndrome. Circulation 1976; 53:749.

50. Winkle RA, Lopes MG, Fitzgerald JW, Goodman DJ, Schroder JS, Harrison DC. Arrhythmias in patients with mitral valve prolapse. Circulation 1975; 52:73.

51. Savage DD, Levy D, Garrison RJ, Catelli WP, Kligfield P, Devereux RB, Anderson SJ, Kannel WB, Feinleib M. Mitral valve prolapse in the general population. 3: Dysrhythmias: The Framingham study. Am Heart J 1983; 106:582.

52. Kreisman K, Kleiger R, Schad N. Arrhythmia in prolapse of the mitral valve (abstr). Circulation 1971; 43(suppl 2):137.

53. Brodsky M, Wu D, Denes P, Kanakis C, Rosen KM. Arrhythmias documented by 24 hour continuous electrocardiographic monitoring in 50 male students without apparent heart disease. Am J Cardiol 1977; 39:390.

54. Sobotka PA, Moyer JH, Bauernfeind RA, Kanakis C, Rosen KM. Arrhythmias documented by a 24-hour continuous ambulatory electrocardiographic monitoring in young women without apparent heart disease. Am Heart J 1981; 101:753.

55. Kligfield P, Devereux RB. Arrhythmias in mitral valve prolapse. Clin Progr Electrophysiol Pacing 1985; 3:403.

56. Kramer HM, Kligfield P, Devereux RB, Savage DD, Kramer-Fox R. Arrhythmias in mitral valve prolapse: effect of selection bias. Arch Intern Med 1984; 144:2360.

57. Gooch AS, Vicencio F, Maranhao V, Goldberg H. Arrhythmias and left ventricular asynergy in the prolapsing mitral leaflet syndrome. Am J Cardiol 1972; 29:611.

58. Chesler E, King RA, Edwards JE. The myxomatous mitral valve and sudden death. Circulation 1983; 67:632.

59. Hutchings GM, Moore GW, Skoog DK. The association of floppy mitral valve with disjunction of the mitral annulus fibrosus. N Engl Med J 1986; 314:535.

60. Shrivastava S, Guthrie RB, Edwards JE. Prolapse of the mitral valve. Mod Concepts Cardiovasc Dis 1977; 46:57.

61. Salazar AE, Edwards JE. Friction lesions of ventricular endocardium: relation to chordae tendinae of mitral valve. Arch Pathol 1970; 90:364.

62. Cobbs BW, King SB. Ventricular buckling: a factor in the normal ventriculogram and peculiar hemodynamics associated with mitral valve prolapse. Am Heart J 1977; 93:741.

63. Gornick CC, Tobler HG, Pritzker MC, Tuna IC, Almquist A, Benditt DG. Electrophysiologic effects of papillary muscle traction in the intact heart. Circulation 1986; 73:1013.

64. Mason JW, Koch FH, Billingham ME, Winkle RA. Cardiac biopsy evidence for a cardiomyopathy associated with symptomatic mitral valve prolapse. Am J Cardiol 1978; 42:557.

65. Bharati S, Granston AS, Liebson PR, Loeb HS, Rosen KM, Lev M. The conduction system in mitral valve prolapse syndrome with sudden death. Am Heart J 1981; 101:667.

66. Wellens HJJ, Duren DR, Lie KI. Observations on mechanisms of ventricular tachycardia in man. Circulation 1976; 54:237.

67. Crawford MH, O'Rourke RA. Mitral valve prolapse: a cardiomyopathic state? Prog Cardiovasc Dis 1984; 27:133.

68. Chesler E, King RA, Edwards JE. The myxomatous mitral valve and sudden death. Circulation 1983; 67:632.

69. Maron BJ, et al. "Malignant" hypertrophic cardiomyopathy: identification of a subgroup of families with unusually frequent premature death. Am J Cardiol 1978; 41:1133.

70. Puddu PE, Pasternac A, Tubau JF, Krol R, Farley L, de Champlain J. QT interval prolongation and increased plasma catecholamine levels in patients with mitral valve prolapse. Am Heart J 1983; 105:422.

71. Bekheit SG, Ali AA, Deglin SM, Jain AC. Analysis of QT interval in patients with idiopathic mitral valve prolapse. Chest 1982; 81:620.

72. Boudoulas H, Reynolds JC, Mazzaferri E, Wooley CF. Mitral valve prolapse syndrome: the effect of adrenergic stimulation. J Am Coll Cardiol 1983; 2:638.

73. Gaffney AF, Karlsson ES, Campbell W, Schutte JE, Nixon JV, Willerson JT, Blomqvist CG. Autonomic dysfunction in women with mitral valve prolapse syndrome. Circulation 1979; 59:894.

74. Coghlan HC, Phares P, Cowley M, Copley D, James TN. Dysautonomia in mitral valve prolapse. Am J Med 1979; 67:236.

75. Winkle RA, Lopes MG, Fitzgerald JW, et al. Propranolol for patients with mitral valve prolapse. Am Heart J 1977; 93:422.

76. Gooch AS, Viccencio F, Maranhao V, Goldberg H. Arrhythmias and left ventricular asynergy in the prolapsing mitral leaflet syndrome. Am J Cardiol 1972; 29:611.

77. Jeresaty RM. Mitral Valve Prolapse. New York: Raven Press, 1979:251.

78. Pratt CM, Young JB, Wierman AM, Borland RM, Seals AA, Leon CA, Raizner A, Quinones MA, Roberts R. Complex ventricular arrhythmias associated with the mitral valve prolapse syndrome. Am J Med 1986; 80: 626.

79. DeMaria AN, Amsterdam EA, Vismara LA, Neumann A, Mason DT. Arrhythmias in the mitral valve prolapse syndrome. Ann Intern Med 1976; 84:656.

80. Levy PS, Blanc A, Clementy J, Dallocchio M, Bricaud H. Prolapsus valvulaire mitral: les troubles du rhythme ontils un substratum electrophysiologique? Arch Mal Coeur 1982; 75:671.

81. Josephson ME, Horowitz LN, Kastor J. Paroxysmal supraventricular tachycardia in patients with mitral valve prolapse. Circulation 1978; 57:111.

82. Gallagher JJ, Gilbert M, Svenson RH. Wolff-Parkinson-White syndrome. The problem, evaluation and surgical correction. Circulation 1975; 57:767.

83. Wit AL, Fenoglio JJ, Wagner BM, Bassett AL. Electrophysiological properties of cardiac muscle in the anterior mitral valve leaflet and the adjacent atrium in the dog. Possible implications for the genesis of atrial dysrhythmias. Circ Res 1973; 32:731.

84. Wit AL, Fenoglio JJ, Hordof AJ, Reemtsma K. Ultrastructure and transmembrane potentials of cardiac muscle in the human anterior mitral valve leaflet. Circulation 1979; 59:1283.

85. Dobmeyer DJ, Stine RA, Leier CV, Schaal SF. Electrophysiologic mechanisms of provoked atrial flutter in mitral valve prolapse syndrome. Am J Cardiol 1985; 56:602.

86. Leichtman D, Nelson R, Gobel FL, Alexander CS, Cohn JN. Bradycardia with mitral valve prolapse: a potential mechanism of sudden death. Ann Intern Med 1976; 85:453.

87. Ware JA, Magro SA, Luck JC, Mann D, Nielson AP, Rosen KM, Wyndham CR. Conduction system abnormalities in symptomatic mitral valve prolapse: an electrophysiologic analysis of 60 patients. Am J Cardiol 1984; 53: 1075.

88. Andre-Fouet X, Tabib A, Jean-Louis P, Anne D, Dutertre P, Gayet C, De Mahange AH, Loire R, Pont M. Mitral valve prolapse, Wolff-Parkinson-White syndrome, His bundle sclerosis and sudden death. Am J Cardiol 1985; 56:700.

89. Schaal SF, Fontana MB, Wooley CF. Mitral valve prolapse: spectrum of conduction defects and arrhythmias (abstr). Circulation 1974; 50(suppl 3):97.

90. Chandraratna PA, Ribas-Meneclier C, Littman BB, Samet P. Conduction disturbances in patients with mitral valve prolapse. J Electrocardiol 1977; 10:233.

91. Bharti S, Rosen KM, Miller LB, Strasberg B, Lev M. Sudden death in three teenagers (abstr). Circulation 1981; 64(suppl 4):71.

92. Coghlan HC, Phares P, Cowley M, Copley D, James TN. Dysautonomia in mitral valve prolapse. Am J Med 1979; 67:236.

93. Gaffney FA, Bastian BC, Lane LB, Taylor WF, Horton J, Schutte JE, Graham RM, Pettinger W, Blomqvuist G. Abnormal cardiovascular regulation in the mitral valve prolapse syndrome. Am J Cardiol 1983; 52:316.

94. Devereaux RB, Perloff JK, Reichek N, Josephson MD. Mitral valve prolapse. Circulation 1976; 54:2.

95. Wood P. Aortic stenosis. Am J Cardiol 1958; 1:553.

96. Hancock EW. Valvular heart disease. In: Rubenstein E, Federman DD, eds. Scientific American Medicine. New York: Scientific American, Inc., 1985; 1:XI.

97. Schwartz LS, et al. Syncope and sudden death in aortic stenosis. Am J Cardiol 1969; 23:647.

98. Eddleman EE Jr, et al. Critical analysis of clinical factors in estimating severity of aortic valve disease. Am J Cardiol 1973; 31:687.

99. Siegel RJ, Roberts WC. Electrocardiographic observations in severe aortic valve stenosis: correlative necropsy study to clinical, hemodynamic and

ECG variables demonstrating relation of 12-lead QRS amplitude to peak systolic transaortic pressure gradient. Am Heart J 1982; 103:201.

100. Jones RC, Walker WJ, Jahnke EJ, Winn DF. Congenital aortic stenosis. Correlation of clinical severity with hemodynamic and surgical findings in forty-three cases. Ann Intern Med 1963; 58:486.

101. Romhilt DW, Bove KE, Norris RJ. A critical appraisal of the electrocardiographic criteria for the diagnosis of left ventricular hypertrophy. Circulation 1969; 40:185.

102. Bruns DL, van der Hauwaert LG. Aortic systolic murmur developing with increasing age. Br Heart J 1958; 20:370.

103. Roberts WC, et al. Congenitally bicuspid aortic valve causing severe, pure aortic regurgitation without superimposed infective endocarditis. Analysis of 13 patients requiring aortic valve replacement. Am J Cardiol 1981; 47: 206.

104. Rosenbaum M, Elizari M, Lazari J. Los Hemibloques. Buenos Aires: Paidos, 1968:363.

105. Gooch AS, Calatayud JB, Rogers PA, Garman PA. Analysis of the P wave in severe aortic stenosis. Dis Chest 1966; 49:459.

106. Sutnick AI, Soloff LA. P wave abnormalities as an electrocardiographic index of hemodynamically significant aortic stenosis. Circulation 1963; 28: 814.

107. Klein RC. Ventricular arrhythmias in aortic valve disease: analysis of 102 patients. Am J Cardiol 1984; 53:1079.

108. Olshausen KV, Schwarz F, Apfelbach J, Rohrig N, Kramer B, Kubler W. Determinants of the incidence and severity of ventricular arrhythmias in aortic valve disease. Am J Cardiol 1983; 51:1103.

109. Gaasch WH. Left ventricular radius to wall thickness ratio. Am J Cardiol 1979; 43:1189.

110. Strauer BE. Myocardia oxygen consumption in chronic heart disease: role of wall stress, hypertrophy and coronary reserve. Am J Cardiol 1979; 44: 730.

111. Peterson KL, Tsuji J, Johnson A, Didonna J, Le Winter M. Diastolic left pressure-volume and stress-strain relations in patients with valvular aortic stenosis and left ventricular hypertrophy. Circulation 1978; 58:77.

112. Johnson LL, Sciacca RR, Ellis K, Weiss MB, Cannon PJ. Reduced left ventricular myocardial blood flow per unit mass in aortic stenosis. Circulation 1978; 57:582.

113. Vincent WR, Buckberg GD, Hoffman JIE. Left ventricular subendocardial ischemia in severe valvar and supravalvar aortic stenosis: a common mechanism. Circulation 1974; 49:326.

114. Buckberg G, Eber L, Helman M, Gorlin R. Ischemia in aortic stenosis hemodynamic prediction. Am J Cardiol 1975; 35:778.

115. Shipley RA, Shipley LJ, Wearn JT. The capillary supply in normal and hypertrophied hearts of rabbits. J Exp Med 1937; 65:29.

116. Roberts JT, Wearn JT. Quantitative changes in the capillary-muscle relationship in human hearts during normal growth and hypertrophy. Am Heart J 1941; 21:617.

117. Gunther S, Grossman W. Determinants of ventricular function in pressure-overload hypertrophy in man. Circulation 1979; 59:679.

118. Brodie BR, McLaurin LP, Grossman W. Combined hemodynamic-ultrasonic method for studying left ventricular wall stress. Am J Cardiol 1976; 37:964.

119. Thompson R, Mitchell A, Ahmed M, Towers M, Yacoub M. Conduction defects in aortic valve disease. Am Heart J 1979; 98:2.

120. Rasmussen K, Thomsen PEB, Bagger JP. H V interval in calcific aortic stenosis. Relation to left ventricular function and effect of valve replacement. Br Heart J 1984; 52:82.

121. Nair CK, Aronow WS, Stokke K, Mohiuddin SM, Thomson W, Sketch MH. Cardiac conduction defects in patients older than 60 years with aortic stenosis and without mitral annular calcium. Am J Cardiol 1984; 53:169.

122. Hohn AR, van Praagh S, Moore AAD, Vlad P, Lambert EC. Aortic stenosis. Circulation 1965; 32(suppl):111.

123. Flamm MM, Braniff BA, Kimball R, Hancock EW. Mechanism of effort syncope in aortic stenosis (abstr). Circulation 1967; 35(suppl II):109.

124. Leake D. Effort syncope in aortic stenosis. Br Heart J 1959; 21:289.

125. Dhingra RC, Amat-y-Leon F, Pletras RJ, Wyndham C, Deedwania PC, Wu D, Denes P, Rosen KM. Sites of conduction disease in aortic stenosis. Significance of valve gradient and calcification. Ann Intern Med 1977; 87: 275.

126. Campbell M. Calcific aortic stenosis and congenital bicuspid aortic valves. Br Heart J 1968; 30:606.

127. Smith N, McAnulty JG, Rahimtoola SH. Severe aortic stenosis with impaired left ventricular function and clinical heart failure: results of valve replacement. Circulation 1978; 58:255.

128. Rahimtoola SH. Valvular heart disease: a perspective. J Am Coll Cardiol 1983; 1:199.

129. Blackstone EH, Kirklin JW. Death and other time-related events after valve replacement. Circulation 1985; 72:735.

130. Konish Y, Matsuda K, Mishiwaki N, et al. Ventricular arrhythmias late after aortic and/or mitral valve replacement. Jap Circ J 1985; 49:576.

131. Estes EH. Left ventricular hypertrophy in acquired heart disease: a comparison of the vectorcardiogram in aortic stenosis and aortic insufficiency. In Hoffman I, ed. Vectorcardiography. Amsterdam: North Holland, 1976.

132. Toone EC, Pierce EL, Hennigar GR. Aortitis and aortic regurgitation associated with rheumatoid spondylitis. Am J Med 1959; 26:255.

133. Perloff JK, Harvey WP. Clinical recognition of tricuspid stenosis. Circulation 1960; 52/346.

134. Gibson R, Wood P. The diagnosis of tricuspid stenosis. Br Heart J 1955; 17:552.

135. Salazar E, Levine HD. Rheumatic tricuspid regurgitation. The clinical spectrum. Am J Med 1962; 33:111.
136. Sodi-Pillares D, Bisteni A, Herrmann GR. Some views on the significance of R and QR type of complexes in right precordial leads in the absence of myocardial infarction. Am Heart J 1952; 43:716.
137. Marvin RF, Schrank JP, Nolan SP. Traumatic tricuspid insufficiency. Am J Cardiol 1973; 32:723.
138. Silverman BK, et al. Pulmonary stenosis with intact ventricular septum. Correlation of clinical and physiological data, with review of operative results. Am J Med 1956; 20:53.
139. Campbell M. Simple pulmonary stenosis. Pulmonary valvular stenosis with a closed ventricular septum. Br Heart J 1954; 16:273.
140. Abrahams DG, Wood P. Pulmonary stenosis with normal aortic root. Br Heart J 1951; 13:519.
141. Deverall PB, Roberts NK, Start J. Arrhythmias in children with pulmonary stenosis. Br Heart J 1970; 32:472.
142. Holmes JC, Fowler NO, Kaplan S. Pulmonary valvular insufficiency. Am J Med 1968; 44:851.

15

Pregnancy and Valvular Heart Disease

Celia M. Oakley
Hammersmith Hospital and The Royal Postgraduate Medical School, London, England

I. INTRODUCTION

Management of pregnancy in women with valvular heart disease requires understanding of the major hemodynamic changes in the cardiovascular system which occur during pregnancy, labor, and delivery, and of the likely effects of these changes on the valve disease so that the hemodynamic consequences of pregnancy can be anticipated.

A. Cardiorespiratory Changes in Pregnancy, Labor, and the Puerperium

Pregnancy induces changes in blood volume and cardiac output (1,2). The blood volume starts to rise very early in pregnancy, secondary to hormonally induced relaxation of smooth muscle, which increases the capacitance of the venous bed. Both plasma and red cell volume rise, and a greater rise in plasma volume than in red cell volume accounts for the physiological anemia of pregnancy (3). With the gradual rise in blood volume is an accompanying rise in the stroke volume with negligible increase in the resting heart rate. By the last trimester of pregnancy the blood volume and the stroke volume are increased by 30–50% above the nonpregnant value. The increase in both blood volume and stroke volume is even greater in multiple pregnancies. Echocardiographic imaging with Doppler has been used serially in healthy women with documentation of increases in left ventricular cavity size, indices of contractility and stroke output (4–6). These changes revert to normal after delivery, rapidly in the first week but then more slowly, taking up to a month in all.

In the last trimester of pregnancy the uterus causes mechanical obstruction to venous return to the heart through the inferior vena cava (7). This obstruction is present only in the supine position and results in a fall in right atrial pressure and in stroke volume compared with measurements made with the mother in the lateral position. Measurements of cardiac output made in the supine position gave rise to the myth that the cardiac output rises to a maximum at around 20–24 weeks but then does not rise further during the rest of the pregnancy (7). The cardiac output continues to rise through pregnancy, with an increasing proportion of the increase going to the uterine circulation.

1. Respiratory Response to Pregnancy

Other changes in pregnancy are an increase in oxygen uptake (8) and an increase in ventilation (9). Tidal volume is reduced in late pregnancy, and respiratory frequency is increased. During pregnancy, the functional residual capacity of the lungs is reduced by the raised diaphragm but vital capacity is unchanged and there is a fall in airway resistance (10). The increase in cardiac output is greater than the increase in oxygen consumption in normal healthy women. Resting oxygen consumption increases by about 30% and is caused largely by the requirement of the pregnant uterus and the increased work of breathing. Oxygen consumption rises more during exercise than in the nonpregnant state due to diminished efficiency from the added weight. Pregnant women hyperventilate, and arterial PCO_2 is 10 mmHg lower than in the nonpregnant state. This persists during exercise. Arterial pH is maintained at 7.40 by a compensatory drop in bicarbonate (11).

2. Cardiovascular Symptoms and Signs in Pregnancy

Symptoms of normal pregnancy may mimic those of cardiopulmonary disease. These include diminished exercise tolerance with complaint of dyspnea and fatiguability. Peripheral edema is common in late pregnancy due to increased sodium and water retention, mechanical compression of the inferior vena cava, and increased venous pressure in the legs. Physical signs include hot hands with dilated veins, sometimes "hepatic" palms, venous pressure increased up to 5 cm above the clavicle with prominent pulsation, slightly reduced blood pressure (but an increased blood pressure response to exercise), sometimes basal crackles in the lungs, and leg edema in later pregnancy. The heart is displaced upward and to the left. Changes in the heart sounds include a loud first heart sound, exaggerated splitting of the second heart sound, and a third heart sound at the apex which is nearly always audible (12). A fourth heart sound is less frequently heard. Systolic ejection murmurs are almost universal, best heard at the apex and left sternal edge and often remarkably loud. As with innocent murmurs in childhood, these vary with posture and are unaccompanied by any other pathological finding. Thrills and diastolic murmurs are always pathological. These changes in the cardiovascular signs in pregnancy most closely simulate those of atrial septal defect—which is easily excluded or confirmed by echocardiography.

The electrocardiographic response to change in cardiac position and hyperventilation include axis shift and repolarization changes.

3. Labor, Delivery, and the Puerperium

Cardiovascular changes during labor and delivery are influenced by pain and anxiety levels, posture, analgesia and anesthesia, mode of delivery, and by drugs and anesthetic agents.

Cardiac output increases with each contraction during labor, systolic and diastolic blood pressure rises, and the heart rate may swing widely. The rise in cardiac output and blood pressure which increase as labor progresses is attenuated by pain relief and further reduced by epidural analgesia and by supine position (13,14). Epidural or spinal anesthesia causes a fall in blood pressure and cardiac output. General anesthesia is associated with minimal change in heart rate, blood pressure, and cardiac output except during intubation and extubation (14).

A further increase in cardiac output occurs immediately postpartum, with a rise in central venous pressure (15). This is caused by increased blood volume, decreased uterine blood flow, and absence of inferior vena caval compression. This usually lasts less than an hour and is dependent on the amount of blood lost and the oxytocic agent used. These changes rapidly return toward normal with fall in blood volume and cardiac output but take up to 4 to 5 weeks to complete (3).

Prostaglandins given to induce labor have little effect on hemodynamics (16), but oxytocic drugs cause vasoconstriction, increase of central blood volume, and swings in heart rate and blood pressure (17).

Failure to increase stroke volume in pregnancy will be revealed by an increase in heart rate. Tachycardia thus indicates a reduction in cardiovascular reserve (18). This does not matter in cardiac disorders with rapid ventricular filling and normal coronary flow demand, but in mitral valve disease, aortic stenosis or hypertrophic cardiomyopathy tachycardia is likely to cause a rise in left atrial pressure, and in aortic stenosis or hypertrophic cardiomyopathy, tachycardia may give rise to angina (19).

The reduction in venous return to the heart when the mother sits or lies supine in later pregnancy has been utilized unknowingly by obstetricians, who have traditionally kept their pregnant cardiac patients at bed

Table 1   Changes in the Blood in Pregnancy

Increase in red cell mass
Greater increase in plasma volume (so-called physiological anemia)
Increase in concentration of clotting factors II, VI, VIII, IX, and X
Increase in concentration of fibrinogen
Increase in blood velocity
Decreased deformability of erythrocytes
Increase in platelet turnover

---

rest. They had observed that mitral stenosis might be well tolerated in these supine resting patients, and they knew that uterine blood flow is optimized by rest, so the same strategy was adopted for patients with valve disease as in patients with hypertension and preeclampsia. The disadvantages of such classic management were an increase in the tendency to varicose veins and venous thrombosis and the fact that these women were separated from their families for long periods.

B. Changes in the Blood in Pregnancy

Apart from the increased plasma and red cell volume, the other pregnancy induced change which is important to patients with valvular heart disease is the hypercoagulable state (20,21). Pregnancy is associated with increased concentration of circulating clotting factors, increased platelet turnover, and reduced fibrinolytic activity (Table 1). The theoretically increased tendency to thrombosis caused by these changes is counteracted by the more rapid circulation, but there is still a heightened risk of leg vein thrombosis in later pregnancy (22,23), of left atrial thrombus formation in mitral stenosis, and of thrombosis on artificial heart valves (18,19).

C. Valvular Heart Disease in Pregnancy

Valvular heart disease seen in pregnancy may be congenital or acquired, rheumatic or nonrheumatic. While rheumatic heart disease remains the most frequently seen valve disease in young adults in the developing world, congenital disease, aortic and pulmonary stenosis or mitral regurgitation, and acquired nonrheumatic valve disease such as mitral leaflet prolapse are now more prevalent in the West.

As a general rule, most patients who are in New York Heart Association Classification Class I or IIA before pregnancy will manage pregnancy without difficulty, but there are exceptions, particularly patients with mitral stenosis (18,19).

II. RHEUMATIC HEART DISEASE

Rheumatic fever is still common in the Middle and Far East, parts of Southern Europe, and South America. Acute rheumatic fever is a serious complication of pregnancy and may be fatal during labor. Active carditis may precipitate failure in patients with established valve disease. Rheumatic fever is rare in the indigent population of Northern Europe and North America, but the large immigrant population to these territories ensures that rheumatic heart disease remains a frequently encountered problem in pregnancy. While cardiac abnormalities are usually identified in childhood or at preemployment medical examinations, heart disease in young women from medically unmonitored communities may have been unknown until they are first seen in pregnancy.

A. Mitral Valve Disease

In mitral valve disease, symptoms may have been absent or unnoticed before pregnancy or may have increased in severity since a previous pregnancy. Mitral stenosis is the dominant lesion in 90% of women with rheumatic heart disease seen in pregnancy (24) and remains the most common potentially lethal heart condition seen in pregnancy (19).

Mitral stenosis may have been missed during routine medical examination in pregnancy because the murmur is diastolic and submammary. Sinus rhythm is usual in the age group. Many patients do well, but mitral stenosis is treacherous and most complications of rheumatic heart disease in pregnancy relate to it.

Symptoms sometimes develop rapidly in patients with moderately severe but previously asymptomatic mitral stenosis (25). The first sign of impending trouble is a rise in the sinus rate without any change in rhythm and often without antecedent contributory factors such as anemia or infection. Exertion or simple anxiety may be sufficient. Tachycardia reduces the time for left atrial emptying, so that as the pressure rises, left ventricular stroke volume falls and a reflex rise in sinus rate follows (19). A vicious circle of increasing heart rate and increasing left atrial pressure is thus initiated and can lead to pulmonary edema within hours or even within minutes of the onset of shortness of breath, the anxiety caused by the dyspnea adding to the tachycardia and thus to acceleration of the problem (Fig. 1). It is noteworthy that patients with long-established mitral stenosis complicated by pulmonary hypertension are less vulnerable and may accomplish pregnancy safely though with increasing pulmonary hypertension and often the development of right-sided failure.

Most young women with mitral stenosis during pregnancy have simple commissural fusion with a well-preserved valve structure and are suitable

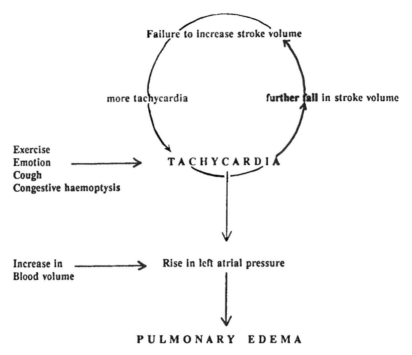

Figure 1   Mechanism of sudden development of breathlessness and pulmonary edema in mitral stenosis in pregnancy.

either for balloon angioplasty or for closed mitral valvotomy. The problem may be availability of expertise for either of these procedures, but the first need is for recognition of the situation and its immediate relief.

The patient in trouble from a rising left atrial pressure has a sinus tachycardia, low pulse pressure, usually normal venous pressure in the neck, and very often no crackles or abnormalities upon ausculation of the lungs because the edema is interstitial. The opening snap is early, usually loud (but may have been mistaken for a pulmonary closure sound), and the diastolic murmur is virtually all presystolic, leading on to a loud first sound. The ECG shows left atrial P waves, usually right-axis deviation, but not necessarily any evidence of right ventricular hypertrophy (because patients with marked pulmonary hypertension sometimes do not get into trouble in pregnancy despite severe mitral stenosis). A chest X-ray shows a small heart with a small left atrium, though with some prominence of the left atrial appendage and pulmonary venous congestion which may have been underestimated because of the pulmonary plethora of pregnancy and heavy breast shadows.

Echocardiography is a certain means of diagnosis, providing both quantitative information on severity and qualitative information concerning the anatomy of the mitral valve.

A first measure is to slow the sinus tachycardia. Relief of anxiety with a sedative plus the administration of a beta-adrenergic blocking drug such as atenolol, 50 mg, repeated as necessary, are needed first (18,19). A small dose of diuretic should be given but gives only marginal relief, and larger doses are apt to cause serious dehydration in these patients who have no overall fluid retention.

Balloon valvuloplasty has shown itself to be a very effective means of opening the mitral valve in young people with mitral stenosis, but the irradiation involved provides a relative contraindication to this method of relief during pregnancy. While it may be the method of choice in early pregnancy, closed mitral valvotomy is preferable later on in pregnancy, provided a suitably experienced surgeon is available. Open mitral valvotomy is practiced almost exclusively now in the West but is associated with a high chance of fetal loss. The skill of closed mitral valvotomy is rapidly being lost to surgeons trained in the West because it is rarely done, there being little or no indication except during pregnancy. Transesophageal echocardiography during the operation of closed mitral valvotomy provides the surgeon with a wonderful pictorial progress report, rendering the procedure no longer "blind." The Tubbs dilator can be manipulated into the mitral orifice under ultrasonic vision and the commissural split judged also by ultrasonic means. The risk of closed mitral valvotomy carried out in pregnancy is low and no higher than in the nonpregnant state. The risk of unseating the pregnancy is also remarkably small. Following operation the patient will be fit to return home to her family for the remainder of the pregnancy, can look forward to a safe delivery, and will be relieved of her symptoms to look after the new baby and the rest of her family afterwards.

If the valve is unsuitable for valvotomy or valvuloplasty or if for any reason it is not possible to relieve a stenosed mitral valve in pregnancy, then administration of a beta-blocking drug in sufficient dosage to maintain the heart rate below 90 can be used in order to secure the lowest possible left atrial pressure and prevent sudden rises in it associated with tachycardia. Digoxin should be used if atrial fibrillation occurs, but it does not slow the heart in sinus rhythm when increased sympathetic drive easily overcomes the mild vagal slowing effect of this drug. Beta-blockers should also be used prophylactically in any patient with moderately severe mitral stenosis in pregnancy, even if intervention does not seem to be required.

When the mitral valve is unsuitable for valvotomy because of regurgitation or multiple valve disease, then medical treatment is usually preferable to valve replacement or open repair during pregnancy. If it is essential, this has to be done, but there is a considerable risk of fetal loss.

Vaginal delivery with epidural anesthesia is chosen with caesarian section only for obstetric indications. The patient should be sat up promptly after delivery, and oxytocic agents, which have important vasoconstrictor effects, should be used under cover of diuretic.

B. Mixed and Multivalve Disease

Patients with more severe rheumatic heart disease, mitral regurgitation, or multiple valve disease often go through pregnancy without problems and more safely than patients with pure mitral stenosis (26). Such patients are more likely to be in atrial fibrillation, have larger left atria, and a tendency also to congestive heart failure, but the risk of pulmonary edema is less (18). It is preferable for these patients to have their babies before valve replacement rather than after.

C. Aortic Regurgitation

Aortic regurgitation is well tolerated in pregnancy. Tachycardia with its reduced diastolic interval limits regurgitant flow. The left atrial pressure does not rise because, in the absence of mitral stenosis, left ventricular filling is rapid.

Patients with severe aortic regurgitation who are going to need valve replacement should, if possible, complete their families first.

D. Mitral Regurgitation

The same arguments apply to severe mitral regurgitation without mitral valve obstruction. Systemic vasodilatation will tilt the balance in favor of forward flow. There is therefore a tendency for the patient with mitral regurgitation to improve in pregnancy when the systemic vascular resistance falls. It is doubtful whether a systemic vasodilator such as hydralazine, which is safe in pregnancy, will offer any further advantage. The patient with mitral regurgitation may suffer an increase in left atrial pressure with tachycardia because of high V waves together with diminished time for the increased mitral inflow volume to leave the left atrium during diastole.

III. NONRHEUMATIC VALVE DISEASE

A. Congenital Aortic Valve Stenosis

Isolated aortic valve stenosis is usually caused by a congenitally bicuspid aortic valve and is rarely if ever, of rheumatic origin. This congenital malformation is very common but is five times more prevalent in males than in females.

Aortic stenosis may have been asymptomatic in childhood and young adult life but is readily recognized by the loud aortic ejection systolic murmur preceded by an ejection click and followed by a loud closure sound usually without a regurgitant murmur. It tends to increase in severity through childhood because of differential growth and because of the early onset of degenerative changes in the valve even in the first decades of life and leading to calcification by the fourth or fifth decade.

Aortic stenosis is potentially serious in pregnancy because an increase in stroke output will cause an increase in left ventricular systolic pressure (27), therefore in left ventricular work, and this may not be matched by a commensurate increase in coronary blood flow to the left ventricle, which, in aortic stenosis, is entirely diastolic. If stroke volume does not increase, a reflex increase in heart rate will reduce diastolic coronary flow time and may well lead to the development of left ventricular ischemia. The shortened diastolic time may also lead to an increase in left atrial pressure because of prolonged isovolumic relaxation and prolonged left ventricular filling time. The vasodilation of pregnancy may predispose to syncope on effort, always a dangerous symptom with a risk of sudden death.

Severe aortic valve stenosis is treated by open valvotomy during childhood, and this may widen the valve orifice sufficiently for aortic valve replacement to be delayed until a woman has completed her family. Open aortic valvotomy is often still useful in a young woman, but previous valvotomy in childhood will preclude further conservative surgery should the need arise in a woman, either anticipating pregnancy or because of trouble during pregnancy. Because of the nature of the malformation, open valvotomy tends to reduce rather than remove stenosis, and the surgeon has to trade off the possible advantages of increasing the orifice size against the chance of causing aortic regurgitation. Persistence of turbulent flow ensures that deterioration of the cusps with eventual calcification continue after valvotomy. Restenosis after valvotomy carried out early in childhood may be caused by differential growth, with inevitable degenerative changes eventually reducing mobility. Balloon aortic valvuloplasty carries a high risk of inducing severe regurgitation and is an unsatisfactory procedure for congenital aortic stenosis but may give relief in emergency.

Even severe aortic valve stenosis may not have given rise to any symptoms before pregnancy. Angina and breathlessness caused by inadequate coronary flow and a rising left atrial pressure may develop during pregnancy in the absence of deterioration in systolic function. Indeed, the development of systolic left ventricular failure is uncommon in pregnancy except in cases in which congenital aortic valve stenosis was combined with disease of the ventricle such as endocardial fibroelastosis. Evidence of left ventricular hypertrophy on the ECG with marked repolarization changes indicate severe stenosis with left ventricular compromise or, occasionally, associated endocardial fibroelastosis. More often the ECG shows only voltage changes of left ventricular hypertrophy, and in such cases the new development of ST-segment depression with T-wave flattening or inversion during pregnancy gives clear evidence of new subendocardial ischemia.

If the patient is first seen in pregnancy and is asymptomatic, every effort should be made to bring the pregnancy to a successful conclusion without intervention until after delivery. Open aortic valvotomy or valve replacement will be needed if the pregnancy is still early and the patient has developed syncope, angina, or left ventricular failure. These procedures carry no additional maternal risk in pregnancy but threaten the fetus. If the pregnancy is further advanced when symptoms or evidence of left ventricular ischemia or failure develop, rest in bed will often alleviate symptoms. As most of these patients have good left ventricular systolic function with mainly diastolic failure, the use of a beta-adrenergic blocking drug slows the ventricular rate, promotes better coronary blood flow and left ventricular filling, so relieving angina and pulmonary congestion. Nitrates may be used in addition to further lower left atrial pressure and are preferable to the use of diuretics during pregnancy.

If operation can no longer be deferred and the baby is viable, the correct order of procedure is for the baby first to be delivered by caesarian section and for this to be followed by aortic valve replacement. This is because the baby can be delivered very quickly and this will be followed by some improvement in the mother's condition. On no account should the aortic valvotomy or valve replacement be carried out before delivering a viable fetus. This is because of a high risk of intrauterine fetal death during induction of anesthesia or during the period of bypass. Delivery of the baby also improves operating conditions for the surgeon and reduces the risk of postoperative respiratory problems in the mother.

B. Other Congenital Heart Disease

Mild or moderate pulmonary valve stenosis is well tolerated in pregnancy. Pulmonary valve stenosis is well treated by balloon valvuloplasty, and this can be carried out in pregnancy but only if stenosis is very severe, with syncope or right ventricular failure.

More complex congenital heart disease must be considered individually. Patients with valve-bearing conduits for complex pulmonary atresia or corrected truncus arteriosus who are in Class I or II are likely to tolerate pregnancy, but the risk of congenital heart disease in their offspring may be as high as 20% (compared to 4% for simple defects and 1% for the normal population). Patients with a Fontan circulation after operation for tricuspid atresia may not tolerate pregnancy, although at least one successful pregnancy has been reported.

Patients with Ebstein's anomaly of the tricuspid valve who are acyanotic tolerate pregnancy well, but patients with preexcitation may have more frequent episodes of tachycardia during pregnancy. Choice of drug treatment may be a problem.

C. Hypertrophic Cardiomyopathy (HOCM)

Pregnancy is usually well tolerated in HOCM (28), the hemodynamic changes with increased blood volume and stroke output tending to reduce outflow tract obstruction and the risk of syncope. Although sudden death in pregnancy has been reported in a patient being treated with verapamil, most patients do well. Beta-blocking drugs are given for angina or breathlessness, but not routinely. Amiodarone is avoided where possible, but has been used through pregnancy without abnormality or even thyroid dysfunction occurring in the offspring. Genetic counseling has not usually deterred patients from pregnancy, even when the family history included cases of sudden and early death.

D. Marfan's Syndrome and Other Hereditary Connective Tissue Disorders

Women with Marfan's syndrome may first develop complications during pregnancy (29). They run a risk of aortic dissection or of rupture of a dilated aortic root, of the development or increase in aortic or mitral regurgitation, and of heart failure. This is particularly likely when cardiovascular complications of Marfan's syndrome are already apparent and in patients with a bad family history. Dissection of the ascending aorta should be treated by immediate surgery, because death is usually caused by rupture into the pericardium.

Genetic counseling against pregnancy in families with a bad history may be necessary, and in any case, the patient with Marfan's syndrome should always have the benefit of genetic counseling in this dominantly inherited condition.

In patients with isolated aortic regurgitation or mitral valve prolapse, the possibility of Marfan's syndrome should always be considered, and Marfan's syndrome may be present even in patients who have no external ocular or skeletal stigmata or family history to suggest this diagnosis.

Patients with the dominant form of osteogenesis imperfecta with blue sclerae and a history of multiple fractures in childhood also carry a risk of developing aortic regurgitation due to aortic root dilatation or of dissection. Similar complications may occur in Ehlers-Danlos syndrome.

E. Mitral Leaflet Prolapse

Mitral leaflet prolapse became a very common diagnosis soon after the development of M-mode echocardiography, and many young women were incorrectly diagnosed as having this abnormality. This was shown in an echocardiographic study carried out in Framingham in which the incidence of mitral leaflet prolapse was up to 30% in young underweight women but down to 3%, the same as in young or middle-aged men, by the time the young underweight woman had become older and stouter. This indicated that the condition was either fatal or that the echo criteria were flawed.

At the present time, mitral leaflet prolapse is diagnosed only in patients who have physical signs of a nonejection click or clicks with a late-systolic or pansystolic murmur or evidence of prolapse with a structurally abnormal valve shown on echocardiography (30).

The "click murmur syndrome" may be due to chordal lengthening or leaflet redundancy (the floppy or ballooning mitral valve). Both tend to occur together in Marfan's syndrome, in which massive ballooning of the mitral leaflets even toward the posterior wall of the left atrium may be seen despite only slight mitral regurgitation. Dilatation of the annulus also occurs in Marfan's syndrome, as it does also in some of the other inherited abnormalities of connective tissue such as Ehler's-Danlos syndrome, osteogenesis imperfecta, pseudoxanthoma elasticum, and Morquio's syndrome. Mitral prolapse may be associated with pectus excavatum, straight back syndrome, or a long thin bodily habitus without other stigmata of Marfan's syndrome.

In the absence of Marfan's syndrome or other hereditary conditions, mitral prolapse usually carries a good prognosis even when associated with structural abnormality in the valve. The well-publicized complications of atrial and ventricular arrhythmias, atypical chest pain, and systemic embolism are in fact uncommon. Electrocardiographic abnormalities with inverted T waves in leads II, III, and AVF are sometimes seen, usually in patients with more florid prolapse.

Most patients are asymptomatic, and no problems are to be anticipated during pregnancy, when the low blood pressure and increased blood volume tends to cause disappearance of nonejection clicks and late-systolic murmurs and lessening of regurgitation. Mitral leaflet prolapse associated with mitral regurgitation is of course at risk from infective endocarditis. More severe mitral regurgitation associated with mitral prolapse should be treated by valve repair whenever possible, but the pregnancy can usually be completed safely before this is needed.

Mitral regurgitation is also seen in systemic lupus due to Libman-Sacks endocarditis. It occasionally becomes severe or may rarely progress to stenosis. It is very uncommon in pregnancy.

IV. VALVULAR PROSTHESES

A. Choice of Prosthesis

In order to avoid a need for anticoagulant treatment in pregnancy, there has been wide advocacy of the use of bioprostheses for young women with severe valve disease who need surgery and who may later wish to raise a family (15,45). Unfortunately, bioprostheses show poor durability, and this is even further diminished in children and young adults (31). Rapid deterioration is likely to occur during pregnancy because of increased calcium turnover. Moreover, bioprostheses are not immune from thromboembolism or, indeed, from valve thrombosis. Should atrial fibrillation develop, the use of oral anticoagulants through pregnancy is mandatory, and any advantage of the bioprosthesis is lost.

In countries with a continuing incidence of rheumatic heart disease in the young, mitral valve prostheses are required more often than aortic valve prostheses. Where rheumatic fever no longer occurs, the valve prostheses are more often required for congenital disease, in treatment of congenital aortic valve stenosis, with valve-bearing conduits in complex atresia, or for congenital and acquired nonrheumatic mitral valve disease in which atrial fibrillation is less likely. In patients with rheumatic mitral valve disease, atrial fibrillation will eventually develop, bringing a need for long-term use of anticoagulants to prevent embolism.

Although in justification of the practice of advising bioprostheses for young women, it is said that the risk of a second operation for valve replacement is not increased, this statement needs to be examined carefully. It is true that some published series show that the risk of a second valve replacement is no greater than the risk of a first operation, but this excludes patients requiring emergency re-replacement. Although bioprostheses usually degenerate quietly, with a gradual development of regurgitation or mixed stenosis and regurgitation, these valves can split, producing sudden massive regurgitation requiring emergency operation, and such operations carry a high risk (32). The procedure of removing a degenerated valve and replacing it with a new valve is inherently more difficult technically than the first operation, and carries a higher risk both to life and of complications. Moreover, the risk of the second operation has to be added to that of the first operation. This second operation is carried out after the woman has used the good years of her bioprosthesis to have her pregnancies, and she faces the second operation with young children. At best this means that she cannot look after her home and family for a time, but at worst, death or a major complication may deprive them of a mother who might have been fit and well for many years if she had been given a mechanical prosthesis.

Our practice is to recommend mechanical prostheses for children and young people regardless of their sex (18,19,34,35), in order to provide the best prognosis for life and health. Regardless of the question of pregnancy, it has now been shown that with longer follow-up the prognosis for patients with mechanical prostheses is better than for patients in whom bioprostheses have been implanted, and this is because of the greater need for reoperation in patients with bioprostheses (32,33). Young women with mechanical prostheses who desire pregnancy are not advised against it (60,35a,45a).

B. Management of Patients with Mechanical Prostheses During Pregnancy (Table 2)

Oral anticoagulants are continued throughout pregnancy until 2 weeks before the estimated time of delivery, when the patient is admitted to hospital and transferred to intravenous heparin in full anticoagulant doses. While mother and fetus are under continued observation, problems can be recognized immediately (19,34,35). The baby can be delivered expeditiously should a retroplacental hemorrhage occur. Intravenous heparin loses its effect within an hour of stopping the infusion. It is more easily controlled and therefore to be preferred to subcutaneous calcium heparin.

Table 2 Management of Pregnancy After Replacement with a Mechanical Valve Prosthesis

---

Continue warfarin until 2 weeks before delivery
Meticulous control (INR 2.0–2.5)
Aspirin (300 mg alternate days)
Change to IV heparin in hospital in last 2 weeks (partial thromboplastin time 1.5 to 2.0) or elective caesarian section at 38 weeks
Normal delivery
Resume IV heparin
Antibiotic cover
Back to warfarin immediately after delivery (continuing IV heparin until INR 2.5)

Elective caesarian section at 38 weeks is an alternative that avoids the need for heparin (35a). There is no need to reverse intravenous heparin before vaginal delivery, because the contracting uterus reduces blood loss and the heparin effect is quickly lost. It is more important to ensure that there is minimal break in the continuity of anticoagulation. Once the baby is delivered, oral anticoagulants are immediately restarted and heparin continued until the INR is back in the therapeutic range. In the case of emergency surgical delivery, heparin can be briefly reversed immediately before caesarian section, then restarted without pause and continued until warfarin takeover is completed.

1. Heparin

Transfer from oral anticoagulants to heparin in pregnancy has been widely advocated, particularly for the first trimester, in order to avoid the warfarin embryopathy (15,36–40), but the risk of embryopathy is low, less than 5% (41–44), and can be minimized by optimal control of the INR, which should be kept below 3.0. The use of heparin for anticoagulation during pregnancy has not been justified by evidence of safety and efficacy (45–50). A Med Line Search has revealed no published series to justify the practice, and there are numerous reports of serious problems. High doses over a prolonged period carry a risk not only of serious maternal hemorrhage (50,51,58), but a considerable risk of fetal death or prematurity due to retroplacental hemorrhage (41). Lesser complications of long-term heparin include thrombocytopenia (which adds to the haemorrhagic risk), osteopenia, and alopecia (36). The patient cannot be retained in hospital for observation throughout the pregnancy, so complications are not likely to be noticed quickly and action taken. Lower doses of heparin may be followed by thrombosis of the prosthesis (45,47,49,50,52,54,56). There is thus no justification for this practice.

2. Oral Anticoagulants

The coumarin anticoagulants have a bad reputation in pregnancy because of the observation of skeletal abnormalities and central nervous system defects in some infants born to mothers who had been given oral anticoagulants in pregnancy (41,53). These reports led to the practice of implanting bioprostheses in young women, to the practice of transferring women with mechanical prostheses to heparin either during the first 3 months of pregnancy or throughout pregnancy, and to frequent advice against contemplating pregnancy at all (15,41). These practices have so limited the experience of most cardiologists and obstetricians that, while continuing to advocate the use of bioprostheses or of heparin, most of them have no personal experience of pregnancy in women with mechanical prostheses taking oral anticoagulants.

Oral anticoagulants cross the placenta, where their anticoagulant effect is greater than in the mother. This is because of the immature fetal liver and the inability of large-molecular-size maternal liver enzymes to cross the placental barrier. The enhanced anticoagulant effect may cause hemorrhage in developing vascular cartilaginous bone, giving rise to the so-called warfarin embryopathy. The risk is greatest toward the end of the first trimester, and its magnitude is dose-dependent. The central nervous system is vulnerable to possible hemorrhage throughout the pregnancy (38,40,53).

The risk of fetal damage by coumarin drugs in pregnancy has almost certainly been exaggerated by anecdotal cases that reported disaster preferentially (41,46,54,56). Moreover, most of the anecdotal reports which were put together in the review by Hall et al. in 1980 (41) had come from the United States, where anticoagulant control was and still is much poorer than it is in Europe. This was because of the American use of thromboplastins of low responsiveness, which caused less prolongation of the prothrombin time than a standard thromboplastin for any given dose of warfarin, and their failure to adopt the international normalized ratio (INR) (57). American use of similar prothrombin time ratios to the INR used in Europe led to an increased number of major bleeding complications, which was only corrected two or three years ago with the recommendation for lower warfarin dosage aiming at prothrombin ratios of 1.5–1.7 instead of 2–2.5 as previously and equivalent to INRs of 2.5–3.5.

Most single-center series reporting the outcome of pregnancy for patients with prosthetic valves have come from countries which still have a high incidence of rheumatic heart disease and large numbers of young women with mainly mitral prostheses (42,43,45,48–50,56–59,60,61). In these countries anticoagulant control is often difficult, with a high incidence of both hemorrhagic and thromboembolic events (59) in the mothers as well as of fetal prematurity (44). Despite these difficulties, reports from the developing world have been encouraging (42–44,48,50,51,55,56,59), and outcome is likely to be even better with more meticulous anticoagulant supervision and antenatal care in the developed nations. However, no major cardiac center in the West sees a sufficient number of young women with prosthetic valves to be able to gain a large experience in the use of oral anticoagulants in pregnancy (63,64,66,68).

3. Conclusion

Risks to the mother from the use of anticoagulant drugs in pregnancy are no higher than outside pregnancy (62), and risks to the fetus are minimized when patient cooperation is maximal and anticoagulant control is precise (65). The risks of thromboembolic events in pregnant women treated with oral anticoagulation are no greater than are reported in the nonpregnant population with prosthetic mechanical heart valves (45). A recent survey confirmed the greater safety and efficacy of warfarin over heparin anticoagulation for women with valvular prostheses as well as the accelerated deterioration of bioprostheses during pregnancy (45a). The INR should be maintained at between 2.0 and 2.5, and in such circumstances the chances of oral anticoagulants damaging the fetus are small. It has been suggested that fetal risk is related to maternal dose requirement and that women requiring less than 5 mg warfarin per day to achieve a therapeutic INR pose minimal risk to the fetus. In asymptomatic or mildly symptomatic patients with prosthetic heart valves who are willing and able to follow a strict regime of medical care, pregnancy is not associated with increased morbidity in the mother or fetus (45).

V. INFECTIVE ENDOCARDITIS IN PREGNANCY

Infective endocarditis is rare in pregnancy (70), but when it is encountered it presents particularly difficult management problems. The diagnosis is made in the usual way by the presence of fever and of cardiac abnormality. Positive blood cultures may follow, and echocardiography may show vegetations, although the diagnosis can never be excluded if vegetations are not seen. Use of the transesophageal window for echocardiography greatly increases the sensitivity of the technique in the detection of vegetations.

If the cardiac reserve was seriously compromised before the infection, any fever or deterioration in the valve caused by the infection is likely to cause heart failure. Surgical treatment of endocarditis may be indicated to save the mother's life, and in this instance the fetus has to take its chance. The basic principles of diagnosis and of management of endocarditis (69) are not different in pregnancy from in the nonpregnant state. (See Chapter 12.)

In suspected infective endocarditis, antibiotics are started immediately after the blood cultures have been taken, without waiting for bacteriological confirmation. The drugs are selected by the usual educated guess as to the likely organism. This is most likely to be a sensitive streptococcus unless the patient has had a recent skin infection or any kind of surgical skin incision. In patients with a recently inserted valve prosthesis, staphylococci remain common and must be considered likely for the first postoperative year, during which nosocomial *Staphylococcus epidermidis* may still make its appearance.

The use of tetracyclines is contraindicated because they cause discoloration of the deciduous teeth, but these drugs are used only for endocarditis caused by coxiella, and in pregnancy rifampicin should be preferred. Aminoglycosides can be ototoxic to the fetus, and therefore gentamicin should be avoided except when it is considered to be life-saving. Its use should never be extended for periods longer than 2 weeks, and meticulous attention should be given to peak as well as to trough blood levels. When gentamicin is given for its synergistic effect with penicillin, the doses required are small, aiming for peak levels of no more than 5 mg/L and troughs of under 1 mg/L. Angiotensin-converting enzyme inhibitors cause fetal renal failure, and oligohydramnios and should not be given for relief of heart failure caused by valve regurgitation. Such patients need surgical treatment.

Surgery is indicated for sudden or increasing hemodynamic compromise caused by deterioration in the valve, for infection by a resistant organism, or for infection by a sensitive organism with failure of response caused by a paravalvular abscess (69). A softer indication is recurrent embolism with recognition of new vegetations. Echocardiography plays a major part in assessing response and progress.

The need for prophylactic antibiotics to prevent infective endocarditis after normal delivery in women with susceptible heart disease has been questioned (67), but most continue to use a combination of amoxycillin and gentamicin. Prophylaxis is certainly indicated for patients with prosthetic valves.

VI. EFFECT OF DRUGS GIVEN IN PREGNANCY TO WOMEN WITH VALVE DISEASE

The physiological adaptations of pregnancy tend to alter the pharmacokinetics of drugs by affecting absorption or metabolism (65). Nearly all antibiotics cross the placenta by simple diffusion. The rate of transfer is related to the concentration gradient and the diffusion constant of the drug. This is inversely related to its molecular weight. Information is limited, most having come from estimates on cord blood after giving parenteral antibiotic to the mother during labor.

As a general principle, only essential drugs are given during pregnancy, and the choice is made from established drugs with well-authenticated safety records whenever possible (Table 3). Some may affect the fetus adversely or alternatively be given to the mother to treat the fetus. They may be potential teratogens. They may be secreted in breast milk with possible continuing effect on the child.

EDITOR'S COMMENTS

Dr. Oakley acknowledges that both heparin and oral anticoagulation have potential complications for both mother and fetus. The author recommended continuing oral anticoagulation with warfarin during the first trimester of pregnancy—keeping the INR between 2.0 and 2.5, which is

Table 3 Drugs Used During Pregnancy

Drug class	Use in pregnancy	Comments
Digitalis	Indications as in nonpregnant women. May need higher dose. Reaches fetus in reduced concentration.	Alleged to shorten duration of labor
Diuretics	Indicated only for treatment of heart failure.	May reduce uterine blood flow and cause deterioration in preeclampsia
Vasodilators	Nitrates for preload reduction. Hydralazine for afterload reduction.	
	ACE inhibitors contraindicated.	May cause fetal renal failure and oligohydramnios
Antiarrhythmic agents	Avoid phenytoin.	Causes fetal abnormalities
	Disopyramide, lignocaine, and quinidine appear to be safe.	
	Amiodarone—insufficient data.	Two successful pregnancies reported without neonatal thyroid or other anomalies.
Beta-adrenergic blocking drugs	Very safe; in wide usage despite theoretical hazards to the fetus.	Neonatal hypoglycemia, bradycardia, hypotension, and low Apgar scores not seen. Normal intrauterine growth.
Calcium channel blocking drugs	Verapamil appears afe. Too little information on newer drugs.	But myocardial depressant and vasodilator.
Anticoagulants:		
Heparin	Does not cross placenta.	May cause maternal or retroplacental bleeding, prematurity, or still birth.
Warfarin	Crosses placenta.	Teratogenic effect 4% in first trimester; continued risk of fetal cerebral bleeding because of greater anticoagulant effect in fetus than in mother.
Antiplatelet agents	Aspirin is safe in pregnancy; No information with other agents.	Reduces fetal loss from placental insufficiency.

equivalent to a prothrombin ratio (PT) of 1.5–1.7. This practice is not advised in the majority of medical centers in the United States (see below). Dr. Oakley implies that fetal complications, namely skeletal and neurological abnormalities, may be related to the bleeding tendency which is associated with intense anticoagulation regime (PT 2.0–2.5), rather than due to the intrinsic teratogenic effect of warfarin. The outmoded test of PT, using the available commercial thromboplastin reagents in the United States, has a marked variation in responsiveness, and this makes an optimal and safe anticoagulation therapy rather a difficult task [Hirsh et al., Chest 1992; 102 (suppl 4):312–26]. Therefore the author suggests that using a less intense anticoagulation regime (INR 2.0–2.5), and a more sensitive technique (adopting the standardized international normalized ratio, INR) to control the anticoagulation state of the pregnant patients may reduce the fetal complication. This relative decrease in the fetal complication rate may be comparable to or even better than the maternal risk of thromboembolism which is associated with the regime of subcutaneous heparin.

The U.S. recommendation for the use of the anticoagulation agents during pregnancy has been recently revised [Ginsberg JS, Hirsh J, Chest 1992; 102 (suppl 4):385–90]. It advises discontinuing oral anticoagulation during the first trimester and particularly between the 6th and the 12th weeks of gestation. This is the period during which the fetal skeleton is suspected to be vulnerable to the side effect of oral anticoagulation agents. It is recommended that a low dose of 5000 U or an adjusted dose of subcutaneous heparin is given 12-hourly throughout pregnancy, prolonging activated partial thromboplastin time (APTT) to one and a half times control. Alternatively, as soon as pregnancy is diagnosed, warfarin is discontinued and subcutaneous heparin is given until the 13th week of gestation. Warfarin is restarted until the middle of the third trimester, and finally subcutaneous heparin recommenced until delivery.

In our area of practice, i.e., Saudia Arabia, the prevalence of rheumatic heart disease in the young is relatively high. Thus it is common to encounter pregnant patients with mitral stenosis or mechanical valvular prostheses that require long-term anticoagulation. Pregnancy is frequently diagnosed at a relatively late date, i.e., during 10 to 12 weeks of gestation. In such patients, warfarin anticoagulation is continued, though INR is checked more often. If a pregnancy is, diagnosed early, however, we use the subcutaneous heparin regime between the 8th and 13th weeks. In our practice, we have been using the low INR of 2.0–2.5 for a long period of time, and prior to the recent publication which advocates the use of a less intense anticoagulation regime (INR 2.0–2.5 or PT 1.5–1.7). This policy was implemented in our institution because of the high rate of bleeding complications and because many of our patients live far away from major hospitals. Although we have not conducted a formal study to examine the issue of warfarin (coumadin) embryopathy and the neurological complications of such a regime with low INR, our questionnaire to our obstetricians and pediatricians indicated that they have rarely come across such birth anomalies. It is conceivable that in order to diagnose such congenital anomalies, an expert neonatologist is required, and this may explain the marked variation in the reporting incidence of fetal skeletal complication from 5% (as indicated by Dr. Oakley) to 28% (Iturbe-Allesio et al., N Engl J Med 1986; 315:1390–3).

During the breast-feeding period, warfarin (coumadin) can be reintroduced. It has been shown that warfarin (coumadin) is not secreted into breast milk (Orme et al., Br Med J 1977; 1:1564–65; and McKenna et al., J Pediatr 1983; 103:325–7).]

REFERENCES

1. Walters WAW, MacGregor WG, Hills M. Cardiac output at rest during pregnancy and the puerperium. Clin Sci 1966; 30:1.
2. Ueland K, Metcalfe J. Circulatory changes in pregnancy. Clin Obstet Gynecol 1975; 18:41.
3. Lung CJ, Conovan JC. Blood volume during pregnancy. Significance of plasma and red cell volume. Am J Obstet Gynecol 1967; 98:393.
4. Rubler S, Damani PM, Pinto ER. Cardiac size and performance during pregnancy estimated with echocardiography. Am J Cardiol 1977; 40:534.
5. Katz R, Karliner JS, Resnik R. Effects of a natural volume overload state (pregnancy) on left ventricular performance in normal human subjects. Circulation 1978; 58:434.
6. Robson SC, Hunter S, Boys R J, Dunlop W. Serial study of factors influencing changes in cardiac output during human pregnancy. Am J Physiol 1989; 25b:H1060–50.
7. Lees MM, Taylor SH, Scott DB, et al. A study of cardiac output at rest throughout pregnancy. J Obstet Gynaecol Br Commonw 1967; 74:319.
8. Pernoll ML, Metcalfe J, Schlenker TL, et al. Oxygen consumption at rest and during exercise in pregnancy. Respir Physiol 1975; 25:282.
9. Gee JB, Packer BS, Millen JE, et al. Pulmonary mechanics during pregnancy. J Clin Invest 1967; 46:945.
10. Knuttgen HG, Emerson K Jr. Physiological response to pregnancy at rest and during exercise. J Appl Physiol 1974; 36:549.
11. Lucius H, Gahlenbeck H, Kleine HO, et al. Respiratory functions, buffer system and electrolyte concentrations of blood during human pregnancy. Respr Physiol 1970; 9:311.
12. Cutforth R, MacDonald CB. Heart sounds and murmurs in pregnancy. Am Heart J 1966; 71:741.
13. Ueland K, Hansen JM. Maternal cardiovascular dynamics II: Posture and uterine contractions. Am J Obstet Gynaecol 1969; 103:1–7.

14. Ueland K, Metcalfe J. Circulatory changes in pregnancy. Clin Obstet Gynaecol 1975; 18:41.
15. Perloff JK. Pregnancy and cardiovascular disease. In: Braunwald E, ed. Heart Disease. Philadelphia: Saunders, 1984; 1763–81.
16. Karim SMM, Hiller K, Somers K, et al. The effects of prostaglandin E_2 and F_2 administered by different routes on uterine activity. J Obstet Gynaecol Br Commonw 1971; 78:172.
17. Hendricks CH, Brenner WE. Cardiovascular effects of oxytocic drugs used postpartum. Am J Obstet Gynecol 1970; 108:751.
18. Oakley CM. Pregnancy in heart disease. In: Douglas P, ed. (Brest A, series ed.). Heart Disease in Women, Cardiovascular Clinics 14/3. Philadelphia: FA Davis, 1989:57–80.
19. Oakley CM. Heart disease in pregnancy. In: Sleight P, Vann Jones J, eds. Cardiology. London: Heinemann, 1983:121–6.
20. Todd ME, Thompson JH Jr, Bowie ETJ, Owen LA. Changes in blood coagulation during pregnancy. Mayo Clin Proc 1965; 40:370–83.
21. Shaper AG: The hypercoagulable states. Ann Intern Med 1985; 102:814–28.
22. Ullery JC. Thromboembolic disease complicating pregnancy and the puerpartum. Am J Obstet and Gynaecol 1954; 68:1243–60.
23. Badaracco MA, Vessey M. Recurrence of venous thromboembolic disease and use of oral contraceptives. Br Med J 1974; 1:215–7.
24. Szekely P, Smith L. Heart Disease and Pregnancy. Edinburgh and London: Churchill-Livingstone, 1974.
25. Clark SL, Phelan JP, Greenspoon J, Aldah LD, Horenstein J. Labor and delivery in the presence of mitral stenosis: central haemodynamic observations. Am J Obstet Gynaecol 1985; 152:984.
26. Szekely P, Turner R, Smith L. Pregnancy and the changing pattern of rheumatic heart disease. Br Heart J 1973; 35:1293.
27. Avias F, Pineda J. Aortic stenosis and pregnancy. J Reprod Med 1978; 20: 229.
28. Oakley GDG, McGarry K, Limb DC, Oakley CM. Management of pregnancy in patients with hypertrophic cardiomyopathy. Br Med J 1979; 1:1749.
29. Pyeritz RE. Material and fetal complications of pregnancy in the Marfan syndrome. Am J Med 1981; 71:784.
30. Oakley CM. Mitral valve prolapse. Quart J Med 1985; 56:317.
31. Rupprath G, Theur O, Vogt J, et al. The durability of bioprostheses in young people. Long-term results with intra- or extra-cardiac implanted porcine valves. J Cardiovasc Surg 1985; 26:251–7.
32. Bortolotti U, Milano A, Mazzucco A, et al. Results of re-operation for primary tissue failure of porcine bioprostheses. J Thorac Cardiovasc Surg 1985; 90:564–9.
33. Bloomfield P, Kitchin AH, Wheatley DJ, Walbaum PR, Lutz W, Miller HC. A prospective evaluation of the Bjork-Shiley, Hancock and Carpentier-Edwards heart valve prostheses. Circulation 1986; 73:1213–22.
34. Oakley CM. Pregnancy in patients with prosthetic heart valves. Br Med J 1983; 286:1680.

35. Oakley CM. Valve prostheses and pregnancy. Br Heart J 1987; 58:303.
35a. Cotrufo M, deLuca TSL, Calabro R, et al. Coumarin anticoagulation during pregnancy in patients with mechanical valve prostheses. Eur J Cardiothorac Surg 1991; 5:300–305.
36. Howie PW. Anticoagulants in pregnancy. Clin Obstet Gynaecol 1986; 13: 349–64.
37. Ginsberg JS, Hirsh J. Optimum use of anticoagulants in pregnancy. So Drugs 1988; 34:505–12.
38. Ginsberg JS, Hirsh J. Anticoagulants during pregnancy. Ann Rev Med 1989; 40:79–86.
39. Wehrmacher WH, Messmore HL. Thromboembolic disease during pregnancy: problems with anticoagulant therapy. Compr Ther 1990; 16:31–5.
40. Hirsh J, Cade JF, O'Sullivan EF. Clinical experience with anticoagulant therapy during pregnancy. Br Med J 1970; 1:270–3.
41. Hall JG, Pauli RM, Wilson KM. Maternal and fetal sequelae of anticoagulation during pregnancy. Am J Med 1980; 68:122–40.
42. Pavunkumar P, Venugopal P, Kaul U, et al. Pregnancy in patients with prosthetic cardiac valves. A 10 year experience. Scan J Thorac Cardiovasc Surg 1988; 22:19–22.
43. Chen WWC, Chan CS, Lee PK, Wang RYC, Wong VCW. Pregnancy in patients with prosthetic heart valves: an experience with 45 pregnancies. Quart J Med 1982; 51:358–65.
44. Sareli P, England MJ, Berk MR, et al. Maternal and fetal sequelae of anticoagulation during pregnancy in patients with mechanical heart valve prostheses. JACC 1989; 63:1462–65.
45. Elkayam U, Gleicher N. Letter, N Engl J Med 1987; 316:1664.
45a. Sbarouni E, Oakley CM. Outcome of pregnancy in women with valvular prostheses. Br Heart J (in press).
46. Bennett GG, Oakley CM. Pregnancy in a patient with a mitral valve prosthesis. Lancet 1968; 1:616–9.
47. Larrea JL, Nunez L, Reque JA, Gil Aguardo M, Matarros R, Mingues JA. Pregnancy and mechanical valve prostheses in a high risk situation for the mother and the fetus. Ann Thorac Surg 1983; 36:459–63.
48. Ibarra-Perez C, Aravalo-Toledo N, Alvarez-de la Cadena O, Noriega-Guerra L. The course of pregnancy in patients with artificial heart valves. Am J Med 1976; 61:504–12.
49. Lutz DJ, Nollar KL, Spittal JA Jr, Danielson GK, Fish CR. Pregnancy and its complications following cardiac valve prostheses. Am J Obstet Gynecol 1978; 131:460–8.
50. Salazar E, Zajarias A, Guitarrazn Iturbe I. The problem of cardiac valve prostheses: anticoagulants and pregnancy. Circulation 1984; 70:169–77.
51. Iturbe-Alessio I, Delcarmen Fonseca M, Mutchinik D, Santos MA, Zajarias A, Salazar E. Risks of anticoagulant therapy in pregnant women with artificial heart valves. N Engl J Med 1986; 27:1390–3.
52. Tapanainen J, Ikaheimo M, Jouppila P, Kortelainen ML, Salmela P. Thrombosis in a mechanical aortic valve prosthesis during subcutaneous heparin

therapy in pregnancy. A case report. Eur J Obstet Gynaecol Reprod Biol 1990; 36:175–7.

53. Villasanta V. Thromboembolic disease in pregnancy. Am J Obstet Gynaecol 1965; 93:142–60.

54. McLeod AA, Jennings KP, Townsend ER. Near fatal puerperal thrombosis on Bjork-Shiley mitral valve prosthesis. Br Heart J 1978; 40:934–7.

55. Vitali E, Donatelli F, Quaini E, Gropelli G, Pellegrini A. Pregnancy in patients with mechanical prosthetic heart valves: our experiences regarding 98 pregnancies in 57 patients. J Cardiovasc Surg 1986; 27:221–7.

56. Gonzalez-Santos JM, Vallejo JL, Rico MJ, Gonzales-Santos ML, Horno R, Garcia-Dorado D. Thrombosis of a mechanical valve prosthesis late in pregnancy. Case report and review of the literature. Thorac Cardiovasc Surg 1986; 34:335–7.

57. Hirsh J, Poller L, Deykin D, Levine M, Dalen JE. Optimal therapeutic range for oral anticoagulants. Chest 1989; 95:5S–11S.

58. Casanegra P, Aviles G, Maturana G, Dubernet J. Cardiovascular management of pregnant women with a heart valve prosthesis. Am J Cardiol 1975; 36:802–6.

59. Ben Ismail M, Fekih M, Taktak M, et al. Prostheses valvulaires cardiaques et grossesse. Arch Mal Coeur 1979; 2:192.

60. Guidozzi F. Pregnancy in patients with prosthetic cardiac valves. S Africa Med J 1984; 65:961–3.

61. Lee PK, Wang RYC, Chow JSF, Cheung KL, Wong UCW, Chan TK. Combined use of warfarin and adjusted subcutaneous heparin during pregnancy in patients with artificial heart valves. JACC 1986; 8:221–4.

62. Oakley C, Doherty P. Pregnancy in patients after valve replacement. Br Heart J 1976; 38:1140–8.

63. McColgin S. Gynecology, University of Mississippi Medical Center, Jackson. Pregnant women with prosthetic heart valves. Clin Obstet Gynaecol 1989; 32:76–89.

64. Morris DC. Management of patients with prosthetic heart valves. Curr Prob Cardiol 1982; 7:1–56.

65. Hawkins DF. Drug treatment of medical disorders in pregnancy. In: Hawkins E, ed. Drugs and Pregnancy. 2d ed. London: Churchill Livingstone, 1987: 90–114.

66. Fillmore SJ, McDevitt E. Effects of coumarin compounds on the foetus. Ann Intern Med 1970; 73:731.

67. Stevenson RE, Burton OM, Firlanto GS, et al. Hazards of oral anticoagulants during pregnancy. JAMA 1980; 243:1549.

68. Noller KL. Pregnancy after cardiac surgery. In: Elkyam U, Gleicher N. Cardiac Problems in Pregnancy. New York: USS, 1982: 5–22.

69. Nihoyannopoulos P, Oakley CM, Exadactylos N, et al. Duration of symptoms and the effects of a more aggressive policy: two factors influencing prognosis of infective endocarditis. Eur Heart J 1985; 6:380.

70. Sugrue D, Blake S, Troy P, et al. Antibiotic prophylaxis against infective endocarditis after normal delivery—is it necessary? Br Heart J 1980; 44:499.

16

Assessment of Left and Right Ventricular Function in Valvular Heart Disease

Ramesh C. Bansal
Loma Linda University Medical Center, Loma Linda, California

K. Chandrasekaran
Hahnemann University Hospital, Philadelphia, Pennsylvania

Muayed Al Zaibag
Armed Forces Hospital, Riyadh, Saudi Arabia, and Loma Linda University Medical Center, Loma Linda, California

I. INTRODUCTION

Accurate assessment of ventricular function is essential in the evaluation of patients with valvular heart disease. The prognosis of a patient with ischemic or valvular heart disease is profoundly influenced by the status of left ventricular performance. Timing of surgical therapy and preoperative prediction of surgical outcome often depend on measurement of global left ventricular systolic function. As a general rule, the valve replacement surgery is postponed late enough in the course of the disease to justify the surgical risk, yet early enough to avoid irreversible deterioration of left ventricular contractility. For this reason, there is a continuing search for easily measured variables which will distinguish reversible from irreversible myocardial abnormality and allow surgery to be undertaken at the correct time. Before discussing the role of various imaging modalities in assessment of ventricular function, it will be useful to review basic concepts regarding determinants of overall left ventricular performance and commonly utilized clinical indices of left ventricular contractility and their limitations.

Examination of the pressure–volume loop of the left ventricle shows that there are two phases of both systole and diastole (Fig. 1). The isovolumic contraction phase begins at point A when the mitral valve closes. Point A (end-diastole) represents preload of the left ventricle. During the isovolumic contraction phase, the left ventricular pressure rises without volume change until the aortic valve opens and ejection begins at point B. During the ejection phase of systole, left ventricular volume decreases. At the end of systole (point C), the aortic valve closes and the isovolumic relaxation begins. The mitral valve opens at point D, and left ventricular filling occurs during the remainder of the diastole.

Although the largest body of work concerning left ventricular function has focused on systolic performance, the importance of diastolic function in causing cardiac symptoms has become increasingly clear. Impaired diastolic function may cause congestive heart failure in patients with significant left ventricular hypertrophy, even in the presence of normal or supernormal systolic function. Furthermore, evaluation of right ventricular performance is even more complex, partly because of the unusual shape of the right ventricle.

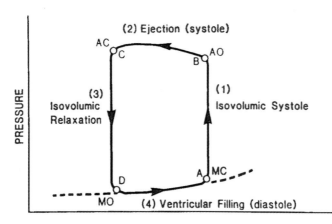

Figure 1 Illustration of the left ventricular pressure volume loop for a single cardiac cycle. At point A, mitral valve closes (MC), and this point represents end-diastole or preload of the left ventricle. The segment AB represents isovolumic systole (1). At point B, aortic valve opens (AO); and at point C, aortic valve closes (AC). The segment BC represents the ejection phase of systole (2). Isovolumic relaxation is the phase between C to D (3). At point D, mitral valve opens (MO) and ventricular filling takes place during segment D to A (4).

The first section of this chapter will focus on the principal determinants and indices to measure the systolic and diastolic performance of both the left and right ventricles. The second section of this chapter will review the role of various imaging techniques which can be utilized for assessment of ventricular function in patients with valvular heart disease.

II. LEFT VENTRICULAR SYSTOLIC FUNCTION

A. Principal Determinants of Left Ventricular Systolic Performance

It is important to gain a detailed understanding of left ventricular performance and the various factors that can alter it. In the simplest terms, left ventricular function in systole depends on the mass of left ventricular muscle available for contraction, preload, afterload, heart rate, and contractility (1,2) (Fig. 2).

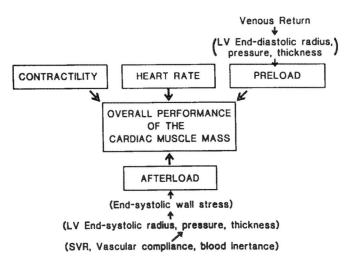

Figure 2 Overall left ventricular performance during systole depends on the cardiac muscle mass available to contract. Besides the muscle mass, the intrinsic contractility, preload, afterload, and heart rate affect the overall systolic performance. Preload is affected by pulmonary venous return, left ventricular (LV) end-diastolic radius, pressure, and wall thickness. Afterload is best approximated by the end-systolic wall stress. End-systolic wall stress depends on the end-systolic radius of the left ventricle, end-systolic pressure, and wall thickness. The vascular parameters which affect the afterload include systemic vascular resistance (SVR), vascular compliance, and blood inertance.

1. Left Ventricular Muscle Mass

The overall mass of healthy myocytes is responsible for generating systolic contractile force. Muscle mass may be decreased in patients with mitral stenosis, due to atrophy of myocardial fibers. The left ventricle is a "protected" chamber and carries no added hemodynamic burden in this valvular lesion. In aortic stenosis, there may be *concentric* left ventricular hypertrophy in response to increased systolic pressure from outflow obstruction and the mass is increased. Increased systolic wall stress from chronic pressure overload leads to thickening of individual myocytes and of the ventricular wall as a result of parallel replication of sarcomeres and myofibrils (3). In chronic aortic regurgitation, there is diastolic volume overload as the blood leaks back into the left ventricle through the incompetent aortic valve. This leads to dilatation and mild hypertrophy of the left ventricle. This lesion can produce the largest and the heaviest hearts encountered by pathologists. This pattern of hypertrophy is called *eccentric* left ventricular hypertrophy. Mitral regurgitation, like aortic regurgitation, causes diastolic overload of the left ventricle due to excessive amounts of blood returning from the left atrium in diastole through the mitral valve. This lesion also causes left ventricular dilatation and eccentric hypertrophy. The eccentric type of left ventricular hypertrophy probably results from the development of longer myocytes or fibers. The length of myofiber may be increased due to replication of sarcomeres in series and possibly by slippage between adjacent myofibrils.

In acute aortic and mitral regurgitation, there is no significant left ventricular dilatation. Myocardial sarcomeres exhibit an increase in end-diastolic stretch, and this finding may account for increased systolic function. In contrast, in the compensated state of chronic pressure and volume overloading, these adjustments in chamber size and mass (hypertrophy) allow enhancement of overall cardiac performance. In long-standing left ventricular hypertrophy (exhaustion phase), there may be deterioration of systolic function because of increased myocardial oxygen demand and interstitial fibrosis. Left ventricular mass can be measured by angiographic, echocardiographic, and various other imaging modalities. The changes of left ventricular wall thickness and muscle mass will affect the preload and afterload.

2. Preload

Preload is defined as the force or load acting to stretch the left ventricular fibers at end-diastole. Preload determines the maximal resting length of the sarcomeres. Higher preload is therefore associated with better left ventricular performance (decrease in end-systolic volume, increase in stroke volume, and increase in ejection fraction), presumably through the Frank-Starling mechanism. Decreases in preload have the opposite effects. The optimal sarcomere length for maximum tension development is about 2.2 μm. Preload is reflected by the left ventricular (LV) end-diastolic pressure, volume, and stress. Left ventricular *end-diastolic stress* is probably the best available indicator of preload; it is calculated as the force per cross-sectional area, according to the LaPlace relation:

Left ventricular end-diastolic stress

$$= \frac{\text{left ventricular end-diastolic pressure} \times \text{end-diastolic radius}}{2 \times \text{wall thickness}}$$

A more precise calculation of LV end-diastolic stress uses Mirsky's variation (4) of the LaPlace relationship:

$$\text{LV end-diastolic stress} = P \times \frac{b}{h}\left(1 - \frac{h}{2b} - \frac{b^2}{2a^2}\right) \quad \text{in mmHg}$$

or

LV end-diastolic stress

$$= P \times \frac{b}{h}\left(1 - \frac{h}{2b} - \frac{b^2}{2a^2}\right) \times 1.332 \quad \text{in kdyne/cm}^2$$

where P = left ventricular end-diastolic pressure (mmHg); b = midwall semiminor axis (half of the sum of the minor axis diameter and the wall thickness) at end-diastole; a = midwall semimajor axis (half of the sum of the length and wall thickness) at end-diastole; and h = end-diastolic left ventricular wall thickness. The results obtained by this formula are in millimeters of mercury and are converted to kilodynes per square centimeter by multiplying the result by a conversion factor of 1.332 kdyne/cm²/mmHg. Because of the complexity of this calculation, preload is clinically often estimated as left ventricular end-diastolic pressure, volume, or diameter. In the absence of mitral stenosis, pulmonary artery wedge pressure can be used as an indirect measurement of left ventricular end-diastolic pressure. Preload is often decreased in mitral stenosis, normal to decreased in well-compensated aortic stenosis, but increased at the time of left ventricular decompensation. Preload is increased in chronic mitral and aortic regurgitation. There is also a slight increase in preload in acute mitral and aortic regurgitation.

3. Afterload

Afterload is defined as the load that the left ventricle encounters during ejection. This is the force resisting systolic shortening of the myofibrils. It depends on aortic systolic pressure, peripheral vascular resistance, left ventricular systolic dimension, and systolic wall thickness. An isolated increase in afterload can produce an increase in left ventricular end-diastolic volume and end-systolic volume, and a decrease in stroke volume and ejection fraction.

Decreases in afterload usually have the opposite effects. Afterload is measured by calculating the systolic left ventricular wall stress. Three different types of systolic wall stresses have been described which act in three different directions: circumferential, meridional, and radial. In most instances, *circumferential systolic wall stress* is used as the preferred measure of left ventricular afterload. Because of the changing nature of left ventricular pressure, volume, and wall thickness during systole, the wall stress is complex to calculate and is not constant. Left ventricular catheterization and angiography can be utilized to calculate the systolic pressure, volume, and wall thickness on a frame-by-frame basis throughout systole. End-systolic, mean systolic, and peak systolic wall stresses can then be calculated by using Mirsky's variation of the LaPlace relationship (4–6). Peak systolic stress is the greatest stress in each beat. In general, peak systolic stress occurs during the first one-third of ejection. This stress is a major modulator of ventricular hypertrophy. Mean systolic stress is the mean of stress calculation in each angiographic frame from aortic valve opening to aortic valve closure. *End-systolic stress* is the afterload that determines the overall extent of LV fiber shortening. Calculation of end systolic stress uses the end-systolic aortic pressure at the dicrotic notch, the systolic minor axis diameter (D), the systolic major axis (L), and the end-systolic wall thickness (h):

End-systolic left ventricular wall stress

$$= P \times \frac{b}{h}\left(1 - \frac{h}{2b} - \frac{b^2}{2a^2}\right) \times 1.332 \text{ kdyne/cm}^2$$

where P = end-systolic aortic pressure, h = end-systolic wall thickness, a = midwall semimajor axis ($L/2 + h/2$) at end-systole, and b = midwall semiminor axis ($D/2 + h/2$) at end-systole. Afterload measured by end-systolic wall stress is increased in patients with hypertension (increased systolic pressure), aortic stenosis (high left ventricular systolic pressure), and chronic aortic regurgitation (high systolic pressure and high LV sys-

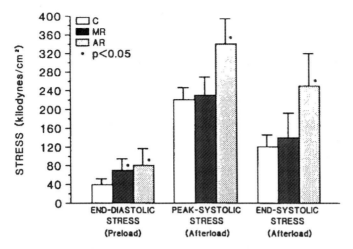

Figure 3 Comparison of preload measured as end-diastolic wall stress and afterload measured as peak or end-systolic wall stress in patients with aortic regurgitation (AR), mitral regurgitation (MR), and control subjects (C). Values are mean ± standard deviation. the symbol * indicates a significant difference from the control group with a P value of <0.05. (Reproduced with permission from Ref. 8.)

tolic diameter), and is normal to minimally increased (Fig. 3) even in chronic mitral regurgitation (high left ventricular systolic diameter) (5–8). Left ventricular systolic wall stress alone, however, does not reflect all the forces resisting systolic ejection of the blood in the setting of low-impedance leak, as seen in patients with mitral regurgitation (5–8). Vascular factors that impede the forward flow of blood during ventricular ejection also should be considered in the concept of afterload. The most widely used of these vascular impedance parameters is systemic vascular resistance (SVR). Other vascular factors include arterial compliance, viscoelasticity, and blood inertance. In mitral regurgitation, the left ventricle ejects blood both in the high-impedance systemic circulation and the low-impedance left atrium. The regurgitation occurs predominantly during the isometric contraction phase and the early portion of the ejection phase.

4. Heart Rate

It is well known that cardiac output and other measures of overall left ventricular performance are highly heart rate-dependent. With increasing heart rate, time available for left ventricular filling during diastole is also shortened. In normal subjects this is not a major problem, since most of the filling occurs in early diastole. However, in pathological conditions such as left ventricular hypertrophy and decreased compliance, as in patients with aortic stenosis, an increase in heart rate can result in a fall in left ventricular preload. When heart rate increases to greater than 160 beats/min, it may produce reduction in end-diastolic volume, end-systolic volume, ejection fraction, and stroke volume. Cardiac output, however, may remain unchanged.

5. Contractility

Contractility is defined as the intrinsic ability of the myocardium to alter its performance which is independent of changes in preload, afterload, and heart rate. An augmentation of contractility leads to a decrease in end-diastolic volume and end-systolic volume, and an increase in stroke volume and ejection fraction. A number of indices have been developed to measure contractility, but the majority of them are affected by the loading conditions. The differentiation between decreased overall left ventricular systolic performance due to depressed contractility and that due to abnormal loading conditions is an important issue. The challenge is to develop a noninvasive parameter which is not affected by loading conditions and which reflects changes in contractility.

B. Indices to Measure Systolic Left Ventricular Performance and Contractility

This section will discuss the commonly utilized approaches to evaluate the global left ventricular performance during various phases of systole (1,2).

1. Isovolumic-Phase Indices

The simplest and most commonly utilized isovolumic-phase index is the peak rate of left ventricular pressure rise (dP/dt). This is calculated from high-fidelity catheter recordings of the left ventricle during isovolumic systole. Peak dP/dt is largely independent of changes in afterload. In the presence of marked peripheral vasodilation, peak dP/dt may occur at the time of aortic valve opening and result in underestimation of true contractile state. However, an increase in preload can cause increase in dP/dt. Peak dP/dt is useful in assessing directional changes in contractility during acute interventions. The peak of dP/dt ranges from 841 to 1696 mmHg/s. It increases in response to exercise, tachycardia, and following administration of atropine, B-agonists, and digitalis glycosides. Peak dP/dt increases slightly by increase in preload and changes little by methoxamine-induced increase or nitroprusside-induced decrease in afterload. The dP/dt for a developed pressure of 40 mmHg (dP/dt/DP) is measured during the isovolumic contraction phase of the ventricle during the time left ventricular systolic pressure rises by 40 mm above the end-diastolic pressure. This generally occurs before opening of the aortic valve and is thus unaffected by changes in afterload and is also less sensitive to changes in preload (1). This index can also be derived noninvasively by the mitral regurgitation signal obtained by continuous-wave Doppler recordings (9). (See echocardiography section.)

2. Ejection-Phase Indices

Ejection-phase measures of left ventricular fiber shortening are based on data which is acquired during ventricular ejection. These indices are extensively used in clinical practice, but they are affected by changes in loading conditions, particularly increased by higher preload and decreased by higher afterload (1,2). The following are the commonly used ejection-phase indices.

   a. Left Ventricular Volumes and Output. Left ventricular stroke volume, cardiac output, and stroke work can be measured at the bedside in the coronary-care unit or in the cardiac catheterization laboratory. Left ventricular stroke work index (SWI) is a measure of external work performed by the left ventricle. Stroke work is determined as gram-meters/meter^2 (g-m/m^2) and is calculated as follows:

$$\text{LVSWI}\left(\frac{\text{g-m}}{\text{m}^2}\right) = \frac{\begin{array}{c}(\text{mean LV systolic pressure}) - \\ (\text{mean LV end-diastolic pressure}) \times \text{SV} \times 0.0136\end{array}}{\text{body surface area in m}^2}$$

   Mean arterial pressure (sum of one-third of systolic and two-thirds of diastolic pressure) can be substituted for the mean LV systolic pressure, and mean pulmonary artery wedge pressure can be substituted for the mean LV end-diastolic pressure. A constant 0.0136 is used to convert mmHg into the g-m system (2). The normal LV stroke work index is 50 ± 20 g-m/m^2 (mean ± SD)^2. This parameter is not reliable in patients with volume or pressure overload. LV stroke work of less than 20 g-m/m^2 indicates severe LV dysfunction (2). Cardiac output can also be measured by Doppler echocardiography. Ventricular function curves (Frank-Starling) can be constructed by plotting the left ventricular preload (pulmonary artery wedge pressure) on the *x* axis and cardiac output or stroke work index along the *y* axis. It is well known that through the use of compensatory mechanisms, cardiac output, and stroke work index can be nearly normal, even in patients with dilated cardiomyopathy with poor function and marked depression of contractility.

   b. Extent of Left Ventricular Fiber Shortening. *Ejection fraction* (EF)
is one of the most common clinically used measures of left ventricular
function. It can be determined by angiography or other noninvasive methods. The normal value of EF is 72 ± 8% (2). By echocardiography, percent
fractional shortening (FS) of the minor diameter can be calculated, and
this gives information similar to ejection fraction. Ejection fraction will
increase with increase in preload and decrease in afterload. An increase
in afterload for a given contractile state leads to incomplete emptying of
the left ventricle and increase in end-systolic volume. This initially increases the end-diastolic volume, which maintains the stroke volume.
However, with further increase in afterload, the preload reserve is exhausted and there is a fall in left ventricular ejection fraction due to afterload mismatch (10). A fall in left ventricular ejection fraction therefore
may be noted in patients with aortic stenosis and aortic regurgitation despite reasonable and stable contractile state due to excessive afterload
(afterload mismatch). Similarly, reduced afterload due to low-impedance
leak into the left atrium in patients with mitral regurgitation may spuriously
maintain ejection fraction in the normal range despite decreased left ventricular contractility (10).

   *c. Left Ventricular Velocity of Circumferential Fiber Shortening
(Vcf).* Vcf can be determined by angiography or echocardiographic
methods (1). It is calculated as percent fractional shortening divided by
LV ejection time in seconds. Vcf appears to be independent of preload
but is highly dependant on afterload, contractility, and heart rate.

3. End-Systolic Indices of Left Ventricular Function

A variety of end-systolic indices to assess contractility have been described (11–13).

   a. End-Systolic Dimension and End-Systolic Volume Index. End-
systolic volume is independent of preload. End-systolic diameter reflects
end-systolic volume and can be measured by M-mode and two-dimensional echocardiography. Henry et al. (14) used the end-systolic diameter
(ESD) in patients with aortic regurgitation and found that in asymptomatic
patients, an end-systolic diameter of greater than 5.5 cm predicted the
onset of symptoms within an average of 39 months if the aortic valve was
not replaced. Four of five (80%) patients with ESD >5.5 cm developed
symptoms during the follow-up period and required operation. In contrast,
4 of 20 (20%) patients with initial ESD of <5.0 cm developed symptoms
and required operation. Henry et al. (15) also reported their observation
in 49 symptomatic patients with severe chronic aortic regurgitation. They
observed that 9 of 13 (69%) with preoperative ESD ≥5.5 cm and FS <25%
died either at operation (2 patients) or died late postoperatively of conges-

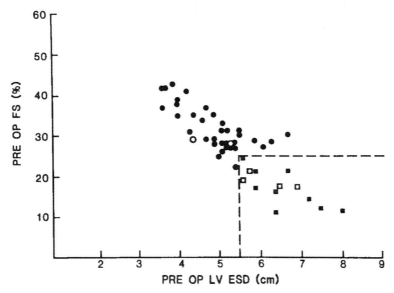

Figure 4 Plot of preoperative left ventricular fractional shortening (PRE OP FS) along the vertical axis and preoperative left ventricular end-systolic diameter (PRE OP LV ESD) in centimeters along the horizontal axis in 49 patients with symptomatic severe aortic regurgitation. Nine of 13 patients in the high-risk group (filled and open squares) with ESD of >5.5 cm and FS of <25% died due to congestive heart failure (filled squares), and there were only four survivors (open squares) in this high-risk group. In contrast, only 2 of 36 patients with ESD of <5.5 cm and FS of >25% (filled and open circles) died of congestive heart failure (open circles). (Redrawn and reproduced with permission from Ref. 15.)

tive heart failure (7 patients). In contrast, 2 of 36 (6%) patients with ESD <5.5 cm and FS >25% died either at operation (1 patient) or late from congestive heart failure (1 patient) (Fig. 4). Schuler et al. (16) observed that all 12 patients with chronic mitral regurgitation and preoperative ESD <4 cm and normal ejection fraction who underwent mitral valve replacement maintained their postoperative ejection fraction. In contrast, all 4 patients with preoperative ESD >5 cm showed deterioration of left ventricular ejection fraction following mitral valve replacement (Fig. 5). Similarly, Zile et al. (17) observed that all 4 patients with chronic severe mitral regurgitation, with preoperative ESD >4.5 cm (2.6 cm/m^2) had poor postoperative outcome (Fig. 6).

Borow et al. (18) correlated preoperative left ventricular angiographic end-systolic volumes with postoperative outcome in patients with aortic

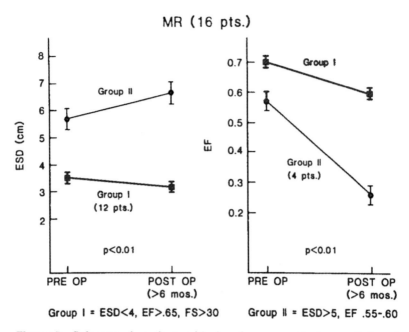

Figure 5 Subgroups in patients with chronic severe mitral regurgitation showing the changes in left ventricular ejection fraction (EF) calculated from echocardiography and end-systolic diameter (ESD) before the operation and at late follow-up of more than 6 months. Group I (12 patients) with ESD of <4 cm, EF >0.65 and fractional shortening (FS) >30% showed preservation of left ventricular ejection fraction and systolic dimension postoperatively. Group II (4 patients) with preoperative ESD of >5 cm and preoperative EF of <0.60 showed enlargement of left ventricular size at end-systole and decrease in ejection fraction postoperatively. (Redrawn and reproduced with permission from Ref. 16.)

(20 patients), mitral (16 patients), and combined valvular (5 patients) regurgitation. All 7 patients with aortic regurgitation and preoperative LV end-systolic volume index of less than 60 cc/m² had excellent symptomatic relief and normal postoperative function (echocardiographic fractional shortening or FS >34%) after aortic valve replacement. Three of 4 patients with end-systolic volume index between 61 to 90 cc/m² had mild symptoms and mild depression of left ventricular function postoperatively (FS 25–34%). In contrast, 2 of 9 patients with LV end-systolic volume index of >90 cc/m² died, and all the others had persistent symptoms and severe depression of left ventricular function postoperatively (FS <25%) (Fig. 7). These investigators also noted that all 3 patients with mitral regurgita-

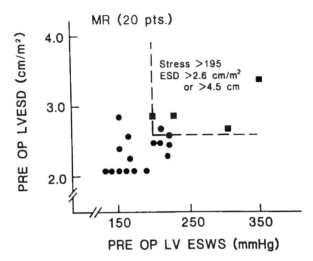

Figure 6 Plot showing correlation of left ventricular end-systolic diameter (LVESD in cm/m²) along the vertical axis and preoperative left ventricular end-systolic wall stress (PRE OP LVESWS in mmHg) along the horizontal axis from 20 patients with chronic mitral regurgitation who underwent mitral replacement. There are 16 patients who had optimal postoperative left ventricular performance with normalization of left ventricle size (filled circles). Four patients had persistent enlargement of the left ventricle and systolic dysfunction postoperatively (filled squares). The combination of end-systolic diameter of >2.6 cm/m² or >4.5 cm and end-systolic stress of >195 mmHg identifies all 4 patients with suboptimal outcome, and there is only one false positive. (Redrawn and reproduced with permission from Ref. 17.)

tion and preoperative LV end-systolic volume index of <30 cc/m² had normal postoperative left ventricular function (echocardiographic fractional shortening >34%). All 4 patients with mitral regurgitation and LV end-systolic volume index between 31 and 60 cm³/m² had mildly depressed postoperative left ventricular function (FS 25–30%). Five of six patients with LV systolic volume index of 61–90 cm³/m² either had persistent symptoms and moderate to severe postoperative left ventricular dysfunction (FS 20–25%), and 1 patient died. Two of 3 patients with LV systolic volume index of >90 cm³/m² died, and the remaining 1 patient had severe left ventricular dysfunction (Fig. 8). In another study of 48 patients with chronic mitral regurgitation, by Crawford et al. (19), end-systolic volume index of more than 50 cm³/m² was predictive of postoperative left ventricular dysfunction. Data from these studies indicates that valve replacement should be performed in chronic severe aortic regurgitations when

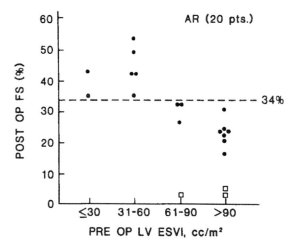

Figure 7 Plot of preoperative left ventricular end-systolic volume index (PRE OP LVESVI cm³/m²) along the horizontal axis and postoperative echocardiographic fractional shortening (POST OP FS %) from 20 patients with chronic aortic regurgitation (AR). All patients with LVESVI <60 cm³/m² showed preservation of left ventricular systolic function postoperatively. One out of four patients with LVESVI between 61 and 90 cm³/m² died (open square), and remaining three patients had mild postoperative LV dysfunction (filled circles). Two patients with LVESVI >90 cm³/m² (open squares) died, and others had mild to moderate postoperative LV dysfunction (filled circles). (Redrawn and reproduced with permission from Ref.18.)

LVESD, FS, and ESVI index are <5.5 cm, >25%, and <90 cm³/m², respectively. Mitral valve surgery for chronic regurgitation should be undertaken when LVESD, FS, and ESVI are <4.5 cm, >30%, and <50 cm³/m², respectively.

It should be noted, however, that besides contractility, afterload also affects the end-systolic volume or dimension. Patients with high end-systolic wall stress or afterload may have increased end-systolic volume, even in the presence of relatively preserved contractile function. This finding may explain the fact that most patients with aortic regurgitation, in whom afterload is increased, have good prognosis despite increased end-systolic dimension. In contrast, in patients with chronic mitral regurgitation, in whom afterload is normal or reduced, even mild elevation of end-systolic volume may reflect depression of contractility (4–7). It is therefore necessary to correct end-systolic volume for afterload to gauge contractile function properly. This concept has led to the development of

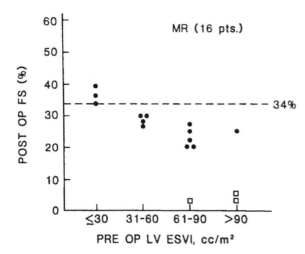

Figure 8 Plot of preoperative left ventricular end-systolic volume index (PRE OP LVESVI cm³/m²) along the horizontal axis and postoperative echocardiographic fractional shortening (POST OP FS %) from 16 patients with chronic mitral regurgitation (MR) who underwent surgery. Patients with end-systolic volume index of <60 cm³/m² had either normal or mild postoperative LV dysfunction. Patients with LVESVI >60 cm³/m² had mild to moderate LV dysfunction postoperatively, and there were three deaths (open squares). (Redrawn and reproduced with permission from Ref. 18.)

several end-systolic indices which are sensitive to contractility, incorporate afterload, and are independent of preload. (See next paragraph.)

b. The Ratio of End-Systolic Stress to End-Systolic Volume Index (ESWS/ESVI). Carabello et al. (6) have utilized this ratio in patients with chronic mitral regurgitation to predict postoperative outcome. Left ventricular end-systolic wall stress and end-systolic volume indices can be calculated from angiographic studies. This group of investigators found that this ratio was marginally better than end-systolic volume index alone in predicting postoperative results in patients with mitral regurgitation. They calculated the ratio of end-systolic stress to end-systolic volume index in 21 patients with chronic mitral regurgitation and 30 normal subjects. Normal value for this ratio was 5.6 ± 0.9. A low ratio suggests a high end-systolic volume for a given end-systolic wall stress (afterload) and indicates relatively less ventricular shortening (decreased contractility) for a given afterload. Four of the 5 patients in this series with mitral regurgitation who were found to have a ratio of less than 2.5 died postoperatively, and the fifth had persistent symptoms. On the other hand, the group of other 16 patients with mitral regurgitation and preoperative end-systolic wall stress to end-systolic volume index ratio of more than 2.6 did well postoperatively (Fig. 9). In contrast, Kontos et al. (20) in a study of 28 patients with mitral regurgitation undergoing surgical correction at the Mayo Clinic, were unable to confirm these findings. Moreover, these stress-to-volume ratios require invasive studies with calculation of frame-by-frame stress throughout systole and incorporate assumptions regarding

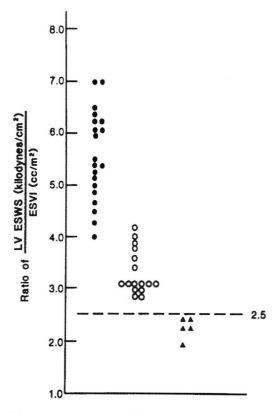

Figure 9   Ratio of left ventricular end-systolic wall stress (LV ESWS in kdyne/cm²)/and systolic volume index (ESVI in cm³/m²) for normal subjects (filled circles), 16 patients with mitral regurgitation who had optimal postoperative left ventricular function (open circles), and 5 patients with mitral regurgitation with poor postoperative outcome (filled triangles). Four out of five patients with ratio <2.5 died, and the fifth patient had postoperative left ventricular dysfunction. (Redrawn and reproduced with permission from Ref. 6.)

the shape of the ventricle. Calculation and use of these ratios in clinical practice is generally not feasible.

c. *End-Systolic Stress–Ejection Fraction Relations*. Ejection fraction or fractional shortening by echocardiography and wall stress can be plotted along the *y* and *x* axis, respectively, for an individual patient, and upward shift of this relationship generally indicates a positive inotropic intervention. This relationship is, however, affected by preload (21).

d. *End-Systolic Stress–Velocity of Fiber Shortening Relationship*. Velocity of fiber shortening (Vcf) is not dependent on preload but is sensitive to contractilty and afterload. Vcf is also sensitive to heart rate and can be corrected for heart rate, when it is called Vcf_c. Vcf_c can be plotted along the *y* axis and left ventricular end-systolic stress along the *x* axis, and this index of left ventricular performance is sensitive to inotropic state, incorporates afterload, and is independent of preload. Colan et al. have used echocardiographic techniques to plot this relationship between Vcf_c and end-systolic stress. For an individual patient, an upward shift in this relationship indicates a positive inotropic intervention (22). Plotting of these relationships requires inotropic (intravenous dobutamine infusion) and/or afterload (methoxamine infusion) interventions. These are also based on assumptions and are difficult to calculate on a day-to-day basis.

4. Left Ventricular Performance During Exercise

Effect of dynamic exercise on left ventricular performance and ejection fraction has been studied in patients with valvular heart disease with the hope of assessing contractility and contractile reserve (23). Normally, exercise increases left ventricular ejection fraction as a result of peripheral vasodilation (decreased afterload), increase in sympathetic tone (increased contractility), and increased venous return. In patients with volume overload due to aortic regurgitation, however, exercise can decrease ejection fraction despite normal left ventricular contractility. This abnormal ejection-fraction response to dynamic exercise in these patients may be due to abnormal interaction of left ventricular compliance, preload, and afterload (23). Most clinicans, however, continue to use exercise radionuclide angiography or echo-Doppler studies to assess patients' symptomatic status and effects of exercise on LV function and pulmonary artery pressure. This information can be used in clinical decision making.

III. LEFT VENTRICULAR DIASTOLIC FUNCTION

Traditionally, cardiologists have focused their attention on assessment of systolic function, and evaluation of diastolic function has largely been ignored. Recently, however, isolated diastolic dysfunction has been demonstrated to be the cause of heart failure. Diastolic dysfunction is frequently associated in conditions that produce systolic dysfunction as well. Abnormalities of diastolic dysfunction have been demonstrated in conditions associated with left ventricular hypertrophy (hypertension, aortic stenosis), myocardial ischemia, and infarction (24,25). Abnormalities of left ventricular filling are also seen in patients with aortic and mitral regurgitation. Diastolic function has proved to be a difficult parameter to assess quantitatively in the clinical setting.

A. Principal Determinants of Left Ventricular Diastolic Function

For clinical purposes, duration of left ventricular diastole is from aortic valve closure to mitral valve closure. Ventricular diastole is subdivided into four components: (1) the isovolumic relaxation time (IVRT); (2) an early rapid filling phase (RFP); (3) diastasis or slow filling phase (SFP) and; (4) filling during atrial contraction. In the intact heart, left ventricular filling during these phases of diastole is controlled by interaction of processes of active myocardial relaxation, chamber and myocardial compliance, diastolic suction, atrial contractility, left ventricular diastolic pressure prior to atrial contraction, and ventricular interaction or interdependence. Alteration in left ventricular filling or diastolic dysfunction may occur due to abnormalities of: (1) active ventricular relaxation; (2) chamber or myocardial compliance; and (3) enhanced ventricular interdependence. Active myocardial relaxation is an energy-dependent process which is assumed to begin with aortic valve closure and completes shortly after mitral valve opening.

B. Indices to Measure Left Ventricular Diastolic Function

Myocardial relaxation may become slow and prolonged with left ventricular hypertrophy due to hypertension, aortic stenosis, and hypertrophic cardiomyopathy. Myocardial relaxation is described by isovolumic relaxation indices, such as negative rate of rise in pressure ($-dP/dt$), the time constant of relaxation or tau, and isovolumic relaxation time (IVRT). The first two parameters require the use of high-fidelity, manometer-tipped catheters. IVRT is the time interval between aortic valve closure and mitral valve opening. This time interval is prolonged when the relaxation is slow and can be measured by dual M-mode and Doppler techniques. *Chamber compliance* is the change is pressure relative to a change in volume (dP/dV). Diastolic stiffness is not constant and increases with high diastolic volume with a curvilinear relationship between pressure and volume. Increased chamber stiffness means low compliance. Chamber stiffness is increased or compliance decreased when a relatively high intracardiac pressure is present for a given volume. Chamber compliance is decreased in patients with aortic stenosis, hypertrophic cardiomyopathy, and with the normal aging process. Compliance is increased in chronic mitral regurgitation, chronic aortic regurgitation, and dilated cardiomyopathy.

Enhanced ventricular interdependence between the two ventricles due to excessive pericardial restraint is the probable underlying mechanism of diastolic dysfunction seen in patients with sudden dilatation of the left heart chambers due to acute aortic and mitral regurgitation. This phenomenon is also responsible for abnormalities in patients with constrictive pericarditis and cardiac tamponade. In addition to the various disease processes, diastolic function can be affected by cardiac rhythm, heart rate, end-diastolic volume, left ventricular systolic performance, and the patient's age. At present, diastolic function can be evaluated by using several techniques: left ventricular angiography, radionuclide ventriculography, Doppler echocardiography, ultrafast computed tomography, and magnetic resonance imaging. Doppler echocardiography allows examination of transmitral and pulmonary venous flow velocities and provides insight into the abnormalities of diastolic function.

IV. RIGHT VENTRICULAR FUNCTION (SYSTOLIC AND DIASTOLIC)

The determinants of right ventricular systolic and diastolic function are basically similar to those of the left. Assessment of right ventricular performance, however, is more complex due to its unusual shape. Multiple imaging techniques have been utilized to measure right ventricular function. Right ventricular wall thickness can be measured by two-dimensional echocardiography, but the mass is more accurately assessed by ultrafast computed tomography. Currently, gated first-pass radionuclide imaging using a region of interest of variable size, appears to be the most widely available and reliable method of calculating right ventricular ejection fraction. Ultrafast computed tomography is also accurate but more expensive. Ultrafast computed tomographic and echocardiographic studies have shown that the thickness of the right ventricular wall is 3–4 mm, whereas left ventricular wall thickness is 9–12 mm (26). The end-diastolic and end-systolic volumes of the right ventricle are larger than those of the left ventricle by 18% and 76%, respectively. The stroke volume of the left and right ventricle are, however, nearly equal. Left ventricular stroke volume is 2–3% higher than that of the right due to bronchial flow (27). The right ventricular ejection fraction in normal adults is, therefore, lower than that of left (normal RVEF 57 ± 6; LVEF 65 ± 8%) ventricular ejection fraction. Two-dimensional echocardiography is another acceptable and practical method for evaluating overall right ventricular size, wall thickness, wall motion, and ejection fraction. Information regarding right ventricular systolic pressure can be obtained by Doppler-derived tricuspid regurgitation signal (28). Diastolic function can be assessed by examination of the flows across the tricuspid valve and hepatic veins using pulsed Doppler methods.

V. IMAGING METHODS TO ASSESS LEFT AND RIGHT VENTRICULAR FUNCTION

Comprehensive quantitative assessment of left (or right) ventricular function would include information regarding mass, volume (end-diastolic and end-systolic), systolic and diastolic performance, perfusion, and metabolism of the muscle. A variety of techniques have been utilized to accomplish these goals. These methods include cardiac catheterization and contrast angiography, echocardiography, radionuclide angiography, ultrafast computed tomography, and magnetic resonance imaging (MRI). Thallium-201 scintigraphy is clinically available to study myocardial perfusion. Positron emission tomography (PET) and MRI using phosphorus-31 spectroscopy are some of the emerging methods for obtaining information on the myocardial metabolism. Thallium-201 scintigraphic and position emission tomographic techniques will not be discussed in this chapter.

A. Cardiac Catheterization and Contrast Angiography

Over the last several decades, catheterization and angiographic techniques have been utilized to study systolic and diastolic performance of the left ventricle (1,29).

1. Left Ventricular Mass

Left ventricular mass can be calculated by angiographic methods. Biplane area–length methods are used to calculate the total (cavity plus the muscle) and the left ventricular cavity volume. The difference between the total and the cavity volume equals the muscle volume. The muscle volume is multiplied by the specific gravity of cardiac muscle (1.05) to obtain the left ventricular muscle mass. In this method, wall thickness is assumed to be homogenous and is measured along the anterior wall of the left ventricle. This assumption would cause error in patients with regional thinning due to infarction and asymmetric hypertrophy of the myocardium.

2. Isovolumic-Phase Indices

The maximal rate of left ventricular pressure rise (dP/dt) can be calculated from high-fidelity catheter recordings of the left ventricle during isovolumic systole. The normal value of dP/dt is more than 1200 mmHg/s. This parameter is not routinely used in patient management.

3. Ejection-Phase Indices

Right and left heart catheterization allow assessment of intracardiac pressures. Thermodilution and angiographic methods are utilized to measure stroke volume (SV), cardiac output (CO), end-diastolic volume (EDV), end-systolic volume (ESV), and ejection fraction (EF). In patients with valvular regurgitation, these methods can be used to measure forward cardiac output and regurgitant volume. The normal values for these parameters are as follows: CO 3.0 ± 0.5 L/min/m²; EDV 70 ± 20 mL/m²; ESV 24 ± 10 cm³/m²; EF 67 ± 0.8. Ejection fraction and end-systolic volume indices are the most commonly utilized parameters in patients with valvular heart disease.

4. End-Systolic Indices

End-systolic left ventricular volume index has been utilized in several studies to predict the postoperative outcome in patients with mitral and aortic regurgitation. Left ventricular end-systolic volume index of >90 cm³/m² was predictive of postoperative left ventricular dysfunction in patients with aortic regurgitation (18). In contrast, left ventricular end-systolic volume index of >60 cm³/m² in one study (18) and >50 cm³/m² in another study (19) was predictive of postoperative left ventricular dysfunction in patients with mitral regurgitation. End-systolic volume index is independent of preload but is influenced by afterload. Therefore, a certain group of investigators has studied the ratio of end-systolic stress to end-systolic volume index. This ratio can also be calculated by complete angiographic studies.

B. Echocardiography

A variety of echocardiographic techniques are routinely utilized to evaluate and follow biventricular function in patients with valvular heart disease. All these techniques will be discussed at length in this section. M-mode echocardiography continues to be a valuable tool to assess wall thickness, dimension, and evaluate systolic left ventricular function. M-mode recording should be obtained by directing the cursor line through the largest diameter of the left ventricle using parasternal short- or long-axis views. The cursor should be aligned perpendicular to the walls and the cavity. A cursor line directed obliquely through the left ventricular cavity will provide erroneous wall thickness and cavity dimension. In some patients, it is not possible to obtain accurate left ventricular cavity dimensions from the M-mode recording due to the position of the left ventricle. In these cases, the measurements should be made directly from the two-dimensional echocardiographic views. Figures 10 and 11 illustrate the technique of measuring the left ventricular end-diastolic diameter (LVEDD), left ventricular end-systolic diameter (LVESD), fractional shortening (FS), posterior wall thickness in diastole (PWTD), ventricular septal thickness in diastole (VSTD), posterior wall thickness in systole (PWTS), and ventricular septal thickness in systole (VSTS). End-diastolic left ventricular radius (half of LVEDD) can be divided by the average end-diastolic wall thickness (half of the sum of PWTD and VSTD) to obtain the end-diastolic radius/thickness (R/T) ratio. The end-diastolic R/T ratio can be multiplied by systolic blood pressure, and this product has been shown to correlate with the peak systolic wall stress and has been found to be useful in clinical decision making in patients with valvular

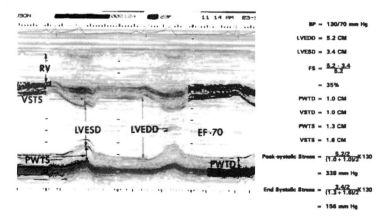

Figure 10 This M-mode recording was obtained from a 28-year-old asymptomatic female with moderate aortic regurgitation due to aneurysm of the ascending aorta. Ejection fraction was normal at 0.70. Left ventricular end-diastolic diameter (LVEDD) and left ventricular end-systolic diameter (LVESD) and fractional shortening (FS) were normal. Posterior wall thickness at end-diastole (PWTD), ventricular septal thickness at end-diastole (VSTD), posterior wall thickness at end-systole (PWTS), and ventricular septal thickness at end-systole (VSTS) are reported on the illustration. Calculation of peak and end-systolic stresses are also shown.

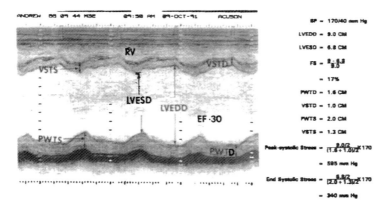

Figure 11 This M-mode recording was obtained from a 32-year-old patient with severe aortic regurgitation due to rheumatic heart disease. Left ventricular end-systolic diameter (LVESD) is markedly increased to 6.8 cm, and fractional short-ening (FS) is markedly reduced to 17%. Peak systolic stress is increased to 595 mmHg, and end-systolic stress is markedly increased to 340 mmHg. This patient was in severe congestive heart failure; he underwent successful open-heart sur-gery, and his aortic valve was replaced with a St. Jude prosthesis. The patient improved markedly from symptoms of congestive heart failure in the postoperative period. However, a postoperative echocardiogram taken 1 month after surgery showed persistent left ventricular enlargement and no significant change in ejec-tion fraction (EF). His pre- and postoperative ejection fraction was approximately 0.30.

regurgitation. End-systolic left ventricular radius (half of LVESD) can be divided by the average end-systolic wall thickness (half of the sum of PWTS and VSTS) to obtain the end-systolic radius/thickness (R/T) ratio. This end-systolic R/T ratio can be multipled by systolic blood pressure, and this product correlates with end-systolic wall stress and also has been found to be useful in decision making regarding surgery in patients with valvular regurgitation (17,30–32). Fractional shortening (FS) is calculated by dividing the difference between LVEDD and LVESD by LVEDD. Figures 10 and 11 illustrate the technique of obtaining various M-mode measurements from two patients with aortic regurgitation. The normal value for fractional shortening is >30%. E-point septal separation (EPSS) of >8 mm on the M-mode recordings of the mitral valve generally indicates reduced ejection fraction. This finding, however, is not reliable in patients with mitral stenosis, aortic regurgitation, and apical asynergy with com-pensatory hyperdynamic motion at the base of the left ventricle. Poor mitral valve excursion, systolic convergence of the aortic valve, and reduced aortic root motion are several other features of poor cardiac output and function.

Gaasch et al. (31) noted that LV end-systolic diameter (LVESD) of >5 cm or 2.6 cm/m² and peak systolic stress of >600 mmHg were predictive of postoperative dysfunction in patients with chronic severe aortic regurgitation (Fig. 12). Kumpures et al. (32) studied 43 patients with chronic aortic regurgitation who underwent surgery. They observed normalization of left ventricular size and function in 28 patients and persistent left ventricular enlargement and systolic dysfunction in 15 patients. Fractional shortening of >28%, end-systolic diameter of <5 cm, and end-systolic wall stress of <235 mmHg were the most predictive indices for postoperative normalization of left ventricular size and function (Fig. 13). In a study of 20 patients with chronic mitral regurgitation who underwent surgery (17), 16 patients had normalization of LV size and function postoperatively. All 4 patients with suboptimal outcome had LVESD >4.5 cm (2.6 cm/m²), FS <31%, and end-systolic wall stress >195 mmHg (Fig. 6).

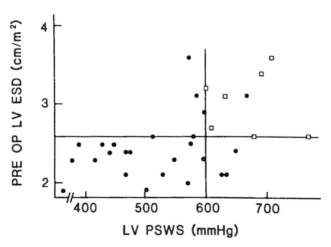

Figure 12 Plot of preoperative left ventricular end-systolic diameter (PRE OP LV ESD in cm/m²) on the vertical axis and left ventricular peak systolic wall stress (LV PSWS in mmHg) along the horizontal axis from 32 patients with aortic regurgitation who underwent arotic valve replacement (filled circles and open squares). There were seven patients with persistent postoperative left ventricular enlargement and dysfunction (open squares). All of these seven patients are correctly identified by combination of preoperative LV ESD of >2.6 cm/m² and LV PSWS of >600 mmHg. There is only one false positive. (Redrawn and reproduced with permission from Ref. 31.)

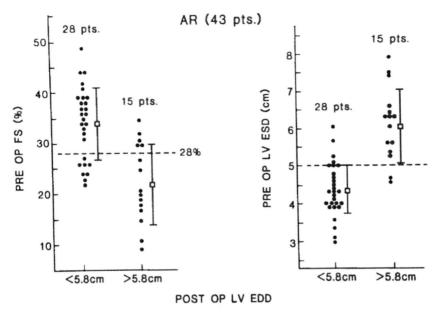

POST OP LV EDD

Figure 13 Findings of a study of aortic valve replacement in 43 patients with chronic aortic regurgitation (AR). There were 28 patients in whom postoperatively left ventricular end-diastolic diameter (POST OP LV EDD) normalized to <5.8 cm and 15 patients in whom there was persistent left ventricular enlargement with size >5.8 cm. The left panel shows the preoperative fractional shortening in the two groups of patients, and the horizontal broken line indicates the cutoff value that best separates the two groups. The majority of patients with preoperative fractional shortening (PRE OP FS) <28% appear to have postoperative LV enlargement. The right panel shows that the majority of patients with preoperative left ventricular end-systolic diameter (PRE OP LV ESD in cm) >5 cm have persistent postoperative LV enlargement. (Redrawn and reproduced with permission from Ref. 32.)

All the tomographic two-dimensional echocardiographic views should be obtained to reliably assess the regional and global wall motion and function (33). From the two-dimensional echocardiographic views, left ventricular volumes and ejection fraction can be calculated. Pulsed Doppler techniques can be utilized to calculate stroke volume and cardiac output. Continuous-wave Doppler methods can be used to record the mitral regurgitation signal. From this signal, dP/dt can be measured (Fig. 14). Thus combination of various echo-Doppler techniques allow us to evaluate left ventricular mass, dP/dt, volumes, and ejection fraction.

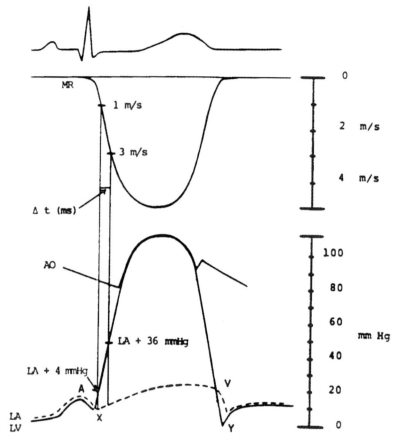

Figure 14 This diagram shows the method of calculation of left ventricular $\Delta p/ \Delta t$ or dP/dt from the continuous-wave Doppler-derived mitral regurgitation signal. Δt is the time taken for the mitral regurgitation (MR) signal to rise from 1 to 3 m/ s. Δp is the magnitude of rise in left ventricular pressure when the MR velocity increases from 1 to 3 m/s.

$$\frac{\Delta p}{\Delta t} \text{ or } \frac{dP}{dt} = \frac{32}{\Delta t \text{ in ms}} \times 1000 \text{ mmHg/s}$$

(Reproduced with permission from Ref. 9.)

1. Left Ventricular Mass

Hypertensive patients with increased left ventricular mass (>125 g/m^2 for males; and >110 g/m^2 for females) have three times higher incidence of morbid events (death, myocardial infarction, stroke, and need for coronary bypass surgery) as compared to patients without left ventricular hypertrophy (LVH). In concentric hypertrophy (aortic stenosis), wall thickness is increased but the chamber size is normal. In eccentric hypertrophy (patients with aortic and mitral regurgitation), left ventricular dimension is increased with minimal increase in wall thickness. In both types of hypertrophic patterns, the left ventricular mass is increased. Ideally, the systolic function and left ventricular mass should be close to normal following surgery in patients with mitral and aortic regurgitation. Left ventricular mass can be estimated simply from measurement of septal and posterior wall thickness by M-mode echocardiography (normal <12 mm). Devereux and Reichek (34) developed a method to estimate the left ventricular mass using M-mode echocardiography. This group of investigators utilized the Penn convention for measuring the wall thickness (excluding the endocardial thickness from the thickness of the septum and posterior wall):

$$Mass = 1.04 \left[(LVEDD + VSTD + PWTD)^3 - (LVEDD)^3 \right] - 14 \text{ g}$$

Other investigators have had equally good results with the standard method of measuring wall thickness (35):

$$1.05 \left[(LVEDD + VSTD + PWTD)^3 - (LVEDD)^3 \right] \text{ g}$$

M-mode echocardiographic techniques can be applied to hearts with wall thicknesses uniformly increased, as in patients with valvular heart disease. However, in patients with regional wall motion abnormalities in the presence of ischemic heart disease and nonuniform thickening of the walls (hypertrophic cardiomyopathy), two-dimensional echocardiographic methods should be used to calculate the left ventricular mass. Two-dimensional echocardiographic methods for measuring left ventricular wall thickness use one of two algorithms based on area–length and the truncated ellipsoid models (36). The area–length algorithm assumes the left ventricular shape to be like a bullet and calculates the mass by the following equation:

$$LV \text{ mass} = 1.05 \times \frac{5}{6} (A_{EP} \times L + T) - (A_{EN} \times L)$$

Where A_{EP} = epicardial area of the left ventricle from the short-axis view at the level of the papillary muscle in diastole (including the area of the muscle as well as the cavity); A_{EN} = endocardial left ventricular area from the two-dimensional short-axis view at the level of the papillary muscle in diastole (only the area of the left ventricular cavity); L = length of the left ventricle from midpoint of the mitral valve to the apex from the apical four- or two-chamber view; T equals wall thickness; $\frac{5}{6}$ is a factor utilized in the bullet formula to calculate the volume (volume = area $\times L \times \frac{5}{6}$); and 1.05 is the special gravity of the heart muscle.

2. Isovolumic-Phase Indices of Left Ventricular Function

A variable degree of mitral regurgitation is frequently present in patients with valvular heart disease. A continuous-wave Doppler-derived mitral regurgitation signal can be used to calculate the rate of left ventricular pressure rise in systole. This parameter is an index of left ventricular dP/dt. The time (Δt) taken for the continuous-wave Doppler mitral regurgitation signal to increase from 1 to 3 m/s is measured in milliseconds (ms). Left ventricular dP/dt can be calculated by the following equation (Fig. 14):

$$\frac{dP}{dt} = \frac{32}{\Delta t \text{ in ms}} \times 1000 \text{ mmHg/s}$$

This parameter is relatively independent of afterload but is influenced by preload. In a study performed from our laboratory (9), preoperative dP/dt of >1343 mmHg/s in patients with mitral regurgitation predicted postoperative ejection fraction of >50%.

3. Ejection-Phase Indices of Left Ventricular Function

Various ejection-phase indices can be derived from echo-Doppler methods.

a. Stroke Volume and Cardiac Output. A number of studies have successfully used echo-Doppler methods for determination of stroke volume and cardiac output. Pulsed Doppler examination allows measurement of velocity across different valves. The integral of this velocity signal is known as stroke distance. Stroke volume can be calculated by multiplying the stroke distance with the area of the valve where the velocity is being measured. Lewis et al. (37) successfully used left ventricular outflow tract and mitral inflow region to measure the stroke volume and cardiac output. In patients with mitral and aortic regurgitation, forward and regurgitant volumes can be calculated by estimating the flows across the left ventricular inflow and outflow regions. Regurgitant fraction in aortic regurgitation equals flow across the aortic valve in systole (total stroke output), minus flow across the mitral valve in diastole (forward output), divided by flow across the aortic valve in systole (total stroke output). In mitral regurgitation, regurgitant fraction equals flow across the mitral valve in diastole (total stroke output), minus flow across the aortic valve in systole (forward output), divided by flow across the mitral value in diastole (total output).

b. *LV Volumes and Ejection Fraction.* Left ventricular end-diastolic diameter (LVEDD) from M-mode echocardiogram provides a measure of left ventricular dilatation and size (normal <5.6 cm). Left ventricular end-systolic diameter (LVESD) reflects left ventricular size in systole (normal <3.5 cm). Fractional shortening (FS) calculated from these diameters (LVEDD − LVESD/LVESD; normal >30%) in a symmetrically contracting left ventricle can be used as an index of ejection fraction. Teichholz method (38) can be used to calculate the volumes (*V*) from these M-mode echocardiographic measurements:

$$V = D^3 \times \frac{7}{2.4 + D}$$

where V = volume, and D = end-diastolic or end-systolic diameter. Using this method, end-diastolic volumes, end-systolic volumes, and ejection fraction can be calculated. The Teichholz method is reasonably accurate in a symmetrically contracting left ventricle.

A variety of methods can be used to calculate the volumes and ejection fraction more accurately using two-dimensional echocardiography (36,39). These methods include single-plane area–length, biplane area–length, bullet formula, single-plane modified Simpson's rule, and biplane modified Simpson's rule disk summation methods.

Single-plane area–length method: $V = 0.85 \times A^2/L$, where A = planimetered endocardial area of the apical four- or two-chamber view and L = length. If endocardium cannot be traced using computer software, then volume can be calculated by measuring the length and the short-axis diameter from apical four- or two-chamber views. In this formula, volume = $0.52 \times L \times D^2$.

Biplane area–length method: $V = 0.85 \times A_1 \times A_2/L$, where A_1 = planimetered area of the endocardium from the apical four-chamber view, A_2 = area from the apical two-chamber view, and L = longest length from either four- or two-chamber views. If the endocardium cannot be traced, then short-axis diameters from four (D_1) and two-chamber (D_2) views can be used. In this equation, $V = 0.52 \times L \times D_1 \times D_2$.

Bullet formula: $V = \frac{5}{6} \times A \times L$, where A = planimetered endocardial area of the left ventricle from the parasternal short-axis view at the level of the papillary muscle and L = length of the left ventricle from apical views.

The Modified Simpson's rule formula treats the left ventricle as a stack of multiple short cylinders. The ventricular volume is then calculated as the sum of the volumes of each individual cylinder. This calculation can be performed by using a single (apical four- or two-chamber view) or biplane approach (both apical four- and two-chamber views). This disk summation method, using the modified Simpson's rule, is preferred over other methods because it is less sensitive to geometric distortions and can be used in left ventricles of different size and shapes. Both left ventricular end-diastolic volume (EDV) and end-systolic volume (ESV) can be calculated using these two-dimensional volumetric methods. Ejection fraction (EF) = EDV − ESV/EDV (normal = 0.70 ± 8). The volumes calculated by these echocardiographic methods are generally lower than those obtained by angiography. Ejection fraction calculated by echocardiography, however, correlates reasonably well with angiographic methods. Quinones and associates (40) have developed a simplified method of measuring left ventricular ejection fraction from parasternal and apical two-dimensional echocardiographic images without the need of planimetry and/or computer processing. Multiple endocardial diameters are measured from parasternal (diameter just below the mitral valve leaflets and at the level of the papillary muscle) and apical (three diameters, one just below the mitral valve leaflets, second at the level of the papillary muscle in the midventricle, and third in the apical region) views. An average is made of all these five diameters at end-diastole (D_d) and at end-systole (D_s). Ejection fraction then can be calculated by the following formula:

$$EF = \frac{D_d{}^2 - D_s{}^2}{D_d{}^2} + \left(1 - \frac{D_d{}^2 - D_s{}^2}{D_d{}^2}\right)(\%\Delta L)$$

where $\%\Delta L$ is the fractional shortening of the long axis of the left ventricle and is estimated from subjective assumption of the motion of the apex (normal apical contraction, plus 15%; hypokinetic, plus 5%; akinetic, 0%; mild dyskinesis, −5%; and severe dyskinesis, −10%). The estimated ejection fraction by this simplified method agrees well with the ejection fraction determined by radionuclide or contrast angiographic techniques.

In the clinical setting, visual estimation of left ventricular ejection fraction by experienced echocardiographers has become a common practice. The correlations between visual estimates and other methods are quite good. Left ventricular diastolic function can be assessed by measuring pulsed Doppler flow across pulmonary veins and the mitral valve. The

transmitral flow recording shows decreased E velocity, prolonged deceleration time (DT), increased A velocity and lower E/A ratio in patients with
diastolic dysfunction due to impaired relaxation, as seen in patients with
left ventricular hypertrophy. In patients with elevated left atrial pressure
(mitral regurgitation, restrictive hemodynamics, and decreased compliance), transmitral flow shows increase in E velocity, decrease in deceleration time, decrease of A velocity, and increase in E/A ratio. Pulmonary
vein recording shows predominant systolic filling in the former and the
diastolic filling in the latter pattern of diastolic dysfunction (24,25).

Echocardiography can also be used to estimate right ventricular size,
wall thickness, motion, and ejection fraction. Watanabe and associates
(41) calculated right ventricular volume and ejection fraction using two
orthogonal apical views, applying the modified Simpson's rule. This
method, however, consistently underestimated the volumes as compared
to angiographic techniques. Right ventricular diastolic dysfunction can be
evaluated using transtricuspid and hepatic venous flow velocities (25).

C. Radionuclide Angiography

The radionuclide techniques provide useful information regarding left and
right ventricular function and severity of valvular regurgitation (42). These
techniques are safe, noninvasive, and permit evaluation of cardiac performance at rest and during a variety of physiological and pharmacological
interventions. Echocardiography and radionuclide angiographic procedures are ideal for serial evaluation of patients with valvular heart disease.

Cardiac performance can be assessed by one of two radionuclide techniques: (1) first-pass radionuclide angiocardiography; or (2) equilibrium
radionuclide angiography or gated blood pool scanning or multigated acquisition (MUGA) scanning technique. Both these approaches employ
scintillation cameras for acquiring cardiac images and radionuclide data.
More recently, several nonimaging probes have been utilized for prolonged ventricular function monitoring. The nonimaging probe, called the
"nuclear stethoscope," is no longer available. Another instrument, called
the VEST, employes the basic principles of equilibrium radionuclide angiography and allows for monitoring over several hours following blood pool
labeling (41). Both first-pass and equilibrium gated blood pool scanning
techniques are capable of providing information about left ventricular end-
diastolic volume (EDV), end-systolic volume (ESV), stroke volume (SV),
and ejection fraction (EF). Right ventricular ejection fraction also can be
calculated. In most laboratories, equilibrium gated blood pool scanning
is the most widely used method. The severity of valvular regurgitation
can be expressed as a ratio between left ventricular to right ventricular

stroke counts or as the *regurgitant index*, which is equal to left ventricular stroke counts minus right ventricular stroke counts/LV stroke counts × 100. Regurgitant fraction can also be calculated. The first-pass technique analyzes the transit of a compact intravenous bolus of a radioisotope (technetium-99m pertechnetate) through the central circulation in the first five to six heart beats. A multicrystal camera was preferred for first-pass studies because of its high counting efficiency. More recently, multicrystal cameras have been replaced with digital cameras. The ejection fraction of both left and right ventricles can be measured from the time–activity curve of each ventricle. The first-pass technique is the modality of choice for evaluation of right ventricular function. A first-pass radionuclide angiogram also can be constructed from the left ventricular time activity curve from the first two to four successive cardiac cycles. The composite image is played back in a cine-loop format for analysis of regional wall motion abnormalities. The presence of major arrhythmias usually invalidates the first-pass data. The more commonly used gated blood pool equilibrium radionuclide angiography is performed by using technetium-99m-labeled red blood cells. These technetium-labeled red blood cells are first allowed to distribute uniformly throughout the patient's blood volume, and then imaged using a standard single-crystal gamma camera. The count collection by the camera is gated to the patient's electrocardiogram. Each cardiac cycle is divided into 16 to 64 equal intervals or frames. Data collected during the same frame of several hundred successive cardiac cycles are then added together to generate an average single cardiac cycle and display the information in a cine-loop format. The left ventricular volumes and ejection fraction can be calculated from the end-diastolic and end-systolic counts. High counting rates obtained with the gated blood pool studies provide superior resolution and assessment of regional and global ventricular performance. High-resolution images can be obtained with gated blood pool scanning for 3 to 5 h, and this strength allows imaging in multiple projections at rest, exercise, and during various interventions. Atrial fibrillation and other arrhythmias, commonly present in patients with valvular heart disease, clearly affect the data acquisition due to wide variation in R-R interval. It should be noted that the ejection fractions determined from the first-pass studies are generally lower than those obtained with the gated blood pool method. Patients with valvular heart disease who are followed serially should be studied with one method to avoid errors because of differences in the techniques.

In patients with aortic regurgitation, the gated blood pool studies are accurate in determination of left ventricular ejection fraction. In patients with mitral regurgitation, however, here may be significant overlap between the left atrium and the left ventricle. In certain patients, this overlap cannot be eliminated, and erroneous left ventricular count and ejection fraction may be calculated. The radionuclide techniques have been utilized to address the issue of timing of aortic valve replacement in patients with aortic regurgitation in a series of published articles from Bonow and co-workers (22). They have demonstrated that a great majority of asymptomatic patients with aortic regurgitation and normal ejection fraction do well on long-term follow-up, and only <4% per year require valve replacement because of symptoms or decrease in resting ejection fraction. In comparison, two-thirds or more of the asymptomatic patients who show evidence of left ventricular dysfunction (ejection fraction <45%) develop symptoms requiring operation within 2 to 3 years. Furthermore, these investigators have also pointed out that the preoperative resting left ventricular ejection fraction is a major determinant of postoperative outcome and survival in patients with severe aortic regurgitation. They found that there was significant improvement in postoperative ejection fraction in patients whose preoperative value was >45%. The majority of patients with preoperative ejection fraction of <30% showed a decrease in postoperative ejection fraction. Survival at 5.5 years was 96% in patients with normal preoperative ejection fraction (30 patients with ejection fraction >45%), compared with 63% in patients with an abnormal preoperative ejection fraction (50 patients with preoperative ejection fraction <45%). Recent data suggest that the ejection-fraction response to maximum exercise is abnormal in many asymptomatic patients with aortic regurgitation, and that the magnitude of decrease in ejection fraction with exercise *does not appear* to predict subsequent clinical outcomes (23). Patients with an increase in ejection fraction during exercise are, however, unlikely to develop symptoms or left ventricular dysfunction.

D. Ultrafast Computed Tomography

Conventional computed tomographic techniques take 1 to 3 s for image acquisition and produce blurred images of cardiac chambers. Ultrafast computed tomography (CT) is made possible by rapid scanning time. The cine CT images of the heart can be obtained by using the Imatron C-100 computed tomography scanners (43). In the standard cardiac mode, the resolution in the imaging plane is 1.5 mm, slice thickness is 8 mm, and temporal resolution is 17 frames per second. In the high-resolution mode, the resolution is 0.7 mm and slice thickness is 3 mm. Radiographic contrast media are used for chamber opacification. The ultrafast CT images of the heart can be used to calculate the mass, end-diastolic volume (EDV), end-systolic volume (ESV), stroke volume (SV = EDV − ESV), and ejection fraction (EF = EDV − ESV/EDV) of both right and left ventricles

(26,27,43). Normally, right ventricular end-diastolic volume is larger than left ventricular end-diastolic volume by an average of 18%. Right ventricular (RV) EF is lower than that of left ventricular (LV) EF by an average of 13% (LVEF = 70 ± 5%; RVEF = 57 ± 6%). Mass of the right ventricular free wall is 27 ± 4 g/m^2 by computed tomographic methods. LV mass (including ventricular septum) is 80 ± 10 g/m^2. CT methods show that the difference between left and right ventricular stroke volume is minimal (LV stroke volume 0 to 10 cm^3 larger than right ventricular stroke volume). In patients with aortic or mitral regurgitation, left ventricular stroke volume is higher and the difference between left- and right-sided stroke volumes provides an estimate of regurgitant volume (43). Current data suggest strongly that cine CT can provide reproducible and precise measurement of biventricular chamber volume, mass, and ejection fraction. Limitations of CT include lack of portability, cost, use of contrast agents, and X-rays. Further work needs to be done to define its value in clinical practice.

E. Magnetic Resonance Imaging

Magentic resonance imaging (MRI) is quite different from the other imaging modalities. Ultrasound and conventional X-ray techniques utilize either ultrasound or X-ray beams to create the images. However, no beam is used in magentic resonance imaging. Instead, the images are created from the radio signals received from the hydrogen nuclei on the water and fat molecules of the cardiac tissue when the characteristics of their rotation in a magnetic field are changed by radiofrequency pulses. MRI techniques can use different imaging pulse sequences to produce cardiac images (44). The standard *spin echo sequence* approach displays the blood pool as dark, and the myocardium has an intermediate signal intensity. The second common approach for cardiac imaging uses the *gradient reversal sequence*. In the images obtained by gradient reversal sequence technique, the appearance of the blood pool is brighter and that of the myocardium darker. Multislice technique allows one to obtain multiple tomographic slices of the heart from apex to base. These images are gated to the electrocardiogram. These gated multislice images permit measurement of volumes by using the Simpson's rule method. In cine MRI, multiple images of a single slice obtained during different portions of the cardiac cycle are displayed rapidly by the computer, like the frames of a movie. Gradient reversal sequence is used in most cine MRI approaches. Mitral regurgitation is visualized as a region of signal loss in the left atrium and aortic regurgitation as a region of signal loss in the left ventricular outflow tract on these gradient-reversal cine MRI images. The MRI techniques allow assessment of left ventricular mass, volumes, ejection fraction and degree of regurgitation. At present, it takes a long time to acquire these images. The widespread clinical application of these methods will definitely require considerable reduction of study time. High-speed planar imaging technique is currently being developed. This technique allows the acquisition of cardiac images in a fraction of a second.

VI. CONCLUSIONS

Serial assessment of left ventricular function by various imaging modalities (particularly echocardiography) has become extremely valuable for proper timing of surgery in patients with mitral and aortic regurgitation. In acute symptomatic mitral and aortic regurgitation, surgery is generally performed on an urgent basis. However, in chronic aortic and mitral regurgitation, the following guidelines may be used.

A. Chronic Severe Aortic Regurgitation (AR)

1. Chronic Severe AR with Minimal or No Symptoms

In this group of patients, combined LV size and performance parameters obtained from serial echocardiographic, radionuclide, and exercise studies should be utilized in decision making. Aortic valve replacement should be performed if multiple criteria are met:

   a. LVESD approaches 5.5 cm (echo).
   b. FS decreases toward 25% (echo).
   c. LV peak systolic wall stress <600 mmHg (echo).
   d. LV end systolic wall stress <235 mmHg (echo).
   e. LV end systolic volume index <90 c/m^2 (angio).
   f. EF decreases to 50% range on serial studies (echo/angio).
   g. Decreased exercise capacity on serial exercise studies.

2. Chronic Severe Aortic Regurgitation with Significant Symptoms

   a. If preoperative LV size is moderately enlarged (LVESD 5.5 cm) and LV performance is normal to moderately impaired (FS ≥25%, EF 50%), ventricular size and function usually improve after valve replacement.
   b. If preoperative LV size is markedly enlarged (ESD >6.0) and performance is significantly impaired (FS ≤ 25%, EF 30–40%), the surgery should be performed but risk of persistent postoperative LV enlargement and moderate LV dysfunction is expected.
   c. If preoperative LV size is markedly enlarged (ESD >6 cm, ESVI

>150 cm³/m²), and LV performance is markedly impaired (FS <25%, EF <30%), surgery may be performed at higher surgical risk. The potential for irreversible LV dysfunction is markedly increased as well.

d. Surgery should be individualized if EF <25%. The operative risk and postoperative LV dysfunction is extremely high.

B. Chronic Severe Mitral Regurgitation (MR)

1. Chronic Severe MR with Minimal or No Symptoms
The following parameters of LV size and function on serial studies should be utilized for timing of mitral valve surgery. As a rule, reparative technique should be used when possible.

a. LVESD ≤4.5 cm (echo)
b. FS ≥30% (echo)
c. LVESS ≤195 mmHg (echo)
d. LVESVI ≤50–60 cm³/m² (angio)
e. LVEF ≥65% (echo, angio)
f. LV dP/dt from MR Doppler signal ≥1350 mmHg
g. Ratio of LVESWS/ESVI ≥2.5 (angio)
h. Decreasing exercise capacity and increase in exercise-induced pulmonary hypertension.

2. Chronic MR with Severe Symptoms
a. If there is moderate dilation (LVESD 4.5–5.5 cm) and mild LV dysfunction (EF 45–60%), the surgery can be performed at low risk. The risk of persistent LV enlargement and severe dysfunction is high, however. Patients will generally experience relief from congestive symptoms.
b. If there is severe dilation of LV (LVESD ≥5.5 cm) and reduced function (EF 30–45%), the risk of surgery is moderately increased. Postoperative severe LV enlargement and poor systolic function are expected.
c. If the EF is <30%, the decision regarding surgery should be individualized. It can be accomplished in patients with ischemic heart disease with obstructive coronary disease when bypass grafting and MV replacement can be performed. Feasibility of mitral valve repair should be assessed and done whenever possible. Mitral valve repair helps preserve the overall left ventricular performance (45).

REFERENCES
1. Braunwald E. Assessment of cardiac function. In: Braunwald E, ed. Heart Disease. Philadelphia: Saunders, 1992:419–43.

2. Grossman W. Evaluation of systolic and diastolic function of the myocardium. In: Grossman W, ed. Cardiac Catheterization and Angiography. Philadelphia: Lea and Febiger, 1986:301–19.
3. Grossman W, Jones D, McLaurin P. Wall stress and patterns of hypertrophy in human left ventricle. J Clin Invest 1975; 56:56–64.
4. Mirsky I, Corin WJ, Murakami T, Grimm J, Hess OM, Krayenbeuhl HP. Correction for preload in assessment of myocardial contractility in aortic and mitral valve disease: application of the concept of systolic myocardial stiffness. Circulation 1988; 78:68–80.
5. Corin WJ, Monrad ES, Murakami T, Nonogi H, Hess OM, Krayenbeuhl HP. The relationship of afterload to ejection performance in chronic mitral regurgitation. Circulation 1987; 76:59–67.
6. Carabello BA, Nolan SP, McGuire LB. Assessment of preoperative left ventricular function in patients with mitral regurgitation: value of the end-systolic wall stress–end-systeolic volume ratio. Circulation 1981; 64:1212–7.
7. Peterson KL. Timing of cardiac surgery in chronic mitral valve disease: implications of natural history studies and left ventricular mechanics. Sem Thoracic Cardiovasc Surg 1989; 1:106–17.
8. Wisenbaugh T, Spann JF, Carabello BA. Differences in myocardial performance and load between patients with similar amounts of chronic aortic versus chronic mitral regurgitation. J Am Coll Cardiol 1984; 3:916–23.
9. Pai RG, Bansal RC, Shah PM. Doppler-derived rate of left ventricular pressure rise. Its correlation with postoperative left ventricular function in mitral regurgitation. Circulation 1990; 82:514–20.
10. Ross J Jr. Afterload mismatch in aortic and mitral valve disease: implications for surgical therapy. J Am Coll Cardiol 1985; 5:811–26.
11. Suga H, Sagawa K, Shoukas AA. Load independence of the instantaneous pressure–volume ratio of the canine left ventricle and effects of epinephrine and heart rate on the ratio. Circ Res 1973; 32:314–20.
12. Sagawa K. The end-systolic pressure–volume relation of the ventricle: Definition, modifications and clinical use. Circulation 1981; 63:1223–30.
13. Carabello BA, Spann JF. The uses and limitations of end-systolic indexes of left ventricular function. Circulation 1984; 69:1058–64.
14. Henry WL, Bonow RO, Rosing DR, Epstein SE. Observations on the optimum time for operative intervention for aortic regurgitation. II. Serial echocardiographic evaluation of asymptomatic patients. Circulation 1980; 61:484–92.
15. Henry WL, Bonow RO, Borer JS, et al. Observations on the optimum time for operative intervention for aortic regurgitation. I. Evaluation of the results of aortic valve replacement in symptomatic patients. Circulation 1980; 61:471–83.
16. Schuler G, Peterson KL, Johnson A, et al. Temporal response of left ventricular performance to mitral valve surgery. Circulation 1979; 59:1218–31.
17. Zile MR, Gaasch WH, Carroll JD, Levine HJ. Chronic mitral regurgitation: predictive value of preoperative echocardiographic indexes of left ventricular function and wall stress. J Am Coll Cardiol; 1984; 3:235–42.

18. Borow KM, Green LH, Sloss LJ, et al. End-systolic volume as a predictor of post-operative left ventricular performance in volume overload from valvular regurgitation. Am J Med 1980; 68:655–63.

19. Crawford MH, Souchek J, Oprian CA, et al. Determinants of survival and left ventricular performance after mitral valve replacement. Circulation 1990; 81:1173–81.

20. Kontos GS, Schaff HV, Gersh BJ, et al. Left ventricular function in subacute and chronic mitral regurgitation (abstr). J Am Coll Cardiol 1986; 7:11.

21. Borow KM, Green LH, Grossman W, Braunwald E. Left ventricular end-systolic stress-shortening and stress-length relations in humans: normal values and sensitivity to inotropic state. Am J Cardiol 1982; 50:1301–8.

22. Colan SD, Borow KM, Neumann A. Left ventricular end-systolic wall stress-velocity of fiber shortening relation: a load-independent index of myocardial contractility. J Am Coll Cardiol 1984; 4:715–24.

23. Bonow RO. Radionuclide angiography in the management of asymptomatic aortic regurgitation. Circulation 1991; 84(suppl I):296–302.

24. Nishimura RA, Housmans PR, Hatle LK, Tajik AJ. Assessment of diastolic function of the heart: background and current applications of Doppler echocardiography. Part I: Physiologic and pathophysiologic features. Mayo Clin Proc 1989; 64:71.

25. Nishimura RA, Abel Md, Hatle LK, Tajik AJ. Assessment of diastolic function of the heart: background and current applications of Doppler echocardiography. Part II: Clinical studies. Mayo Clin Proc 1989; 64:181.

26. Hajduczok ZD, Weiss RM, Marcus ML. Right ventricular mass can be accurately assessed by ultrafast computed tomography (abstr). J Am Coll Cardiol 1989; 13:8A.

27. Reiter SJ, Rumberger JA, Feiring AJ, et al. Precision of measurements of right and left ventricular volume by cine computed tomography. Circulation 1986; 74:890–5.

28. Currie PJ, Seward JB, Chan K-L, et al. Continuous wave Doppler examination of right ventricular pressure. A simultaneous Doppler-catheterization study in 127 patients. J Am Coll Cardiol 1985; 6:750–6.

29. Sheehan FH. Cardiac angiography. In: Marcus ML, Schelbert HR, Skorton DJ, Wolf GL, eds. Cardiac Imaging. Philadelphia: Saunders, 1991:110–48.

30. Quinones MA, Mokotoff DM, Nouris S, Winters WL, Miller RR. Noninvasive quantitation of left ventricular wall stress. Validation of method and application to assessment of chronic pressure overload. Am J Cardiol 1980; 45:782–90.

31. Gaasch WH, Carroll JD, Levine HJ, Criscitiello MG. Chronic aortic regurgitation: prognostic value of left ventricular end-systolic dimension and end-diastolic radius/thickness ratio. J Am Coll Cardiol 1983; 1:775–82.

32. Kumpuris AG, Quinones MA, Waggoner AL, Kanon DJ, Nelson JG, Miller RR. Importance of preoperative hypertrophy, wall stress and end-systolic dimension as echocardiographic predictors of normalization of left ventricular dilation after valve replacement in chronic insufficiency. Am J Cardiol 1982; 49:1091–100.

33. Bansal RC, Tajik AJ, Seward JB, et al. Feasibility of detailed two-dimensional echocardiographic examination in adults: prospective study of 200 patients. Mayo Clinic Proc 1980; 55:291–308.
34. Devereau RB, Reichek N. Echocardiographic determination of left ventricular mass in man. Anatomic validation of the method. Circulation 1977; 55: 613–618.
35. Woythaler JN, Singer SL, Kwan OL, Demaria AN. Accuracy of echocardiography versus electrocardiography in detecting left ventricular hypertrophy: comparison with post mortem mass measurements. J Am Coll Cardiol 1983; 2:305–11.
36. Schiller NB. Two-dimensional echocardiographic determination of left ventricular volumes, systolic function, and mass: summary and discussion of the American Society of Echocardiography. Circulation 1991; 84(suppl I):I-280–7.
37. Lewis JF, Kuo LC, Nelson JG, Limacher MC, Quinones MA. Pulsed Doppler echocardiographic determination of stroke volume and cardiac output: clinical validation of two new methods using the apical window. Circulation 1984; 70:425–31.
38. Teichholz LE, Kreulen T, Herman MV, Gorlin R. Problems in echocardiographic volume determinations: echocardiographic-angiographic correlations in the presence or absence of asynergy. Am J Cardiol 1976; 37:7–11.
39. Wahr DW, Wang YS, Schiller NB. Left ventricular volumes determined by two-dimensional echocardiography in a normal adult population. J Am Coll Cardiol 1983; 3:863–8.
40. Quinones MA, Waggoner AD, Reduto La, et al. A new, simplified and accurate method for determining ejection fraction with two-dimensional echocardiography. Circulation 1981; 64:744.
41. Watanabe T, Katsume H, Matsukubo H, et al. Estimation of right ventricular volume with two dimensional echocardiography. Am J Cardiol 1982; 49: 1946–53.
42. Zaret BL, Wackers FJT, Soufer R. Nuclear cardiology. In: Braunwald E, ed. Heart Disease. Philadelphia: Saunders, 1992:276–311.
43. Marcus ML, Weiss RM. Evaluation of cardiac structure and function with ultrafast computed tomography. In Marcus ML, Schelbert HR, Skorton DJ, Wolf GL, eds. Cardiac Imaging. Philadelphia: Saunders, 1991:669–81.
44. Peshock RM. Magnetic resonance imaging of the heart: quantitation. In: Marcus ML, Schelbert HR, Skorton DJ, Wolf GL, eds. Cardiac Imaging. Philadelphia: Saunders, 1991:811–27.
45. Goldman ME. Mora F, Guarino T, Fuster V, Mindich BP. Mitral valvuloplasty is superior to valve replacement for preservation of left ventricular function: an intraoperative two-dimensional echocardiographic study. J Am Coll Cardiol 1987; 10:568–75.

17

Timing of Surgery in Chronic Aortic and Mitral Regurgitation

Daniel L. Kulick and Shahbudin H. Rahimtoola
University of Southern California, Los Angeles, California

I. INTRODUCTION

Cardiac valve replacement, pioneered by the work of Starr and Harken and their colleagues in the early 1960s, has had a lasting impact in patients with valvular heart disease. Results following cardiac valve replacement have continued to improve, with decreased operative and late mortality, because of: (1) improved operative technique, including better methods of myocardial protection; (2) improved patient selection, including earlier identification of patients before the development of severe, irreversible left ventricular, pulmonary, renal, and hepatic dysfunction; and (3) improved perioperative and long-term medical management. The goals of valve replacement are (1) relief of symptoms caused by severe valvular heart disease with improved exercise capacity and quality of life; (2) prevention of the development of severe, irreversible left ventricular dysfunction; (3) prevention of the occurrence of potentially life-threatening episodes of acute pulmonary edema; (4) prevention of the development of severe pulmonary hypertension and secondary right ventricular failure; and (5) prevention of cardiac death.

The optimal timing of valve replacement is of importance (1,2). In patients who are severely symptomatic, the marked improvement in symptomatic status observed following successful valve replacement in most patients warrants consideration for prompt surgical intervention. In patients with no or only mild symptoms, the decision is more difficult. Per-

---

Adapted from Ref. 1, by permission of the editors, E. Braunwald, M. D., and the publisher, W. B. Saunders Company.

formance of operation "too late" may result in the development of severe, irreversible left ventricular dysfunction, which may fail to improve or actually worsen following valve replacement; the outcome may be one of increased operative mortality, impaired long-term survival, and severe congestive heart failure in operative survivors. Conversely, performance of early valve replacement, before it is clearly necessary, places the patient at unnecessary risk of the many complications of prosthetic heart valves.

II. NATURAL HISTORY

A. Aortic Regurgitation

Chronic severe aortic regurgitation is often tolerated for many years without symptoms, as progressive left ventricular dilatation and hypertrophy occur to accommodate the volume overload condition. With time, left ventricular failure may occur, resulting in symptomatic congestive heart failure. The expected 10-year survival of patients with mild to moderate aortic regurgitation is 85–95% in the United States (3). Of patients with mild aortic regurgitation, 75% of patients may be alive without need for valve replacement at 10 years; among patients with moderate aortic regurgitation, only 22% of patients may be alive without need for valve replacement at 10 years (4). Of patients with chronic severe aortic regurgitation, an asymptomatic latent period of variable duration may ensue, but once symptoms develop, the long-term prognosis with medical therapy alone may be unfavorable; prognosis is adversely affected by the presence of symptomatic heart failure, angina pectoris, or abnormal left ventricular function (4). Among patients with severe heart failure due to chronic aortic regurgitation, mortality is 50% at 2 years, and approaches 100% at 10 years with medical therapy alone. Asymptomatic patients with severe aortic regurgitation and normal left ventricular function progress to requirement for aortic valve replacement (due to development of symptoms or worsening left ventricular function) at a rate of 4%/year or less; early progression to aortic valve replacement is more commonly observed in patients with markedly elevated left ventricular volumes (5). A small number of patients with severe aortic regurgitation may develop sudden cardiac death prior to the development of other symptoms (4).

B. Mitral Regurgitation

In chronic mitral regurgitation the chronically volume-overloaded left ventricle may be well tolerated for many years, due in large part to the ability of the left ventricle to empty blood into the low-impedance left atrium throughout the entire duration of systole. Eventually, severe left ventricular dysfunction may result, with inability to maintain an adequate forward cardiac output; severe left atrial hypertension may develop as well, with late development of pulmonary hypertension and eventual right heart failure. Many of these severe hemodynamic abnormalities may develop in an occult fashion over many years, and symptoms may not result until severe, irreversible left ventricular dysfunction is already present.

The most common etiology of severe mitral regurgitation in parts of the United States necessitating mitral valve surgery is myxomatous valve disease or other connective tissue disorders, followed by mitral regurgitation secondary to coronary artery disease; a smaller number of cases are secondary to rheumatic mitral valvular involvement or infective endocarditis (6). The prognosis of patients with chronic mitral regurgitation is dependent more on the symptomatic and hemodynamic status of the patient than on the underlying cause of mitral regurgitation, although mitral regurgitation caused by coronary artery disease is associated with a less favorable prognosis. With medical therapy, patients with chronic mitral regurgitation which has come to medical attention may have a 5-year survival of 53%, and a 10-year survival of only 22% (7).

III. VALVE REPLACEMENT

A. Operative Mortality

Operative mortality following valve replacement surgery (defined as mortality within 30 days of surgery) depends on many factors; overall, the operative mortality following single valve replacement is generally ≥2-5%, and for double valve replacement is ≥5-10% (8). Recent series of valve replacement surgery have observed lower operative mortality rates than earlier series from the late 1960s and early-mid 1970s (9–11). Reasons for improved results of valve replacement are multifactorial, including: (1) improved surgical and myocardial protection techniques; (2) improved patient selection; and (3) improved medical care of the patient in the immediate postoperative period. These variables are often grouped together, and considered to represent a "time factor" in the evolution of results of valve replacement surgery. Operative results following valve replacement depend more on patient-related factors than on the type of valve implanted (12,13). Moreover, other factors that influence the results of valve replacement, that is, health-care delivery factors, are listed in Table 1.

Numerous clinical variables confer increased risk of early mortality following cardiac valve replacement. These include the following. (1) Se-

Table 1 Health-Care Delivery Factors That Influence Results of Surgery

Preoperative management
  Time patient seeks medical care
  Patient acceptance of and compliance with diagnostic and therapeutic measures
  Expertise of care provided by family practitioners, internists, and cardiologists
  Timing of referral for specialized cardiac investigation and interventional
    treatment
  Expertise in nonsurgical intervention treatment
Quality of surgical management
  Expertise of anesthesia team
  Expertise of surgical team
  Surgical techniques
  Expertise in perioperative care
Postoperative management
  Expertise in long-term care of patients after interventional therapy
    Early diagnosis and treatment of complications
    Specialized care with certain treatments (e.g., anticoagulants)
  Patient cooperation and compliance with long-term care

Source: From Ref. 52.

vere congestive heart failure, as manifested by severe symptomatology (functional classes III or IV) and/or severe depression of left ventricular function, markedly increases operative risk in patients undergoing valve replacement (10,11,14,15). Salomon et al. (16) observed a nearly 10-fold increase in operative mortality in patients undergoing mitral valve replacement who were in functional class IV, as opposed to patients in classes I or II (21.3% vs. 2.2%). (2) Severe pulmonary hypertension also confers increased risk, as does (3) associated coronary artery disease. In patients with significant coronary artery disease, performance of valve replacement without concomitant myocardial revascularization results in markedly increased operative mortality (10,14,17); for this reason, all patients with significant coronary artery disease undergoing valve replacement should receive concomitant myocardial revascularization. In patients with severe mitral regurgitation due to coronary artery disease, the operative mortality for mitral valve replacement may be more than threefold higher than in patients with mitral regurgitation not caused by coronary artery disease (10,16). (4) Other factors include the need to perform emergency surgery (14), reoperations (10,14) and advanced age (>65–70 years of age) (10,14–16).

In addition to procedure-related mortality, valve replacement may be associated with significant morbidity, including perioperative myocardial damage, cerebrovascular accidents, low cardiac output syndromes with multiorgan system failure, and need for repeat operation due to postoperative bleeding or early prosthetic valve endocarditis. Perioperative myocardial infarction may occur in ≥2% of patients following valve replacement (8), and may be particularly ominous in patients with marginal or poor left ventricular function prior to valve replacement.

B. Late Results of Valve Replacement

Among operative survivors, the late results of valve replacement are generally excellent. In reviewing the earliest cohorts of patients treated with valve replacement, overall survival (including operative mortality) is similar for aortic and mitral valve replacement, being 56% at 10 years and 44% at 15 years (8). In later cohorts of patients, benefitting from improved surgical and medical techniques, late survival is even better. For example, in a large group of patients with chronic severe aortic regurgitation treated with aortic valve replacement, Bonow et al. (18) observed a 5-year survival of 83% for patients operated on between 1976 and 1983, as contrasted to a 5-year survival of only 62% for those operated on prior to 1976.

Major determinants of late results following valve replacement are as follows:

1. The preoperative presence of severe congestive heart failure and/or left ventricular dysfunction. Heart failure, particularly that which is chronic in duration, results in diminished long-term survival following both mitral and aortic valve replacement (3,9,15,16,19).
2. Associated coronary artery disease. In patients with severe coronary artery disease who undergo valve replacement without concomitant myocardial revascularization, late mortality is markedly increased; conversely, the performance of myocardial revascularization with valve replacement results in late survival rates comparable to those of patients without significant coronary artery disease undergoing valve replacement (8,17).
3. Etiology of valve disease. In patients with severe mitral regurgitation caused by coronary artery disease, late survival following valve replacement is less than that of patients with mitral regurgitation caused by other etiologies (8,16,20,21).

Following valve replacement, the majority of patients have marked reduction in symptoms, with many returning to previous employment (3,9,16). Causes of late morbidity and mortality following valve replacement are diverse. Among cardiac causes of poor clinical status following valve replacement are severe congestive heart failure, sequelae of perioperative myocardial infarction, tachy- and bradyarrhythmias, and sudden cardiac death. Valve prosthesis-related complications may adversely affect late outcome as well; such complications include thromboembolic events, sequelae of valve dysfunction, anticoagulant-related bleeding, and prosthetic valve endocarditis. Some deaths following valve replacement may also be due to noncardiac etiologies, particularly in the older patient population.

IV. LEFT VENTRICULAR FUNCTION

As discussed above, the preoperative status of left ventricular function is a major determinant of the ultimate results of valve replacement.

A. Aortic Regurgitation

Chronic severe aortic regurgitation presents a significant volume overload to the left ventricle, with this chamber undergoing progressive dilatation. Elevated systolic pressures present a degree of pressure overload as well; the combination of elevated left ventricular volume and systolic pressure results in marked increases in left ventricular wall tension. To achieve a reduction in wall stress, the left ventricle undergoes eccentric hypertrophy (22–24). Eventually, the degree of left ventricular hypertrophy fails to correct for the increased ventricular volumes, and the left ventricular radius-to-wall thickness ratio increases, as does left ventricular wall stress (i.e., afterload mismatch) (22,23).

The initial response to afterload mismatch is a further increase in left ventricular volumes in order to maintain a normal resting ejection fraction (preload reserve). When the upper limit of preload reserve is attained, further increases in left ventricular afterload result in a decline in resting left ventricular performance. When resting left ventricular dysfunction is present in patients with chronic aortic regurgitation, some left ventricular dysfunction may be recoverable following aortic valve replacement due to correction of afterload mismatch. Nonetheless, long-standing severe aortic regurgitation may result in irreversible left ventricular dysfunction, reflected in depressed intrinsic contractility and a downward shift of the end-systolic stress–volume relation. At this stage, much of the decrease in left ventricular performance may be permanent, with myocardial biopsy specimens demonstrating myofibril loss and fibrosis; left ventricular function may fail to improve at this stage following aortic valve replacement.

Ricci (24) has demonstrated that left ventricular preload reserve in patients with chronic aortic regurgitation was exhausted above a left ventricular end-diastolic volume of 160 cm³/m². Below this value, an increase in left ventricular afterload resulted in further increase in diastolic volume to maintain a normal left ventricular ejection fraction; when end-diastolic volume was >160 cm³/m², further increase in left ventricular afterload resulted in a fall in resting ejection fraction.

In patients with chronic severe aortic regurgitation, elevated left ventricular diastolic pressures and low diastolic coronary perfusion pressures may result in myocardial ischemia in the absence of atherosclerotic coronary artery disease. Resting myocardial ischemia may further contribute to resting left ventricular dysfunction in such patients and may be reversible following aortic valve replacement.

As symptoms are often likely to occur much later in the course of chronic aortic regurgitation than in aortic stenosis, the development of severe, irreversible left ventricular dysfunction in patients with chronic aortic regurgitation is far more insidious. Krayenbuehl et al. (25) have demonstrated that for any given degree of symptoms, more preoperative depression of intrinsic left ventricular contractility is present in patients with aortic regurgitation compared to those with aortic stenosis. For this reason, improvement in left ventricular performance following aortic valve replacement may be less in patients with chronic aortic regurgitation than in those with aortic stenosis.

Long-term results following aortic valve replacement in patients with aortic regurgitation are dependent largely on the status of preoperative left ventricular function. Patients with only moderate cardiomegaly and normal or mildly depressed left ventricular ejection fraction demonstrate marked reduction of left ventricular volumes and mass, and improvement in ejection fraction, 6–12 months following aortic valve replacement (22); improvement in mild left ventricular systolic dysfunction following aortic valve replacement for chronic aortic regurgitation suggests that this dysfunction is due primarily to afterload mismatch and not intrinsic contractile failure. While increased left ventricular volumes and mass improve soon following aortic valve replacement, these values still remain greater than normal in most patients (25–29). Monrad et al. (30) observed continued reduction in left ventricular mass and volume for up to 8 years following aortic valve replacement in patients with chronic aortic regurgitation (Table 2).

Patients with chronic aortic regurgitation, marked cardiomegaly, and severe depression of left ventricular function are far less likely to exhibit hemodynamic improvement following aortic valve replacement, due to the presence of irreversible left ventricular damage. Persistent left ventricular dilatation and systolic dysfunction following aortic valve replacement is associated with a poor long-term prognosis (19). Patients with aortic regur-

Table 2   Effect of Aortic Valve Replacement on Left Ventricular Function in
Patients with Aortic Regurgitation

		Before operation	After AVR[a]	
	Controls		1.6 ± 0.5 yr	8.1 ± 2.9 yr
LV end-diastolic volume index (mL/m²)	93 ± 14	225 ± 49	123 ± 36	111 ± 53
LV end-systolic volume index (mL/m²)	31 ± 9	99 ± 35	51 ± 30	46 ± 47
LV ejection fraction (%)[b]	67 ± 7	57 ± 11	61 ± 9	64 ± 14
LV muscle mass index (8/m²)	85 ± 9	191 ± 36	128 ± 29	113 ± 35

[a] AVR = aortic valve replacement.
[b] Changes not statistically significant.
Source: From Ref. 30.

gitation and intermediate degrees of cardiomegaly and left ventricular dysfunction exhibit variable responses following aortic valve replacement,
with some patients showing marked improvement and others having persistent left ventricular dysfunction, congestive heart failure, and poor late
survival (2,22). In making decisions about the timing and appropriateness
of aortic valve replacement in patients with chronic aortic regurgitation,
preoperative parameters of left ventricular systolic function are much
more effective in prediction of expected postoperative results than are
measurements of preoperative diastolic volumes and pressures (18,29,
31,32).

As the prognosis following aortic valve replacement in patients with
chronic aortic regurgitation is closely interrelated to the resultant postoperative left ventricular function, recommendations for aortic valve replacement are facilitated by knowledge of anticipated postoperative ventricular function based on preoperative parameters. Resting preoperative
left ventricular ejection fraction is an excellent predictor of postoperative
left ventricular function following aortic valve replacement in patients
with aortic regurgitation (18,26). Patients with mild depression of ejection
fraction due to aortic regurgitation often normalize their ejection fraction
following aortic valve replacement (33,34), whereas patients with severe
preoperative left ventricular dysfunction generally suffer from persistent
ventricular dysfunction following valve replacement (18,34). In patients
demonstrating improvement in left ventricular ejection fraction in the first
months following aortic valve replacement, further improvement may be
observed as late as 3–7 years following surgery (35).

Recoverability of left ventricular function following aortic valve replacement in patients with chronic aortic regurgitation is more likely when the duration of left ventricular dysfunction prior to valve replacement is brief. Bonow et al. (36) observed all patients with resting left ventricular dysfunction of no more than 14 months in duration prior to valve replacement to develop normal ventricular function 6 months following surgery (mean increase in left ventricular ejection fraction from 0.42 to 0.63); conversely, 64% of patients with left ventricular dysfunction of 18 months or longer in duration had no change or a fall in ejection fraction following aortic valve replacement. These findings suggest that close follow-up of asymptomatic patients with chronic aortic regurgitation is safe; if occult left ventricular dysfunction should develop during the follow-up interval, detection and valve replacement within no more than about 1 year is likely to result in improvement of ventricular function postoperatively.

In addition to predicting postoperative left ventricular dysfunction, depression of left ventricular ejection fraction in patients with chronic aortic regurgitation is predictive of diminished late survival following aortic valve replacement. Patients with preoperative left ventricular dysfunction have been demonstrated to have reduced 3-year survival following aortic valve replacement, when compared to patients with normal preoperative ventricular function (19,37).

Left ventricular dysfunction associated with severe clinical heart failure in patients with chronic aortic regurgitation may be associated with a particularly poor prognosis following aortic valve replacement. In patients with chronic severe aortic regurgitation and resting left ventricular ejection fraction <0.50, Greves et al. (32) demonstrated a 5-year survival following aortic valve replacement of only 63% in patients with severe preoperative symptoms (functional class III or IV), as opposed to 88% in patients with milder symptoms (functional class I or II).

While resting left ventricular ejection fraction is useful in predicting results following aortic valve replacement for chronic aortic regurgitation, many patients with abnormal preoperative ejection fraction will develop normal ventricular function following valve replacement, and some with normal preoperative function will first develop abnormal left ventricular function only after aortic valve replacement (18,26,27). Some of the poor results following aortic valve replacement in patients with abnormal preoperative ventricular function in early series may have been related to perioperative myocardial damage, with further reduction in borderline left ventricular function; with improved surgical techniques, the majority of patients with impaired left ventricular function due to chronic aortic regurgitation may still benefit from aortic valve replacement (18).

Left ventricular ejection fraction is dependent on ventricular loading conditions, and is not an independent measure of intrinsic contractility. If preload reserve is not exhausted, a normal ejection fraction may be observed even in the presence of a decrease in intrinsic myocardial contractility, at the expense of increased diastolic volumes. Similarly, a ventricle with normal myocardial contractility may exhibit a reduced ejection fraction in the presence of increased afterload. Despite these limitations, measurement of resting left ventricular ejection fraction is a valuable index in the evaluation of patients with chronic severe aortic regurgitation; it is widely available, relatively easy to obtain, reproducible, and is generally predictive of expected clinical and hemodynamic results following aortic replacement; moreover, it has stood the test of time. Other hemodynamic and volumetric variables, several of which are discussed below, have been evaluated for their preoperative predictive value for results following aortic valve replacement in patients with aortic regurgitation; none of these variables has been clearly demonstrated to be of greater value than resting left ventricular ejection fraction. Moreover, many of these variables may be poorly reproducible or more difficult to measure accurately, limiting their general value. While these other variables are physiologically sound, and provide valuable information for the evaluation of patients with chronic aortic regurgitation, clinical decisions regarding the optimal timing for aortic value replacement may generally be made based on clinical status of the patient and the resting left ventricular ejection fraction.

M-mode and two-dimensional echocardiography affords a noninvasive method of serially evaluating patients with chronic aortic regurgitation. Echocardiographic parameters of left ventricular function have been examined as preoperative predictors of results following aortic valve replacement. Increased preoperative end-systolic (≥ 55 mm) and end-diastolic ($\geq 75-80$ mm) dimensions and decreased fractional shortening (≤ 0.25) have been correlated with poor outcome following aortic valve replacement in patients with chronic aortic regurgitation (3,19,33,38). Unfortunately, M-mode echocardiographic measurements may be less reliable in patients with chronically dilated, hypertrophied left ventricles; M-mode echocardiographic measurements in such patients may correlate poorly with angiographic ventricular volumes and dimensions, due to changes in ventricular geometry and regional contraction abnormalities (19,23).

Serial echocardiographic measurements of ventricular dimensions are valuable in following individual patients over time, but may exhibit poor reproducibility, due to changes in patient position, transducer angulation, gain settings, and other factors. Intraobserver variability over a 3-month interval may be as high as 8 mm for end-systolic and end-diastolic dimensions, and 0.12 for fractional shortening (39); variability may be higher if different observers interpret serial studies. For this reason, a single abnormal echocardiographic measurement should not be used as a sole criterion for the recommendation of valve replacement; any abnormal measures should be confirmed with repeated measurement, and placed in overall clinical context.

Left ventricular end-systolic volume may also be used to predict residual left ventricular function following aortic valve replacement for aortic regurgitation; preoperative values >60–90 cm^3/m^2 are associated with persistent left ventricular dysfunction and poor clinical outcome following surgery (3,34,40). The *ratio of left ventricular end-diastolic radius to wall thickness* reflects the effective degree of compensatory left ventricular hypertrophy in normalizing wall stress in patients with chronic aortic regurgitation; an increase in this ratio reflects inadequate hypertrophy, and may be associated with persistent left ventricular dilatation and congestive heart failure following aortic valve replacement (19). Abnormal shifts of the *left ventricular end-systolic wall stress–volume relation* are similarly predictive of poor results following aortic valve replacement in patients with aortic regurgitation (40). While this load-independent relationship is theoretically quite attractive in evaluating intrinsic left ventricular contractility, this measure is not obtained routinely, and may be difficult to assess reliably; if it is not measured meticulously, with proper attention to detail, this relationship may not be a truly load-independent index of intrinsic left ventricular contractility (31).

An abnormal *exercise response of left ventricular ejection fraction* may be a very sensitive marker of occult left ventricular dysfunction in patients with chronic aortic regurgitation and normal resting ejection fraction (3,19). The response of ejection fraction to exercise is highly load-dependent, however, and cannot be used to interpret ventricular function without knowledge of the change in systemic resistance with exercise; this measurement may also be affected by the mode of exercise employed (i.e., upright versus supine). An abnormal response of left ventricular ejection fraction during exercise may be present for many years in asymptomatic patients with chronic aortic regurgitation and normal resting ejection fraction; the clinical implications of this finding remain uncertain (2). In such patients, an abnormal response of ejection fraction during exercise should not be used as an indication for aortic valve replacement, but may suggest a need for closer follow-up in asymptomatic patients, observing for a decline in resting left ventricular function.

Measurement of *exercise cardiac hemodynamics* may provide useful information about ventricular function in patients with chronic aortic regurgitation. Elevated exercise pulmonary artery wedge pressures correlate with abnormal rest and exercise left ventricular ejection fraction in patients with aortic regurgitation (41,42); peak exercise wedge pressures ≥15 mmHg correlate with decreased peripheral oxygen uptake, reflecting inadequate oxygen delivery to working muscles (42).

Objective determination of *exercise capacity* provides valuable information in patients with chronic aortic regurgitation. In patients with mild to moderate impairment of resting left ventricular function, results of aortic valve replacement are more favorable in patients with normal preoperative exercise capacity than in those with abnormal exercise tolerance (19). Ideally, objective exercise testing should be part of the evaluation in asymptomatic patients with severe aortic regurgitation, as some patients may not perceive symptoms due to a chronic subconscious reduction in activity level as a response to chronic disease.

A critical issue in the management of patients with chronic severe aortic regurgitation is whether there is a level of preoperative left ventricular dysfunction so severe that the results of valve replacement may be so poor as to preclude recommendation for surgery; very little data are available in such patients. The few series of aortic valve replacement including patients with resting left ventricular ejection fraction <0.30–0.35 suggest that many such patients may have poor late survival and persistent depression of left ventricular function following valve replacement. Although some such patients may benefit from valve replacement (18,26,28,32,35), no data are available that carefully compare surgical to nonsurgical therapy in patients with aortic regurgitation and severe left ventricular dysfunction. The decision to recommend aortic valve replacement in patients with severe left ventricular dysfunction must be carefully individualized.

B. Mitral Regurgitation

Chronic mitral regurgitation is a highly insidious, slowly progressive lesion which may result in severe, irreversible left ventricular dysfunction prior to clinical detection. Chronic volume overload in mitral regurgitation results in the development of eccentric left ventricular hypertrophy in an attempt to normalize wall stress. Much of what has been described above on the response of the left ventricle to chronic aortic regurgitation applies to chronic mitral regurgitation as well, but there are important differences. Left ventricular afterload in patients with chronic mitral regurgitation is less than that in those with aortic regurgitation (43). The major cause of the lower afterload in patients with chronic mitral regurgitation is the ability to eject blood into the low-impedance left atrium throughout systole; the absence of an isovolumic contraction phase, with as much as half of the regurgitation occurring prior to aortic valve opening, reduces left ventricular systolic wall stress. Similarly, lower left ventricular systolic pressure in patients with mitral as opposed to aortic regurgitation tends to result in lower wall stress; conversely, the increased left ventricular volumes in patients with chronic mitral regurgitation adversely affects left ventricular afterload.

Early in the course of chronic mitral regurgitation, left ventricular ejection fraction may be increased, due to favorable afterload conditions (discussed above) as well as utilization of preload reserve secondary to elevated ventricular volumes (44). With time, insidious irreversible left ventricular contractile dysfunction may develop, with a downward and rightward shift of the left ventricular end-systolic stress–volume relation (22,23). Due to the above favorable left ventricular loading conditions, irreversible intrinsic contractile dysfunction may be present despite a resting ejection fraction in the low-"normal" range (0.50–0.60) (43). When resting left ventricular ejection fraction is <0.50 in patients with chronic mitral regurgitation, irreversible left ventricular dysfunction may already be present.

Mitral valve replacement in patients with chronic mitral regurgitation and abnormal intrinsic left ventricular function (even if the resting ejection fraction is in the "normal" range) may result in marked worsening of left ventricular performance. Mitral valve replacement in such patients eliminates the intrinsic afterload reduction afforded by systolic emptying into the left atrium, and presents an acute postoperative increase in afterload to the left ventricle. As all left ventricular stroke volume must now be delivered into the high-impedance aorta, and the left ventricle must now undergo isovolumic contraction, marked afterload mismatch may develop following mitral valve replacement; if intrinsic left ventricular contractility is abnormal, a marked fall in left ventricular performance may be noted postoperatively. The response of left ventricular function in patients with chronic mitral regurgitation following mitral valve replacement is markedly different than that of patients with chronic aortic regurgitation following aortic valve replacement; in patients with aortic regurgitation, left ventricular ejection fraction may be depressed due to preoperative afterload mismatch, and improved loading conditions following aortic valve replacement may result in improved left ventricular performance.

Series of patients with chronic mitral regurgitation and normal preoperative left ventricular ejection fraction have demonstrated a fall in ejection fraction of 0.09–0.16 following mitral valve replacement (45–47); in such patients, despite reduction in left ventricular end-diastolic volumes following mitral valve replacement, no changes are observed in end-systolic volumes. Hemodynamic and angiographic changes following mitral valve

Table 3 Hemodynamic and Angiographic Changes Following Mitral Valve
Replacement in Patients with Chronic Mitral Regurgitation[a]

	Pre-op	Post-op
Mean PAP (mmHg)	29 ± 11	22 ± 9[b]
LVEDP (mmHg)	18 ± 8	12 ± 6[b]
LVEDVI (mL/m^2)	117 ± 51	89 ± 27[b]
LVESVI (mL/m^2)	54 ± 42	50 ± 25
LVEF	0.56 ± 0.15	0.45 ± 0.13[b]
RV/EDV	0.49 ± 0.31	0.12 ± 0.17[b]

[a] EDP = end diastolic pressure; EDVI = end diastolic volume index; EF = ejection fraction; ESVI = end systolic volume index; LV = left ventricular; RV = regurgitant volume.
[b] $p < 0.001$ (versus pre-op).
Source: From Ref. 46, used with permission.

replacement in patients with chronic mitral regurgitation in the Veterans
Administration Cooperative Study (46) are presented in Table 3.

Patients with chronic mitral regurgitation and borderline left ventricular
ejection fraction (0.50–0.60) may have significant impairment of left ventricular function following mitral valve replacement (34,46,47). If resting
left ventricular ejection fraction is very much below 0.50 in patients with
chronic mitral regurgitation, severe postoperative left ventricular dysfunction may follow mitral valve replacement, with persistent congestive heart
failure and impaired long-term prognosis (34,40,46,48). While an abnormal
preoperative resting left ventricular ejection fraction has an excellent specificity for predicting impaired left ventricular function following mitral
valve replacement in patients with chronic mitral regurgitation, the sensitivity of this index is poor, as many patients with abnormal postoperative
left ventricular function have normal preoperative ejection fractions (46).
Recommendation for valve replacement in patients with chronic mitral
regurgitation should be made before any impairment of left ventricular
performance develops, if maximal clinical and hemodynamic benefit is to
be observed following surgery.

In addition to preoperative ejection fraction, left ventricular volumes
in patients with chronic mitral regurgitation are predictive of anticipated
results following mitral valve replacement. Elevated preoperative left ventricular end-systolic volumes (>60 cm^3/m^2) are correlated with severe
postoperative left ventricular dysfunction, persistent congestive heart failure, and poor late survival (34,40,46,48); even mild elevation of preoperative end-systolic volumes (31–60 cm^3/m^2) may be associated with postoperative left ventricular dysfunction (34). Significant elevation of left

ventricular end-diastolic volumes in patients with chronic mitral regurgitation is also associated with poorer results following mitral valve replacement (34,40,46,48). In a series of patients with chronic mitral regurgitation, "normal" left ventricular function (mean ejection fraction 0.57; ejection fraction in all patients >0.50), and markedly dilated left ventricles (end-diastolic and end-systolic dimensions >70 mm and >50 mm, respectively), Schuler et al. (47) observed a fall in left ventricular ejection fraction to 0.26 following mitral valve replacement.

In an effort to achieve a more reliable and precise predictor of postoperative left ventricular function following mitral valve replacement in patients with chronic mitral regurgitation, the left ventricular end-systolic stress–volume relation has been evaluated. The advantage of this load-independent measurement is its ability to detect early intrinsic depression of left ventricular contractility, such that valve replacement may be performed at the earliest stages of left ventricular dysfunction, before severe damage has developed. While this measure has been demonstrated to be a reliable predictor of postoperative left ventricular function (40,48), reliable measurement of the relation must be made, with meticulous attention to detail.

It is apparent, therefore, that patients with chronic severe mitral regurgitation must be carefully followed by their physicians, and interventions performed at the earliest, and often when the signs of left ventricular systolic dysfunction are subtle. If valve replacement is performed after the onset of severe intrinsic left ventricular dysfunction, the results of valve replacement are likely to be less than ideal. While serial noninvasive follow-up of patients (with echocardiographic or radionuclide techniques) is practical and effective, the limitations of these techniques (discussed above in the section on patients with aortic regurgitation) must be kept in mind. It remains uncertain if there is a lower limit of left ventricular dysfunction, below which the results of mitral valve replacement in patients with chronic mitral regurgitation may be so poor that valve replacement is contraindicated; if such a limit exists, selected patients with extremely poor left ventricular function due to chronic mitral regurgitation (ejection fraction <0.25–0.30) might be potential candidates for cardiac transplantation.

Newer techniques of mitral valve repair, as opposed to valve replacement, may result in better preservation of left ventricular function following surgery in patients with chronic mitral regurgitation. In patients with mitral regurgitation caused by coronary artery disease with depressed left ventricular function, both early and late survival may be improved following mitral valve repair, when compared to replacement with a prosthetic valve (49,50). In a series of patients with severe coronary artery disease, mitral regurgitation, and severe depression of left ventricular function (ejection fraction 0.21–0.40), Kay et al. (50) demonstrated a late (>6-year) survival following mitral valve repair and coronary bypass surgery of 32%, as opposed to only 12% following mitral valve replacement and coronary bypass surgery. However, the numbers of patients in this series was small, and it is uncertain whether the patients treated by the two methods were identical or comparable.

Improved results following mitral valve repair in patients with mitral regurgitation and depressed left ventricular function may be related to the important role of the subvalvular apparatus, including chordal structures and papillary muscles, on left ventricular function; preservation of these structures results in more favorable left ventricular contraction patterns and regional loading conditions. When mitral valve replacement is necessary, preservation of these subvalvular structures may result in less postoperative depression of left ventricular function than when these structures are excised (51). While mitral valve repair may be preferable for patients with severe mitral regurgitation and left ventricular dysfunction, the ability to repair the mitral valve can usually not be guaranteed preoperatively, and the surgeon may still be required to replace the valve, with the resultant potentially deleterious effects described above; for this reason, all patients referred for surgical treatment of chronic mitral regurgitation should be considered to be potential candidates for valve replacement.

V. COMPLICATIONS OF PROSTHETIC HEART VALVES

Insertion of a prosthetic heart valve may alleviate many of the adverse manifestations of chronic valvular heart disease but exposes the patient to a life-long risk of prosthesis-related morbidity and mortality. In addition to possible adverse hemodynamic results following valve replacement, due both to preoperative left ventricular dysfunction and perioperative myocardial damage, many complications may be related directly to the prosthetic device. These complications are listed in Table 4, and several are discussed briefly below.

Prosthetic valve endocarditis is observed with an incidence of ≤1%/ year but presents a life-long risk to the patient; the incidence of this complication is similar for mechanical and bioprosthetic valves.

Malfunction of prosthetic valves may be related to dehiscence of the prosthesis from surrounding cardiac structures, structural failure of the valve, sudden thrombosis of the valve, or severe hemolysis related to the prosthetic device. Clinical manifestations of valve dysfunction are those of obstruction or regurgitation, or severe anemia in the case of hemolysis.

Table 4   Potential Complications of Prosthetic Heart Valves

Operative mortality
Operative morbidity
  Myocardial infarction
  Cerebrovascular accident
  Low cardiac output state
  Damage to conducting system, requiring permanent pacemaker insertion
Prosthetic valve endocarditis
Prosthetic valve malfunction
  Dehiscence
  Structural failure
  Thrombosis, hemolysis
  Obstruction, regurgitation
Thromboembolic complications
Anticoagulant-related bleeding
Valve prosthesis–patient mismatch
Need for prosthetic valve replacement
Late mortality, including unexplained sudden death

Source: Modified from Ref. 8.

The occurrence of *thromboembolic events* in patients with prosthetic heart valves may result in serious, life-long clinical sequelae or even mortality. The incidence of thromboembolic events is approximately 1–2%/year for patients with aortic prostheses, and 2–5%/year for patients with mitral prostheses (8). While the incidence of thromboembolic events is similar for patients with either mechanical or bioprosthetic valves, all patients with mechanical prostheses require life-long anticoagulation, while most patients with bioprosthetic valves, particularly in the aortic position, do not require long-term anticoagulation.

Anticoagulant-related *bleeding* represents a clinical threat to patients with prosthetic heart valves. The observed incidence of major bleeding in patients with prosthetic heart valves taking oral anticoagulants is 1–2%/year, and that of minor bleeding is 4–8%/year (8). Prothrombin time should be maintained between 1.6 and 1.9 times control valves; values greater than this do not confer added protection against thromboembolic events, but are associated with an increased risk of bleeding (52). Certain patients are at increased risk of bleeding during anticoagulation therapy and may require consideration for insertion of bioprosthetic devices.

Valve prosthesis–patient mismatch occurs when the effective orifice of the prosthetic valve is insufficient to allow normal valvular function for the patient. All prosthetic valves are inherently stenotic, with in-vitro orifices less than that of native valves; the effective orifice may be further compromised in the patient by tissue ingrowth and endothelialization following implantation. The problem may be particularly magnified in patients with small valve annuli, requiring placement of smaller prosthetic devices. While prosthesis–patient mismatch may be observed with any prosthetic device, certain valves have better hemodynamic qualities than others, particularly in the smaller sizes; in patients with very small valve annuli, the St. Jude bivalve prosthesis may be particularly advantageous. Most cases of prosthesis–patient mismatch are generally mild and clinically insignificant, although severe prosthetic valve stenosis may occasionally result, necessitating repeat surgery with implantation of a larger, more hemodynamically favorable valve.

VI. MITRAL VALVE REPAIR

The beneficial effects of mitral valve repair as opposed to valve replacement on left ventricular function in patients with chronic mitral regurgitation have already been discussed in detail. Many other aspects of valve repair instead of replacement in patients with mitral regurgitation are very favorable. First and foremost, valve repair spares the patient from having a prosthetic device implanted and the need for anticoagulation; thromboembolic events, bleeding complications, and endocarditis are less frequent following mitral valve repair (51,53). Following mitral valve repair, the incidence of thromboembolism is only 3–6% at 5–10 years (50,54).

In most series, the operative mortality following mitral valve repair is less than or equivalent to that following mitral valve replacement (51,53,54); patients receiving valve repair in these series are highly selected, however, rather than randomized, and may not be exactly comparable to those receiving valve replacement. Durability of mitral valve repair has been good during relatively limited follow-up. The need for reoperation is low in the first 5 years following mitral valve repair, being well under 10% (51,53); by 7–10 years, 6–19% of patients may require mitral valve replacement (54). Reoperation is generally required due to residual mitral valve stenosis or regurgitation following valve repair, or late recurrent mitral regurgitation following valve repair (53). Some patients develop left ventricular outflow obstruction, which is usually mild but may require surgical correction if it is severe.

Feasibility of mitral valve repair depends on several factors, including (1) valve morphology, (2) experience of the surgeon with the procedure, and (3) desire of the surgeon to perform the procedure. Mitral valve repair may be a technically difficult procedure and requires an experienced surgeon willing to devote the time necessary to learn and to perform the procedure. Experienced surgeons with intention to perform mitral valve repair may be able to successfully repair as many as 80% of valves in patients with chronic mitral regurgitation (49,51). Successful mitral valve repair is most likely when mitral regurgitation is caused by coronary artery disease or myxomatous degeneration; valve repair is less often feasible in patients with a rheumatic etiology of mitral regurgitation. While mitral valve repair may appear feasible based on preoperative assessment of valve morphology, findings during surgery may necessitate replacement of the valve instead. For this reason, patients with chronic mitral regurgitation referred for mitral valve surgery should be considered potential candidates for mitral valve replacement.

In summary, the potential advantages of mitral valve repair, as opposed to replacement, in patients with chronic mitral regurgitation include (1) better preservation of left ventricular function, (2) reduced thromboembolic and bleeding complications, and (3) reduced risk of endocarditis. The long-term (>10–20 years) durability of mitral valve repair remains to be defined.

VII. SELECTION OF PATIENTS FOR VALVE REPLACEMENT

Based on the above discussion of the natural history and physiology of chronic left-sided cardiac valvular lesions and the response of patients to valve replacement, recommendations for appropriate selection of patients for valve replacement may be suggested. These recommendations are summarized in Table 5 and discussed below.

A. Aortic Regurgitation

In patients with symptomatic chronic severe aortic regurgitation, improvement in clinical status and long-term survival following aortic valve replacement suggest this to be appropriate therapy. Little data are available following aortic valve replacement in patients with very severe left ventricular dysfunction (ejection fraction <0.20) and chronic aortic regurgitation; as the outcome of valve replacement may be less favorable in this subset of patients, decisions regarding aortic valve replacement in such patients should be individualized. Most patients with symptoms and severe left ventricular dysfunction due to chronic aortic regurgitation should probably undergo aortic valve replacement.

In patients with chronic severe aortic regurgitation and no symptoms, timing of valve replacement is a more challenging issue. The goal in the asymptomatic patient, therefore, is to perform aortic valve replacement at the earliest sign(s) of left ventricular dysfunction, before severe, irrever-

Table 5 Selection of Patients for Valve Replacement[a]

Aortic regurgitation
  Symptoms (individualize if resting LV EF < 0.20)
  No symptoms: EF < 0.50 (individualize if < 0.20)
              EF > 0.50 + (1) Marked LV dilatation (EDD > 70–75 mm,
                                ESD > 55 mm) *and*
                          (2) Abnormal exercise capacity or abnormal in-
                                crease in PAWP with exercise
Mitral regurgitation[b]
  Symptoms: Normal or abnormal LV function (individualize if EF < 0.30)
  No symptoms: EF < 0.55–0.60 (individualize if EF < 0.30)
              Marked LV dilatation (EDD > 70–75 mm; ESD > 50 mm) *and*
              Decreased exercise capacity or abnormal increase in PAWP with
              exercise.
              Resting pulmonary hypertension

[a] AVA = aortic valve area; EDD = echocardiographic end-diastolic dimension; EF = ejection fraction; ESD = echocardiographic end-systolic dimension; LV = left ventricular; MVA = mitral valve area; PA = pulmonary artery pressure; PAWP = pulmonary artery wedge pressure.
[b] Mitral valve repair is preferable to replacement whenever feasible.
Source: Modified from Ref. 1.

sible dysfunction results. As many patients with chronic valvular heart disease may either deny symptoms or adapt to adverse hemodynamic conditions by subconsciously "down-regulating" their activity level, asymptomatic patients should be assessed objectively with formal exercise testing. Of the many parameters of left ventricular function which have been examined in patients with chronic aortic regurgitation, resting left ventricular ejection fraction is the most practical to follow.

In asymptomatic patients with chronic severe aortic regurgitation and normal resting left ventricular ejection fraction, valve replacement may be considered in those patients with markedly dilated left ventricles (echocardiographic end-diastolic dimension >70–75 mm, end-systolic dimension >55 mm) *and* evidence of abnormal exercise physiology (objective decrease in exercise capacity or an abnormal increase in pulmonary artery wedge pressure during exercise).

Patients with asymptomatic chronic severe aortic regurgitation should be followed noninvasively at intervals of approximately 12 months; when evidence develops that left ventricular function is becoming adversely affected (marked increase in left ventricular volumes or dimensions; left ventricular ejection fraction which is still "normal" but has decreased from prior values to ≤0.60), patients should be evaluated carefully, possibly with exercise hemodynamics, and the follow-up interval should be decreased to 6 months. When overt resting left ventricular dysfunction is observed or when marked left ventricular dilatation is accompanied by abnormal exercise capacity or physiology, complete left and right heart catheterization should be performed to assess fully the severity of aortic regurgitation and any other associated valvular lesions, as well as the status of left ventricular function and the coronary arterial circulation. At this stage, valve replacement should be strongly considered, before severe, irreversible left ventricular dysfunction develops. In all asymptomatic patients, the risks of valve surgery, including operative morbidity and mortality and long-term cardiac and prosthesis-related morbidity and mortality, must be considered. If the risks of surgery are quite high due to markedly advanced age or poor medical condition of the patient, or because of the need for a complex operation secondary to severe disease of the proximal ascending aorta, the decision for valve replacement in the asymptomatic patient should be carefully individualized.

B. Mitral Regurgitation

In patients with symptomatic mitral regurgitation and normal left ventricular function, significant improvement in symptoms and possibly survival may be expected following mitral valve replacement. As chronic mitral regurgitation may mask intrinsic left ventricular dysfunction by virtue of favorable effects on left ventricular loading conditions, "normal" left ventricular function is likely only when resting left ventricular ejection fraction is $\geq 0.55–0.60$; even above this range, intrinsic left ventricular function may be impaired, and resting left ventricular ejection fraction may fall to abnormal levels in some patients following successful mitral valve replacement. When resting preoperative left ventricular ejection fraction is $<0.55–0.60$, significant intrinsic left ventricular dysfunction is likely, and postoperatively, ejection fraction may well be <0.40; this may be associated with congestive heart failure and a less favorable long-term prognosis. When resting left ventricular ejection fraction is >0.30 in patients with symptomatic chronic mitral regurgitation, mitral valve replacement should be performed in most patients, to prevent further worsening of left ventricular function, making later valve replacement even less favorable. When symptomatic patients with chronic mitral regurgitation first present with a resting left ventricular ejection fraction <0.30, the likelihood of a poor outcome following mitral valve replacement may be quite high; the decision to perform valve replacement in such patients must be individualized.

In asymptomatic patients with chronic severe mitral regurgitation, the insidious and often inapparent progression of left ventricular dysfunction make the decision for optimal timing of valve replacement difficult. While valve replacement performed "too early" clearly exposes patients to unnecessary risks of prosthesis-related morbidity and mortality, excessive delay in valve replacement may result in very poor operative results. Unlike patients with chronic aortic regurgitation in whom mild–moderate depression of left ventricular ejection fraction is often associated with excellent clinical results following aortic valve replacement, an abnormal ejection fraction in patients with chronic mitral regurgitation portends potentially poor results following mitral valve replacement. In patients with mitral regurgitation and resting left ventricular ejection fraction ≤0.55–0.60, mitral valve replacement should be strongly considered before left ventricular function further declines or pulmonary hypertension develops at rest; at this early stage, the results of valve surgery offer maximal potential benefit. Mitral valve replacement should also be considered if left ventricular ejection fraction is above this range, but is clearly decreasing on serial examination, or if marked left ventricular dilatation is present (echocardiographic end-diastolic dimension >70–75 mm; end-systolic dimension >50 mm); valve surgery may be particularly indicated when such findings are associated with objective decrease in exercise capacity or when associated with resting pulmonary hypertension. When it is available and reliable, analysis of the left ventricular end-systolic wall stress–volume relation may permit early detection of intrinsic left ventricular dysfunction.

In patients with chronic severe mitral regurgitation, the lower incidence of thromboembolic and infectious complications, and better preservation of left ventricular function observed following mitral valve repair as opposed to replacement, make this the procedure of choice whenever possible. As discussed earlier, the feasibility of mitral valve repair is dependent on many factors, and mitral valve replacement may ultimately be required in many patients. For this reason, all patients with severe mitral regurgitation referred for surgical therapy should be considered candidates for valve replacement.

REFERENCES

1. Kulick DL, Rahimtoola SH. Selection of patients for cardiac valve replacement. In: Braunwald E, ed. Heart Disease, A Textbook of Cardiovascular Medicine. 3d ed., Philadelphia: Saunders, 1990:257–72.
2. Rahimtoola SH. Perspective on valvular heart disease: an update. J Am Coll Cardiol 1989; 14:1–23.
3. Nishimura RA, McGoon MD, Schaff HV, Giuliani ER. Chronic aortic regurgitation: indications for operation—1988. Mayo Clin Proc 1988; 63:270–80.

4. Turina J, Hess O, Sepulcri F, Krayenbuehl HP. Spontaneous course of aortic valve disease. Eur Heart J 1987; 8:471–83.

5. Siemienczuk D, Greenberg B, Morris C, et al. Chronic aortic insufficiency: factors associated with progression to aortic valve replacement. Ann Intern Med 1989; 110:587–92.

6. Waller BF, Morrow AG, Maron BJ, et al. Etiology of clinically isolated, severe, chronic, pure mitral regurgitation: analysis of 97 patients over 30 years of age having mitral valve replacement. Am Heart J 1982; 104:276–88.

7. Hammermeister KE, Fisher L, Kennedy JW, Samuels S, Dodge HT. Prediction of late survival in patients with mitral valve disease from clinical, hemodynamic, and quantitative angiographic variables. Circulation 1978; 57: 341–9.

8. Rahimtoola SH. Valvular heart disease: a perspective. J Am Coll Cardiol 1983; 1:199–215.

9. Samuels DA, Curfman GD, Friedlich AL, Buckley MJ, Austen WG. Valve replacement for aortic regurgitation: long-term follow-up with factors influencing the results. Circulation 1979; 60:647–54.

10. Sethi GK, Miller DC, Souchek J, et al. Clinical, hemodynamic, and angiographic predictors of operative mortality in patients undergoing single valve replacement. J Thorac Cardiovasc Surg 1987; 93:884–97.

11. Scott WC, Miller DC, Haverick A, et al. Determinants of operative mortality for patients undergoing aortic valve replacement: discriminant analysis of 1,479 operations. J Thorac Cardiovasc Surg 1985; 89:400–13.

12. Bloomfield P, Kitchin AH, Wheatley DJ, Walbaum PR, Lutz W, Miller HC. A prospective evaluation of the Bjork-Shiley, Hancock, and Carpentier-Edwards heart valve prostheses. Circulation 1986; 73:1213–22.

13. Hammermeister KE, Henderson WG, Burchfield CM, et al., and Participants in the Veterans Administration Cooperative Study on Valvular Heart Disease. Comparison of outcome after valve replacement with a bioprosthesis versus a mechanical prosthesis: initial 5 year results of a randomized trial. J Am Coll Cardiol 1987; 10:719–32.

14. Fremes SE, Goldman BS, Ivanov J, Weisel RD, David TE, Salerno T, and the Cardiovascular Surgeons at the University of Toronto. Valvular surgery in the elderly. Circulation 1989; 80(suppl I):I-77 to I-90.

15. Acar J, Luxereau P, Ducimetiere P, Cadilhac M, Jallut H, Vahanian A. Prognosis of surgically treated chronic aortic valve disease: predictive indicators of early postoperative risk and long-term survival, based on 439 cases. J Thorac Cardiovasc Surg 1981; 82:114–26.

16. Salomon NW, Stinson EB, Griepp RB, Shumway NE. Patient-related risk factors as predictors of results following isolated mitral valve replacement. Ann Thorac Surg 1977; 24:519–30.

17. Mullany CJ, Elveback LR, Frye RL, et al. Coronary artery disease and its management: influence on survival in patients undergoing aortic valve replacement. J Am Coll Cardiol 1987; 10:66–72.

18. Bonow RO, Picone AL, McIntosh CL, et al. Survival and functional results after valve replacement for aortic regurgitation from 1976 to 1983: impact of preoperative left ventricular function. Circulation 1985; 72:1244–56.

19. Bonow RO, Rosing DR, Kent KM, Epstein SE. Timing of operation for chronic aortic regurgitation. Am J Cardiol 1982; 50:325–36.

20. Cheitlin MD. The timing of surgery in mitral and aortic valve disease. Curr Probl Cardiol 1987; 12:69–149.

21. Pinson CW, Cobanoglij A, Metzdorff MT, Grunkemeier GL, Kay PH, Starr A. Late surgical results for ischemic mitral regurgitation: role of wall motion score and severity of regurgitation. J Thorac Cardiovasc Surg 1984; 88: 663–72.

22. Ross J. Left ventricular function and the timing of surgical treatment in valvular heart disease. Ann Intern Med 1981; 94:498–504.

23. Ross J. Afterload mismatch in aortic and mitral valve disease: implications for surgical therapy. J Am Coll Cardiol 1985; 5:811–26.

24. Ricci DR. Afterload mismatch and preload reserve in chronic aortic regurgitation. Circulation 1982; 66:826–34.

25. Krayenbuehl HP, Turina M, Hess OM, Rothlin M, Senning A. Pre- and postoperatively left ventricular contractile function in patients with aortic valve disease. Br Heart J 1979; 41:204–13.

26. Hwang MH, Hammermeister KE, Oprian C, et al. Preoperative identification of patients likely to have left ventricular dysfunction after aortic valve replacement. Participants in the Veterans Administration Cooperative Study on Valvular Heart Disease. Circulation 1989; 80(suppl I):I-65 to I-76.

27. Mirsky I, Henschke C, Hess OM, Krayenbuehl HP. Prediction of postoperative performance in aortic valve disease. Am J Cardiol 1981; 48:295–303.

28. Kennedy JW, Doces J, Stewart DK. Left ventricular function before and following aortic valve replacement. Circulation 1977; 56:944–50.

29. Fioretti P, Roelandt J, Sclavo M, et al. Postoperative regression of left ventricular dimensions in aortic insufficiency: a long-term echocardiographic study. J Am Coll Cardiol 1985; 5:856–61.

30. Monrad ES, Hess OM, Murakami T, Nonogi H, Corin WJ, Krayenbuehl HP. Time course of regression of left ventricular hypertrophy after aortic valve replacement. Circulation 1988; 77:1345–55.

31. Borow KM. Surgical outcome in chronic aortic regurgitation: a physiologic framework for assessing preoperative predictors. J Am Coll Cardiol 1987; 10:1165–70.

32. Greves J, Rahimtoola SH, McAnulty JH, et al. Preoperative criteria predictive of late survival following valve replacement for severe aortic regurgitation. Am Heart J 1981; 101:300–8.

33. Carabello BA, Usher BW, Hendrix GH, Assey ME, Crawford FA, Leman RB. Predictors of outcome for aortic valve replacement in patients with aortic regurgitation and left ventricular dysfunction: a change in the measuring stick. J Am Coll Cardiol 1987; 10:991–7.

34. Borow KM, Green LH, Mann T, et al. End-systolic volume as a predictor of postoperative left ventricular performance in volume overload from valvular regurgitation. Am J Med 1980; 68:655–63.

35. Bonow RO, Dodd JT, Maron B J, et al. Long-term serial changes in left ventricular function and reversal of ventricular dilatation after valve replacement for chronic aortic regurgitation. Circulation 1988; 78:1108–20.

36. Bonow RO, Rosing DR, Maron BJ, et al. Reversal of left ventricular dysfunction after aortic valve replacement for chronic aortic regurgitation: influence of duration of preoperative left ventricular dysfunction. Circulation 1984; 70: 570–9.

37. Forman R, Firth BG, Barnard MS. Prognostic significance of preoperative left ventricular ejection fraction and valve lesion in patients with aortic valve replacement. Am J Cardiol 1980; 45:1120–25.

38. Grossman W. Aortic and mitral regurgitation: how to evaluate the condition and when to consider surgical intervention. JAMA 1984; 252:2447–9.

39. Szlachcic J, Massie BM, Greenberg B, Thomas D, Cheitlin M, Bristow JD. Intertest variability of echocardiographic and chest X-ray measurements: implications for decision making in patients with aortic regurgitation. J Am Coll Cardiol 1986; 7:1310–7.

40. Carabello BA, Williams H, Gash AK, et al. Hemodynamic predictors of outcome in patients undergoing valve replacement. Circulation 1986; 74: 1309–16.

41. Massie BM, Kramer BL, Loge D, et al. Ejection fraction response to supine exercise in asymptomatic aortic regurgitation: relation to simultaneous hemodynamic measurements. J Am Coll Cardiol 1985; 5:847–55.

42. Boucher CA, Wilson RA, Kanarek DJ, et al. Exercise testing in asymptomatic or minimally symptomatic aortic regurgitation: relationship of left ventricular ejection fraction to left ventricular filling pressure during exercise. Circulation 1983; 67:1091–100.

43. Corin WJ, Monrad ES, Murakami T, Nonogi H, Hess OM, Krayenbuehl HP. The relationship of afterload to ejection performance in chronic mitral regurgitation. Circulation 1987; 76:59–67.

44. Berko B, Gaasch WH, Tanigawa N, Smith D, Craige E. Disparity between ejection and end-systolic indexes of left ventricular contractility in mitral regurgitation. Circulation 1987; 75:1310–9.

45. Kennedy JW, Doces JG, Stewart DK. Left ventricular function before and following surgical treatment of mitral valve disease. Am Heart J 1979; 97: 592–8.

46. Crawford MH, Souchek J, Oprian CA, et al. Determinants of survival and left ventricular performance following mitral valve replacement. Circulation 1990; 81:1173–81.

47. Schuler G, Peterson KL, Johnson A, et al. Temporal response of left ventricular performance to mitral valve surgery. Circulation 1979; 59:1218–31.

48. Carabello BA, Nolan SP, McGuire LB. Assessment of preoperative left ventricular function in patients with mitral regurgitation: value of the end-systolic wall stress–end-systolic volume ratio. Circulation 1981; 64:1212–7.

49. Kay JH, Zubiate P, Mendez MA, Vanstrom N, Yokoyama T. Mitral valve repair for significant mitral insufficiency. Am Heart J 1978; 96:253–62.

50. Kay GL, Kay JH, Zubiate P, Yokoyama T, Mendez M. Mitral valve repair for mitral regurgitation secondary to coronary artery disease. Circulation 1986; 74(suppl I):I-88 to I-98.

51. Cosgrove DM, Stewart WJ. Mitral valvuloplasty. Curr Probl Cardiol 1989; 14:353–416.

52. Rahimtoola SH. Lessons learned about the determinants of results of valve surgery. Circulation 1988; 78:1503–7.

53. Carpentier A, Chauvaud S, Fabiani JN, et al. Reconstructive surgery of mitral valve incompetence: ten-year appraisal. J Thorac Cardiovasc Surg 1980; 79:338–48.

54. Galloway AC, Colvin SB, Baumann FG, Harty S, Spencer FC. Current concepts of mitral valve reconstruction for mitral insufficiency. Circulation 1988; 78:1087–98.

Part III

18

Conservative Valve Surgery

Carlos M. G. Duran
King Faisal Specialist Hospital, Riyadh, Saudi Arabia

I. INTRODUCTION

Conservative surgery of the cardiac valves has as long a history as that of cardiac surgery. In fact, successful closed commissurotomies (1,2) were performed well before the first closure of the patent ductus (3) and resection of the coarctation of the aorta (4). Before the advent of cardiopulmonary bypass, the inventiveness of the surgeons proposed many and generally unsuccessful procedures for regurgitant lesions (5). Cardiopulmonary bypass, by making possible the direct visualization of the cardiac valves, stimulated further attempts which were soon overtaken by the new valve prostheses. Their ease of implantation and guaranteed immediate competence displaced the unpredictable repair technique. Only a few surgeons, probably because of their continuous exposure to the diseased mitral valve, maintained an interest in attempting repair in a young population. The enlightened approach of John Kirklin, who, in 1980, as president of the American Association for Thoracic Surgery, organized a symposium on mitral valve repair, can be considered the turning point for valve repair. Today the longer patient follow-up available showing the stability of repair and the problems of the prostheses, particularly in the mitral position, have established the desirability of valve conservation wherever possible. The degree of development of this reparative surgery is, however, not homogeneous for all cardiac valves. The tricuspid valve is nearly universally repaired, the mitral valve is often conserved, while the aortic valve is still reconstructed occasionally and in only a few centers. This chapter is an attempt at reviewing the present situation of this moving field, where there is still considerable room for development, not only in the surgical techniques but also in the establishment of precise indications.

II. PRINCIPLES OF VALVE REPAIR

Surgeons must change considerably their traditional approach to valve surgery when considering valve conservation. If a valve is going to be replaced, there is no great need for its detailed study. Valve conservation requires an excellent exposure and a conscious effort to carefully observe every valve, even if a replacement is anticipated. Every element of the valve apparatus must be analyzed and its lesions identified when planning which surgical maneuvers will be applied. A maximum time for observation must be mentally established before a final replacement decision is undertaken. An intraoperative method for the visual testing of the repair must also be selected among the many already described, none of which is yet fully reliable. Although intraoperative echocardiography has become an essential tool in valve repair, this visual evaluation is still essential, since it allows further repair maneuvers within the same aortic cross-clamp period and before cavity closure and weaning of the patient from bypass.

This change of attitude of surgeons must be accompanied by a similar change in the mentality of cardiologists, who must understand the requirements and limitations of valve conservation. The standard evaluation of valve areas and gradients, however useful, is not sufficient. Annulus diameter, leaflet size and mobility, direction of regurgitant jets, etc., are essential data not only to establish the feasibility of repair, but also to direct the surgeon's attention during his or her mandatory intraoperative analysis of the lesions. The cardiologist must be aware of the limitations of intraoperative echocardiography and understand and often participate in the difficult decision of whether to accept a less than perfect result or proceed to a valve replacement. In any case, both the surgeon and the cardiologist must have an a-priori conviction that repair, whenever possible, is far superior to valve replacement for the patient and therefore worth the effort. This positive attitude toward repair is based on the advantages that conservation of the patient's own tissues entails. The fact that it is a living tissue covered with endothelium reduces very significantly its thrombogenicity, avoiding the need for permanent anticoagulation. Because the natural design is maintained, the valve hemodynamics and the function of the cardiac chambers are superior to that obtained with present-day prostheses.

III. MITRAL VALVE REPAIR

Mitral valve surgery, because of its historical development, has traditionally been divided into surgery for mitral stenosis (commissurotomy), followed by valve replacement and more recently by repair for regurgitant lesions. This still often-used classification is no longer valid, particularly after the advent of the very successful percutaneous mitral balloon dilatation. The degree of success and therefore the indications for mitral balloon dilatation depend directly on the anatomic situation of the valve and are exactly the same as those necessary for a successful closed commissurotomy. Those cases of mitral stenosis with a very deteriorated valvular apparatus should undergo open-heart surgery and again, according to the pathology encountered, will be amenable to a repair or if very abnormal will end with a replacement. Mitral surgery, therefore, should be considered a continuum that stretches from a single conservative maneuver, such as an annuloplasty, to valve replacement, passing through progressively more complex repair maneuvers often necessary in stenotic lesions. The only possible modern classification for mitral surgery is replacement and conservation.

A. Evolution of Mitral Repair

The possibility of opening a stenotic mitral valve by digital splitting of the fused commissures was apparently suggested by Samways as early as 1898 (6). On May 20, 1923, Cutler inserted a valvulotome through the left ventricle to cut both cusps. The operation was temporarily successful (1). The first successful finger-splitting closed mitral commissurotomy was done in England by Henry Souttar in 1925, who surprisingly did not attempt to repeat it (2). In 1929, Cutler and Beck in the United States presented their final report on 5 patients treated surgically, with one survivor at 4.5 years (7). It was only 20 years later that Baily (8), Harken et al. (9), and Brock (10) again started digitally dilating the stenotic mitral valve through the left atrial appendage. The results were in some cases spectacular, although in others it became apparent that some valves were impossible to split under finger pressure alone, and resulted during the 1950s in a number of instruments designed to achieve dilatation. The transventricular Tubbs dilator became the most popular and is still used today in many centers (11). At the present time, the development and wide use of cardiopulmonary bypass in most Western countries has led to the performance of mitral commissurotomy under direct vision. Few young cardiac surgeons have been exposed to the technique of closed commissurotomy. Today, when echocardiographic studies can provide a clear picture of the anatomical situation of the mitral apparatus, it is possible to select those cases traditionally sent for surgery and direct them toward balloon dilatation if this is technically or economically available.

The surgical treatment of insufficiency also has a long history of attempts to reduce the dilated annulus, even in the days of closed surgery (5). The advent of extracorporal circulation made possible the plication of the annulus under direct vision of the valve (5,12–17). The use of sutures placed in the posterior aspect of the annulus close to the commissures is credited to Wooler et al. (18), Kay et al. (19), and Reed et al. (20). This concept remains valid today, although it has been displaced by the more precise prosthetic ring annuloplasties initially described by Carpentier et al. (21). In 1971 they described a rigid ring designed to remodel the mitral annulus. The area of the anterior leaflet is maintained while the posterior aspect of the annulus is plicated, reducing the overall annulus circumference. Duran and Ubago (22) subsequently proposed the use of a flexible ring, which follows the principles of the rigid ring but whose flexibility allows for the normally occurring continuous movements of the annulus during the cardiac cycle.

A different approach to reducing the size of the annulus was suggested by Shumway and Lewis (23), who proposed, as early as 1954, the use of autologous tissue to increase the surface area of the leaflets. This method was later studied experimentally and used clinically by Sauvage and Wood (24), Frater et al. (25), and Ross and Olsen (26). The long-term fate of this fresh tissue in the mitral area has not been reported, and there is concern that it probably will shrink. In the hope that glutaraldehyde-treated pericardium would not undergo a similar process, Gallo and Duran (27) and Deac et al. (28) proposed the use of glutaraldehyde porcine pericardium for posterior leaflet advancement; more recently, short-term glutaraldehyde-treated autologous pericardium has also been reported (29).

The surgery of chordae tendineae was initiated by McGoon (30), who in 1959 described a method for correction of ruptured chordae in which the flail segment of the leaflet is excluded by plication. This procedure, which decreases the length of the free edge of the involved leaflet, is not consistently satisfactory when applied to the anterior leaflet, due to the loss of tissue area. Its greatest application is the rupture of chordae to the posterior leaflet. Merendino et al. (14) in the same year, suggested the triangular resection of the unsupported segment and resuturing of the leaflet tissue. This technique, although more elegant and frequently used today, has the same advantages and limitations as McGoon's plication. In 1963 Kay and Egerton (31) proposed the suture of the flail segment to the nearest papillary muscle head. More recently, Carpentier et al. (32) and Duran (33) have described a method for the transfer of normal chords to the unsupported area of a leaflet secondary to rupture of its chordal attachments.

Regurgitation due to leaflet prolapse secondary to elongation of its chordae can now be treated by a variety of chordal shortening techniques (34,35). They all reduce the excess of the affected chord by plicating the redundant chord on to the parent papillary muscle or repositioning its papillary head.

B. Surgical Anatomy

The mitral valve complex consists of a continuous curtain of cusp tissue attached proximally to the junction of the left atrium and ventricle and distally by chordae teninae to the wall of the left ventricle. It consists of various structures.

1. Annulus

The fibrous annulus surrounds the base of the left ventricle, encompassing both its inlet (mitral) and outlet (aortic) orifices. The mitral portion of the cardiac skeleton is D-shaped, with its straight part dividing the aortic and mitral valves. At each extremity, two thickenings form the right and left fibrous trigones of the heart. The intertrigonal distance is constant during the cardiac cycle and very seldom becomes distorted by pathological processes. The left atrial wall is attached to this intertrigonal sheet, as well as to both fibrous trigones and to the curved part of the skeleton. This part of the mitral annulus thins out as it separates from the trigones, and since the base of the left ventricle is attached to it, both its size and shape change continuously during the cardiac cycle in the normal subject. Multiple pathological processes affect this thinner part of the annulus, giving rise to mitral annular dilatation. The posterior or mural cusp of the mitral valve is attached to this curved portion of the skeleton. Morphological studies in the normal adult postmortem heart have shown that the mitral annulus has a circumference between 8.5 and 10 cm.

2. Leaflets

The mitral cusps are inserted at their base along the whole perimeter of the orifice. Their central or free edge presents multiple indentations; the two constant ones are called commissures, or, better, commissural areas: the anterolateral or anterior and posteromedial or posterior. Their recognition is essential, since they define the anterior and posterior leaflets and must be identified when performing an open commissurotomy. The limits of the commissural zones correspond to the limits of insertion of these chords and range from 5 to 13 mm with a depth of 8 mm.

3. The Chordae Tendineae

The very thin chordae tendineae attach the leaflet tissue to the papillary muscles. In spite of their apparent variability. Raganathan et al. (36) and Acar and Deloche (37) have described and classified them in terms that are very useful to the surgeon. The commissural chords arise from the anterior and posterior papillary muscles and branch in a fanlike manner to be inserted into both commissural areas. The anterior leaflet chords are inserted on the rough or contact area of the anterior cusp and have a length between 10 and 15 mm (37).

The posterior leaflet chords can be classified into (1) chords attached to the free edge at each of the indentations of the posterior leaflet, (2) free-edge chords similar but thinner and more numerous than their corresponding anterior leaflet chords, and (3) basal or third-order chords which arise directly from the ventricular wall and are inserted into the ventricular aspect of the posterior leaflet far from the contact area. These chords are specific to this leaflet. The length of the posterior leaflet chords varies between 13 and 17 mm (37).

4. Papillary Muscles

There are two groups of papillary muscles: the anterolateral or anterior and the posteromedial or posterior. Approximately half of the chordae from each group attach to the corresponding commissure, while the other half attach to both anterior and posterior leaflets. The blood supply to the anterior muscle is from the left anterior descending coronary artery, one of its diagonal branches, or even from a marginal branch. The posterior muscle is supplied by the posterolateral branches of either the circumflex or the right coronary artery and is the most frequently affected by coronary disease.

C. Pathology

Until recently, discussion of the etiology and pathology of mitral disease, and particularly regurgitation, would have been academic, since in all cases a valve replacement was the only accepted therapy. With the advent of reconstructive techniques, the etiology of mitral disease assumes more importance in selecting the most appropriate corrective procedure. Although a catalog of all the possible etiologies of mitral disease can be enumerated, its surgical usefulness is doubtful. We will rather follow, as suggestive by Davies (38), a more practical method based on the alterations found in each valve component.

1. Annular Disease

Mitral annular dilatation can occur either due to connective tissue disorders such as Marfan's syndrome, Ehlers-Danlos syndrome, or osteogenesis imperfecta, or may be secondary to chronic left ventricular dilatation. Spontaneous mitral ring calcification develops in the elderly, particularly women, as a bar of calcium at the hinge of the posterior leaflet.

2. Leaflets

Rheumatic disease produces thickening and retraction of the cusps, leading to lack of coaptation and regurgitation. This fibrosis is usually more intense in the posterior cusp and particularly in its posteromedial aspect. Bacterial endocarditis affects the leaflets initially with vegetations. Increase in leaflet surface area is a typical feature of the "mitral prolapse syndrome." The often weakened, whitish and opaque cusps are redundant and balloon into the left atrium, giving rise to the "billowing valve syndrome." Mitral prolapse can be secondary to rheumatic, ischemic, traumatic, or degenerative processes and therefore represents a final pathway which, if severe, results in mitral regurgitation and needs a specific surgical treatment.

3. Chords

The chords probably represent the most critical element in the mitral complex. Basically, chords might be shortened, elongated, or ruptured. Rheumatic fibrosis is the main cause of chordal shortening. Fibrous fusion of adjacent chords, along with progressive shortening until their practical disappearance, lead to both stenosis and regurgitation. Chordal elongation is typical of the degenerative disease mentioned above, resulting in leaflet prolapse. The posterior cusp chords are more frequently involved, particularly those attached to the middle scallop. Chordal rupture is usually associated with the degenerative mitral prolapse or bacterial endocarditis.

4. Papillary Muscles

The main pathological processes involving the papillary muscles that result in mitral incompetence are ischemia and the cardiomyopathies. The muscle can completely rupture close to the tip of one of its heads shortly after an acute myocardial infarction, resulting in sudden, severe mitral incompetence. In other cases, necrosis may lead to fibrosis of the muscle tip, resulting in an elongated fibrous band. Following an ischemic episode, some patients develop transient mitral regurgitation due to papillary dysfunction (39).

D. Surgery

1. Indications

The choice of the appropriate procedure must be based primarily on the anatomical situation of each individual valve, which can be accurately

Table 1 Factors Influencing the Indications for Mitral Repair

---

A. Major
   Valve pathology
   Valve lesions (annulus, leaflet, subvalvar)
   Etiology (rheumatic, degenerative, ischemic)
B. Minor
   Cardiac:
      Left atrial size
      Thrombus
      Associated surgery
      Left ventricular function
   Noncardiac:
      Age, sex
      Geographic
      Socioeconomic
      Lifestyle

---

determined preoperatively with two-dimensional color Doppler echocardiography. Basically, each structure (annulus, leaflets, chords, and papillary muscles) can have either normal, restricted, or increased mobility. Restriction is due to fibrosis or calcification and laxity to degeneration. A combination of situations is often the case. A completely destroyed valve due to severe fibrosis or calcification will require replacement. Other extravalvular cardiac and noncardiac factors which also play an important role in the selection of the procedure are summarized in Table 1. Extracardiac factors to be considered are age, sex, socioeconomics, geography, and lifestyle of the patient. Clearly, in young patients and women who desire to have children, every effort should be made to repair the valve, even at the price of not achieving a perfect result. The same applies for patients whose geographic or social situation makes anticoagulation an exercise in utopian thinking.

2. Technique

All procedures are performed through a median sternotomy with cardiopulmonary bypass. Careful identification of each element of the mitral complex is essential, and requires good visibility, patience, and judgment. Excellent visibility is achieved with cardioplegia and a wide atriotomy. The incision is carried just behind the interatrial groove and continued upward beyond and behind the superior vena cava and curved backward behind the inferior vena cava.

The efficacy of mitral closure must be checked and the cause of regurgitation identified. The mitral valve must be observed through the open atrium while the left ventricle is filled under pressure. The simplest way is to inject saline into the ventricle under pressure with a syringe through a catheter across the mitral valve. Another method is to inject cardioplegia through a cannula introduced via the ascending aorta and crossing the aortic valve. The method we favor is the injection of cardioplegia or blood through a small cannula introduced into the left ventricle through a small stab wound in the apex, which is also used as a left vent.

If reconstruction is considered appropriate, each lesion should be treated individually (Table 2; Figs. 1 and 2). Fused commissures should be sectioned with a scalpel under continuous observation of the underlying commissural chords. Fibrosis of the subvalvular apparatus calls for longitudinal splitting, which often extends down the corresponding papillary muscle. Even if the lesion is regurgitant and no gradient has been detected preoperatively, if the commissures are fused, they should be split to increase leaflet mobility. Posterior leaflet mobility can also be improved by splitting secondary chords that tether it to the ventricular wall. Occasionally, the retraction of this posterior leaflet is so severe that the only conservative solution is to perform a longitudinal incision in the leaflet parallel and close to the annulus, with insertion of a lozenge of autologous or xenogeneic pericardium to increase the surface of the leaflet.

The amount of chordal elongation present and therefore how much needs to be shortened is determined by elevating the affected leaflet and

Table 2 Repair Techniques According to the Lesion at Each Level of Mitral Apparatus

Level	Lesion	Repair
Annulus	Dilatation	Annuloplasty
Commissures	Fusion	Commissurotomy
	Calcification	Resection
Leaflets	Billowing	Resection
	Prolapse	Resection
	Retraction	Enlargement
	Calcification	Excision
Chords	Fusion	Separation
	Elongation	Shortening
	Rupture	Chord Transfer
		New Chord
Papillary muscles	Elongation	Repositioning
	Malposition	Annuloplasty
	Dysfunction	Annuloplasty

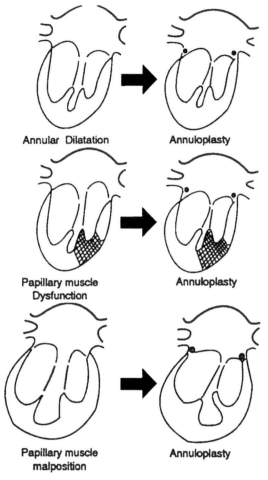

Figure 1 Repair of regurgitant mitial lesion with normal leaflet mobility.

comparing it to the opposite normal leaflet. Shortening is done by plication
of the papillary end of the chord by burrowing it into its corresponding
split papillary muscle. Posterior chordal rupture is treated by quadrangular
resection of the affected portion of the leaflet and resuture. Surprisingly,
up to one-third of the posterior leaflet can be excised without harm. The
leaflet edges are sutured with interrupted, nonreabsorbable sutures supported by the prosthetic ring that must always be implanted. Rupture of
one of the main chords to the anterior leaflet has been treated in the same
fashion. However, in our experience, resection of even relatively small

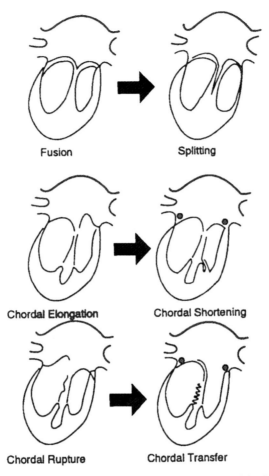

Figure 2 Repair or regurgitant mitial lesion with abnormal leaflet mobility.

portions of this leaflet often results in significant residual stenosis. Recently, we have found that transposition of the corresponding opposite chord of the posterior leaflet onto the anterior can solve this problem. A quadrangular area of the posterior cusp carrying its chordae is transposed and sutured on to the atrial surface of the anterior. The resulting gap is closed as in posterior chordal rupture.

Annular dilatation giving rise to regurgitation is treated by selective annular constriction by means of a prosthetic ring. Although a number of such rings are available commercially, they are all based on the principle that the annulus does not dilate uniformly and that the intertrigonal distance remains constant. Based on this distance, the appropriate ring is selected and the annulus sutured onto it so that a plication of the commissural and posterior leaflet areas is achieved without reducing the base of the anterior leaflet. Prosthetic ring annuloplasty has become a very standardized and popular method, which is being used even in cases where the annulus is not very dilated but to compensate for the lack of tissue due to leaflet retraction. The limit to this technique is the possibility of solving regurgitation but inducing stenosis.

E. Results

Generally, the clinical results of mitral valve repair are superior to those of mitral valve replacement. A recent review by David (40) of the literature showed a compounded hospital mortality for mitral stenosis of 0.9% for repair versus 7.3% for replacement, and in mitral regurgitation 3.4% for repair versus 10.6% for replacement. This significant difference is probably due to the better left ventricular function following mitral repair, where the annulo-ventricular continuity is preserved (41,42). It remains to be seen whether this difference is maintained when the results of replacement with conservation of the chordal attachments become available.

The incidence of thromboembolism, hemorrhagic complications, and infective endocarditis is definitely lower after mitral valve repair than after replacement (43–58). The actuarial survival after mitral valve repair is greater than after valve replacement (48,50,53,55,56). All these figures however, do not take into account that these are not randomized studies and therefore the different patient populations might be biased toward performing repairs in less evolutioned patients. The possibility of an unsuccessful repair requiring immediate replacement during the same operation, or at a later date, is the only negative factor of mitral valve reconstruction and probably constitutes the main reason for the reluctance of some surgeons to embark on a systematic conservative approach to mitral surgery. The possible causes of failure of a repair are (1) a wrong indication, where the degree of valve destruction should have precluded any attempt at conservation; (2) a technical error due to either misjudgment in the assessment of the lesions or in the performance of a particular maneuver; (3) an instability of the repair technique, which although theoretically possible, our experience has shown is always related to an incorrect technique; (4) progression of the underlying pathology. The etiology plays a very important role in the overall results, not only because it determines the predominant type of lesions and consequently their difficulty for correction, but also in terms of late results affected by the progression of the disease (57,58,59).

The incidence of unsuccessful attempts at reconstruction followed by immediate valve replacement is seldom mentioned in the literature and more rarely are the consequences discussed. These cases are usually included in the replacement group, compounding its already higher mortality. Only recently Craver et al. (51), mentioned that of a group of 78 patients, 65 had a repair and 13 (16.6%) an unsuccessful repair followed by replacement in the same operation. Four of these died in hospital (30.7%). In a group of 203 young rheumatic patients operated on during a 2-year period for mitral regurgitation at our institution, 49 (24.1%) required a mitral valve replacement, 136 (67%) had a successful repair, and 18 (8.9%) had an unsuccessful attempt at repair. The hospital mortality was 4% for replacement, 1.4% for repair, and 16.6% for the unsuccessful repairs. This last group of patients, when studied a posteriori, were found to have pre- and intraoperative findings closer to those who underwent replacement than to those with a successful repair (60). Further similar studies and more attention to the preoperative echocardiographic data should identify those patients who are unsuitable for repair on anatomical grounds.

The etiology of the mitral lesion determines both the rate of repair versus replacement and the stability of the reconstruction. Rheumatic lesions, although historically the first to be repaired, have been shown to be more difficult to treat conservatively and have a higher rate of reoperation for early and late valve dysfunction, which oscillates between 10 and 27% (58–62). The younger the age group, the less stable the repair will be, probably due to the ongoing rheumatic process (60). Degenerative lesions are far easier to repair and so far have shown a very high degree of stability (50,53,58).

Mitral regurgitation secondary to ischemia is still an area where experience is limited (63–69). Attempts at the evaluation of the results are severely hampered by the very different mitral pathologies encountered in patients requiring revascularization. It is not yet clear in which patients the mitral regurgitation cannot be ignored and, if so, whether a repair or a replacement is the appropriate solution. We recently (69) reviewed 169 consecutive patients with coronary artery disease and varying degrees of mitral insufficiency. The hospital mortality was 7% among the 87 patients who underwent repair and 13.4% among the 82 who had valve replacement. No difference in late mortality was apparent between the two groups (±14%) at 5 years maximum follow-up. Analysis of the mitral pathology encountered at surgery revealed that all patients could be classified into three distinct categories very useful for the evaluation of the results and consequently for establishing indications (Table 3). Patients in category I ("associated MR"), in whom the mitral pathology is independent from

Table 3   Classification and Treatment of Mitral Regurgitation in Ischemic
Disease

Type	Definition	Pathology	Treatment
I	Associated	Independent of ischemia (degenerative, rheumatic)	Repair/replace
II	Functional	Papillary muscle dysfunction (normal looking mitral)	Annuloplasty
III	Organic	Papillary muscle rupture	Replace

the ischemic problem, should be treated like any other mitral patient, i.e., with repair or replacement according to the valve status. The results should be reasonably good. In the second or "functional" group the surgeon, although aware of the presence of significant regurgitation, does not find any anatomical mitral anomaly with the exception of an occasional annular dilatation. This group, with obvious similarities to functional tricuspid regurgitation, should be treated with a ring annuloplasty. Patients with type III regurgitation have a visibly abnormal mitral valve due to ischemic events affecting the leaflets or subvalvular apparatus ("organic MR"). Because of the usually acute presentation, deteriorated ventricular function, poor mitral valve visibility, and technical difficulty of repair, these patients in general should be treated with a chordal-saving valve replacement. Given the advanced age of these patients (in our case a mean of 69 years), it is likely that a bioprosthesis will last the patient's expected life span (70), while failure of a valve repair, leading to reoperation, is unacceptable.

In summary, mitral valve repair can now be considered an established surgical procedure for the treatment of mitral valve disease. It is superior to valve replacement although not always possible. The rate of repair versus replacement is greatly influenced by the underlying pathology, which in the case of degenerative disease should be close to 80–90% of the cases. In rheumatic disease this rate depends on the age of the patient, oscillating between 40% and 60%. Its application to other pathologies such as infective and ischemic pathologies, although encouraging, is still awaiting further study. The advent of modern Doppler echocardiography will define precisely the indications and limits of this surgery. Better myocardial protection will enlarge its scope.

IV. AORTIC VALVE RECONSTRUCTION

Conservative surgery of the aortic valve has as long a history as mitral repair. In fact, the first aortic commissurotomy was performed by Tuffier

(71) in 1913, well before a similar successful attempt was done in the mitral area (1). Before the advent of cardiopulmonary bypass, aortic regurgitation was treated by bicuspidization (72) and circumclusion (73). Once open-heart surgery was available, the rather unpredictable aortic valve repair maneuvers were soon abandoned in favor of new prostheses. Nowadays, the vast majority of surgeons treat all aortic lesions, with the exception of congenital stenotic lesions in the very young and regurgitations secondary to septal defects, with replacement. More recently, the successful and universally accepted repair of the atrioventricular valves, coupled with the awareness of the problems inherent to all prostheses, has encouraged a new interest in aortic valve reconstruction.

A. Surgical Anatomy

The aortic valve should be considered as a complex structure that includes the annulus, leaflets, and sinuses of Valsalva (Fig. 3). The annulus, which is scalloped, corresponds to the insertion of the three cusps and is anchored to the fibrous skeleton of the heart. The left trigone corresponds to the lowest point of the left coronary sinus and the right trigone to the right coronary sinus, which in some animals, e.g., the bovines, is a bony structure. The base of the annulus at the level of the right sinus is situated immediately above the interventricular septum.

The three leaflets or semilunar cusps are of different sizes and are inserted into the annulus following an elliptical line. Their free edges present a contact area or lunnulae, which at their center is thickened or nodules of Arantzius and peripherally is very thin at the level of the commissures, inserted into a thickening of the aortic wall.

Corresponding with each cusp, the aorta bulges into three sinuses of Valsalva. The lower limit of each sinus corresponds with the line of insertion of each leaflet and its upper limit is clearly delineated by a curved thickening of the aortic wall or supraaortic ridge or crest. At variable points of the right and left sinuses the corresponding origins of the coronary arteries are situated. The actual relative dimensions of each part of the aortic valve complex are important and have been studied extensively by Swanson and Clark (74) (Fig. 4).

B. Pathology

The aortic valve lesions have traditionally been classified as stenotic, regurgitant, and mixed. This clinically useful clarification, however, does not address the problems encountered when repair surgery is contemplated. A better grouping of pathologies should be used based on the mobility of the cusps. Although the whole aortic complex should be ana-

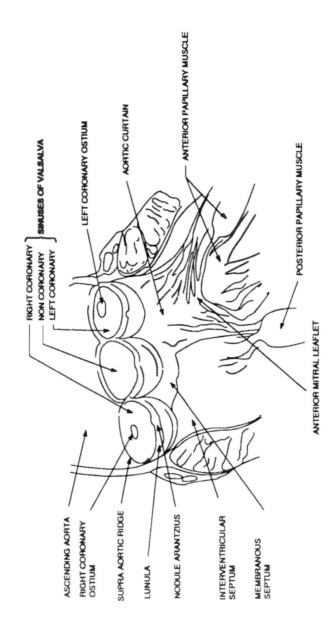

Figure 3 Aortic valve anatomy.

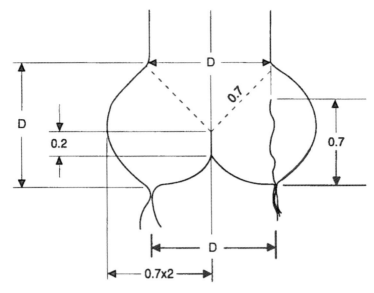

Figure 4   Dimensions of the aortic valve elements in relation with the annulus diameter (D). (Modified from Ref. 74.)

lyzed observing the annulus, sinuses, leaflets, and commissures, the state of the cusps will determine the type of surgical maneuver to be applied. The aortic cusp mobility can be normal, restricted, or prolapsed. Normal cusp mobility is present in cases of aortic regurgitation due to annular dilatation, cusp perforations, or ruptures. Restricted cusp movement is secondary to commissural fusion and/or thickening and retraction. Increased mobility results in cusp prolapse due to elongation of the free edge or sagging of the leaflet body.

C. Surgery

The same general principles of repair mentioned above apply to the aortic valve. The lesions must be carefully analyzed and treated individually. Intraoperative echocardiography is mandatory. Excellent exposure is easier to achieve in the aortic than in the mitral area.

We always perform a transverse aortotomy initiated close to the aortic cross clamp, away from the commissures, and then down the center of the noncoronary sinus and stop a few millimeters from the annulus. Closure of this aortotomy after a repair is always easy due to the absence of a rigid prosthesis. This is done with two single over-and-over 4/0 prolene continuous sutures, started at both ends of the incision and tied at the most anterior aspect of the ascending aorta.

A variety of surgical maneuvers are nowadays available for aortic valve conservation. The choice of technique depends on the surgical findings and, as in mitral repair, in most cases more than one maneuver is required to achieve competence. According to the pathological clarification described above, the following techniques are available.

The most frequent cause of regurgitation in the presence of *normal cusp mobility* is the dilatation of the annulus in the presence of normal leaflets (Fig. 5). Two annuloplasty techniques are available, encircling suturing of the whole aortic circumference ("circumclusion") and subcommissural annuloplasty. Circumclusion of the aortic valve was first described by Taylor et al. in 1958 (73), and was used by several surgeons with and without cardiopulmonary bypass. Recently, Chauvand et al. (75) reported its use in 35 patients with ages ranging between 5 and 65 years (mean 26). The etiology was rheumatic in 15, congenital in 10, idiopathic dilatation in 7, and endocarditis in 3. There was one operative death (3%), and with a mean follow-up of 1.9 years, 3 patients (9%) required reoperation and 15% had moderate residual regurgitation.

Subcomissural annuloplasty consists of the placement of three pledgeted "U" sutures through the aortic wall of the sinus of Valsalva close to each commissure. These sutures, by plicating the aortic wall, reduce its total circumference. This technique, which we described as original

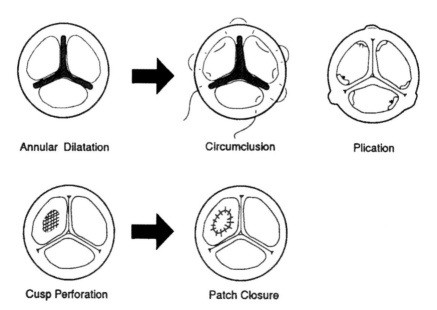

Annular Dilatation   Circumclusion   Plication

Cusp Perforation   Patch Closure

Figure 5   Aortic valve repair principles in lesions with normal cusp mobility.

(76), had in fact been reported by Cabrol et al. in 1966 (77). We have used this technique for over 15 years with very satisfactory results (78), and Cosgrove et al. (79) recently reported its use in 21 consecutive patients.

The other cause of aortic regurgitation in the presence of normal cusp mobility is leaflet perforation, secondary to healed infective endocarditis. These very discrete orifices can be closed with a patch of glutaraldehyde-treated pericardium. Direct closure should not be used, as it will reduce the cusp area. For the same reason, interrupted sutures should be preferred to a running suture, which tends to reduce the leaflet size.

Increased cusp mobility, giving rise to aortic insufficiency, is due to prolapse of one or more cusps (Fig. 6). Two techniques again have been described: cusp resuspension and cusp resection. Cusp resuspension, originally described by Garamella et al. (80) and popularized by Trusler et al. (81), consists of the plication of the free edge of the prolapsing cusp close to its commissure with a pledgeted suture, which is anchored to the adjacent aortic wall. Cusp resection consists of the triangular resection of the leaflet with its base in the free edge and apex toward its line of attachment. While Cosgrove et al. (79) have used this technique, we rather favor resuspension as an easier and safer maneuver.

Reduced cusp mobility is due to commissural fusion and/or leaflet thickening (Fig. 7). Aortic commissurotomy must always be performed, even if

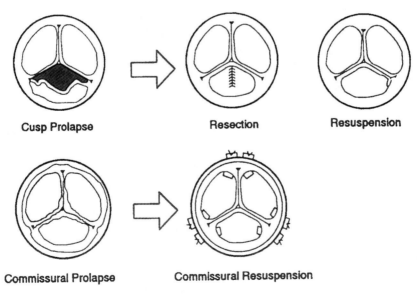

Cusp Prolapse   Resection   Resuspension

Commissural Prolapse   Commissural Resuspension

Figure 6 Aortic valve repair in lesions with increased cusp mobility.

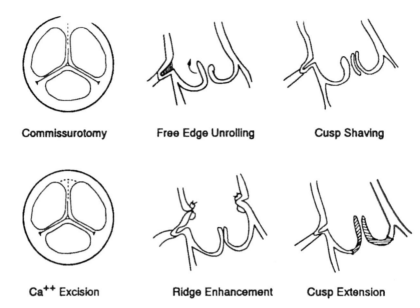

| Commissurotomy | Free Edge Unrolling | Cusp Shaving |

| Ca⁺⁺ Excision | Ridge Enhancement | Cusp Extension |

Figure 7   Aortic valve repair principles in lesions with reduced cusp mobility.

minimal fusion is present, in order to increase cusp mobility. Occasionally, isolated calcification of the commissural area is found. A commissorotomy through the calcified nodule can be performed followed by shaving of the calcium from each cusp. Thickened leaflets are very often found, but the degree of thickening and retraction is very viable. In the young rheumatic patient, a typical finding is fairly normal leaflets with only their free edges thickened and retracted. In these cases, free-edge unrolling is possible. Repeat incisions are made on the sinus aspect of the leaflet and, by forceful pull with forceps, the free edge unrolls, gaining a few millimeters. In older patients, a fibrous bar corresponding to the lunnulae, which immobilizes the cusp, can be resected (82). It must be emphasized that each of these maneuvers very seldom achieves competence and requires reinforcement by others. In those cases of free-edge unrolling, we perform an enhancement of the supraaortic ridge by placement of two pledgeted "U" sutures at the level of each crest. We showed in the experimental animal that this simple technique induces an early closure of the aortic valve, probably due to an increase in normally occurring vortices within the sinuses of Valsalva (83). It can be postulated that this vortex increase reduces the tendency toward inward rolling of the leaflet free edges. In any case, it is a very fast surgical maneuver that at worst is innocuous.

In the presence of very severe cusp retraction, these maneuvers cannot be used, and extension of all three cusps is performed with a single strip of fashioned glutaraldehyde-treated pericardium. Originally we used commercially available glutaraldehyde-treated bovine pericardium, following the technique described by Batista et al. (84). Experience progressively changed our technique and choice of material. At present we use a strip of the patient's own pericardium, which is resected according to the aortic annulus diameter as measured intraoperatively by transesophageal echocardiography. The pericardium is placed for 10 min in 0.5% glutaraldehyde in an appropriate-sized container, which has the shape of the three leaflets. This single strip is sutured to the leaflet remnants with 4/0 prolene continuous sutures starting at the midpoint of each leaflet and stopping at each native commissure. The new commissure is sutured to the aortic wall and tied outside onto a pledget.

Two main questions must be addressed when considering the use of this approach. The first is the need for a standard surgical technique that ensures a correct, reproducible, and safe result in terms of immediate competence. The second is the long-term durability of the selected material. We recently reviewed our experience in a group of 45 patients who had a cusp extension with pericardium. There was no hospital mortality and, with a maximum follow-up of 3 years, there were no late deaths nor embolic events, although none was anticoagulated. The mean preoperative degree of regurgitation was 3.24 ± 0.8 (graded 0–4+). The mean intraoperative regurgitation post repair was 0.59 ± 0.5, which was maintained throughout the follow-up period. There were two reoperations in this group of patients, but both due to dysfunction of the simultaneously performed mitral repair. In both of them the aortic valve was inspected, revealing pliable pericardium at 4 and 8 months postsurgery. This technique can now be considered standardized and reproducible.

The second question is the durability of the pericardium. In the 1960s several authors used nontreated pericardium with poor results (85–89). The small number of cases and lack of adequate myocardial protection probably resulted in poor anatomical results, which invalidate any conclusion. The larger but negative experience with fresh autologous fascia lata described by Senning (90) emphasizes the importance of tissue pretreatment. More recently, Batista (91) and Yacoub et al. (92) have reported satisfactory long-term results with the use of glutaraldehyde-treated bovine pericardium. On the other hand, the rather limited durability of the Ionescu-Shiley pericardial bioprosthesis (93), particularly in the young patient (94), casts some doubt on the long-term results of glutaraldehyde-treated bovine pericardium. The absence of a rigid stent used in cusp extension, however, not only reduces the transvalvular gradient, which is especially important in patients with small roots, but also reduces the tissue stress, hopefully increasing its durability. This hypothesis is supported by the reports of Angell et al. (95) showing that the free-hand homograft failure is approximately 12 years versus 8 when the homograft is mounted on a stent. Even in the event of failure, the excision of the calcified pericardium should be easy, given that the patient's leaflet remnants have been preserved. The recent report by Chachques et al. (96) of the biological advantages of glutaraldehyde-treated autologous pericardium and its clinical application for cusp extension in the mitral position (29) encouraged us to use it in the last 25 cases with excellent results to date.

The intraoperative testing of the aortic repair is done by direct visualization of the valve through a modified cytoscope, introduced through the partially closed aortotomy while injecting cardioplegia with the aorta cross-clamped. Once the aorta is unclamped, during the rewarming period, the percent of left vent return in relation to the pump output is measured for a full minute. Percentages below 10 are considered satisfactory. These methods, however, do not eliminate the use of transesophageal or epicardial echocardiography once off bypass.

D. Indications

As in the case of mitral valve repair, the indications for aortic valve repair depend primarily on the lesions encountered. Calcified valves are beyond repair, given that the different attempts at decalcification have been shown to be very short-lived. Very thick and rigid valves are also beyond the possibility of present-day reconstruction. Those valves with minimal or moderate fibrosis of the leaflet base are good candidates for repair. If the degree of cusp retraction is too important, cusp extension is indicated. However, because the long-term durability of the glutaraldehyde-treated autologous pericardium is still unknown, we reserve this technique for young patients where anticoagulation is a problem. Cusp prolapse is in fact more frequent than one realizes. These cases are amenable to resuspension always followed by annuloplasty. The occasionally found perforation, secondary to healed infective endocarditis, can be closed with a small patch of pericardium.

The rate of aortic valve repair depends on the etiology and age of the patient, which will influence the type of lesion encountered. We recently reviewed our total surgical experience with aortic regurgitation, treated during a 2-year period. There were 251 patients with a mean age of 23 years. Valve replacement was performed in 144 and reconstruction was possible in 107 patients (42.6%) (97). It is likely that, as happened with mitral repair, the initial surprise and reluctance of the surgeons who thought that repair candidates did not occur in their patient population will be drastically changed when they begin to observe each aortic valve with a conservative attitude.

V. TRICUSPID VALVE REPAIR

Treatment of the tricuspid valve, because it is less often affected, has followed the development in the surgery of the other valves and in particular the mitral valve (98). Closed commissurotomy was first performed in 1952 (99). The danger of inducing severe regurgitation, its frequent association with insufficiency, and the improvements in cardiopulmonary bypass advocated open correction. At present, stenosis is treated by open commissurotomy (100) and regurgitation lesions by annuloplasty. The technique described by Kay et al. (101), which consisted of the transformation of the tricuspid into a bicuspid valve by plication of the posterior leaflet area, has been practically abandoned because the correction does not withstand the test of time. Tearing of the stitches and the fact that the annulus can continue to dilate were implicated (102). The semicircular annuloplasty proposed by Cabrol (103) and DeVega (104) uses a double continuous suture that reduces the annulus at the level of the anterior and posterior leaflets without interfering with the base of the septal leaflet, which is normally not dilated. It is rapidly performed and is efficient in reducing regurgitation. It has the danger of inducing stenosis if it is not carefully measured and has also been blamed for the tendency of the suture to become detached, with recurrence of the insufficiency (105). A different approach was described by Carpentier and co-workers in 1971 (21), in which they used a preshaped rigid prosthetic ring of different sizes, which was sutured to the tricuspid annulus reducing it selectively. We (22) described a flexible ring which follows the same principle, but due to its flexibility adapts better to the continuous changes in the shape and size of the normal tricuspid orifice. At least theoretically, it would be less prone to dehiscence and to induce stenosis because of its ability to become more circular during diastole.

A. Indications

The vast majority of tricuspid valve lesions can be repaired. The problem, rather, lies in diagnosing its presence, degree of regurgitation, and whether it is organic or functional. Two-dimensional color Doppler echocardiography has become a very reliable instrument, provided the tricuspid valve is systematically and carefully analyzed (106,107).

Our present-day indications for tricuspid valve repair are as follows. (1) All organic lesions should undergo a commissurotomy, followed by a flexible ring annuloplasty. Ignoring the lesion on the basis of the small gradient present before surgery is dangerous, as it is likely to become significant due to the postoperative increase in cardiac output, secondary to the repair of the left sided lesions (108). The occasional case of a traumatic rupture of a chord or papillary muscle can be easily treated conservatively. Bacterial endocarditis lesions can seldom be repaired because of the very extensive valve damage that is usually present. (2) Functional regurgitation should be treated by an annuloplasty unless very mild. Those patients with a moderate regurgitation and low pulmonary (arteriolar) resistance should undergo a simple DeVega-type annuloplasty. In these cases it can be expected that the right ventricular failure will improve after the reduction in afterload following the mitral repair. It can be safely presumed that the tricuspid regurgitation will eventually decrease if not disappear altogether. The annuloplasty is directed toward an improved postoperative period. Those patients with severe regurgitation should undergo a ring annuloplasty. It is felt that the degree of annular dilatation would impose too much strain on DeVega suture (109).

B. Results

Because of the characteristics of the tricuspid valve, the results of its repair are very difficult to analyze objectively. The hospital mortality varies between 4% and 31% (110). In a series of 359 patients who underwent tricuspid repair between 1974 and 1979 at our institution, the hospital mortality was 8.4% (108). More recently, in a series of 172 patients who had a tricuspid repair performed between 1988 and 1991, the hospital mortality was 4%. This disparity in mortality rates reported in the literature is not due primarily to the different types of repairs, but rather to the preoperative condition of the patients.

We have also shown that the postoperative functional status and, more important, the cardiac output of the patients, is related directly to the results of the surgery on left-sided lesions and not with the hemodynamic results of the tricuspid surgery (108). Postoperative hemodynamic and Doppler studies have shown residual transvalvular gradients in a significant number of patients after annuloplasty. This incidence was 50–70% after a DeVega annuloplasty (111,112), 33–68% after a Carpentier ring (113,114), and 31% after a Duran flexible annuloplasty (108). The gradients oscillated between 2 and 8 mmHg. Residual insufficiency was also frequent, although clearly related to the presence of postoperative mitral dysfunction. In spite of these problems, tricuspid valve repair is universally accepted as far superior to tricuspid replacement, which carries a much higher risk of endocarditis or thrombosis (115).

The rate of tricuspid repair versus replacement is the highest among the cardiac valves. In our reported series, of 368 patients operated on for tricuspid disease, where 50% had organic disease, only 9 (2.4%) had a replacement (108). It can be concluded that, although it is not yet perfect, repair has become the procedure of choice in tricuspid valve surgery.

REFERENCES

1. Cutler EC, Levine SA. Cardiotomy and valvulotomy for mitral stenosis. Experimental observations and clinical notes concerning an operative case with recovery. Boston Med Surg J 1923; 188:1023.
2. Souttar HJ. The surgical treatment of mitral stenosis. Br Med J 1925; 2: 603.
3. Gross RE, Hubbard JP. Surgical ligation of patent ductus arteriosus: report of first successful case. JAMA 1939; 112:729.
4. Craaford C, Nylin G. Congenital coarctation of the aorta and its surgical treatment. J Thorac Surg 1945; 347:347.
5. Bailey CP. Surgery of the Heart. Philadelphia: Lea & Febiger, 1955:482.
6. Samways DW. Cardiac peristalsis. Its nature and effects. Lancet 1898: 1: 927.
7. Cutler EC, Beck CS. The present status of the surgical procedures in chronic valvular disease of the heart. Arch Surg 1929; 18:403.
8. Bailey CP. The surgical treatment of mitral stenosis (mitral commissurotomy). Dis Chest 1949; 15:377.
9. Harken DE, Ellis LB, Ware PF, et al. The surgical treatment of mitral stenosis. I valvuloplasty. N Engl J Med 1948; 239:801.
10. Baker C, Brock RC, Campbell M. Valvulotomy for mitral stenosis: report of six successful cases. Br Med J 1950; 1:1283.
11. Logan A, Turner R. Surgical treatment of mitral stenosis with particular reference to the transventricular approach with a mechanical dilator. Lancet 1959; 2:874.
12. Lillehei CW, Gott VL, De Wall RA, Varco RL. The surgical treatment of stenotic or regurgitant lesions of the aortic or mitral valves by direct vision utilizing a pump oxygenator. J Thorac Surg 1958; 35:190.
13. Davila JC, Glover RP. Circumferential suture of the mitral valve for the correction of regurgitation. Am J Cardiol 1958; 2:267.
14. Merendino KA, Thomas GI, Jesseph JE, Herron PW, Wintersheid LC, Vetto RR. The open correction of rheumatic mitral regurgitation and/or stenosis. Ann Surg 1959; 150:5.
15. Anderson AM, Cobb LA, Bruce RA, Merendino KA. Evaluation of mitral annuloplasty for mitral regurgitation. Clinical and hemodynamic status four to 41 months after surgery. Circulation 1962; 26:26.
16. Gerbode F, Kerth WJ, Osborn JJ, Selzer A. Correction of mitral insufficiency by open operation. Ann Surg 1962; 155:54.
17. Belcher JR. The surgical treatment of mitral regurgitation. Br Heart J 1964; 25:513.
18. Wooler GH, Nixon PGF, Grimshaw VA, Watson PA. Experiences with the repair of the mitral valve in mitral incompetence. Thorax 1962; 17:49.

19. Kay JH, Egerton WS, Zubiate P. The surgical treatment of mitral insufficiency with use of the heart-lung machine. Surgery 1961; 50:67.
20. Reed GE, Tice DA, Clauss RH. Asymetric exaggerated mitral annuloplasty. Repair of mitral insufficiency with hemodynamic predictability. J Thorac Cardiovasc Surg 1965; 49:752.
21. Carpentier A, Deloche A, Dauptain J, Soyer R, Blondeau P, Piwnica A, Dubost CH. A new reconstructive operation for correction of mitral and tricuspid insufficiency. J Thorac Cardiovasc Surg 1971; 61:1.
22. Duran CG, Ubago JL. Clinical and haemodynamic performance of a totally flexible prosthetic ring for atrioventricular valve reconstruction. Ann Thorac Surg 1976; 22:458.
23. Shumway NE, Lewis FJ. Experimental surgery of the mitral valve under direct vision using hypothermia. Surg Forum 1954; 5:12.
24. LR Sauvage, SJ Wood. Technique for correction of mitral insufficiency by leaflet advancement. J Thorac Cardiovasc Surg 1966; 51:649.
25. Frater RW, Berghius S, Brown AL, Ellis FH Jr. The experimental and clinical use of autogenous procedures for the replacement and extension of mitral and tricuspid valve cusps and chordae. J Cardiovasc Surg 1965; 6: 214.
26. Ross JK, Olsen EGJ. Mitral valve reconstruction by posterior cusp advancement using a pericardial graft. Long term follow-up in nine patients. Thorax 1976; 31(3):324.
27. Gallo JI, Duran CMG. Uso clinco del pericardio heterologo tratado con glutaraldehido para la ampliacion del velo valvular mitral. Rev Cir Esp 1980; 34:63.
28. Deac R, Brate D, Liebhart M, et al. The reconstruction of the mitral valve with stabilized biological tissue in 33 cases. In: Duran C, Angell WW, Johnson AD, Oury JH, eds. Recent Progress in Mitral Valve Disease. London: Butterworths, 1984:436.
29. Chauvaud S, Jebara V, Chachques JC, et al. Valve extension with glutaraldehyde-preserved autologous pericardium. Results in mitral valve repair. J Thorac Cardiovasc Surg 1991; 102-171.
30. McGoon DC. Repair of mitral insufficiency due to rupture chordae tendinae. J Thorac Cardiovasc Surg 1960; 30:357.
31. Kay JH, Egerton WS. The repair of mitral insufficiency associated with rupture of the chordae tendinae. Ann Surg 1963; 157:351.
32. Carpentier A, Relland J, Deloche A, et al. Conservative management of the prolapsed mitral valve. Ann Thorac Surg 1978; 26:294.
33. Duran CG. Repair of anterior mitral leaflet chordal rupture or elongation (the flipover technique). J Cardiac Surg 1986; 1:161.
34. Carpentier A. Valve reconstruction in predominant mitral valve incompetence. In: Duran C, Angell WW, Johnson AD, Oury JH, eds. Recent Progress in Mitral Valve Disease. London: Butterworths, 1984:265.
35. Duran CMG. Surgical management of elongated chordae of the mitral valve. J Cardiac Surg 1989; 4:253.

36. Raganathan N, Silver MD, Wigle ED. Recent advances in the knowledge of the anatomy of the mitral valve. In: Kalmanson D, ed. The Mitral Valve: A Plurdisciplinary Approach. Acton, MA: Publishing Science Group, 1976: 3.

37. Acar C, Deloche A. Anatomie et physiologie des valves mitrale et tricuspide. In: Acar J, ed. Cardiopathies valvulaires acquises. Paris: Flammarion, 1985:3.

38. Davies MJ. Aetiology and pathology of the diseased mitral valve. In: Ionescu MI, Cohn LH, eds. Mitral Valve Disease. Diagnosis and Treatment. London: Butterworths, 1985:27.

39. Raghill SC, Castra L, Niczyporuk MA, et al. Circumflex occlusion alters mitral subvalvular mechanics. Circulation 1991; 4(suppl II):44.

40. David TE. A rational approach to the surgical treatment of mitral valve disease. In: Karp RB, ed. Advances in Cardiac Surgery. Vol. 2 St. Louis, MO: Mosby Year Book, 1990:63.

41. Lillehei CW, Levy MJ, Bonnabeau RC. Mitral valve replacement with preservation of papillary muscles and chordae tendinae. J Thorac Cardiovasc Surg 1964; 47:532.

42. David TE, Burns RJ, Bacchus CM, Druck MN. Mitral valve replacement for mitral regurgitation with and without preservation of chordae tendinae. J Thorac Cardiovasc Surg 1984; 88:718.

43. Krayenbuehl HP. Surgery for mitral regurgitation. Repair versus valve replacement. Eur Heart J 1986; 7:638.

44. Yacoub M, Halim M, Radley-Smith R, McKay R, Nijveld A, Towers M. Surgical treatment of mitral regurgitation caused by floppy valves. Repair versus replacement. Circulation 1981; 64(suppl II):210.

45. Duran CG, Pomar JL, Revuelta JM, et al. Conservative operation for mitral insufficiency. Critical analysis supported by postoperative hemodynamic studies of 72 patients. J Thorac Cardiovasc Surg 1980; 79:3326.

46. Adebo OA, Ross JK. Surgical treatment of ruptured mitral valve chordae. A comparison between valve replacement and valve repair. Thorac Cardiovasc Surg 1984; 32:139.

47. Oliveira DBG, Dawkins KD, Kay PH, Paneth M. Chordal rupture II. Comparison between repair and replacement. Br Heart J 1983; 50:318.

48. Perier P, Deloche A, Chauvaud S, et al. Comparative evaluation of mitral valve repair and replacement with Starr, Bjork and porcine valve prostheses. Circulation 1984; 70(suppl I):187.

49. Sand ME, Naftel DC, Blackstone EH, Kirklin JW, Karp RB. A comparison of repair and replacement for mitral valve incompetence. J Thorac Cardiovasc Surg 1987; 94:208.

50. Galloway AC, Colvin SB, Baumann FG, Harty S, Spencer FC. Current concepts in mitral valve reconstruction for mitral insufficiency. Circulation 1988; 78:1087.

51. Craver JM, Cohen C, Weintraub WS. Case-matched comparison of mitral valve replacement and repair. Am Thorac Surg 1990; 49:964.

52. Antunes MJ, Magalhaes MP, Colsen PR, Kinsley RH. Valvuloplasty for rheumatic mitral valve disease. A surgical challenge. J Thorac Cardiovasc Surg 1987; 94:44.

53. Cosgrove DM, Chavez AM, Lytle BW, et al. Results of mitral reconstruction. Circulation 1986; 74(suppl I):82.

54. Vega JL, Fleitas M, Martinez R, et al. Open mitral commissurotomy. Ann Thorac Surg 1981; 31:266.

55. Eguaras MG, Luque I, Montero A, et al. A comparison of repair and replacement for mitral stenosis with partially calcified valves. J Thorac Cardiovasc Surg 1990; 100:161.

56. Angell WW, Oury JH, Shah P. A comparison of replacement and reconstruction in patients with mitral regurgitation. J Thorac Cardiovasc Surg 1987; 93:665.

57. Reed GE, Pooley RW, Moggio R. Durability of measured mitral annuloplasty. J Thorac Cardiovasc Surg 1980; 79:321.

58. Deloche A, Jebara VA, Relland JYM, et al. Valve repair with Carpentier techniques. The second decade. J Thorac Cardiovasc Surg 1990; 99:990.

59. Duran CG, Revuelta JM, Gaite L, Alonso C, Fleitas MG. Stability of mitral reconstructive surgery at 10–12 years with predominantly rheumatic valvular disease. Circulation 1988; 78(suppl I):91.

60. Duran CMG, Gometza B, Balasundaram S, Al Halees Z. A feasibility study of valve repair in rheumatic mitral regurgitation. Eur Heart J 1991; 12(suppl B):34.

61. Lessana A, Carbone C, Romano M, et al. Mitral valve repair. Results and the decision-making process in reconstruction. Report of 275 cases. J Thorac Cardiovasc Surg 1990; 99:622.

62. Antunes MJ, Kinsley RH. Mitral valve annuloplasty; results in an underdeveloped population. Thorax 1983; 38:730.

63. Cohn LH, Kowalker W, Bhatia S, et al. Comparative morbidity of mitral valve repair versus replacement for mitral regurgitation with and without coronary artery disease. Ann Thorac Surg 1988; 45:284.

64. Rankin JS, Feneley MP, St. Hickey M, et al. A clinical comparison of mitral valve repair versus valve replacement in ischemic mitral regurgitation. J Thorac Cardiovasc Surg 1988; 95:165.

65. Rankin JS, St. Hickey M, Smith R, et al. Ischemic mitral regurgitation. Circulation 1989; 79(suppl I):116.

66. Kay GL, Kay JH, Zubiate P, Yocoyama T, Mendez M. Mitral valve repair for mitral regurgitation secondary to coronary artery disease. Circulation 1986; 74(suppl I):88.

67. Carpentier A, Didier L, Deloche A, Perrier P. Surgical anatomy and management of ischemic mitral valve incompetence (abstr). Circulation 1987; 76(suppl IV):1776.

68. Connolly MW, Gelbfish JS, Jacobwitz IJ, et al. Surgical results for mitral regurgitation from coronary artery disease. J Thorac Cardiovasc Surg 1986; 91:379.

69. Oury JH, Cleveland JC, Angell WW, Duran CG. Ishemic mitral valve disease: classification and systematic approach to management. American Association Thoracic Surgeons Meeting, May 1991.
70. Pupello DF, Bessome LN, Blank RH, Lopez-Cuenca E, Hiro SP, Ebra G. The porcine bioprosthesis: patient age as a factor in predicting failure. In: Bodnar E, Yacoub M, eds. Biologic and Bioprosthetic Valves. New York: Yorke Med Books, 1986:130.
71. Tuffier T. Etat actuel de la chirurgie intrathoracique. SVII Internat Congress Med., Sec VII(Pt II) 1913:247.
72. Starzl TE, Cruzat EP, Walker FB, Lewis FJ. A technique for bicuspidization of the aortic valve. J Thorac Cardiovasc Surg 1959; 188:1023.
73. Taylor WJ, Thrower WB, Black H, Harken DE. The surgical correction of aortic insufficiency by circumclusion. J Thorac Cardiovasc Surg 1958; 35: 192.
74. Swanson M, Clark RE. Dimensions and geometric relationships of the human aortic valve as a function of pressure. Circ Res 1974; 35:871.
75. Chauvand S, Mihailean S, Leca F, Carpentier A. Midterm evaluation of aortic annulus contention for aortic valve insufficiency. European Association of Cardiothoracic Surgeons 4th Annual Meeting, Naples, 1990.
76. Duran CMG. Reconstructive techniques for rheumatic aortic valve disease. J Cardiac Surg 1988; 3:23.
77. Cabrol C et A, Guiraudon G, Bertrand M. Le traitment de l'insufisance aortique par l'annuloplastie aortique. Arch Mal Coeur 1966; 59:1305.
78. Duran CMG, Alonso J, Gaite L, et al. Long term results of conservative repair of rheumatic aortic valve insufficiency. Eur J Cardio-thorac Surg 1988; 2:217.
79. Cosgrove M, Rosenkranz ER, Hendren WG, Bartlett JC, Stewart WJ. Valvuloplasty for aortic insufficiency. J Thorac Cardiovasc Surg 1991; 102:571.
80. Garamella JJ, Cruz AB Jr, Heupel WH, Dahl JC, Jensen NK, Berman R. Ventricular septal defect with aortic insufficiency. Successful surgical correction of both defects by the transaortic approach. Am J Cardiol 1960; 5:266.
81. Trusler GA, Moes CA, Kidd BS. Repair of ventricular septal defect with aortic insufficiency. J Thorac Cardiovasc Surg 1973; 66:394.
82. Shapira N, Fernandez J, McNicholas KW, et al. Hypertrophy of nodules of Arantius and aortic insufficiency: pathophysiology and repair. Ann Thor Surg 1991; 51:969.
83. Duran CMG, Balasundaram S, Bianchi S, Ahmad R, Wilson N. Hemodynamic effect of supraaortic ridge enchancement on the closure mechanism of the aortic valve and its implication in aortic valve repair. Thorac Cardiovasc Surg 1990; 38:6.
84. Batista RJV, Dobrianskij A, Comazzi M, et al. Clinical experience with stentless pericardial monopatch for aortic valve replacement. J Thorac Cardiovasc Surg 1987; 93:19.

85. Bjork VO, Hultquist G. Teflon and pericardial aortic valve prosthesis. J Thorac Cardiovasc Surg 1964: 47:693.

86. Bailey CP. In: Discussion of Senning A. Fascia lata replacement of aortic valves. J Thorac Cardiovasc Surg 1967; 54:486.

87. Kay EB. In: Discussion of Senning A. Fascia lata replacement of aortic valves. J Thorac Cardiovasc Surg 1967; 54:489.

88. Bahnson HT, Hardesty RL, Baker LD Jr, Brooks D II, Gall DA. Fabrication and evaluation of tissue leaflets for aortic and mitral valve replacement. Ann Surg 1970; 171:939.

89. Edwards WS. Aortic valve replacement with autogenous tissue. Ann Thorac Surg 1969; 8:126.

90. Senning A. Fascia lata replacement of aortic valves. J Thorac Cardiovasc Surg 1967; 54:465.

91. Batista RJV. In: Discussion of David TE, Pallick C, Boss J. Aortic valve replacement with stentless porcine aortic bioprosthesis. J Thorac Cardiovasc Surg 1990; 99:113.

92. Yacoub M, Khaghani A, Dhalla N, et al. Aortic valve replacement using unstented dura or calf pericardium: early and long term results. In: Bodnar E, Yacoub M, eds. Biologic and Bioprosthetic Valves. New York: Yorke Medical Books, 1986; 684.

93. Duran CG. Tissue valves. In: Yacoub M, ed. Current Opinion in Cardiology. London: Gower Academic Journals, 1986:69.

94. Odell JA, Gillmer D, Whitton ID, Vythilingum SP, Vanker EA. Calcification of tissue valves in children: occurrence in porcine and pericardial bioprosthetic valves. In: Bodnar E, Yacoub M, eds. Biological and Bioprosthetic Valves. New York: Yorke Medical Books, 1986:259.

95. Angell WW, Oury JH, Lamberti JJ, et al. Durability of the viable aortic allograft. J Thorac Cardiovasc Surg 1989; 98:48.

96. Chachques JC, Vasseur B, Perrier P, et al. A rapid method to stabilize biological materials for cardiovascular surgery. Ann NY Acad Sci 1988; 529:184.

97. Duran CMG, Kumar N, Gometza B, Halees Z. Indications and limitations of aortic valve reconstruction. Ann Thorac Surg 1991; 52:447.

98. Cohen SR, Sell JE, McIntosh CL, et al. Tricuspid regurgitation in patients with acquired, chronic, pure mitral regurgitation. Prevalence, diagnosis and comparison of preoperative clinical and hemodynamic features in patients with and without tricuspid regurgitation. J Thorac Cardiovasc Surg 1987; 94:481.

99. Bailey ChP. Tricuspid stenosis. In: Bailey CP, ed. Surgery of the Heart, Philadelphia: Lea & Febiger, 1955:846.

100. Revuelta JM, Garcia R, Duran CMG. Tricuspid commissurotomy. Ann Thorac Surg 1985; 39:489.

101. Kay JH, Maselli-Campagna G, Isuji KK. Surgical treatment of tricuspid insufficiency. Ann Surg 1965; 162:53.

102. Pluth JR, Ellis FH Jr. Tricuspid insufficiency in patients undergoing mitral replacement. Conservative management, annuloplasty or replacement. J Thorac Cardiovasc Surg 1969; 58:484.
103. Cabrol C. L'annuloplastie valvulaire. Un nouveau procede. Nouv Pres Med 1972; 1:1366.
104. DeVega N. La anuloplastia selectiva, regulable y permanente. Una technica original para el tratamiento de la insuficiencia tricuspide. Rev Esp Cardiol 1972; 25:555.
105. Kirklin JW. Mitral valve disease with or without tricuspid valve disease. In: Kirklin JW, Barratt-Boyes BG, eds. Cardiac Surgery. Morphology, Diagnostic Criteria, Natural History, Techniques, Results and Indications. New York: Wiley, 1986:323.
106. Chopra HK, Nanda NC, Fan P, et al. Can two-dimensional echocardiography and Doppler color flow mapping identify the need for tricuspid valve repair? J Am Coll Cardiol 1989; 14:1266.
107. Fawzy ME, Mercer EN, Dunn B, Amri M Al, Andaya W. Doppler echocardiography in the evaluation of tricuspid stenosis. Eur Heart J 1989; 10:985.
108. Duran CMG, Pomar JL, Colman T, Figueroa A, Revuelta JM, Ubago JL. Is tricuspid valve repair necessary? J Thorac Cardiovasc Surg 1980; 80:849.
109. Chidambaram M, Abdulali JA, Bahiga G, Ionescu MI. Long term results of DeVega tricuspid annuloplasty. Ann Thorac Surg 1987; 43:185.
110. De Paulis R, Bobbio M, Ottino G, et al. The DeVega tricuspid annuloplasty. Preoperative mortality and long term follow-up. J Cardiovasc Surg 1990; 31:512.
111. Haerten K, Seipel L, Loogen F, Herzer J. Haemodynamic studies after DeVega's tricuspid annuloplasty. Circulation 1978; 58(suppl I):28.
112. Hatle L, Angelsen B. Pulsed and Continuous wave Doppler in diagnosis and assessment of various heart lesions. In: Hatle L, Angleson B, eds. Doppler Ultrasound in Cardiology. Physical Principles and Clinical Applications. 2nd ed. Philadelphia: Lea & Febiger, 1985: 97.
113. Hanania G, Sellier P, Deloche A, et al. Resultats a moyen terme de l'annuloplastie tricuspide reconstructitutive de Carpentier. A propos de 25 cas avec catheterisme postoperatoire. Arch Mal Coeur 1974; 67:895.
114. Lambertz H, Minale C, Flachskampf FA, et al. Long-term follow-up after Carpentier tricuspid valvuloplasty. Am Heart J 1989; 117:615.
115. Thorburn CW, Morgan JJ, Shanahan MX, Chang VP. Long-term results of tricuspid valve replacement and the problem of prosthetic valve thrombosis. Am J Cardiol 1983; 51:1128.

19

Prosthetic Valve Replacement

Mario Albertucci
Albany Medical College, Albany, New York

Robert B. Karp
University of Chicago Hospitals, Chicago, Illinois

I. HISTORICAL DEVELOPMENT

In the late 1950s and early 1960s pioneers of cardiac valve implantation developed and used three distinct types of prosthetic valves. Mechanical valves made entirely of synthetic material were developed and implanted in the orthotopic position by Harken and by Starr in 1960 (1,2). Between 1962 and 1965, clinical experience with homograft aortic valves was established independently by Ross in England and by Barratt-Boyes in New Zealand (3,4). In 1965 Binet and Carpentier implanted the first unstented, formaldehyde-preserved porcine xenograft (5). Subsequently, Carpentier developed the new glutaraldehyde-treated porcine xenograft (6). Despite enormous progress in valve design and characteristics, the ideal valve is still to be developed, and what Harken defined as the 10 characteristics of ideal valve replacement still remain elusive (Table 1) (7).

II. MECHANICAL VALVES

A. Caged-Ball Valve Design

In the 20 years following its introduction, the Starr-Edwards (S-E) type of prosthesis has attained widespread use. The prosthesis is durable, resists thrombosis, and is relatively easy to implant. There is no design-related regurgitation and, in general, the hemodynamic performance is adequate. There are some drawbacks associated with this type of prosthesis:

Table 1   Characteristics of the Ideal Valve Replacement

1. It must not propagate emboli
2. It must be chemically inert and not damage blood elements.
3. It must offer no resistance to physiological flows.
4. It must close promptly (less than 0.05 s).
5. It must remain closed during the appropriate phase of the cardiac cycle.
6. It must have lasting physical and geometric features.
7. It must be inserted in a physiological site (generally the normal anatomical site).
8. It must be capable of permanent fixation.
9. It must not annoy the patient.
10. It must be technically practical to insert.

Source: From Ref. 7.

1. The high cage profile may abut the intraventricular septum in patients with small left ventricular outflow tract, perhaps causing left ventricular outflow tract obstruction or leading to arrhythmias.
2. There is a relatively small secondary orifice in patients with small aortas, the resultant crowding leading to outflow gradients.
3. In small sizes, the prosthesis is somewhat obstructive.
4. There remains an important embolization rate.
5. There is hemolysis in some patients.

Modifications to the original caged-ball design were attempted in order to correct some of these problems. The Smeloff-Cutter offered longer ball travel distance and a smaller poppet to increase effective orifice. Cloth-covered struts were suggested by Braunwald et al. (8) to decrease thromboembolism and diminish poppet wear. Despite these modifications, the most successful and durable design proved to be the simple Silastic ball valve with bare struts and Teflon sewing ring, which was developed in 1967 and continues to enjoy some popularity today.

B. Tilting-Disk Design

The introduction of the concept of hingeless, freely floating, durable disk that could pivot into the open position characterized the era of tilting-disk valve design. In the late 1960s, Lillehei-Kaster (L-K) and Bjork-Shiley (B-S) valves were introduced with the intent of reducing the transvalvular gradient, particularly in small-sized prostheses, and reducing the thromboembolic rate. Extensive research to improve the Lillehei-Kaster valve culminated in the Omniscience I valve. The disk diameter-to-tissue annulus diameter ratio was increased. There was reduced disk wear, presumably by optimizing disk curvature to pivot axis eccentricity with an opening angle of 80°. Further improvements were introduced in 1981 with a thicker Teflon sewing ring and the recommendation that anterior orientation of the larger orifice was necessary in the mitral position to avoid interference between the disk and the posterior structures. The latest model of this valve is the Omnicarbon, which features a change in the housing material from titanium to pyrolyte carbon in an attempt to further decrease thromboembolism.

The Bjork-Shiley valve has been a very effective prosthesis over the years. As a tilting-disk device, it is characterized by good hemodynamics, low hemolysis, low profile, and relatively low rate of thromboembolism. The earlier models of the Bjork-Shiley were plagued with a high (3.25%) (9) rate of valve thrombosis in mitral position. This was probably due to an area of stasis behind the valve (the lesser orifice). The 60° convexo-concave model was developed to prevent this problem by permitting the disk to slide out 2.5 mm from the ring in open position. The low-flow area was reduced by 50%, resulting in a decrease in valve thrombosis in the first year to 0.28%.

However, in this 60° convexo-concave model, there was a major manufacturing flaw, resulting in the problem of strut fracture and poppet escape. Recommendations for managing patients with 60° Bjork-Shiley valves have been published by Hiratzka et al. (10). Their conclusions and those of others are that risk of prophylactic re-replacement continues to exceed the risk of fatal strut fracture.

To correct the problem of strut fracture, the 70° Convexo-Concave prosthesis was developed. This model further improved the valve hemodynamic performance but did not correct completely the problem of strut fracture. The 70° CC was not used in the United States and was withdrawn from the market in 1983.

The Monostrut 70° convexo-concave valve was introduced in 1982. Structural failure of this valve has not been reported. The Monstrut valve is not yet approved for clinical use in the United States, but has excellent hemodynamic characteristics and low rates of thromboembolism (9).

Hall of Norway attempted to improve the characteristics of the tilting-disk valve by:

1. Moving the disk pivot centrally to enlarge the minor orifice and avoid stasis and thrombosis
2. Introducing a sliding motion of the doughnut-shaped disk away from the tapered guide rod housing in full opening to wash away any potential platelet aggregates on the disk or struts

3. Combining a pyrolyte disk with a titanium housing incorporating no welds to enhance durability
4. Using a Teflon sewing ring to reduce fibrous overgrowth or pannus formation at the sewing ring–valve interface
5. Using a nonocclusive, nonoverlapping disk to allow for maximum orifice area

The maximum opening angle is 75° in aortic and 70° in mitral position. This valve is marketed as the Medtronic-Hall (M-H) and has not undergone any structural design modification since clinical implantation began in 1977.

C. Bileaflet Valves

In 1976 prototypes of the St. Jude Medical (SJM) valve were developed with the objective of providing a central-flow, all-pyrolytic-carbon, bileaflet valve. Each leaflet opens to an 85° maximum. In the closed position, the valve leaflet resides at a 25–30° angle. The sewing cuff is a double-velour Dacron. The SJM valve was first implanted in 1977 and since then has undergone no design modification. Leaflet escape has been reported in 10 patients out of 320,000 implants in 13 years. Eighty-two intraoperative leaflet breakage or dislodgements have been reported (11). In 5 of the 10 reported leaflet escape instances, damage to the leaflet was documented, possibly relating to intraoperative trauma. These observations underscore the importance of extreme care in handling the prostheses during implantation.

Two additional bileaflet valves have been developed. The Duromedics-Edwards is an all-carbon valve with leaflet opening angles of 73° and closing angles of 2°. The leaflets are curved rather than flat and thicker than SJM leaflets. The Duromedics valve was withdrawn from the market after 12 leaflet escapes were reported in 20,000 implants. The Carbomedics valve offers a rotatable valve housing with a carbon-coated Dacron sewing ring conceived to reduce tissue ingrowth and pannus formation. The opening angle of the leaflet is 78° and the closing angle is 25°. Implantation began in 1986 and approximately 25,000 implants have been reported outside the United States. Only limited information is available on this valve.

The SJM valve remains the prosthetic valve most often selected in North America. Its hemodynamic performance has been validated in vitro and in vivo. It is durable, quiet, and has an acceptably low rate of thromboembolism.

III. TISSUE VALVES

A. Porcine Xenograft

Two porcine xenograft prostheses are available: the Carpentier-Edwards (C-E) and the Hancock. The Edwards Laboratories valve utilizes 0.625% glutaraldehyde in phosphate-buffered saline at pH 7.4 to sterilize and treat the porcine aortic valves. The strut is totally flexible and made from Elgiloy, a corrosive-resistant alloy of cobalt and nickel. The flexibility of the frame allows the orifice of the bioprosthesis some movement which resembles the natural valve annulus. Because of this flexibility, it is important to avoid distortion at the time of implantation. The ring is not circular but asymmetric, to provide additional support to the right coronary cusp. The asymmetry also allows the use of larger porcine valves by incorporating the muscular portion of the porcine valve in the sewing ring rather than occupying part of the primary orifice. The current models of CE aortic and atrioventricular valves differ in the shapes of their sewing rings, but each includes a silicone sponge rubber insert to enhance coaptation to the patient's valve annulus.

The Hancock Laboratories valve utilizes cold balanced electrolyte solution to store the valve after procurement. The valve is then immersed in 0.2% glutaraldehyde. A pressurized system holds the leaflets in their normal position during the tanning process. The valve is then sutured to a symmetrical, semiflexible strut which contains a silicone rubber insert. The aortic and atrioventricular valves differ only in the shape of their sewing margins. Because of the asymmetry of the porcine bioprosthesis due to the intimate attachment of the right coronary cusp to the septal myocardium, Hancock Laboratories has developed a so-called modified orifice valve. This is accomplished by excising only the muscle-based right coronary leaflet and replacing it with a cusp from another valve, resulting in the modified orifice valve.

The porcine grafts were a major improvement in valve replacement surgery. For the most part, long-term anticoagulation is not necessary. We give patients with the mitral bioprosthesis 6 weeks of coumadin anticoagulation. Aortic replacements receive no anticoagulation. The rate of thromboembolism in porcine bioprosthesis patients not anticoagulated is similar to that seen in mechanical prosthesis patients who are anticoagulated (12) (Table 2). The hemodynamic performance of the porcine valves is satisfactory. The major drawback to porcine bioprostheses is tissue degeneration. That flaw in durability is most apparent in younger subjects (13) (Table 3).

Table 2 Thromboembolism Rates for Mitral and Aortic Valve Replacement:
Literature Review, 1983–1987

Type	Model	Patient years	TE rate
	Mitral Valve Replacement		
Mechanical	Starr-Edwards	19,949	4.4
	Bjork-Shiley	6,188	3.3
	St. Jude	4,104	1.5
	Medtronic Hall	4,053	2.6
	Omniscience	1,017	2.8
Tissue	Carpentier	3,368	2.0
	Hancock	4,831	2.4
	Ionescu	3,702	1.8
	Aortic Valve Replacement		
Mechanical	Starr-Edwards	21,780	2.3
	Bjork-Shiley	7,753	1.9
	St. Jude	5,418	1.4
	Medtronic Hall	6,570	1.8
	Omniscience	753	2.7
Tissue	Carpentier	3,513	1.4
	Hancock	1,890	1.0
	Ionescu	9,296	0.8

Source: Modified from Ref. 12.

Table 3 Age Versus Incidence of Bioprosthesis Degeneration (B.D.) (Percent
Freedom from B.D. at 10 years)[a]

	≤ 40	41–69	≥ 70	P value
AVR	68 ± 9	86 ± 2	94 ± 3	(p = 0.001)
MVR	68 ± 10	84 ± 3	84 ± 3	(p = NS)
DVR	89 ± 10	87 ± 5	100	(p = NS)
All	69 ± 7	85 ± 2	92 ± 3	(p = 0.001)

[a] AVR = aortic valve replacement; MVR = mitral valve replacement; DVR = double valve
replacement.
Source: From Ref. 13 Used with permission of L. H. Cohn.

B. Pericardial Bioprosthesis

Two pericardial valves have been marketed, the Ionescu-Shiley and the Edwards. Each uses glutaraldehyde-treated bovine pericardium, prepared in slightly different configuration. The most attractive characteristic of these bioprostheses is the excellent orifice-to-annulus ratio. However, tissue degeneration is a major concern, and the Ionescu-Shiley has recently been withdrawn from the market due to poor durability.

IV. HOMOGRAFTS

In the early 1960s, homografts were taken under sterile conditions soon after death of the donor and stored at 4°C in Hank's balanced salt solution for 1 to 25 days. Early results reported by Barratt-Boyes were encouraging, showing no incidence of thromboembolism in 8 of 12 functioning homografts during a 12-year period. Transvalvular gradient was trivial. Difficulties of retrieving and storing prompted development of new techniques by which valves were harvested unsterilely, sterilized with either beta-propiolactone or ethylene oxide, and stored in Hank's solution at 4°C or by freeze-drying. Irradiation followed by nitrogen freezing was also used for sterilization and storage. Results with those techniques were disappointing. Although function was excellent for up to 4 years postimplant, there was an intermediate-term and long-term failure rate estimated at 10% at 5 years and 35% at 10 years. The mode of failure was cusp rupture and calcification. Barratt-Boyes and others introduced antibiotic sterilization and cold storage. Valves removed from cadavers unsterilely within 48 hours of death were processed in antibiotic solutions enriched with tissue culture medium. They were stored in tissue culture medium at 4°C until implantation.

Presently there are good data to suggest that the "fresh" or antibiotic-refrigerated state can be reproduced by cryopreservation. Cadaver valves are removed sterilely, processed in antibiotics, and then subjected to cryopreservation at −1°C/min to −140°C. Protection during freezing is provided by the controlled rate and cryoprotectant (DMSO or glycerol) (14). Cryopreserved homografts may remain viable and can be stored 5 years or so (15).

V. SURGICAL TECHNIQUE

A. Thoracic Incision

For successful valve surgery, adequate exposure is mandatory. Median sternotomy leads to optimal exposure of the heart and unobstructed view of all pericardial structures. Cannulation is easy, and multiple alternative modalities of myocardial protection are available. Venting and de-airing are optimally done through this approach. Approach to the aortic, tricuspid, and pulmonary valves is straightforward, but exposure of the mitral valve can occasionally be difficult. Right thoracotomy, either anterior or posterolateral, offers an excellent view of the mitral (and tricuspid) valves, but the rest of the heart is relatively inaccessible. Cannulation through the groin is often necessary, and de-airing and venting is difficult. Myocardial protection may be cumbersome. Despite definite disadvantages, this approach can be very helpful in difficult situations such as mitral valve operations in patients with patent coronary artery bypasses.

B. Perfusion Cannula Sites

The ascending aorta is the most convenient cannulation site. In the presence of severe calcification or aneurysmal disease of the ascending aorta, femoral or iliac, cannulation is necessary. Surgeons should position the aortic cannula in such a way as to avoid a sandblast effect or a Coanda phenomenon. The beveled cannula tip should point downstream of the head vessels.

C. Venous Drainage Cannula and Sites

The two-stage right atrial cannula is suited for most aortic procedures. When extensive manipulation of the heart is needed, for exposure in mitral valve operations, or opening of the right atrium is planned, cannulation of the superior and inferior vena cavae is necessary.

D. Left Ventricular Venting

A venting line has several functions during valve operation:

1. Decompression of the left side of the heart during arrest time
2. Removal of blood to allow a clear operative field
3. Maintenance of lower myocardial temperature by removing the warmer blood returning to the heart

A venting line can be inserted via the ventricular apex, but problems may occur in obtaining a secure closure at the venting site. The right superior pulmonary vein is adequately accessible and safer, and more secure closure can be accomplished. The left atrial appendage or pulmonary artery can also be used for the venting site.

E. Myocardial Protection

Several techniques of myocardial protection are available to allow flexibility in myocardial management:

1. Coronary perfusion without aortic cross-clamping offers good protection when operating on the tricuspid, pulmonary, or mitral valves, particularly when the latter is approached through a right thoracotomy incision.
2. The most common technique employs myocardial cooling with cardioplegic arrest. Blood and various concentrations of substances are infused intermittently in the aortic root or directly in the coronary ostia (in aortic valve surgery).
3. Retrograde coronary sinus cardioplegia infusion offers equally good protection as antegrade infusion and has a distinct advantage in aortic valve surgery.

F. Aortic Incision

Transverse, longitudinal, or "hockey stick" incisions can be employed to expose the aortic valve. Transverse incision can be useful at times in small aortas but limits the options for root enlargement. The "hockey stick" incision offers excellent exposure and allows flexibility in case of need for root enlargement. Longitudinal incision can be useful in large aortas or when aorto-ventriculo-septoplasty is anticipated.

G. Atrial Incision

Incision of the left atrium posterior to the interatrial groove and anterior to the right pulmonary veins offer good exposure of the mitral valve and is adequate in most situations. Attention especially to the sinus node artery is important. The incision through the interatrial septum introduced by Dubost et al. (16) is particularly useful in reoperation and in patients with a small left atrium. This approach is also useful if combined mitral and tricuspid valve operation is necessary. Incisions through the roof of the left atrium between the superior vena cava and the aorta are used by some, but closure must be precise. Standard oblique right atriotomy is adequate for the vast majority of operations on the tricuspid valve.

H. Excision of the Valves and Preparation of the Annulus

Several principles are important to obtain good reproducible results.

1. Aortic Valve

1. The diseased valve must be completely excised, leaving only 1 or 2 mm of annular tissue as a sewing cuff.

2. The annulus must be pliable. Calcifications must be removed gently. We prefer removal of calcification with forceps and not with Rongeurs.
3. Careful irrigation with saline is done before implanting the valve to remove loose debris.

2. Mitral Valve

1. A generous cuff of mitral valve can be left in place, particularly in the vicinity of the intraventricular septum and the posterior leaflet.
2. When removing the posterior leaflet and the chordal attachment, it is important not to transect the papillary muscle too widely so as not to weaken the posterior ventricular wall.
3. Chordal attachment should be removed completely, particularly when using tilting-disk valves. Loose chordae can potentially entangle the prosthetic valve mechanism.
4. Conservation of the mitral tensor apparatus may result in improved left ventricular function postoperatively (17). Most low profile mechanical and bioprosthetic valves can be inserted leaving at least the posterior leaflet and chordae. Special techniques are indicated when saving the anterior leaflet (18).

I. De-airing

Air can become entrapped in the left ventricle, particularly at the apex and under the mitral value, in the left atrium and appendage, and in the pulmonary veins. A systematic approach to ridding the heart of air is very important to prevent significant morbidity in an otherwise successful operation.

With the patient in Trendelenburg position:

1. Aortic root venting is used to remove air while the heart starts to fill. Temporary occlusion of the right coronary artery will prevent air embolism in right coronary distribution. This vent line suction is increased as the heart ejection becomes more effective.
2. If mitral valve operation has been done, the left atrial incision is left partially open to allow blood to escape freely. The incision is closed before the heart is ejecting and before strong suction is applied to the aortic vent line, since this can actually create negative pressure and aspirate air into the heart.
3. Allow blood to circulate through the right ventricle, pulmonary arteries, and veins by inflating the lung.

4. Elevate the ventricular apex (except in mitral valve replacement operations) and invert the left atrial appendage.
5. Fill the heart by decreasing the venous return to dislodge the residual air before discontinuing CPB. If it is available, TEE is useful intraoperatively to assess the adequateness of de-airing.
6. Needle aspiration of the left ventricle and left atrium during progressive manipulation of central blood volume is also effective.
7. Above all, vigorous contraction of the heart is the most important element to adequate clearance of intracardiac air.

VI. TECHNIQUES OF OPERATION

A. Mitral Valve Replacement

The continuous suture technique is used for primary replacement when a mechanical valve is indicated. Because manipulation of the bioprosthesis during insertion may damage the tissue valve, we prefer interrupted sutures in those cases. Also, the bulkier configuration of the tissue prosthesis makes the continuous suture technique more difficult. Interrupted suture technique is also used for secondary replacements, or when a "soft annulus" is present, as in mitral valve replacement for idiopathic hypertrophic subaortic stenosis. Sizing the annulus is done more accurately by eye rather than with a sizer, which can distort the anatomy.

1. Continuous Suture Technique (Fig. 1)

A double-armed 0 polypropylene pledgetted than mattress suture is started at the level of the anterolateral commissure (9 o'clock position). The suture is then passed through the valve sewing ring, and the valve without the holder is lowered in place. The suture line is continued first superiorly up to the midpoint of the anterior leaflet, then inferiorly down to the midpoint of the posterior leaflet. A similar double-armed 0 polypropylene pledgetted mattress suture is started at the level of the posteromedial commissure (3 o'clock position) and carried out superiorly and inferiorly last. About three throws for each quadrant are necessary. The sutures are tied behind the pillar guards of the SJM valve.

2. Interrupted Suture Technique (Fig. 2)

Zero Tycron pledgetted sutures are used. The first suture is placed at the posteromedial commissure. Only one-half of the mattress suture is placed, as this is used as a reference suture to facilitate equal placement of the sutures around the annulus. The second suture is a full mattress placed at the anterolateral commissure with the pledgets on the atrial side. All the other posterior-row sutures are then placed (usually six sutures are

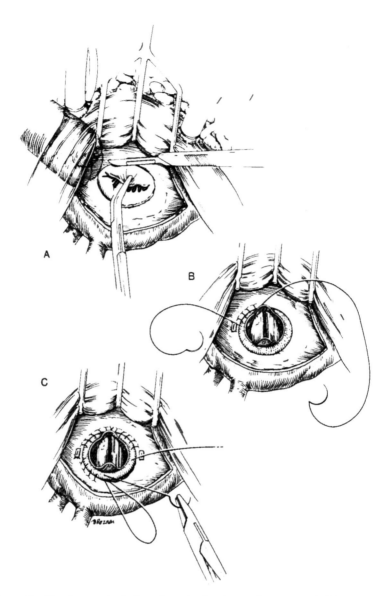

Figure 1 Continuous technique for mitral valve replacement. A. The excision of the valve is facilitated by applying traction to the anterior leaflet. A knife incision in the midportion of the leaflet allows precise initiation of the excision, which is usually completed by scissors. Position of the aorta, circumflex coronary artery, and conduction system should always be kept in mind. B. A 0-polypropylene double-armed pledgetted mattress suture is started in the anterolateral commissure. The valve without the holder is lowered in place at this point. C. The second 0-polypropylene pledgetted mattressed suture is started at the posteromedial commissure. The two suture lines meet at one-half the distance in the anterior and posterior leaflet. The sutures are tied behind the pillar guard of the SJM prosthesis.

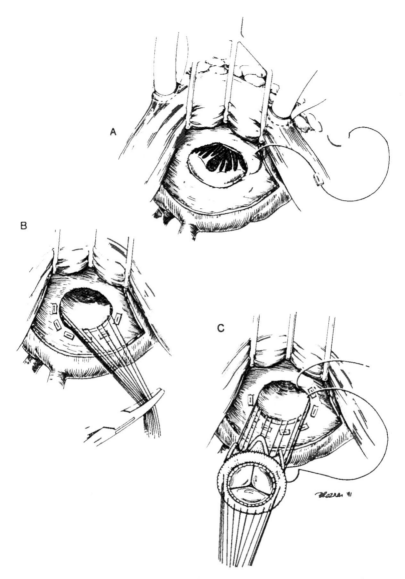

Figure 2 Interrupted technique for mitral valve replacement. A. The first suture is one-half mattress placed at the posteromedial commissure and serves as a reference point. B. Starting with the suture at the anterolateral commissure, the posterior row is placed through the annulus before insertion into the prosthetic sewing ring. C. The anterior row is completed placing the sutures through the annulus and then directly through the prosthesis's sewing ring.

necessary) in the annulus before placing in the valve sewing ring. The second half of the reference suture at the posteromedial commissure is placed and the anterior row is then completed. Here the sutures are placed directly in the valve sewing ring, held at distance by an assistant. The valve is then lowered in place. The pillars of the bioprosthesis are positioned in the ventricle so as not to create left ventricular outflow destruction.

B. Aortic Valve Replacement

The interrupted and continuous suture techniques apply equally well to both mechanical valves and bioprostheses. If the annulus is calcified or quite dilated, the interrupted technique is preferred. For routine valve replacement, continuous suture technique is selected. It is important to size the prosthesis moderately conservatively so as to avoid too large a prosthesis, which can lead to hemorrhage.

1. Interrupted Suture Technique (Fig. 3)

Two-0 pledgetted Tycron mattress sutures are used. The pledgets are placed on the aortic side and the first suture is started at the left coronary–right coronary commissure. The annulus is divided in thirds, and about four mattress sutures are placed for each third. The valve is held at about 15 cm distance, and the sutures are placed directly in its sewing ring. After all sutures are placed, the valve is lowered in place and the sutures are tied in the same order as they were placed. The valve is then inspected for proper function and fit.

2. Continuous Suture Technique (Fig. 4)

Three 2-0 double-armed pledgetted polypropylene sutures are used. One suture is started at each sinus between the residual commissures. The prosthetic valve is held at distance, and the continuous suture line is started with sutures as the midpoint of the base of the right coronary sinus and carried on toward the commissure between the right and left sinuses and then toward the right noncoronary commissure. The same process is repeated for the other thirds of the annulus, each double-armed suture beginning at the midpoint of the sinus. When all sutures are placed, the prosthesis is lowered into place. A blunt nerve hook is used to tighten the polypropylene suture throws to secure the valve in the annulus, and the sutures are then tied. After the valve is inspected for proper function and for fit, the operation is completed as described previously.

C. Enlargement of Aortic Root (Fig. 5)

Several options exist when faced with a small aortic root and need for aortic valve replacement. In the elderly population, simple decalcification

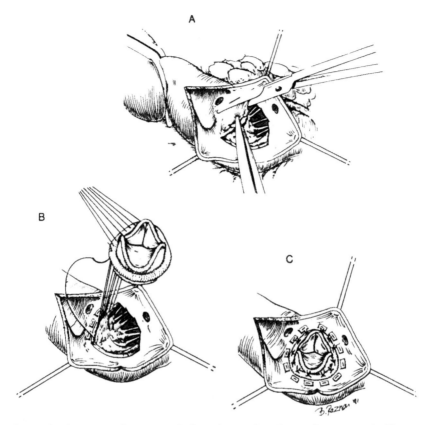

Figure 3 Interrupted suture technique for aortic valve replacement. A. The aortic valve is excised, leaving 1 or 2 mm of annular tissue as a sewing cuff. B. Pledgetted Tycron mattress sutures (2-0) are placed with the pledget on the aortic side. Sutures are placed in the aortic ring and passed directly onto the prosthetic valve sewing ring held at distance. C. After all sutures are placed, the valve is lowered in place and the sutures tied. The valve is then inspected for proper function and fit.

with CUSA has given us satisfying results (19). Alternatively, if a number 19 or larger size can be accommodated in the annulus, an SJM valve is selected for replacement because of the good orifice-to-annulus ratio. When the annulus is smaller than size 19, then an annular-enlarging approach should be selected. The Nicks technique (20) allows enlargement of about 2–3 mm annulus diameter and employs an incision carried through the middle of the noncoronary sinus. The reconstruction uses a

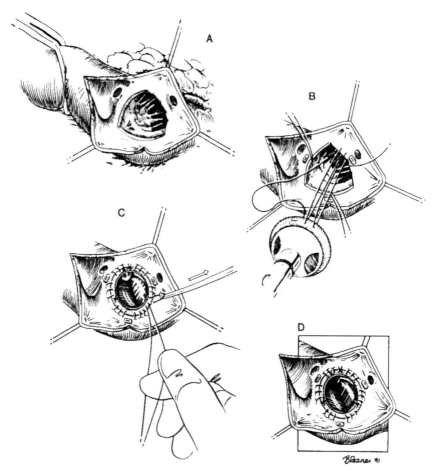

Figure 4 Continuous suture technique for aortic valve replacement. A. The native aortic valve is excised, with attention paid to removing calcific deposits on the annulus so that pliable tissue is left for appropriate placement of the sutures. B. Double-armed pledgetted sutures (2-0 polypropylene) are placed in the middle of each sinus of Valsalva. The sutures are started at the right coronary sinus. The sutures are passed directly into the prosthetic valve sewing ring held at distance. C. After all sutures are placed, the valve is lowered in place. A blunt nerve hook is used to tighten the suture line and secure the valve in place. D. The sutures are then tied and the valve is inspected for proper function and fit.

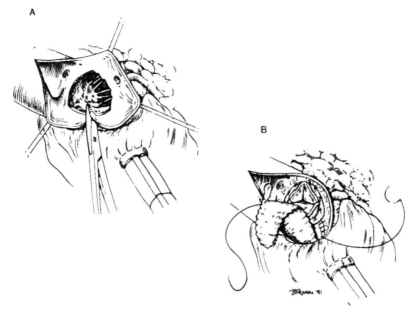

Figure 5   Enlargement of the aortic root. A. The "hockey stick" incision is carried out in the middle of the noncoronary sinus. Usually, division of the anterior leaflet of the mitral valve is not necessary. B. The valve is secured in place with the pledgets sutured at the site of the patch passed from the outside. A continuous suture line anchors the patch to the edges of the aortotomy.

Dacron or pericardial patch to which part of the sewing ring is attached. The Manougian approach (21) allows enlargement of 1½ to 2 valve sizes, and employs an incision carried exactly in the middle of the noncoronary–left coronary commissure. The incision may be carried onto the roof of the left atrium and to the anterior leaflet of the mitral valve. Repair is completed by sewing a Dacron or pericardial patch to the edges of the resulting defect. In both Nicks and Monougian techniques, the pledgetted sutures at the site of the enlargement are passed from outside the patch to inside the lumen of the aorta and then through the prosthesis's sewing ring so that the pledgets are outside the aortic wall. In situations such as a very small aortic root, or in young patients, aortic root replacement using a homograft is indicated. We prefer to a technique similar to the one popularized by Donaldson & Ross (22), which employs interrupted 4-0 polypropylene and sutures and a Teflon felt gasket for the upstream (root) anastomosis. The distal anastomosis is done with running 4-0 polypropylene sutures. Then the coronary arteries are reimplanted with a cuff of aortic wall of about 4–5 mm left around each coronary button, using 5-0 polypropylene

D. Aortic Homograft

The aortic ring is measured with a prosthetic valve sizer. It may not be until this point that the appropriate aortic valve allograft can be delivered from the nitrogen freezer. However, we now employ preoperative sizing utilizing expert transthoracic echocardiography. The allograft has been sized using a Hegar dilator. The size as measured corresponds to the internal orifice of the aortic valve allograft. The appropriate dimension, therefore, for the valve allograft will be 2 or 3 mm smaller than the measured internal annulus diameter of the aortic root. The graft is delivered to the operating room and the surgeon begins the rinsing and thawing process. The valve is then trimmed to debulk the tissue, leaving appropriate support for suturing and for commissural attachment to the valve cusps. The muscle at the base of the donor left ventricle and ventricular septum is trimmed from the allograft aortic ring (Fig. 6). Care must be taken not to buttonhole the aortic wall, particularly in the area of attachment of the anterior leaflet of the mitral valve or in the area of the membranous ventricular septum. The anterior mitral leaflet is trimmed and short-

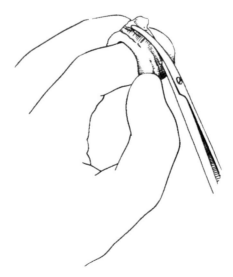

Figure 6   The allograft is trimmed by removing the ventricular muscle and mitral leaflet.

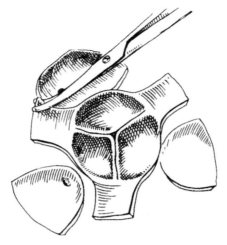

Figure 7   The coronary and noncoronary sinuses are resected, leaving appropriate tissue for suturing of the commissural pillars.

ened, and the ventricular muscle is smoothed using a scissor. Finally, the tubular portion of the ascending aorta is transected and the sinus portions removed so as to leave three columns of aorta supporting the commissures of the aortic cusp (Fig. 7). The valve is sutured in place using two rows (upstream and downstream) of continuous sutures of 4-0 polypropylene.

For the small aortic root, interrupted technique with the valve held at distance is preferred; otherwise, a continuous suture is used. The aortic allograft is rotated 120° counterclockwise for its insertion, so that the remaining muscle on the graft does not appose the ventricular septal muscle of the recipient. The first row of sutures is placed upstream of the aortic ring. This places the bulky portion of the graft upstream (away from) to the narrowest portion of the left ventricular outflow tract; thus, the base of the aortic cusps of the graft lies in the same horizontal plane as did the native aortic valve. To accomplish this suture line, three sutures are placed 120° apart and started in a position midway between the commissural pillars of the graft. The graft at this time is held at distance with a noncrushing vascular clamp (Fig. 8). The graft is then delivered into the aortic root and inverted within itself. The continuous suture line is placed such that the upstream edge of the valve is below the aortic ring. This suture should be made with an effort to place the needle parallel to the long axis of the left ventricular outflow tract. In the area of the membranous ventricular septum, the suture can be slightly more downstream and more superficial to avoid the conduction system (Fig. 9). When this upstream

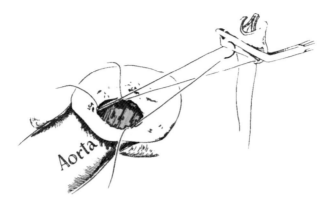

Figure 8 The graft is rotated 120° counterclockwise so that residual allograft muscle does not abut outflow tract muscle, and the three stay sutures are placed into the graft.

suture line is completed, two of the three commissural pillars are everted and positioned against the old commissural attachment of the native valve. It is crucial that the commissural pillar not be placed on tension and that the suture line be allowed to sink into the bulbous sinus portion of the aortic root. A double-armed suture is used, placing the initial suture in

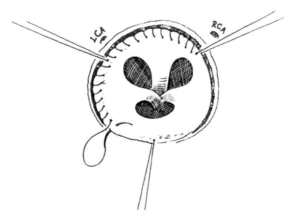

Figure 9 The graft is delivered into the aortic root and inverted within itself. The upstream continuous suture line is completed.

the midpoint of the sinus and keeping the suture line, for the first few bites, very close to the native valve annulus. The suturing is done in such a way that this downstream suture line has a U-shaped (rather than a V-shaped) configuration as it moves up and out of the sinus of Valsalva, positioning the commissural pillars against the aortic wall. The suture ends are tied to one another at the top of the commissural pillars (Fig. 10). An alternative technique can be used to secure the aortotomy closure, that

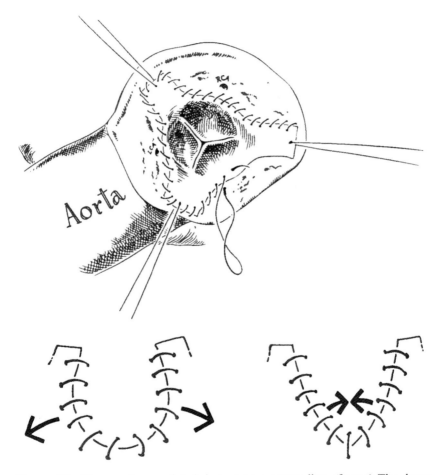

Figure 10 The nearly completed downstream suture line. (Insert) The downstream suture line conforms to the U-shaped spherical configuration of the native aortic sinus. A V-shaped configuration places excessive tension on the commissural attachments and cusps.

is, leaving the noncoronary sinus in place in the allograft and not rotating it. For valve sizes more than 30 mm, we prefer root replacement (15).

E. Tricuspid Valve Replacement (Fig. 11)

Tricuspid valve replacement is occasionally necessary for severe organic tricuspid valve disease. Because of the high incidence of thromboembolism on the right side of the heart, a porcine xenograft valve is preferred. Either running or interrupted suture technique can be used. The sutures are started at the redundant septal leaflet, which is purposely only partially resected. The sutures are passed at the base of this leaflet, avoiding the bundle of His. Alternatively, if the sutures cannot be placed with certainty in this area, the valve can be placed supraannularly, that is, on the atrial side of the tricuspid ring, with the coronary sinus draining into the right ventricle. This technique avoids the conduction system altogether.

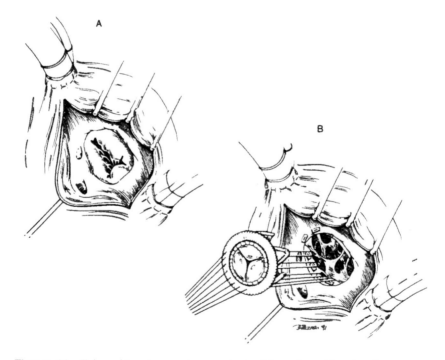

Figure 11 Tricuspid valve replacement. A. The tricuspid valve is exposed through a standard right atriostomy. Bicaval cannulation is necessary. B. The septal leaflet is not excised completely and the sutures are started at this level. In this way, possibility of injury to the conduction system is minimized.

Table 4   Sequencing of Multiple Valve Operation

1. Cardioplegia directly into the coronary ostia[a]
2. Resect aortic valve
3. Size aortic valve
4. Open left atrium
5. Resect mitral valve
6. Replace mitral valve
7. Close left atrium
8. Replace aortic valve
9. Close aortic root
Vent/cardioplegia
10. Open right atrium
11. Replace or repair tricuspid valve

[a] Induction or maintenance of cardioplegia may be by retrograde coronary sinus infusion.

Tricuspid valve surgery is usually necessary in the context of multiple valve disease, so an important part of the procedure is the sequencing of the operation. Even though it is possible to perform tricuspid operation at normothermia and empty-beating state, we prefer to perform this operation on arrested heart because this allows more precise and secure placement of the sutures, particularly in the area of the bundle of HIS. Table 4 outlines our sequencing of the operation for multiple valve procedure.

VII. HEMODYNAMICS OF PROSTHETIC VALVES

By FDA convention, in-vitro hemodynamic comparison between valves is usually done on 27-mm valves. Steady and pulsatile pressure drops, flow visualization, measurement of energy losses in systole and diastole, regurgitant volumes, and calculation of shear stresses may all be helpful in comparing different valves but are not always highly correlated with clinical events such as symptomatic improvement, thromboembolism, and hemolysis. Extrapolation to smaller valve size can be misleading. Analysis of in-vivo performance is, however, informative, and is best done by calculation of effective valve areas for comparable valve sizes, rather than single gradients. Horstkotte et al. (23) compared B-S, L-K, S-E, M-H, and SJM at rest and during exercise, respectively, and these are shown in Table 5.

VIII. COMPLICATIONS

A. Hemolysis

For most contemporary mechanical valves (and certainly for all tissue valves), hemolysis is not a problem. The major factor producing severe

Table 5 Hemodynamics of Prosthetic Valves

	Value type	Rest	Exercise
Mitral	SJM	3.1 ± 0.8	3.4 ± 0.7
size 29	BS	2.2 ± 0.5	2.8 ± 0.6
	MH	1.9 ± 0.5	2.3 ± 0.6
	LK	1.7 ± 0.3	2.2 ± 0.4
	SE	1.8 ± 0.4	2.0 ± 0.4
Aortic	SJM	2.2 ± 0.3	2.5 ± 0.3
size 23	BS	1.5 ± 0.3	1.9 ± 0.3
	LK	1.3 ± 0.1	1.6 ± 0.2
	SE (#24)	1.4 ± 0.2	1.7 ± 0.2

Source: Modified from Ref. 23.

hemolysis is paravalvular leakage. Table 6 gives our suggestions to prevent this complication. Although paravalvular leak is the prevailing cause of excessive hemolysis, other factors include incomplete seating of the poppet, and tissue valve cusp rupture, perforation, or retraction. Since flow through the large mitral valve orifice is less rapid, hemolytic anemia usually does not result after mitral valve replacement unless a perivalvular or transvalvular leak if present.

The anemia resulting from prosthetic valve hemolysis is microangiopatic. Reticulocyte count is high and haptoglobin is completely saturated, i.e., absent. There is a variable level of free hemoglobin. Hematuria may occur after exercise, and there is methemoglobinuria. Serum LDH provides a good index of the severity of hemolysis. Mild hemolysis can be tolerated if the hemodynamic performance of the replacement valve is adequate. Treatment consists of steroids (controversial) and transfusion. Recently, treatment with erythropoietin has been suggested (24). More severe hemolysis must be considered an indication for reoperation.

Table 6 Avoidance of Paravalvular Leaks

Quiet heart
Good exposure
Appropriate suture material
Expanded "shock-resistant" sewing cuff
Antibiotics

B. Thromboembolism

To compare different devices with regard to thrombosis and thromboembolic events, linearized rates in events/100 valve year (%/pt-yr) should be sought. Table 2 presents a summary of a literature review for various mechanical and tissue valves (12). There is a wealth of data for each device, but some generalizations are apparent. No mechanical valve can be managed reliably without systemic anticoagulation, even in children. On the other hand, it is appropriate to manage patients with bioprostheses without anticoagulation. Homograft valves do not require anticoagulation and are remarkably free form thromboembolic complications. Thrombosis and thromboembolic events are more common in the mitral position than in the aortic position (3–4%/pt-yr versus 1–2%/pt-yr). Thrombosis and thromboembolism most frequently are a sequelae of a recent previous interval of inadequate anticoagulation. Patient-related factors also play a role. In some but not all series, previous thromboembolism (T.E.), large left atria, and atrial fibrillation are risk factors (25). Older age has also been implicated. It is clear, however, that rigorous attention to anticoagulation regimens will decrease the risk of thromboembolism to an individual patient and lower the incidence in any group of patients. Thrombotic or embolic complications require prompt recognition and intervention. For the first thromboembolic event, generally the only intervention required is adjustment of Coumadin dose. The appropriate prothrombin level is about 3.5 to 4.0 INR. Certainly, other reasons for T.E. should be sought, including left ventricular thrombus, new myocardial infarction, and prosthetic valve endocarditis.

Recurrent T.E. is an indication for reoperation. Although chemical thrombolysis may be appropriate for right-sided valves, valves, its use for left-sided thrombotic problems is quite controversial. Valve thrombosis is usually marked by rapid onset of heart failure, and diminished or absent prosthetic sounds. Diagnosis usually can be confirmed by echocardiography or cinefluoroscopy. As noted previously, caged-ball valves have higher rates of thromboembolism but a lower incidence of thrombosis. SJM and later-generation tilting-disk valves have comparably lower rates of thrombosis and thromboembolism. Finally, previous embolic events and prosthetic valve endocarditis are strong risk factors for future embolic events.

C. Infection

When infection of a prosthetic valve is diagnosed within 60 days of its insertion, the prosthetic valve endocarditis (PVE) is referred to as early

Table 7   PVE, University of Alabama, 1967–1977

	Medical treatment			Surgical Rx			
		Hospital deaths			Hospital deaths		
Degree of heart failure	No. pts	No.	%	No. pts	No.	%	p
Mild	4	1	25	10	4	40	$p = 0.8$
Moderate	4	4	100	17	6	35	$p = 0.03$
Severe	4	4	100	8	5	63	$p = 0.1$
Total	12	9	75	35	15	43	$p = <0.002$

PVE. However, data from Blackstone and Kirklin (26) suggest that the early (perhaps postsurgical) hazard persists for about 10 months. The natural history of the PVE and its prognosis seems to be different in early versus late PVE. The results of treatment in 47 patients with PVE at UAB (1967 to 1977) are shown in Table 7 (27). Mortality has related to the degree of heart failure, and surgical treatment was better than medical treatment. This difference did not hold in patients with early PVE, where overall mortality was high, 71%. However, in late PVE, surgical treatment was clearly superior. Thus, we consider the natural history and the treatment outcome of late PVE to be quite similar to native valve endocarditis and, therefore, indications for reoperation are similar.

In a recent study of 1465 consecutive in-hospital survivors of valve replacement at UAB, Ivert and colleagues (28) found PVE in 3.6% of subjects (53 patients) at 48 months (Fig. 12). Incremental risk factors for developing PVE were a history of native valve endocarditis, black race, mechanical prostheses, male sex, and longer cardiopulmonary bypass time (Table 8).

D. Durability

Structural integrity and durability are the main advantages of mechanical valves. For the SE 1260 or 6000, MH, and OS valves, there have been no reported instances of structural failure. For the SJM, as mentioned before, about 10 instances of disk escape or fracture were reported, but this was probably related to handling of the valve at the time of implantation.

Many reports are available concerning the long-term outcome of porcine valve bioprosthesis with regard to the incidence of structural deterioration. Gallucci et al. (29) demonstrated that the actuarial freedom from

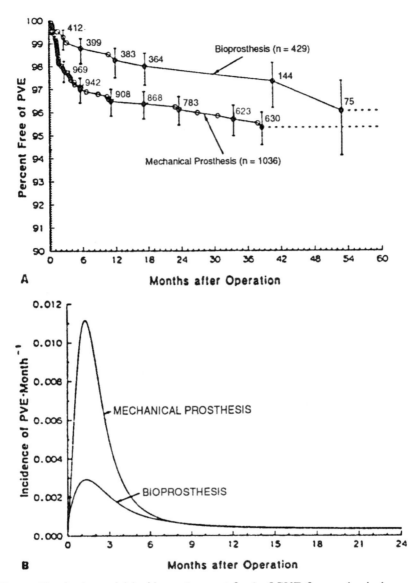

Figure 12 A. Actuarial incidence (percent free) of PVE for mechanical prosthesis versus bioprosthesis. B. Hazard function for incidence of PVE. (From Ref. 28. Used with permission from J. W. Kirklin.)

Table 8 Multivariate Analysis (Cox Proportional Hazard Method) of Incremental Risk Factors for Postoperative PVE

Incremental risk factor	Cox Coefficient (± SD)	Increase in incidence		
		p value	Mean	CL[a]
Presence of NVE (all degrees of activity)	1.7 ± 0.40	<0.0001	5.3	3.5–7.9
Black race	1.3 ± 0.33	<0.0001	3.7	2.7–5.1
Mechanical prostheses	1.0 ± 0.38	<0.005	2.9	2.0–4.2
Male sex	0.7 ± 0.33	<0.04	2.0	1.4–2.8
Longer elapsed time of cardiopulmonary bypass (min)[b]	0.006 ± 0.0033	<0.09	1.4	1.2–1.7[c]

[a] CL = 70% confidence limits.
[b] Or cardiac ischemic time (*p* = 0.03).
[c] 120 versus 60 min.
Source: From Ref. 28. Used with permission of J. W. Kirklin.

primary tissue failure at 15 years was 41% ± 5.5% for mitral valve replacement, 37% ± 10% for AVR. Actuarial freedom from all valve-related complications was 25% ± 4% at 15 years for MVR and 23% ± 7.5% for AVR (Fig. 13). Gallucci et al. concluded that progressive tissue deterioration after 8 years made this type of valve unacceptable after this period of time. Similar results were obtained by Cohen et al., who showed quite reasonable integrity after 10 years but sharp decline in structural integrity between 10 and 15 years after implantation (13). In both Gallucci's and Cohn's series, the age of the patient has significant impact on the durability of the bioprosthesis, i.e., earlier degeneration in younger age. In the elderly (age >70), the incidence of valve degeneration is quite low, particularly in the aortic position (Table 3). Pericardial valves are appreciably less durable than are porcine xenografts.

Durability of aortic homografts is affected by many factors, including procurement technique, preservation technique, storage protocols, and even implantation techniques. Reports suggest that aortic valve homografts perform as well as, if not better than, present-day xenografts. Data presented by O'Brien using cryopreserved "viable" aortic homografts suggest a clear superiority of this technique of valve replacement with a 95% rate of freedom from valve failure at 10 years (15) (Fig. 14).

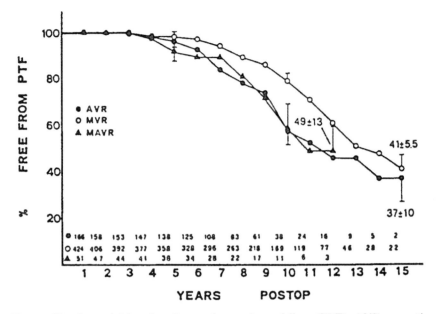

Figure 13 Actuarial freedom from primary tissue failure (PTF). AVR = aortic valve replacement; MVR = mitral valve replacement; MAVR = mitral-aortic valve replacement. (From Ref. 29. Used with permission of V. Bortolotti.)

IX. LONG-TERM RESULTS

Long-term results of valve replacement operation depend only in part on the type of prosthetic device used. Patient-related factors are also of major importance.

Blackstone and Kirklin studied a group of 1533 patients receiving primary aortic and/or mitral valve replacement with or without tricuspid valve surgery or other cardiac procedure (26). The actuarial survival for this group of patients was 74% at 5 years. Several factors were identified as incremental risk for premature death: NYHA preoperative class, any valve operation other than AVR, aortic cross-clamp time, and combined mitral and aortic surgery.

O'Brien reported a 4.8% operative mortality (CL 3.3–67%) for aortic valve replacement using cryopreserved aortic homografts. The actuarial survival at 10 years was 71%, and 99% of the patients were free from reoperation for valve-related problems.

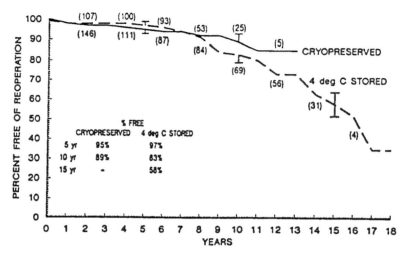

Figure 14 Percent free of reoperation (for any reason) for 4°C stored valve (events = 34) and cryopreserved valve (events = 12). The P value for the difference is 0.37. (From Ref. 15. Used with permission of D. C. McGiffin.)

Based on a multivariate analysis of 2488 patients undergoing valve replacement, the group from the University of Toronto showed that urgent surgery, endocarditis requiring urgent surgery, previous valve surgery, coronary artery disease, and age were important risk factors for long-term survival after aortic valve replacement. For mitral valve replacement, urgent surgery, endocarditis, age, coronary disease, and preoperative ejection fraction were independent predictors of late mortality (30).

The group at Stanford (31) identified functional class, previous myocardial infarction, and hepatic dysfunction as powerful, independent determinants of operative mortality for mitral valve replacement. The type of mitral valve lesion stratified the patient population into different risk subsets, with operative mortality rates of 13% for mitral regurgitation and 8% for mitral stenosis and combined subgroups ($p < 0.004$). In the multivariate analysis employed by the Stanford group, the hemodynamics of the valve lesion did not truly discriminate between operative risk but reflected the fact that more patients with mitral regurgitation were in NYHA class III or IV, were older, had sustained a prior myocardial infarction, or had liver disease. Overall operative mortality for aortic valve replacement has been reported between 5 and 12%; for mitral valve replacement between 4 and 15%; and for double valve replacement between 8 and 16%.

As Blackstone and Kirklin (26) have pointed out, the early phase of higher risk does not end with hospital dismissal or on postoperative day 30, but rather merges with the constant-risk phase at about 3 months after operation. The majority of deaths in this early phase are due to cardiac failure or occur suddenly, and they are associated with preoperative left ventricular dysfunction. In these patients, improved myocardial protection during the operation may be expected to reduce the number of early fatalities. With adequate operative technique, the type of prosthetic valve used for replacement does not appear to have significant impact on operative mortality.

Long-term results for the modern mechanical prostheses are just now beginning to be published. The mechanical valve with the longest follow-up available is the Starr-Edwards. The 5-year survival ranges between 70% and 80%, with somewhat higher survival for aortic valve replacement (80–90%) and lower for mitral valve replacement (65–80%). The same risk factors that affect operative mortality affect long-term survival. Left ventricular dysfunction and the presence of coronary artery disease appear to be particularly important in this regard.

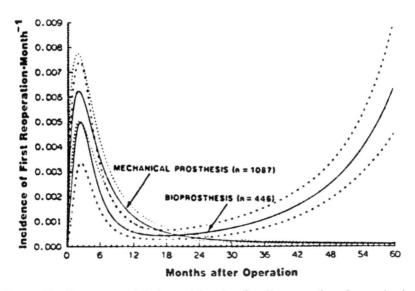

Figure 15 Nomogram of the hazard function for all reoperations for mechanical prostheses and bioprostheses, determined by separate analyses. In the hazard function for mechanical prostheses there is an early peaking phase and a constant phase; in that for bioprostheses there is an early peaking phase and a second rising late phase. (From Ref. 26. Used with permission of J. W. Kirklin.)

The actuarial incidence of reoperation after original valve replacement, as reported by Blackstone and Kirklin (26), is 2.5% (CL 2.2 to 3%) within 6 months; 4.3% (CL 3.8 to 4.8%) within 2 years; and 6.7% (CL 5.9 to 7.7%) within 5 years. The hazard function for reoperation after original operation shows an early peak at 3 months, reflecting the incidence of early prosthetic valve endocarditis and then a descent to a constant hazard function. The shape of the hazard function differs for mechanical valves and bioprostheses, reflecting differences in durability of these two types of valve substitutes (Fig. 15). Finally, the improvement in functional class after valve replacement is present in 80–90% of the patients, with only 5–10% of the patients remaining in functional class III or IV after valve replacement (32,33). After two-thirds of the patients return to class I.

REFERENCES

1. Starr A, Edwards ML. Mitral replacement: a clinical experience with the ball valve prosthesis. Ann Surg 1961; 154:726.
2. Harken R, Soroff HS, Taylor WJ, et al. Partial and complete prosthesis in aortic insufficiency. J Thorac Cardiovasc Surg 1960; 40:744.
3. Barratt-Boyes BG. Homograft aortic valve replacement in aortic incompetence and stenosis. Thorax 1964; 19:131.
4. Ross DN. Homograft replacement of the aortic valve. Lancet 1962; 2:487.
5. Binet JP, Carpentier A, Langlois J, et al. Implantation de valves heterogenes dans le traitment des cardiopathies aortiques. CR Acad Sci Paris 1965; 261: 5733.
6. Carpentier A, Lamaigre CG, Robert L, et al. Biological factors affecting long-term results of valvular heterografts. J Thorac Cardiovasc Surg 1969; 58:467.
7. Harken DE. Heart valves: ten commandments and still counting. Ann Thorac Surg 1989; 48:518.
8. Braunwald NS, Cooper T, Morrow AG. Clinical and experimental replacement of the mitral valve: experience with the use of flexible polyurethane prosthesis. In: Merendino KA, ed. Prosthetic Valves in Cardiac Surgery. Springfield, IL: Charles C Thomas, 1961:307.
9. Bjork VO. The Bjork-Shiley tilting disc valve: past, present and future. In: Crawford FA, ed. State of the Art Reviews: Cardiac Surgery. Current Heart Valve Prostheses. Philadelphia: Hanley & Belfus, 1987:183.
10. Hiratzka LF, Kouchoukos NT, Grunkemeier GL, et al. Outlet strut fracture of Bjork-Shiley 60 degree convexo-concave valve: current information and recommendation for patient care. Am J Coll Cardiol 1988; 11:1130.
11. Odell JA, Durandt J, Shama DM, et al. Spontaneous embolization of a St. Jude prosthetic mitral valve leaflet. Ann Thorac Surg 1985; 39:569.
12. Doty DB. Cardiac Surgery. Chicago: Year Book Medical Publishers, 1985: Aortic A41.

13. Cohn LH, Collins JJ, Disesa VJ, et al. Fifteen-year experience with 1678 Hancock porcine bioprosthetic heart valve replacement. Ann Surg 1989; 40: 435.

14. Angell JD, Christopher BS, Hawtrey CO, Angell WW. A fresh viable human heart valve bank: sterilization, sterility testing, and cryogenic preservation. Transplant Proc 1976; 8(suppl 1):139.

15. McGiffin DC, O'Brien MF, Stafford EG, et al. Long-term results of the viable cryopreserved allograft aortic valve: continuing evidence for superior valve durability. J Card Surg 1988; 3(suppl 1):289.

16. Dubost C, Guilmet D, DeParades B, et al. Chirurgie a coeur ouvent: Nouvelle technique d'ouverture de l'oreillette gauche. L'Abord Biauriculaire. Presse Med 1966; 74:1607.

17. David TE, Uden DE, Strauss HD. The importance of the mitral apparatus in left ventricular function after correction of mitral regurgitation. Circulation 1983; 68(suppl II):II-76.

18. David TE. Mitral valve replacement with preservation of chordae tendineae: rationale and technical considerations. Ann Thorac Surg 1986; 41:680.

19. Scott WJ, Neumann AL, Karp RB. Ultrasonic debridement of the aortic valve with six month echocardiographic follow-up. Am J Cardiol 1989; 64: 1206.

20. Nicks R, Cartmill T, Bernstein L. Hypoplasia of the aortic root. Thorax 1970; 25:339.

21. Manougian S, Seybold-Epting W. Patch enlargement of the aortic valve ring by extending the aortic incision into the anterior mitral leaflet: new operative techniques. J Thorac Cardiovasc Surg 1979; 78:402.

22. Donaldson RM, Ross DN. Homograft aortic root replacement for complicated prosthetic valve endocarditis. Circulation 1984; 70(suppl 1):178.

23. Horstkotte D, Haerten K, Seipe L, et al. Central hemodynamics at rest and during exercise after mitral valve replacement with different prostheses. Circulation 1983; 68(suppl II):II-161.

24. Groopman JE, Molina JM, Scadden DT. Hematopoietic growth factors. Biology and clinical application. N Engl J Med 1989; 321:1449.

25. Edmunds LH. Thrombotic and bleeding complications of prosthetic heart valves. Ann Thorac Surg 1987; 44:430.

26. Blackstone EH, Kirklin JW. Death and other time-related events after valve replacement. Circulation 1985; 72(4):753.

27. Karp RB. Role of surgery in infective endocarditis. In: McGoon DC, ed. Cardiac Surgery. 2d ed. Philadelphia: F. A. Davis, 1987:141.

28. Ivert TS, Dismukes WE, Cobbs CG, et al. Prosthetic valve endocarditis. Circulation (1984); 69(2):223.

29. Gallucci V, Mazzucco A, Bortolotti V, et al. The standard Hancock porcine bioprosthesis: overall experience at the University of Padova. J Card Surg 1988; 3:337.

30. Christakis GT, Weisel RD, David TE, et al. Predictors of operative survival after valve replacement. Circulation 1988; 78(suppl I):I-25.

31. Scott WC, Miller DG, Haverich A, et al. Operative risk of mitral valve replacement: discriminant analysis of 1329 procedures. Circulation 1985; 72(suppl II):II-108.
32. Burckhardt D, Strieber D, Vogt S, et al. Heart valve replacement with St. Jude Medical prosthesis. Circulation 1988; 78(suppl I):I-18.
33. Lindblom D. Long term clinical results after aortic valve replacement with Bjork-Shiley prosthesis. J Thorac Cardiovasc Surg 1988; 95:658.

20

Valvular Surgery in Children

John A. Odell*
University of Cape Town Medical School, and Groote Schuur and Red Cross Children's Hospital, Cape Town, South Africa

Susan M. Vosloo
Groote Schuur and Red Cross Children's Hospital, Cape Town, South Africa

I. INTRODUCTION

Of all the problems facing cardiac surgeons, the greatest is the development of an ideal prosthetic heart valve. Many surgeons would find such a statement hard to accept—surely the development of the artificial heart, the correction of complex congenital heart defects, and the creation of a state of tolerance following cardiac transplantation is more important. But what escapes many cardiac surgeons, because cardiac surgery is expensive, technically demanding, and practiced only in developed countries where social and living standards are high, are the ravages of rheumatic fever and its sequela, rheumatic valvular heart disease. In the developing, underdeveloped, or Third World countries, rheumatic fever is common and large numbers of young patients with valvular heart disease are seen and die of untreated valvular disease. In the disadvantaged Third World, the gap between First and Third World medicine is widening, a population explosion is forecast, and the ability to cope with valvular disease, because of costs of surgery and prosthetic valves, is difficult to imagine.

In addition to the large number of patients and the economic difficulties of treatment in these countries, there is the realization that the perfect

---

* Present affiliation: Division of Thoracic and Cardiovascular Surgery, Mayo Clinic, Rochester, Minnesota.

prosthetic valve has yet to be designed. In children the deficiencies of a prosthetic valve are more obvious than in adults, and the choice of which valve to use is especially difficult. It is extremely difficult to evaluate and compare different series of valve replacement in children. There is no uniform definition of who exactly is a child; some series include patients up to 23 years of age (1), some up to 21 years (2–5), the majority include as children those younger than 16 years (6–9), and some only preteenage children (10). The series are often not comparable in terms of the pathological basis for valve replacement; the large series from the Third World (4,6,11–13) have a preponderance of patients with rheumatic heart disease affecting mainly the mitral valve; the series from the First World are smaller, with a preponderance of younger children with congenital defects, many of which involve the aortic valve or are placed in right-sided conduits (3,5,7–10,14). Facilities to anticoagulate patients who have received prosthetic valves vary from country to country. This influences to some extent valve policy and naturally the risks of thrombosis and thromboembolism; numerous valve types have been used, and many series combine data on various prostheses.

Very few series offer data on emboli in the form of linearized occurrence rates. Others do not report on follow-up, making it impossible to assess the relative risks of complications.

There has been a natural evolution of experience with valve replacement in children; in the early reports the risks were considered so serious it was advised that valve replacement should, if possible, be avoided (15–17); in some series the bioprosthetic valve was recommended as the valve of choice—clearly not now true (10,18)—and more recent experience documents excellent results achieved in infants needing valve replacement (19–21).

II. PROBLEMS WITH VALVE REPLACEMENT IN CHILDREN

The problems associated with valve replacement in adults are shared by children, who also present specific problems related to the size of the prosthesis, the presence of associated congenital defects, the choice of prosthesis, and the need for anticoagulation. In children the deficiencies of a particular heart valve are generally more apparant.

A. Prosthetic Size

The size of the prosthetic valve is an important consideration. Valve replacement with a small-size valve may be necessary, and with development of the child and enlargement of the heart, relative stenosis may occur, necessitating repeated operations. This is more likely the younger the patient. Although at reoperation the insertion of a larger prosthesis may be planned, it may be difficult to insert a significantly larger valve because of a fibrotic annulus. In order to avoid this it may be necessary to consider carefully techniques to enlarge the annulus at the first operation. These techniques are often associated with an increase in morbidity and mortality.

In earlier considerations of the effects of growth on the adequacy of prosthetic valves inserted in small children, it was predicted that the prosthetic valve would accommodate the normal cardiac output of older children or adults (22,23). This is incorrect; relative stenosis does occur. In Kadoba et al.'s series of infants having mitral valve replacement, 55% of survivors needed repeat surgery 3 years later (19). Shore et al., in a series that had few cases of rheumatic valve disease, correlated the effective orifice area of the valve used expressed as a percentage of the calculated area of each valve replaced (24). A wide range of values were obtained, indicating that some valves were severely stenotic at the time of implantation, whereas others had the capacity to accommodate the continued growth of the child.

A disturbing observation by Friedman et al. is that although the introduction of a second prosthesis with a larger orifice area at operation did lower the mean mitral valve diastolic gradient, the pulmonary artery pressure failed to return to normal (25). In adults a prompt fall in pulmonary artery pressure and pulmonary vascular resistance follows prosthetic mitral valve replacement (26,27). Friedman et al. postulated that the elevated pulmonary vascular resistance may represent a persistance of the fetal pattern of pulmonary vasculature resulting from the presence of chronically elevated pulmonary venous pressure due to the congenital mitral deformity or pulmonary venous hypertension and may more readily cause irreversible pulmonary vascular changes in children compared to adults (27). They recommend frequent hemodynamic studies and timely repeat valve replacement prior to the development of cardiac and pulmonary vascular complications (27).

With valvular incompetance the valve annulus is frequently enlarged, and it may be possible to insert a larger-size prosthetic valve. With some prostheses a large valve has the potential to cause varying degrees of obstruction to forward flow (28). It should also be kept clearly in mind that if too large a prosthesis is inserted, with the hemodynamic lesion corrected, postoperative diminution in cardiac size may occur and obstruction of flow may result.

B. Variability in Valve Pathology and Association with Other Cardiovascular Anomalies

A significant proportion of any First World series of valve replacement in children involves congenital abnormalities. These abnormalities are quite variable and may be challenging to repair; occasionally replacement of a valve is necessary. Replacement may not simply be the insertion of the valve in an annulus but may involve the placement of a valve within a conduit, within the atrium, or adjacent to a Dacron patch. The exact siting of the valve may influence results.

An additional compounding consideration may be the presence of associated defects. These defects may need to be corrected before, after, or simultaneously with the valve procedure. It may be advisable in some instances to correct defects which are increasing afterload or preload and observing, over a period of time, the influence the repair has on abnormal valve function. For example, mitral incompetance may be associated with a large patent ductus arteriosus, but incompetance may diminish after ligation of the ductus arteriosus and removal of the volume overload.

The more complex the procedure, the greater is the operative risk. Many of the deaths attributed to valve replacement may in fact not be valve-related but due to the underlying cardiac condition (5).

C. Anticoagulation

The value of anticoagulation to avoid thromboembolic complications in patients with prosthetic heart valves has been well established in adults (29). In children, however, the use of anticoagulants is complicated; children by their nature are active and susceptible to trauma; children resent the taking of blood samples; there may be lack of compliance and difficulties in dosage regulation. Anticoagulation with Warfarin is undesirable in females because of its effects on menstrual and child-bearing function.

In many parts of the world anticoagulant control is virtually nonexistent. A thromboembolic event is particularly devastating in children, but where the infrastructure to support the child through this illness is lacking, it may be life-threatening.

It does appear that thromboembolic episodes are reduced in children (30), although some have documented a high incidence (1,12,18), and the point is frequently made that the risks of bleeding complications because of anticoagulant therapy may be greater than the risk of thrombosis and thromboembolism. The incidence of bleeding with Warfarin remains significant, even though most children do not have underlying medical conditions that predispose to bleeding. Can one afford not to anticoagulate children? Are antiplatelet regimens using aspirin and dipyridamole effective and a safe alternative? Does valve type and position influence thromboembolism in children? Other issues pertaining to valve replacement in children are becoming clearer, but prevention of thrombosis and thromboembolism remains vexing.

1. Is Anticoagulation Necessary?

In some of the large series from the Third World, at least 75% of children were not anticoagulated (6). Unfortunately, because follow-up was incomplete, the exact incidence of thromboembolism is uncertain. Thromboembolism occurred in groups treated with and without Warfarin and in groups treated with aspirin and dipyridamole, suggesting that treatment may not be effective in those in whom it was given or compliance was poor. Pass and colleagues reported on a group of children having valve replacement with the St. Jude Medical valve treated without anticoagulation (2). Their follow-up report was short. No thrombosis or thromboembolism occurred, but in their addendum they reported a thrombosed pulmonary prosthesis and a possible thromboembolic event (2). The same group 5 years later reported late occurrences of thrombosis and thromboembolism (31), attributed by them to chance. Children who did not receive anticoagulants were significantly less free of thrombotic and thromboembolic events than the adults who did receive anticoagulants, but when bleeding complications are added to the risk analysis, there is no significant difference between children and adults. There are thus no present-day studies by which one can confidently answer the question of whether anticoagulation is necessary. The centers in which a policy of no or limited anticoagulation is practiced have incomplete follow-up; in the more sophisticated communities it would be considered unethical not to give anticoagulant or antiaggregate therapy.

Overall thromboembolic rates appear to be lower in children than in adults receiving either a mechanical or bioprosthetic valve, treated in the accepted fashion with Warfarin (9,17) or aspirin either as the sole treatment or combined with dipyridamole. Reported rates of thromboembolism in children approximate 1.0% per 100 patient-years of follow-up (32), compared to adults, which range from 1.8 to 8.0% per 100 patient-years (33), depending on the valve prosthesis and the heart position. Possible reasons may be the infrequent finding of atrial fibrillation in children and the higher basal heart rate compared to adults. Left atrial enlargement is often less prominent, and blood flow velocity across a smaller effective orifice size may be greater. More frequent leaflet cycling may reduce stasis and the consequent risk of thrombus formation.

Avoiding the need for anticoagulants by using bioprosthetic valves is not a satisfactory solution, as these valves are subject to calcific degeneration. Furthermore, bioprosthetic valves are not free from embolic complications, as shown by Wada and colleagues, who demonstrated an embolic rate of 4% per patient-year for the Hancock valve (34).

The question then arises, if one assumes that children have a limited requirement for anticoagulation by Warfarin and accepts the necessity for anticoagulation in adults with prosthetic cardiac valves, when exactly do older children need to be started on such medication? When does the changeover in status occur?

2. Aspirin and Dipyridamole

Aspirin or aspirin with dipyridamole is an attractive alternative to Warfarin therapy in children having mechanical prosthetic valve replacement for the reasons previously mentioned. In particular, these drugs are relatively inexpensive, easy to administer, and do not require monitoring. Antiplatelet agents have been added to stable Warfarin regimens (35,36) in the hope that thromboembolic events that still occur in patients on Warfarin (27) may be eliminated. Unfortunately, although the thromboembolic rate was lowered significantly, the incidence of both major and minor bleeding has been unacceptably high (6.6% per 100 patient-years). Antiplatelet agents used solely in adults with mechanical valves do not adequately protect against thromboembolism. In fact, the rates approach those with no anticoagulation at all (36).

Because of the high incidence of thromboembolic events and bleeding in children receiving Warfarin (12.1% incidence) after a prosthetic valve, the San Francisco group initiated treatment with antiplatelet agents alone (37). A further series by the same group in children with mechanical aortic valves documented no postoperative thrombosis or embolic events (38). Some children were even screened for subclinical cerebral infarcts by magnetic resonance imaging or computed axial tomography.

It is uncertain why antiplatelet agents may be more effective in lowering thromboembolic events in children than in adults. The coagulation cascade is similar, as is platelet adhesion (39).

Hemorrhagic episodes related to Warfarin may be significant in children. Bradley and associates had a 25% incidence compared to a 0% incidence in those treated with aspirin (40). Aspirin is not completely inoccuous, however, and more gastrointestinal events have been noted in adults treated with aspirin compared to Warfarin (41). In children there is always the concern of Reye's syndrome (42).

D. Thromboembolism: Prosthetic Valve Type and Position

1. Starr-Edwards Valve

In the Mayo clinic experience the overall incidence of late thromboembolism is 5.3 per 100 patient-years after aortic valve replacement and 2.0 per 100 patient-years after atrioventricular valve replacement (43). Actuarally determined embolus-free survival after aortic and mitral valve replacement at 10 years was 66 ± 15% and 91 ± 6%, respectively (43).

These results contrast with Odell et al.'s series, where embolus-free survival at 10 years for the mitral position was 60 ± 10% (6). Schaff et al. considered that the difference in time of occurrence and manifestation of thromboembolism in mitral and aortic groups may be the result of different mechanisms of thrombosis (43). Chesebro et al. speculated that fibrin thrombi develop in association with the lower velocity of flow across the mitral prosthesis, whereas in the aortic position, where high-velocity flow occurs, thrombi consist mostly of platelets (35). Attie and associates followed 74 children with Starr-Edwards mitral valves for a mean of 6.4 years and encountered only one instance of valve thrombosis; thromboembolic episodes occurred at a rate of 1.7% per patient-year (13).

Probably the largest series in older children using the Starr-Edwards valve is by John et al. of India (11). Three hundred and one patients had a Starr Edwards valve implanted. One valve thrombosed, and 9 embolic episodes occurred. The linearized rates per 100 patient-years were 0.41, 0.56, and 1.04 for the mitral, aortic, and double valve replacement groups, respectively. All patients were taking coumarin-derived anticoagulants, and the prothrombin time was kept 1.5 times that of the control level. They believe that less stringent anticoagulant control and education of the patient taking anticoagulants offered protection against thromboembolism and anticoagulant-related haemorrhage. Recently they have adopted the policy of aspirin, 300 mg daily, in selected subjects.

2. Bjork-Shiley Valve

Rufilanchas and colleagues reported their experience of 23 children with excellent results (44). They had no episodes of thromboembolism in the short period of follow-up (6–26 months), despite the fact that patients with isolated aortic valve replacement received treatment with aspirin and dipyradamole.

A large group of patients receiving the Bjork-Shiley valve was reported by Iyer et al. from India (30). Of interest were no instances of valve thrombosis in the younger age group compared to 15 instances in adults. Nonfatal embolism, anticoagulant-related hemorrhage, and periprosthetic leak occurred with equal frequency in both groups. At 8 years the embolus-free survival was 98.8 ± 1.1%.

3. St. Jude Medical Valve

The St. Jude Medical valve appears to be associated with a low incidence of thromboembolism, and has even been used in some series without anticoagulants (2). The low incidence may be related to its construction entirely of pyrolytic carbon and better hemodynamics.

4. Valve Position

Patients after aortic valve replacement are less prone to thromboembolic events, probably because the majority are in sinus rhythm. In the mitral area a large left atrium, possible atrial fibrillation, and lower cardiac output predispose the patient toward postoperative thromboembolism (45).

III. SPECIFIC SURGICAL TECHNIQUES

A. Timing of Surgery

Many of the valve replacement operations in children are urgent and life-saving. Included in this category is infectious endocarditis which is progressive despite medical therapy, critical valvular stenosis, massive valvular regurgitation, and fulminant rheumatic valvulitis. For other more chronic and less severe valvular lesions one must consider the risk the valvular defect poses to myocardial function, pulmonary vascular resistance, growth, and development, and compare it with the surgical experience in converting the underlying defect, the operator, and the prosthesis.

In general, valve repair or replacement is indicated when valvular dysfunction is retarding growth or causing significant cardiac symptoms.

B. Technique of Operation

Usually the operative management of children differs little from that of adults or other children having correction of congenital heart defects, with access and cannulation being similar. In small infants and children some surgeons will use circulatory arrest. In using cardioplegia, it is important that the dose given should be sufficient to meet the aim of adequately protecting the heart. Children with valvular heart disease may have markedly dilated and hypertrophied hearts, necessitating judgment by the surgeon in determining the optimal dose of cardioplegia. It is important when using large volumes of cardioplegia in small children not to allow too much cardioplegia to return to the oxygenator. In some patients, it is therefore necessary to snare the cavae and discard the cardioplegic effluent.

C. Surgery in the Acute Phase of Rheumatic Fever

Mitral incompetence is the most common murmur found in the acute phase of rheumatic fever and appears to be related to enlargement of the mitral annulus. In most patients the murmur disappears (46), but in those with significant cardiomegaly it may persist, probably because of progressive dilatation (47). Mitral stenosis usually occurs late after the initial episode of rheumatic fever (48); it is thought that a relatively mild form of rheumatic fever favors the development of pure mitral stenosis (49).

The surgeon who undertakes surgery during the acute phase of the disease will thus be correcting valves that are largely incompetent, unless the acute episode is a recurrent one involving a valve already scarred and deformed. The features of acute carditis are easily recognized at operation. The pericardium is usually adherent and the adhesions may be vascular and edematous, with the inflammatory layer occasionally 1 cm thick. In a few patients there is a large pericardial effusion. The valve leaflets appear edematous but otherwise look surprisingly normal, despite preoperative examination and investigations to the contrary. Jet lesions secondary to regurgitant flow may be seen on the atrial wall (47) and may indicate the site of prolapse or lack of coaption of leaflets. Occasionally, "kissing vegetations" are seen on the line of coaption of the leaflets. These small vegetations are composed of platelets and fibrin. These vegetations may involve the chordae tendinae, and occasionally chordal rupture is found.

From the description of acute rheumatic carditis, it would seem that the mitral valve would be particularly amenable to a conservative procedure, as the incompetence is largely the result of annulus dilatation. The response to corticosteroids and other medical therapy is usually unsatisfactory, and surgery should not be delayed (50).

Our surgical policy is to conserve the valve if at all possible, recognizing, however, that the disease is progressive, that the result may not be optimal, and accepting the need for possible reoperation. In our opinion, any years gained before valve replacement is necessary are beneficial because of the complications associated with valve replacement. Antunes has a different opinion (51) and believes that the pathological changes, characteristic of an early and very unstable inflammatory process, make sutures unsafe; that the pathological changes are still active and the subsequent resolution with scarring would distort the valve, rendering the repair ineffective. Al Kasob et al. also believe that replacement may be preferable to valve repair in the acute phase of the disease (52). Some of our patients are so ill that a path with a more defined result and shorter bypass time (valve replacement rather than repair) is taken. Where there is both aortic and mitral valve involvement, the aortic root often needs to be enlarged because of failure of sufficient dilatation. The incidence of acute carditis is much higher in patients requiring double valve replacement than in those who need aortic or mitral valve replacement alone (6).

Patients needing valve replacement in the acute phase do surprisingly well. Antifailure therapy is still necessary because of myocardial involvement. Prophylaxis against further episodes of rheumatic fever should be maintained.

D. Valvular Surgery Associated with Congenital Defects

It is beyond the scope of this chapter to define all congenital defects that may be associated with a valvular defect that may require surgical correction. Two of the more common defects are mentioned briefly.

1. Atrioventricular Canal Defects

Early repair of complete atrioventricular canal in infancy allows effective mitral and tricupid valve reconstruction in most cases (53,54). There is disagreement whether the so-called cleft should be closed or the valve left as a trileaflet valve. Our own policy is to leave the cleft if the valve is competant; if incompetance is present, single sutures of 4-0 prolene buttressed with autogenous pericardial pledgets are passed through the base of the cleft and the valve tested after each suture is placed. Once competance is achieved, no further sutures are inserted. It is important when repairing the defect that the mitral components of the anterior and posterior bridging leaflets should be approximated at the margin of the interventricular patch so that ample surface for coaption is created along the leaflet edges.

Most children and infants with partial atrioventricular canal associated with significant mitral regurgitation can undergo repair and closure of the primum atrial septal defect. The deficiency of interventricular septum and downward displacement of the mitral valve leaflets may complicate repair. Left ventricular outflow obstruction associated with absence of subaortic septum, downward displacement of the anterior mitral leaflet, or accessory endocardial cushion tissue must be considered. The mitral valve leaflets may need to be detached from the septum, thus creating a "complete" atrioventricular defect. The leaflets are then elevated out of the left ventricular outflow using a patch.

Mitral valve replacement may be necessary in those situations where competance cannot be achieved (this is usually done through the right atrium). Unfortunately, the results of valve replacement in these circumstances are poor (55). Significant left ventricular outflow tract obstruction may be caused by the prosthesis (19).

2. Congenital Aortic Stenosis

Aortic stenosis can result in severe heart failure in the first days or weeks of life. Valvotomy may be undertaken utilizing bypass, inflow occlusion, or blind dilatation. A conservative approach is essential; the surgeon must take care not to be too aggressive and produce catastrophic incompetance.

Although the pressure gradient may be relieved, the procedure must be regarded as palliative (56–60). Most children will have recurrent aortic stenosis and/or incompetance.

When aortic valve replacement is necessary, a large enough valve should be inserted, or techniques such as aortoseptoplasty (60–62), annular augmentation (63,64), or apicoaortic conduit (65) should be considered.

IV. VALVE REPAIR

Repair, even if not perfect, is almost always preferable to valve replacement in the small infant, for whom a good valve substitute simply does not exist (66). Techniques of repair are described elsewhere in this book. In children the use of annuloplasty rings may theoretically, with growth, contribute to secondary valvular stenosis. Absorbable rings are being considered to avoid this problem (67).

A. Choice of Prosthesis

Regardless of which valve is chosen, long-term surveillance is essential. The development of new symptoms should prompt thorough examination of the child to define valvular performance including, if necessary, fluoroscopy, echocardiography, and catheterization. A diagnostic representation of actuarial survival taken from some of the largest series in children is shown in Fig. 1.

1. Bioprosthesis

The seesaw argument—limited durability versus the need for anticoagulation—is maintained in virtually every report comparing mechanical and bioprosthetic valves. Following the enthusiasm for bioprosthetic valves in children which was later dampened by reports of accelerated degeneration due largely to calcification (6), it is generally accepted that a bioprosthetic valve should not be implanted in children. It is worthwhile summarizing the results obtained with bioprosthetic valves in children. Porcine valves survive far longer than bovine pericardial valves (6). Possible reasons are differences in morphology of the leaflets and their response to stress. Extrinsic calcification appears to occur more readily on pericardial valves than porcine valves, and this may be a factor responsible for the increased rate. The mounted, antibiotic, sterilized homograft placed in the mitral position rarely calcifies (7).

Calcification occurs more readily on valves implanted in the mitral position than the aortic. This may be due to increased stress and wear and tear. The triscupid bioprothetic valve rarely calcifies (7); thus, if a

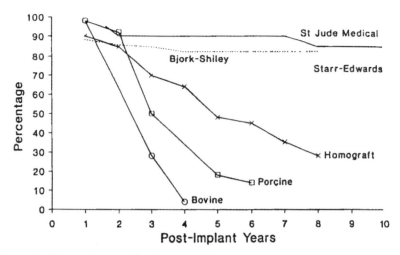

Figure 1 Composite graphic demonstration of actuarial survival curves from the largest and longest valve series in children. All are Third World series except the St. Jude Medical series from Japan (7). The figures relating to the St. Jude Medical valve (7) include all positions; the remainder, the mitral valve position only. The follow-up for the Starr-Edwards valve continues up to 20 years with 59.3% survival (11) and relates, as with the Bjork-Shiley series (30), to patient survival rather than freedom from valve complications—these were minimal in both series. The bioprosthetic valve figures are from Durban, South Africa (6). The striking difference between mechanical and bioprothetic valves is well shown.

homograft is not available, a bioprosthetic valve is preferred to a mechanical valve in the tricuspid position (68,69).

Calcification does not appear to be accelerated because of a previous occurrence involving an implanted valve or lessened because of an increase in the patient's age (70).

2. Antimineralization Processes

In the belief that local treatments may mitigate against calcification, different valve manufacturers have used either surfactant, avoidance of calcium and phosphate ions, incorporation of magnesium ion, various dye compounds, and low-pressure fixation in the hope that their valves may have a lower incidence of calcification. Experiments using the sheep animal model were most encouraging with the porcine valve but not with bovine pericardial valves (71). This may be due to the antimineralization process not affecting extrinsic or surface calcification, which occurs more commonly with the bovine valve.

Clinically, bovine pericardial valves treated with the Hancock T6 process have calcified (6), and porcine valves treated with toludeine blue (Intact) (72) and T6 have also calcified (72).

It does not appear, therefore, that antimineralization processes are effective in children; reports of calcification with these processes are isolated, however, and further series are unlikely to be reported in children because of a natural reluctance by surgeons to implant a bioprosthetic valve, the results of which are unknown in children. In adults a bioprosthetic valve gives reasonable 10-year results, and in this group one would need to wait a considerable period of time and have a large series before any difference between valves treated with or without an antimineralization process is apparent.

In considering the choice of valve, many would favor a bioprosthetic valve in young females (8,73) because of the teratogenic effect of Warfarin, necessary for anticoagulation of a mechanical valve, if used. This argument does not appear to be true (74); it must also be emphasized that pregnancy is probably also a risk factor for bioprosthetic calcification (75).

3. Mechanical Valves

The choice of which mechanical valve to use in children is determined largely by the pathological process requiring valve replacement and the familiarity of the surgeon with the choice of prosthetic valve. The surgeon who deals frequently with the consequences of rheumatic fever, where valvular incompetance and annular dilatation is common, may have completely different needs from the surgeon who is involved with congenital defects, where annular size and the necessity for reoperation are important issues. The former may favor a ball-and-cage valve; the latter a bileaflet valve.

Of the valves used in children, excellent results have been reported in terms of survival and lack of thrombosis and thromboembolism with the use of the Starr-Edwards (6,11,43), with the Bjork-Shiley (6,30), and with the St. Jude Medical valves (6,7). It is difficult to conclude from review of these data which of the currently available valves are superior for generalized paediatric use. We favor the St. Jude Medical valve because of smaller gradients and theoretical risk of less thrombogenicity: Both factors may lessen the need for reoperation. Newly developed bileaflet valves—the Duromedics, Carbomedics, and Sorin bileaflet valves—may also be considered. The Carbomedics and the Shiley monostrut valves are the only mechanical valves manufactured smaller than 19 mm. The ability to rotate the valve is thought to be valuable (19). One should be cautious regarding implantation of a mechanical valve on the right side of the heart (68,69).

B. Management of the Small Annulus

1. The Aortic Annulus

Although no generally accepted standard defining the minimum size of valvular annulus is available, most authors feel that significant gradients are present if small valve prostheses are used. Small-diameter aortic valve prostheses (17 mm and 19 mm) have significant hemodynamic limitations. To some extent, improvements in valve design have lessened this problem. Foster et al. showed acceptable clinical palliation for intervals up to 12 years with 17- and 19-mm-diameter aortic valve prostheses. No annulus-enlargement techniques were used (76).

In most patients (adults or children) with small or hypoplastic annular sizes, it may be preferable to place a larger-size valve combined with an annulus-enlargement procedure. This may be particularly necessary in patients who have undergone valve replacement during childhood and now need implantation of a larger valve.

An assessment of the size of the aortic annulus from the preoperative angiogram is helpful in determining which patients require surgical enlargement of a small annulus. The left ventriculogram is more reliable than root aortography (77). An exact knowledge of the anatomy of the aortic root is essential before operations to enlarge the aortic root are performed (78).

Nicks et al. described an incision made through the midportion of the noncoronary cusp of the aortic valve across the annulus down into the upper part of the anterior leaflet of the mitral valve. Using this technique, the diameter of the aortic annulus is enlarged by approximately 2 mm (63,64). A more radical approach was described by Manougian and Seyhold-Epting (65), where an incision is made down the commissure between the left and noncoronary cusps and deeply into the anterior leaflet of the mitral valve; it may be combined with mitral valve replacement where the mitral annulus is also enlarged (79,80). The defect in the mitral valve is repaired with a patch; the aortic annulus can be enlarged by 5–6 mm (65).

Another, more radical technique to enlarge the annulus is aorto-ventricular septoplasty (60). The aortotomy incision is directed inferiorly through the aortic annulus to the left side of the right coronary ostium. It is extended downward into the upper portion of the adjacent interventricular septum, incising the anterior wall of the right ventricle at its junction with the interventricular septum. The defect in the septum is repaired with a wedge-shaped patch, which continues superiorly onto the ascending aorta. A second patch is used to close the incision made in the anterior right ventricular outflow tract. Using this technique, the diameter of the aortic annulus can be enlarged by more than 6 mm (60–62).

Tilting of the aortic valve prosthesis in order to insert a larger valve was described by Kinsley et al. (81).

2. Left Ventricular Apico-Aortic Conduits

With severe hypoplasia of the aortic annulus or if several aortic valve operations have previously been undertaken, leaving the annulus difficult to reconstruct, a valved conduit between the left ventricular apex and the thoracic or abdominal aorta can be used (66). Other indications for this method are diffuse subaortic stenosis, tubular supravalvular aortic hypoplasia, and severe calcification of the ascending aorta. This technique offers satisfactory relief to left ventricular outflow tract obstruction in adults and children, but long-term results in adults are better (82). In a large series report by Brown et al. in 1988, a high operative mortality was associated with surgery for complex left ventricular outflow tract obstruction. A better outcome is found in patients with obstruction at only a single level (82).

3. The Mitral Annulus

The small mitral annulus can be enlarged only with a technique resembling the Manouguian technique (described above), with which aortic valve replacement is also needed (60–63). The aortic incision is made into the commissure between the left and noncoronary cusps, and extended across the mitral valve annulus. The roof of the left atrium is opened. The incised structures are repaired with patch reconstruction. This provides excellent exposure for concomitant mitral and aortic valve replacement (61–63).

A left-atrial to left-ventricular extracardiac valved conduit may be used to bypass a hypoplastic systemic atrioventricular valve (83–87). The surgical approach is either median sternotomy or left throacotomy. This technique may be used in reoperations where it is not possible to enlarge of the mitral annulus, but it is not advisable if the native mitral valve or previously inserted prosthetic valve is incompetent. Alternatively, it may be used as a primary procedure with the theoretical advantage of allowing the annulus to grow so that an operation on the native mitral valve is still feasible when the patient is older (83–87).

An alternative, less demanding technique is supraannular or intraatrial placement of the prosthetic valve (19,88,89). Results have been variable: some poor (5), some good (19).

C. Reconstruction of the Right Ventricular Outflow Tract

Extracardiac conduits have made repair of many anomalies with right ventricular outflow tract obstruction feasible. Various valved conduits,

including Dacron, polytetrafluoroethylene (PTFE), or fresh aortic allografts, have been used. The valvar component of these included bioprosthetic and mechanical valves as well as aortic allograft valves.

The use of an aortic valve homograft was first reported in 1966 in the
correction of pulmonary obstruction in a patient with underlying tetralogy
of Fallot (90). This patient is still alive and well 22 years following the
operation (91).

The presently available data indicate that the aortic valve homograft,
if well preserved, is the conduit of choice for right ventricular outflow tract
reconstruction. The method of sterilization is thought to be of fundamental
importance (92,93). This is our conduit of choice for both conduit replacement and primary repair of right ventricle pulmonary artery discontinuity.

Early degeneration of xenograft valves and the high incidence of
thombosis on mechanical valves (94) have made these less desirable conduits. Results with the collagen-sealed, knitted Dacron conduit (Tascon
conduit) have been shown to be unsatisfactory (95). Externally stented
polytetrafluoroethylene conduits are preferable to Dacron conduits because of the accelerated rate of neointima formation in Dacron conduits
(96). Presently, nonvalved conduits are favored to the use of Dacron or
PTFE.

Although extracardiac conduits have dramatically improved the results
of complex cardiac surgery corrections, the ideal conduit has not been
found, and efforts to explore alternative extracardiac conduits should continue.

REFERENCES

1. Verrier ED, Tranbaugh RF, Soifer SJ, Yee ES, Turley K, Ebert PA. Aspirin
    anticoagulation in children with mechanical aortic valves. J Thorac Cardiov-
    asc Surg 1986; 92:1013.
2. Pass HI, Sade RM, Crawford FA, Hohn AR. Cardiac valve prostheses in
    children without anticoagulation. J Thorac Cardiovasc Surg 1984; 87:832.
3. Wheller JJ, Hosier DM, Teske DM, Craenen JM, Kilman JW. Results of
    operation for aortic valve stenosis in infants, children and adolescents. J
    Thorac Cardiovasc Surg 1988; 96:474.
4. Antunes MJ. Bioprosthetic valve replacement in children—long-term follow-
    up of 135 isolated mitral valve implantations. Eur Heart J 1984; 5:913.
5. Schaffer MS, Clarke DR, Campbell DN, Madigan CK, Wiggins JW, Wolfe
    RR. The St. Jude Medical cardiac valve in infants and children: role of antico-
    agulant therapy. J Am Coll Cardiol 1987; 9:235.
6. Odell JA, Mitha AS, Vanker EA, Whitton ID. Experience with tissue and
    mechanical valves in the paediatric age group. In: Rabago G, Cooley DA,

eds. Heart Valve Replacement: Current Status and Future Trends. Futura Publishing Company, Inc., Mount Kisco, NY: Futura, 1987: 185.

7. Harada Y, Imai Y, Kurosawa H, Ishihara K, Kadawa M, Fukuwuchi S. Ten year follow up after valve replacement with the St Jude Medical prosthesis in children. J Thorac Cardiovasc Surg 1990; 100:175.

8. Milano A, Vouche PR, Baillot-Vernant F, et al. Late results after left-sided cardiac valve replacement in children. J Thorac Cardiovasc Surg 1986; 92: 218.

9. Rubino M, Stellin G, Mazzucco A, Bortolotti U, Rizzoli G, Faggian G, Dallento L, Milano A, Guerra F, and Gallucci V. Valve replacement in children; early and late results, Thorac Cardiovasc Surgeon. 1989; 37:42.

10. Smith JM, Cooley DA, Ott DA, Ferreira W, Reul GJ. Aortic valve replacement in preteenage children. Ann Thorac Surg 1979; 29:512.

11. John S, Rankumar E, Jairaj PS, Chowdhury U, Krishnaswami S. Valve replacement in the young patient with rheumatic heart disease, review of a twenty-year experience. J Thorac Cardiovasc Surg 1990;99:631.

12. Vidne B, Levy MJ. Heart valve replacement in children. Thorax 1970; 25: 57.

13. Attie F, Kuri J, Zanoniani C, et al. Mitral valve replacement in children with rheumatic heart disease. Circulation 1981; 64:812.

14. Ilbawi MN, Lockhart, CG, Idriss, FS, et al. Experience with St Jude Medical valve prosthesis in children. A word of caution regarding right-sided replacement. J Thorac Cardiovasc Surg 1987; 93:73.

15. Berry BE, Ritter DG, Wallace RB, McGoon DC, Danielson GK. Cardiac valve replacement in children. J Thorac Cardiovasc Surg 1974; 68:705.

16. Mathews RA, Park SC, Neches WH, et al. Valve replacement in children and adolescents. J Thorac Cardiovasc Surg 1977; 73:872.

17. Williams WG, Pollock JC, Geiss DM, Trusler GA, Fowler RS. Experience with aortic and mitral valve replacement in children. J Thorac Cardiovasc Surg 1981; 81:326.

18. Sade RM, Ballenger JF, Hohn AR, Arrants JE, Riopel DA, Taylor AB. Cardiac valve replacement in children. Comparison of tissue with mechanical prostheses. J Thorac Cardiovasc Surg 1979; 78:123.

19. Kadoba K, Jonas RA, Mayer JE, Castenada AR. Mitral valve replacement in the first year of life. J Thorac Cardiovasc Surg 1990; 100:762.

20. Klint RB, Cox WD, Agustsson MH, Horsley BL. Mitral valve replacement in infancy—a case report. J Thorac Cardiovasc Surg 1976; 72:89.

21. Charaf L, Hallberg M, Henze A. Neonatal endocarditis requiring surgery. Scand J Thorac Cardiovasc Surg 1989; 23:79.

22. Freed MD, Bernard WF. Prosthetic valve replacement in children. Prog Cardiovasc Dis 1975; 17:475.

23. Friedberg CK. Diseases of the Heart. 3d ed. Philadelphia: Saunders, 1966; 1033.

24. Shore DF, De Leval MR, Stark J. Valve replacement in children. In: Cohn LH, Gallucci V, eds. Cardiac Bioprosthesis. Proceedings of the Second International Symposium. New York: York Medical Books, 1982: 238.

25. Friedman S, Edmunds H, Cuaso CC. Long-term mitral valve replacement in young children: influence of somatic growth on prosthetic valve adequacy. Circulation 1978; 57:981.

26. Braunwald E, Braunwald NS, Ross J, Morrow AG. Effects of mitral valve replacement on the pulmonary vascular dynamics of patients with pulmonary hypertension. N Engl J Med 1965; 273:509.

27. Dalen JE, Matloff JM, Evans GL, et al. Early reduction of pulmonary vascular resistance after mitral valve replacement. N Engl J Med 1967; 277:387.

28. Roberts WC, Ferrans JT. Complications of replacement either of the mitral or aortic valve or both by either mechanical or bioprosthetic valves. In: Cohn LH, Callucci V, eds. Cardiac Bioprosthesis. Proceedings of the Second International Symposium. New York: York Medical Books, 1982: 331.

29. Cohn LH. Thromboembolism after cardiac valve replacement. In: Matloff J ed. Cardiac Valve Replacement. Berton: Martinus Nijhoff, 1985: 9.

30. Iyer KS, Reddy KS, Rao IM, Venygopal P, Bhatia MI, Gopinath N. Valve replacement in children under twenty years of age. J Thorac Cardiovasc Surg 1984; 88:217.

31. Sade RM, Crawford FA, Fyfe DA, Stroud MR. Valve prostheses in children: a reassessment of anticoagulation. J Thorac Cardiovasc Surg 1988; 95:553.

32. Gardner BTJ, Roland JMA, Neill CA, Donahoo JS. Valve replacement in children. A fifteen year perspective. J Thorac Cardiovasc Surg 1982; 83:178.

33. Edmunds LH. Thromboembolic complications of current cardiac valvular prosthesis. Ann Thorac Surg 1982; 34:96.

34. E.P.S.I.M. Research Group. A controlled comparison of aspirin and oral anticoagulants in prevention of death after myocardial infarction. N Engl J Med 1982; 307:701.

35. Chesebro JH, Fuster V, Elveback LT, et al. Trial of combined Warfarin plus dipyridamole or aspirin therapy in prosthetic heart valve replacement. Danger of aspirin compared with dipyridamole. Am J Cardiol 1983; 51:1537.

36. Altman R, Boullon F, Rouvier J, Raca R, de la Fuente L, Favaloro R. Aspirin prophylaxis of thromboembolic complication in patients with substitute heart valves. J Thorac Cardiovasc Surg 1980; 29:512.

37. Weintstein GS, Mavroudis C, Ebert PA. Preliminary experience with aspirin for anticoagulation in children with prosthetic cardiac valves. Ann Thorac Surg 1982; 33:549.

38. Verrier ED, Tranbaugh RF, Soifer SJ, Yee ES, Turley K, Ebert PA. Aspirin anticoagulation in children with mechanical aortic valves. J Thorac Cardiovasc Surg 1986; 92:1013.

39. Suschke J, Stehr K, Jacobs E. Measurement of thrombocyte adhesions in children. Klin Paediatr 1973; 185:287.

40. Bradley LM, Midgley FM, Watson DC, Getson PR, Scott LP. Anticoagulation therapy in children with mechanical prosthetic cardiac valves. Am J Cardiol 1985; 56:533.

41. Wada J, Yokoyama M, Hashimoto A, et al. Long term follow-up of artificial valves in patients under 15 years. Ann Thorac Surg 1980; 29:519.

42. Hurwitz ED, Barrett MJ, Bregman D, et al. Public Health Service Study on Reye's syndrome and medications. Reports of the pilot phase. N Engl J Med 1985; 313:849.
43. Schaff HV, Danielson GK, DiDonato RM, Puga FJ, Mair DD, McGoon DC. Late results after Starr-Edwards valve replacement in children. J Thorac Cardiovasc Surg 1984; 88:583.
44. Rufilanchas JJ, Juffe A, Miranda AL, et al. Cardiac valve replacement with the Bjork-Shiley prosthesis in young patients. Scand J Thorac Cardiovasc Surg 1977; 11:11.
45. Cohn LH. Thromboembolism in different anatomical positions: aortic, mitral and multiple valves. In: Rabago G, Cooley DA, eds. Heart Valve Replacement: Current States and Future Trends. Mount Kisco, NY: Futura, 1987: 259.
46. Bland EF, Jones TD. Rheumatic fever and rheumatic heart disease. Circulation 1951; 4:836.
47. Edwards JE, Burchell HB. Endocardial and mitral lesions (jet impact) at possible sites of origin of murmur. Circulation 1958; 18:946.
48. Castle RE, Baylin GJ. Severe acquired mitral stenosis in childhood and adolescence. J Paediatr 1961; 58:404.
49. Walsh BJ, Bland EF, Jones TD. Pure mitral stenosis in young persons. Ach. Intern Med 1940; 65:321.
50. Marcus RH, Sareli PU, Pocock WA, et al. Functional anatomy of severe mitral regurgitation in active rheumatic carditis. Ann J Cardiol 1989; 63:577.
51. Antunnes MJ. Mitral Valve Repair. Germany: Schulz, 1989: 129.
52. Al Kasab S, Al Fagih MR, Shahid M, Habbib H, Zaibag MA. Valve surgery in acute rheumatic heart disease. One to four year follow-up. Chest 1988; 94:830.
53. Abbruzzese P, Livermore J, Sunderland CO, et al. Mitral repair in complete atrioventricular canal. J Thorac Cardiovasc Surg 1982; 83:670.
54. Williams WH, Guyton RA, Michalik RE, et al. Individualized surgical management of complete atrioventricular canal. J Thorac Cardiovasc Surg 1981; 81:615.
55. Thiene G, Mazzucco A, Grisolia EF, et al. Post-operative pathology of complete atrioventricular defects. J Thorac Cardiovasc Surg 1982; 83:891.
56. Ankeney L, Tzeng TA, Liebman J. Surgical therapy for congenital aortic valvular stenosis. J Thorac Cardiovasc Surg 1983; 85:41.
57. Presbitero P, Somerville J, Revel-Chion R, et al. Open aortic valvotomy for congenital aortic stenosis: late results. Br Heart J 1982; 47:26.
58. Reid JM, Coleman ED. The management of congenital aortic stenosis. Thorax 1982; 37:902.
59. Sandor GGS, Olley PM, Trusler GA, et al. Long-term follow-up of patients after valvotomy for congenital valvular aortic stenosis in children: a clinical and actuarial follow-up. J Thorac Cardiovasc Surg 1980; 80:171.
60. Konno S, Yasubaru I, Yoshinao I. A new method for prosthetic valve replacement in congenital aortic stenosis associated with hypoplasia of the aortic valve. J Thorac Cardiovasc Surg 1975; 70:909.

61. Misbach GA, Turley K, Ullyot DJ, et al. Left ventricular outflow enlargement by the Kono procedure. J Thorac Cardiovasc Surg 1982; 84:696.
62. Fleming WH, Sarafian LB. Aortic valve replacement with concomitant aortoventriculoplasty in children and young adults: long-term follow-up. Ann Thorac Surg 1987; 43:575.
63. Nicks R, Cartwill T, Bernstein L. Hypoplasia of the aortic root. Thorax 1970; 25:339.
64. Blank RH, Pupello DF, Bessone LN, Harrison EE, Sbar S. Method of managing the small aortic annulus during valve replacement. Ann Thorac Surg 1976; 22:356.
65. Manouguian S, Seyhold-Epting W. Patch enlargement of the aortic ring by extending the aortic incision into the anterior mitral leaflet. J Thorac Cardiovasc Surg 1979; 78:402.
66. Sweeney MS, Walker WE, Cooley DA, Reul GJ. Apico-aortic conduits for complex left ventricular outflow obstruction: 10-year experience. Ann Thorac Surg 1986; 42:609.
67. Chachques TC, Acar C, Fontaliran F, Ponzio O, Bilweis J, Carpentier A. Absorbable rings for paediatric valvuloplasty. Circulation 1989; 80(suppl II): 11.
68. Ilbawi MD, Lockhart CG, Idriss FS, et al. Experience with St Jude medical valve prosthesis in children: a word of caution regarding right-sided placement. J Thorac Cardiovasc Surg 1987; 93:73.
69. Fleming WH, Sarafian LB, Moulton AL, Robinson LA, Kugler JD. Valve replacement in the right side of the heart in children: long-term follow up. Ann Thorac Surg 1989; 48:404.
70. Magilligan DJ, Lewis JA, Heinzerling RH, et al. Fate of a second porcine bioprosthetic valve. J Thorac Cardiovasc Surg 1983; 85:362.
71. Arbustini E, Jones M, Moses RD, et al. Modification of Hancock T6 process of calcification of bioprosthetic cardiac valves implanted in sheep. Am J Cardiol 1984; 63:1388.
72. Williams M. The intact bioprosthesis: the first 4 years. Ann Thorac Surg 1989; 48:587.
73. Deviri E, Levinsky L, Schachner A, Nili M, Levy MJ. Thromboembolism and anticoagulant treatment in patients with heart valve prostheses. In: Rabago G, Cooley DA, eds. Heart Valve Replacement. Mount Kisco, NY: Futura, 1987: 285.
74. Williams M. Personal communication.
75. Bortolotti U, Milano A, Mazzucco A, et al. Pregnancy in patients with a porcine valve bioprosthesis. Am J Cardiol 1982; 50:1051.
76. Foster AH, Tracy CM, Greenberg GJ, McIntosh CL, Clark RE. Valve replacement in narrow aortic roots: serial hemodynamics and long-term clinical outcome. Ann Thorac Surg 1986; 42:506.
77. Imamura E, Tomizawa Y, Hashimoto A, Koyanagi H, Imai Y, Matsumura K. A comparative analysis of left ventriculography and root aortography for estimating aortic annular size. J Thorac Cardiovasc Surg 1987; 93:592.

78. Sud A, Magilligan DJ. Anatomy of the aortic root. Ann Thorac Surg 1984; 38:76.

79. Manouguian S, Kirchoff PG. Patch enlargement of the aortic ring and mitral valve rings with aortic-mitral double-valve replacement. Ann Thorac Surg 1980; 30:396.

80. Rastan H, Atai M, Hadi H, Yazdanyar A. Enlargement of mitral valvular ring: new technique for double valve replacement in children or adults with small mitral annulus. J Thorac Cardiovasc Surg 1981; 81:106.

81. Kinsley RH, Antunes MJ, McKibbin JK. Enlargement of the narrow aortic root and oblique insertion of the St Jude prosthesis. Br Heart J 1983; 50: 330.

82. Brown JW, Stevens LS, Holly S, et al. Surgical spectrum of aortic stenosis in children: a thirty-year experience with 257 children. Ann Thorac Surg 1988; 45:393.

83. Mazzera E, Corno A, Didonata R, et al. Surgical bypass of the systemic atrioventricular valve in children by means of a valved conduit. J Thorac Cardiovasc Surg 1988; 96:321.

84. Corno A, Giannico S, Leibovich S, Mazzera E, Marcelletti C. The hypoplastic mitral valve—when should a Left atrial–left ventricular extracardiac valved conduit be used? J Thorac Cardiovasc Surg 1986; 91:848.

85. Laks H, Hellenbrand WE, Kleinman C, et al. Left atrial-left ventricular conduit for relief of congenital mitral stenosis in infancy. J Thorac Cardiovasc Surg 1980; 80:782.

86. Lansing AM, Elbl F, Solinger RE, et al. Left atrial-left ventricular bypass for congenital mitral stenosis. Ann Thorac Surg 1983; 35:667.

87. Wright JS, Thomson DS, Warner G. Mitral valve bypass by valved conduit. Ann Thorac Surg 1981; 32:294.

88. Gandjbakhch I, Lascar M, Pavie A, Cabrol C, Intra-atrial insertion of a prosthetic mitral valve. J Cardiovasc Surg (Torino) 1988; 29:113.

89. Almeida RS, Elliot MJ, Robinson PJ, et al. Surgery for congenital abnormalities of the mitral valve at the Hospital for Sick Children, London, from 1969–1983. J Cardiovasc Surg (Torino) 1988; 29:95.

90. Ross DN, Somerville J. Correction of pulmonary atresia with a homograft aortic valve. Lancet 1966; 2:1446.

91. Bowman FO, Griffiths SP. Twenty-two years follow-up of an aortic homograft implanted for pulmonary atresia: report of a case. J Thorac Cardiovasc Surg 1989; 98:636.

92. Turley K, Ebert PA. Aortic allografts: reconstruction of right ventricle–pulmonary artery continuity. Ann Thorac Surg 1989; 47:278.

93. Bull C, Macartney FJ, Harvath P, et al. Evaluation of long-term results of homograft and heterograft valves in extracardiac conduits. J Thorac Cardiovasc Surg 1987; 94:12.

94. Ilbawi MN, Lockhart CG, Idriss FS, et al. Experiences with St Jude Medical valve prosthesis in children. A word of caution regarding right-sided placement. J Thorac Cardiovasc Surg 1987; 93:73.

95. Jonas RA, Mayer JE, Castaneda AR. Unsatisfactory clinical experience with a collagen-sealed knitted dacron extracardiac conduit. J Card Surg 1987; 2: 257.
96. Brown JW, Halpin MP, Rescorla FJ, et al. Externally stented polytetrafluoroethylene valved conduits for right heart reconstruction. J Thorac Cardiovasc Surg 1985; 90:833.

21

Valve Surgery in the Elderly

Dennis F. Pupello
St. Joseph's Heart Institute, Tampa, Florida

I. INTRODUCTION

The number of elderly individuals is growing at an unprecedented rate. It is projected that by the year 2030, 22% of the population will be 65 years of age or older (1). Moreover, the number of individuals over 65 is growing faster than the rest of the population. This is a worldwide trend (Fig. 1). Health care for the elderly is, therefore, of utmost importance as one considers the enormous economic impact of providing services for this rapidly expanding segment of our society.

In the United States, the cost of providing health care for the elderly is rising at a rate of approximately 10% per year and exceeds by far the overall inflation rate. Our projected outlay for health-care cost in 1992 is $750 billion. This figure exceeds our annual expenditure for defense (2).

Diseases of the heart represent the most common cause of death for those aged 65 years of age or above. It leads to approximately 50% of all deaths, a rate twice that of the second leading cause, which is malignant neoplasm (3). Cardiac valve pathology represents a significant proportion of this statistic.

Cardiac valve surgery in the elderly thus becomes increasingly important as more patients are reaching advanced age and more are remaining active and demanding an enhanced level of health care. In observing this trend, it is of particular interest to focus on those 85 years of age and older, recently termed the "oldest-old." This group of individuals represents one of the most rapidly growing segments of our population. While the total

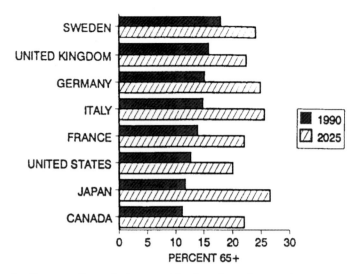

Figure 1   Percent of population age 65+ in selected countries: 1990 and 2025.
(*Source:* U.S. Bureau of the Census. International Data Base.)

U.S. population increased 26% between 1960 and 1980, those aged 85 and above increased by 126% (4).

Our goal in treating valvular lesions in the elderly has been to improve the patients' quality of life in their remaining years and to reduce or minimize the period of senescence near the end of the life cycle. There exists a wealth of data in the literature, in addition to our own experience, documenting acceptable morbidity and mortality for valve surgery in the elderly (5,6). Moreover, there is substantial evidence to support a significant improvement in the patients' quality of life (7,8).

II. AGE-RELATED ALTERATIONS IN PHYSIOLOGY AND ANATOMY

To understand the perioperative management of elderly patients undergoing cardiac valve surgery, one must grasp and appreciate the concept of homeostatic fragility in the elderly. Aging, per se, is accompanied by multiple alterations in the body's physiological function that impede the efficiency or efficacy of the homeostatic regulatory mechanism (9). While day-to-day activities may be only minimally affected, these changes lead to decreased functional reserve in the elderly. As a result, the individual's ability to respond to stress is compromised.

A. Aging and Ventilation

It is well accepted that arterial oxygen tension declines with age in healthy subjects. There is a progressive ventilation–perfusion mismatch. Vital capacity, FEV-1, peak expiratory flow rates, etc., all show an age-dependent decline. Stiffening of the chest wall, weakening of the respiratory muscles, and a decline in pulmonary elastic recoil have all been documented with the aging process (10).

B. Aging and Cardiac Reserve

The rate of diastolic filling in subjects 65 to 80 years of age is approximately 50% of that measured in normal 25- to 45-year-old subjects (11). This is a consequence of the progressive stiffening of the left ventricle with age. The ability to squeeze, however, does not appear to be impaired, although systolic contraction time is increased. With age, the maximum heart rate response to exercise declines. This may be related to the reduced number of beta-adrenergic receptors in the myocardium.

In spite of these physiological changes, the aging human heart can maintain cardiac output by changes in stroke volume, even when a rate increase cannot be achieved. Overall, the aging healthy heart has remarkable functional reserve and is in general not responsible for serious impairment of the homeostatic regulatory mechanism.

C. Aging and Renal Function

Renal physiology is markedly modified as a result of the aging process. Renal blood flow declines with age and may be associated with a reduction in the total number of nephrons. As a result, a gradual decrease in the creatinine clearance occurs. With this decline, the elderly patient is acutely sensitive to changes in plasma volume and to medications with established nephrotoxicity (12).

III. SURGICAL CONSIDERATIONS

As in neonatal cardiac surgery, elderly patients undergoing valve repair or replacement leave little margin for error. Extreme blood pressure fluctuations during induction of anesthesia must be avoided, as patterns of cerebral blood flow are exquisitely sensitive in the elderly. Prolonged operating times while utilizing the pump oxygenator should also be avoided, as elderly patients are more susceptible to the typical derangements in the clotting process caused by cardiopulmonary bypass. In addition, it has been demonstrated that both major arteries and arterioles have less elastic recoil and may bleed excessively. This is especially true in patients undergoing reoperation.

In our experience, we have seen a correlation between excessive oozing postoperatively and core temperatures below 26°C for prolonged periods. This seems to accentuate the pronounced negative effect on the clotting process already produced by the pump oxygenator. Prolonged periods of nonpulsatile flow, coupled with moderate hemodilution, may enhance edema of the alveolar-capillary membrane in the lung. This may increase the chance of a patient suffering an adult respiratory distress syndrome postoperatively. Thus, when complex procedures are encountered and long cardiopulmonary bypass times are anticipated, one should utilize a membrane oxygenator combined with pulsatile flow to minimize the occurrence of these complications.

A. Aortic Stenosis

Aortic stenosis is the most common valvular lesion found in the aged. It is present without symptoms in about 4% of the elderly population (13). Aortic sclerosis, on the other hand, manifested by mild thickening and fibrosis of the valve without significant gradient, is found in approximately 33–50% of all elderly patients; about 20% is rheumatic in origin. In our experience, approximately 50% of elderly patients undergoing aortic valve replacement have a bicuspid aortic valve.

The natural history of severe aortic stenosis is well documented (14). Patients who present with angina have a survival time of approximately 5 years, while those with dyspnea have a grave prognosis. The average survival time for this group of patients is approximately 2 years, and those who present with syncope survive somewhere between 3 and 4 years. Aggressive surgical management is warranted in virtually all patients presenting with severe symptomatic aortic stenosis. Long-term surgical results to date have been excellent (15,16). Moreover, aortic valve replacement in elderly patients is associated not only with improved survival, but with an enhanced quality of life.

Sudden death occurs in 3–5% of asymptomatic patients with aortic stenosis and is usually the result of a malignant arrhythmia. The predominant presenting symptoms include: (1) congestive heart failure, (2) angina with effort, and (3) effort syncope. About one-half of all elderly patients with severe aortic stenosis will develop congestive heart failure, which is usually precipitated by the development of atrial fibrillation. Aortic stenosis is one of the most common causes of syncope in the elderly.

Surgical indications for elderly patients with aortic stenosis include: (1) asymptomatic and symptomatic patients with systolic gradients above

50 mmHg, (2) symptomatic patients with increased heart size or left ventricular mass, (3) symptomatic patients with decrease in their ejection fraction, and (4) patients with a valve orifice of less than 1 cm^2 with symptoms.

The collective surgical mortality for isolated aortic valve replacement is approximately 2% when associated with concomitant coronary artery disease and myocardial revascularization, the mortality ranges from 4% to 6%. If congestive heart failure is present at the time of surgery, the mortality rate rises significantly (to 8-10%). There is a wealth of data that suggest that even after the onset of heart failure, aortic valve replacement in class III and IV elderly patients can be performed with a 10% mortality or less, even if there is evidence of severe impairment of left ventricular function (17).

In recent studies (8,18-20), the 5-year survival rate following isolated aortic valve replacement in the elderly has been approximately 70%. Moreover, these patients have achieved an improved quality of life, which allows them to carry out their activities of daily living independently.

Our surgical experience with elderly patients with isolated aortic valve replacement with a mean age of 75.7 years reveals a hospital mortality of 8%. The 10-year survival of 54.5 ± 5.1% standard error of the mean (SEM) for this group closely parallels that of the normal population corrected for age and sex (Fig. 2). The immediate relief of symptoms and return to

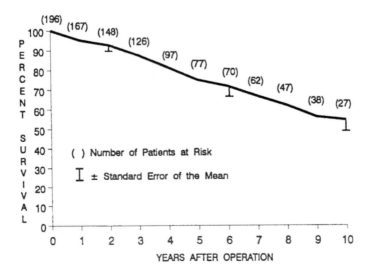

Figure 2 Actuarial survival of aortic stenosis patients 70 years of age and over with valve replacement discharged from the hospital.

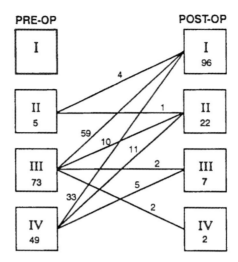

Figure 3 Preoperative and postoperative New York Heart Association functional class of patients 70 years of age and over with valve replacement for aortic stenosis.

an active lifestyle are often dramatic in patients who do not have other complicating chronic illnesses. In this series, 96.1% of the patients were in functional class III or IV preoperatively and at the completion of the current follow-up, 96.7% were in either class I or II (Fig. 3).

B. Aortic Insufficiency

Aortic insufficiency represents the most common diastolic murmur found in elderly patients. Estologies in the past were related to rheumatic fever and syphilis; however, these findings are now decreasing. Presently, connective tissue disorders, anatomic abnormalities, acute aortic dissection, endocarditis, ankylosing spondylitis, and cystic medial necrosis are the most common etiologies of aortic regurgitant lesions (21). Volume overload lesions are usually well tolerated by the left ventricle, even though the heart may be enormous in size. This entity is portrayed usually by electrocardiographic evidence of left ventricular hypertrophy, cardiomegaly on chest X-ray, a hyperactive precordium with a rocking motion, and bounding peripheral pulses with documented wide pulse pressure. The frequently associated systolic murmur is secondary to increase flow along the aortic outflow tract.

It is well recognized that 75% of patients with chronic aortic insufficiency will survive 5 years, and approximately 50% will survive 10 years with medical treatment. If congestive heart failure occurs, 50% are dead within 2 years. Systolic blood pressure above 140 or a diastolic reading of less than 40 is associated with a high risk of death within the ensuing 3 to 6 years, even in asymptomatic patients (13).

Generally, fatigue, dyspnea, and orthopnea are all late symptoms of patients with aortic insufficiency. Although surgical results in patients with chronic aortic insufficiency are not as dramatic as those seen in individuals with severe aortic stenosis, they are acceptable. Perhaps the deleterious effect of long-term volume overloading of the left ventricle and chronic dilatation of this chamber before the patient becomes symptomatic may interfere with obtaining better long-term results. Increasing left ventricular dimensions and decrease of left ventricular ejection fraction with exercise are hallmarks of left ventricular damage. Acute aortic regurgitation as a result of either endocarditis or aortic dissection carries a high operative mortality (22).

Surgical indications for elderly patients with aortic insufficiency include those with: (1) symptomatic chronic aortic insufficiency, (2) asymptomatic aortic regurgitation with left ventricular dysfunction at rest (a systolic volume index of greater than 60 cm^3/m^2), and (3) the inability to increase their ejection fraction with exercise. Surgical mortality of patients with chronic aortic insufficiency and normal coronaries ranges from 1.5% to 2%. If congestive heart failure develops or the patient has associated coronary artery disease, the operative mortality rises abruptly to 5% to 12%.

C. Mitral Stenosis

Historically, the most common etiology for mitral valve disease in the elderly has been rheumatic. However, this is rapidly changing as a result of the declining incidence of rheumatic fever and the increased incidence of mitral valve dysfunction secondary to coronary artery disease.

Clinically, the patient presents well into the long history of mitral valve disease because of the slow, gradual, insidious onset of the stenotic process. Slight changes in daily exercise tolerance or a general decrease in endurance are often difficult to appreciate. In most cases, the onset of atrial fibrillation is what brings the clinical deterioration to the attention of the physician. There is usually a loud S-1, and a diastolic rumble is almost always present. Moreover, the patient will generally have an opening snap. Atrial fibrillation in long-standing mitral valve disease is common, as is systemic arterial embolization. The patient's chest X-ray usually shows left atrial enlargement with increased pulmonary venous vascular markings.

About one-third of all elderly patients with mitral valve disease have mitral stenosis as a result of rheumatic fever. Approximately 50% of elderly patients with mitral valve disease have an associated aortic valve lesion (13). In our surgical experience with 180 consecutive cases of patients 70 years of age and over undergoing mitral valve replacement, 44 had concomitant aortic valve replacement.

D. Chronic Mitral Regurgitation

Regurgitant lesions account for approximately two-thirds of mitral valve disease in elderly patients (13). Papillary muscle dysfunction following myocardial infarction is the most common nonrheumatic etiology. Commonly, atrial fibrillation and associated congestive heart failure are also present. When mitral regurgitation is present, approximately 40% of the patients have congestive heart failure. Mitral valve replacement in this group of patients is usually far less rewarding than aortic valve surgery because of commonly associated left ventricular dysfunction and, frequently, the need for long-term oral anticoagulation (23).

E. Acute Mitral Regurgitation

The most common cause for acute mitral regurgitation in the aged patient is chordal rupture with secondary inadequate leaflet coaptation. This may be secondary to a myocardial infarction, papillary muscle rupture, infective endocarditis, or myxomatous degeneration of the mitral valve cusps. Valve replacement in these types of cases may be a life-saving maneuver. Often, balloon counterpulsation is necessary to support patients during cardiac catheterization and also to wean them from cardiopulmonary bypass when significant damage to the left ventricle has occurred.

Mitral valve prolapse in the elderly is frequently found secondary to myxomatous degeneration. Chordal rupture often results in life-threatening decompensation. Myxomatous degeneration with elongation of chordae increases with age and is often the cause of death in patients presenting with acute mitral regurgitation (24). Emergency surgery under these conditions carries an increased mortality in the elderly. In our experience, the mortality for acute mitral regurgitation as a result of a primary chordal or papillary head rupture has been approximately 28%.

Surgical results with mitral valve replacement in the elderly are less predictable than with aortic valve surgery. The overall operative mortality is higher than that found in aortic valve replacement. When this procedure is combined with coronary revascularization, there is an even further increase in the operative mortality. We are convinced that preserving the posterior leaflet reduces the incidence of A-V groove injury or disruption and may avoid the deleterious effects of the untethered left ventricle.

Our surgical technique in the elderly employs moderate systemic hypothermia (28°C), cold crystalloid cardioplegia for myocardial preservation, and cardiopulmonary bypass employing a membrane oxygenator with relatively low flow rates (35–50 cm³/kg).

F. Selection of a Valve for the Elderly

Although there have been tremendous advances in the design and materials of cardiac prostheses, the search for a more ideal valve continues. Dwight Harkin outlined the optimal criteria for a prosthetic valve (25). These have been recently updated by Bonchek and include: (1) adequate hydraulic characteristics in the normal anatomic position, (2) durable, (3) free of thrombotic problems and require no anticoagulation, (4) biocompatible, nontraumatic to red blood cells or plasma proteins, (5) easy to implant, and (6) silent (26).

Clearly, the ideal valve substitute for all patients has not yet been devised. Mechanical valves offer known durability and predictable performance; however, they require oral anticoagulation indefinitely, and the incidence of systemic embolization has been found to be significant.

Mitral valve repair using standard techniques with ring support, as originally described by Carpentier (27) and Duran and Umbago (28), offer an attractive alternative for patients with nonrheumatic mitral valve disease. This is the treatment of choice and should be attempted in all cases of isolated, noncalcified, mitral valve disease. In younger patients the need for repair, rather than replacement, becomes even more pressing.

When elderly patients present with extensive coronary artery disease requiring concomitant coronary revascularization, controversy exists as to how to best manage these coexisting conditions. The additional ischemic time to complete a repair in this setting may compromise the results. In addition, there is convincing evidence to use the bioprosthesis in this situation because of its superb long-term results.

Bioprosthetic valves offer freedom from anticoagulation for most patients (two-thirds of the patients 70 and over in our series), a very low incidence of thromboembolism, even without anticoagulation, and excellent hemodynamics in the larger sizes. In general, we do not recommend implantation of a bioprosthesis less than 23 mm when the body surface area is greater than 1.7 m². Other alternatives, such as using a homograft or enlarging the aortic annulus, may be necessary. In our experience, each incremental enlargement in valve size increases the cross-sectional area by approximately 20% (29).

The quality of life and expectation for long-term survival with the bioprosthesis in elderly patients exceeds that of mechanical prostheses.

There is a lower rate of thromboembolism and anticoagulant-related hemorrhages, and this results in reduced morbidity and enhanced quality of
life (5). Though valve selection involves a complex process, in our experience the bioprosthesisis the valve of choice for elderly patients (30) and
has been found often to outlive the patient (31).

IV. CLOSING THOUGHTS ON VALVE SURGERY IN THE ELDERLY

Valve surgery in the elderly is a technically demanding procedure. Often,
patients present with reduced left ventricular function, in severe congestive heart failure, and with multiple lesions. The brittle physiology of these
patients requires skilled hands in the operating room, close monitoring,
and precise management of preload, afterload, and myocardial performance in the immediate postoperative period. As a result, there is little
margin for error in this group of patients.

Usually, the surgeon has one opportunity to complete a procedure correctly. Elderly patients are less forgiving; they have compromised myocardial reserve and decreased recuperative powers. One must avoid extremes
of blood pressure fluctuation during induction of anesthesia, avoid prolonged runs on cardiopulmonary bypass, and exercise meticulous attention to detail in the operating room. A recent report showed that in patients
75 years of age and over requiring reoperation to control postoperative
hemorrhage, the hospital mortality tripled (32).

In addition, the tendency for postoperative inertia in the elderly must
be avoided. Early mobilization and other simple prophylactic measures,
such as frequent dorsiflexion of the feet and avoidance of prolonged periods of sitting, preclude the hazards of deep vein thrombosis. The early
initiation of a well-planned cardiac rehabilitation program is essential.

Contraindications to valve surgery in the elderly include: (1) severe
intercurrent disease, (2) physiological abnormalities that increase the risk
so as to preclude a successful outcome, and (3) mental deterioration or
dementia. Chronological age alone cannot be considered a deterrent to
valve surgery in the elderly. In our experience with 104 consecutive cases
of octogenarians with a mean age of 82.4 years, there was a hospital mortality of 13.5%. The long-term survival at 6 years for the hospital survivors
was 54.6 ± 7.7% SEM (Fig. 4). Moreover, these patients experienced an
increased level of functional capacity and an enhanced quality of life. A
significant number have remained active and independent and able to
carry out their activities of daily living with little or no assistance. These

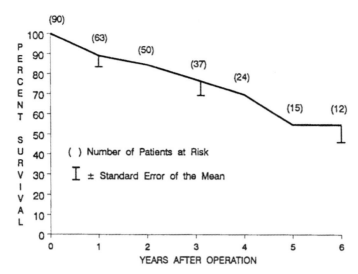

Figure 4 Actuarial survival of valve replacement patients 80 years of age and over discharged from the hospital.

results provide further evidence that age alone cannot be considered a contraindication to valve surgery in the elderly.

Further, the long-term favorable results illustrated by Bessone et al. (18) following valve replacement in the elderly provide a much-needed reference point when alternative therapy, such as aortic balloon valvotomy, is being considered. The controversial results of this experimental method must be used to temper the almost unbridled enthusiasm demonstrated by some authors following the initial report of Cribier and associates in 1986 (33). In addition, the definition of "poor surgical risk" or "inoperable" must be carefully evaluated to avoid denying appropriate surgical treatment to patients who would benefit from valve replacement. Fortunately, the limited benefits of aortic balloon valvuloplasty were put into proper perspective by Francis Robicsek, who, using direct measurements in the operating theater under direct vision, showed no benefit from aortic balloon dilatation (34).

Because of the favorable results of valve replacement in the elderly, advanced age, compromised cardiovascular status, and marginal cardiac reserve should not be viewed as contraindications to valve surgery in this group of patients. Our attention in valve surgery in the elderly has always focused on physiological age rather than chronological age. Our overall goal has always been to enhance the patient's quality of life, rather than the quantity of life.

ACKNOWLEDGMENT

The author wishes to recognize Dr. George Ebra for his excellent technical assistance in the preparation of this work, and Ms. Marilyn Mitchell for typing the manuscript and graphics work.

REFERENCES

1. Aging in America: Trends and Projections. Washington, DC: U.S. Senate Special Committee on Aging, 1991.
2. McKell TE. Under pressure. J Fla Med Assoc 1991; 78(10).
3. Guralnik JM, Fitzsimmons SC. Aging in America: a demographic perspective. Cardiol Clin 1986; 4(2).
4. Suzman R, Riley MW. Introducing the oldest old. Milbank Mem Fund 1985; 63:177–86.
5. Jamieson WRE, Burr LH, Allen P, et al. Quality of life afforded by porcine bioprosthesis. In Rabago G, Cooley DA, eds. Heart Valve Replacement: Current Status and Future Trends. Mount Kisco, NY: Futura, 1987: 225–43.
6. Pupello DF, Bessone LN, Hiro SP, et al. The Carpentier-Edwards bioprosthesis: a comparative study analyzing failure rates by age. J Cardiac Surg 1988; 3(suppl): 369–74.
7. Stephenson LW, MacVaugh H, Edmunds LH. Surgery using cardiopulmonary bypass in the elderly. Circulation 1978; 58:250–4.
8. Arom KV, Nicoloff DM, Linsay WG, et al. Should valve replacement and related procedures be performed in elderly patients? Ann Thorac Surg 1984; 38:466–72.
9. Naftali S, Tuck ML. Homeostatic fragility in the elderly. Cardiol Clin 1986; 4(2):201–12.
10. Holland J, Milic-Emili J, Macklem PT, et al. Regional distribution of pulmonary ventilation and perfusion in elderly subjects. J Clin Invest 1968; 47: 81–92.
11. Gerstenblith G, Fredericksen J, Yin FC, et al. Echocardiographic assessment of a normal adult aging population. Circulation 1977; 56:273–8.
12. Rowe JW, Andres RA, Tobin J, et al. The effect of age on creatinine clearance in man: a cross section and longitudinal study. J Gerontol 1976; 31: 155–63.
13. Wenger NK. Valvular heart disease in the elderly. Cardiol Clin 1986; 4(2): 263–71.
14. Chizner MA, Pearle DL, DeLeon, AC Jr. The natural history of aortic stenosis in adults. Am Heart J 1980; 99:419–24.

15. Cohn LH. The long term results of aortic valve replacement. Chest 1984; 85:387–96.

16. Bessone LN, Pupello DF, Blank RH, et al. Valve replacement in the elderly: a long term appraisal. J Cardiovasc Surg (Torino) 1985; 25:417–25.

17. Smith N, McAnulty JH, Rahimtoola SH. Severe aortic stenosis with impaired left ventricular function and clinical heart failure. Results of valve replacement. Circulation 1978; 58:255–64.

18. Bessone LN, Pupello DF, Hiro SP, et al. Surgical management of aortic valve disease in the elderly: a longitudinal analysis. Ann Thorac Surg 1988; 46:264–9.

19. Copeland JG, Griepp RB, Stinson EB, et al. Isolated aortic valve replacement in patients older than 65 years. JAMA 1977; 237:1578–81.

20. Craver JM, Goldstein J, Jones EL, et al. Clinical hemodynamic and operative descriptors affecting outcome of aortic valve replacement in elderly versus young patients. Ann Surg 1984; 199:733–41.

21. Wong M, Tei C, Shah PM. Degenerative calcific valvular disease and systolic murmurs in the elderly. J Am Geriatric Soc 1983; 31:156–63.

22. Canepa-Anson R, Emanuel RW. Elective aortic and mitral valve surgery in patients over 70 years of age. Br Heart J 1979; 41:493–7.

23. Jamieson, WRE, Dooner J, Monro AI, et al. Cardiac valve replacement in the elderly: a review of 320 consecutive cases. Circulation 1981; 64:II-177–83.

24. Pomerance A. Cardiac Pathology and systolic murmurs in the elderly. Br Heart 1968; 30:687–9.

25. Harken DE. I. A new caged-ball aortic and mitral valve and II. Monitoring and controlled respiration in critically ill patients. Mt Sinai Hosp New York 1965; 32:93–106.

26. Bonchek LI. The basis for selecting a valve prosthesis: cardiac surgery. Cardiovasc Clin 1982; 12(3).

27. Carpentier A. La valvuloplastie reconstitutive, une nouvelle technique de valvuloplastie mitrale. Presse Med 1969; 77:251–53.

28. Duran CMG, Umbago JLM. Clinical and hemodynamic performance of a totally flexible prosthetic ring for atrioventricular valve reconstruction. Ann Thorac Surg 1976: 22(5):458–63.

29. Pupello DF, Blank RH. Valve replacement in the small aortic annulus. In: Roberts AJ, ed. Difficult Problems in Adult Cardiac Surgery. Chicago: Year Book, 1985: 219–7.

30. Pupello DF, Bessone LN, Hiro SP, et al. Bioprosthetic valve durability in the elderly: the second decade. J Card Surg 1991; 6(4)(suppl): 575–9.

31. Jones EL, Weintraub WS, Craver JM, et al. Ten-year experience with the porcine bioprosthetic valve: interrelationship of valve survival and patient survival in 1,050 valve replacements. Ann Thorac Surg 1990; 49:370–84.

32. Paton BC. Review of the indications for coronary artery surgery: 7th Annual Cardiovascular Conference at Hawaii. Am Coll Cardiology, Feb 10–14, 1992.

33. Cribier A, Saovdi N, Berland J, et al. Perutaneous transluminal valvuloplasty of aquired aortic stenosis in elderly patients. Lancet 1986; 63–7.
34. Robicsek F, Harbold NB. Limited value of balloon dilatation in calcified aortic stenosis in adults: direct observations during open heart surgery. Am J Cardiol 1987; 60:857–64.

22

Thromboembolic and Bleeding Complications of Prosthetic Heart Valves

L. Henry Edmunds, Jr.
University of Pennsylvania, Philadelphia, Pennsylvania

I. INTRODUCTION

With the possible exception of free aortic homografts, all prosthetic heart valves are thrombogenic. All activate the coagulation system, but propensity to form thrombi or emboli varies among valves and, to a lesser extent, between the aortic and mitral positions (1). Many variables affect the thrombogenicity of prosthetic heart valves and also the bleeding complications that result from anticoagulation. In normal patients without prosthetic heart valves, blood circulates in a distribution system that is exclusively and universally lined with endothelial cells. Endothelial cells are the only known nonthrombogenic surface and maintain the fluidity of blood by active metabolic processes. Normally there is a dynamic equilibrium between forces initiating and forces inhibiting clotting. In patients with prosthetic heart valves, this dynamic equilibrium is tilted toward thrombosis.

Emboli, thrombi, and bleeding remain the most frequent complications of prosthetic heart valves (1). Thrombotic and bleeding complications represent approximately 50% of all complications in patients with aortic bioprostheses and nearly 75% in patients with aortic mechanical prostheses. For mitral bioprostheses, about 55% of complications are thromboembolic or bleeding; for mitral mechanical prostheses, 67%. Aside from transient platelet emboli and rare instances, free aortic homografts do not cause thromboembolic complications. Thromboembolism and bleeding represent approximately one-third of the complications associated with mitral valve repair (2).

This chapter reviews the subject of thromboembolism and bleeding associated with prosthetic heart valves and to some extent updates my more comprehensive treatise published in 1987 (1).

Pathogenesis: There are no synthetic nonthrombogenic materials; there are some materials which seem to activate the coagulation system more slowly than others (3). These materials are called *thromboresistant* and include inert metallic alloys, pyrolytic carbons, certain segmented polyurethanes, copolymers of polydimethyl siloxane, acrylates and methacrylates, and a few others. The chemical and physical characteristics of thromboresistant materials have not been defined; thromboresistance of any given material must be determined empirically.

Obviously, thromboresistant materials are preferred for prosthetic heart valves, but other manufacturing considerations such as casting or milling properties, hardness, durability, etc., are also important. Hydrogels are not suitable for prosthetic heart valves. Rough surfaces, narrow flow paths, areas of stagnant flow or cavitation, turbulence, and large surface areas are design features that enhance thrombosis. The sewing ring, its relationship with the valve annulus, and the flow patterns around this interface are particularly important early after implantation, before "endothelization" occurs. Smooth surfaces, central flow, minimal turbulence, and the absence of stagnant flow areas are features of successful mechanical heart valves.

The reduced thrombogenicity of bioprosthetic valves is probably related more to central flow, flexible leaflets, and absence of stagnant flow areas and turbulence than to the thromboresistance of chemically preserved, nonviable tissue. Although the question of viable tissue within nutrient or cryopreserved free aortic homografts continues, viability is more likely related to durability than to thrombogenicity. The absence of a sewing ring better explains the low incidence of thromboembolism in patients with these prostheses (4,5).

All prosthetic valves activate factor XII (Hageman factor) and platelets. Factor XII is one of four primary proteins of the contact activation system, and in the presence of the other three proteins is cleaved into two active fragments by contact with nonendothelial cell surfaces. One of these fragments, factor XIIa, activates the coagulation cascade via the intrinsic coagulation pathway. Thrombin is generated near the end of the cascade, and this powerful enzyme converts fibrinogen to fibrin. Fibrin and activated platelets are the nucleus of thrombi.

Platelets are also activated directly by contact with the synthetic surfaces. Activated platelets adhere to surface-adsorbed fibrinogen deposited during the initial moments of blood contact. Activated platelets release a variety of vasoactive and thrombotic substances which contribute to the generation of thrombi.

Both bioprosthetic and mechanical heart valves activate platelets and the coagulation cascade (6,7). Platelets adhere to both types of valves and release beta-thromboglobin from alpha granules and synthesize thromboxane A2, a powerful vasoconstrictor. Both types of prostheses increase plasma concentrations of fibrinolytic enzymes. In general, mechanical valves are associated with higher concentrations of platelet-release markers and fibrinopeptide A (7) than are bioprosthetic valves and therefore are considered more thrombogenic.

Fortunately, natural inhibitors and the massive surface area of the vascular system, which is estimated to be between 1000 and 6300 m^2, counteract activated procoagulant proteins. High flow velocity across small, well-washed synthetic surfaces minimizes activation of factor XII and platelets. Endothelial cells remove thrombin and release tissue plasminogen activator, prostacyclin, and heparan sulfate. Thrombin binds to the endothelial cell surface protein, thrombomodulin, and the complex greatly activates protein C, which with protein S inactivates factors Va and VIIIa. Heparan sulfate accelerates the action of antithrombin III to bind and inactivate thrombin. Prostacyclin inhibits platelets. Tissue plasminogen activator causes the cleavage of plasminogen to plasmin, which lyses fibrin and produces D-dimer, a marker that indicates fibrin has formed and been lysed. Alpha 2-macroglobulin, a protease inhibitor, inhibits both thrombin and plasmin. Constant activation of platelets and factor XII by the synthetic surfaces of prosthetic heart valves forces endothelial cells to establish a new dynamic equilibrium to maintain the fluidity of blood. Coumadin and/or oral platelet inhibitors influence this process, but do not dominate it.

II. DIAGNOSIS OF THROMBOEMBOLISM AND BLEEDING

The diagnosis of a valve-related thromboembolic or bleeding event sometimes requires interpretation; therefore, a set of standard definitions or guidelines is desirable to facilitate comparisons among prostheses, valve locations, and different cardiac groups. A set of guidelines that has received wide support has been published (8). Thromboembolism is defined as any valve thrombosis or embolus that occurs in a patient who has a cardiac valve prosthesis and who does not have endocarditis. Although infection greatly accelerates the incidence of prosthetic valve thrombosis and embolism, such occurrences are considered complications of the infection and are not included in statistics relating to valve thrombosis or emboli.

> Thromboembolism includes any new, permanent or transient, focal or global neurologic deficit (exclusive of hemorrhage) and any peripheral arterial emboli unless proved to have resulted from another cause (e.g., atrial myxoma). Patients who do not awaken postoperatively or who awaken with a stroke or myocardial infarction are excluded. Acute myocardial infarction that occurs after operation is arbitrarily defined as a thromboembolic event in patients with known normal coronary arteries or those who are less than 40 years of age.
>
> Valve thrombosis may be proved by operation, autopsy, or clinical investigation (e.g., endocardiography, angiocardiography, or magnetic resonance imaging) and is listed as a separate subcategory of thromboembolism (8).

Anticoagulant-related hemorrhage is defined as "any episode of internal or external bleeding that causes death, stroke, operation, or hospitalization, or requires transfusion" (8). The definition excludes minor episodes of bleeding, which are often underreported, and is restricted to patients who are receiving anticoagulants and/or platelet inhibitors.

Valve-related thromboembolism is systematically underreported (1). Sudden unexplained death may be due to thromboembolism or other causes; convention recommends that such deaths be considered valve-related unless definitely proved otherwise. Well over 80% of reported thromboemboli involve the central nervous system, which is by far more sensitive to regional ischemia than other organs. Yet the brain receives only 14% of the cardiac output; simple calculation ($0.8 \times 100/14$), assuming that emboli are distributed in proportion to blood flow, indicates that 4.7 emboli are undetected for each detected embolus. Moreover, the fibrinolytic system probably removes many small emboli and perhaps some valve thrombi. These observations, in addition to problems of patient recall and clinical follow-up, strongly suggest that the problem of thromboembolism, and to a lesser extent anticoagulant bleeding, is more common than our statistics indicate.

In reporting instances of valve-related thrombosis, embolism, and anticoagulant-related hemorrhage, data should be stratified by prosthetic valve model and by the location of the prosthesis (aortic, mitral, aortic and mitral, tricuspid). Moreover, the consequences of the complication should be stratified into fatal, nonfatal with residual handicap, and nonfatal without residual disability. From the patients' point of view, a valve that has a relatively high incidence of nonfatal, nonpermanent events is far superior to a valve that produces fatal or permanent strokes.

Thromboembolic and bleeding complications are usually reported as linearized rates or events per 100 patient-years of follow-up. Linearized rates are not applicable unless the risk of the complication can be shown to be constant over the period of interest. Although this may be true for bleeding events, the incidence of valve-related thrombosis and embolism is definitely higher in the first few weeks after operation than it is later (9). Moreover, the incidence of thromboembolism seems less in the current era as compared to the late 1960s and 1970s (9).

Most valve-related thromboembolic and bleeding complications should be reported using time-related statistics starting from operation. The Kaplan-Meier formula provides actuarial estimates of complications and survival and should be reported with standard errors or confidence limits. The Cox proportional hazard model and other parametric statistical methods can provide additional information regarding causes of thromboembolic and bleeding events (8).

III. WARFARIN AND PLATELET INHIBITORS

Warfarin is a water-soluble derivative of coumaric acid and is the most commonly used oral anticoagulant in the United States. For practical purposes, coumaric acids are the only oral anticoagulants available. These drugs competitively block vitamin K epoxidase, which reduces the amount available to carboxylate specific glutamic acid residues required for calcium binding by the four vitamin K-dependent coagulation factors: factors II, VII, IX, and X. The coagulation cascade is slowed by the depletion of these four factors, particularly factor II (prothrombin). Reduced prothrombin prolongs the prothrombin time test, which is widely used to monitor the effectiveness of coumaric acid anticoagulants.

Warfarin is far from an ideal oral anticoagulant. The therapeutic window of the drug (i.e., desired range of prothrombin times) is very narrow, and the mechanism of action is indirect and depends on slowing the coagulation cascade by partially depleting the four vitamin K-dependent coagulation factors, which have different plasma half-lives that vary between 6 and 50 h (10). Therapeutic anticoagulation requires establishing and maintaining a delicate equilibrium between warfarin and vitamin K concentrations within the liver. This is not easy, because a host of variables affect both warfarin and vitamin K concentrations. Although warfarin is completely absorbed from the gut in 2–8 h, 99% is bound to albumin and only 1% is available to suppress vitamin K oxidation in the liver. The drug has a mean half-life in plasma of 40 h and a duration of action of 2–5 days. A huge and growing list of drugs affects the absorption and metabolism of both warfarin and vitamin K. Vitamin K concentrations are also affected by amounts absorbed from foods. The net result is that onset of action is slow and maintenance of therapeutic effectiveness impossible without frequent monitoring of prothrombin times for as long as the drug is used.

Prothrombin times are usually reported in the United States as the patient's prothrombin time in seconds divided by the laboratory control, which varies between batches of commercial thromboplastin used for the test. Increasingly, international normalized ratios (INR units) are being calculated to permit comparisons of prothrombin times between laboratories (10). An exponential correction factor (international sensitivity index, ISI) that is determined for each batch of thromboplastin is used to convert measured prothrombin time ratios to INR units. The ISI indexes the thromboplastin used in the test to a reference thromboplastin maintained by the World Health Organization. In England, the therapeutic range for coumadin anticoagulation is 2.0 to 4.5 INR units (10).

Although the intensity of anticoagulation (high or low prothrombin times) is important in suppressing thrombus formation, difficulties in regulating the drug in patients are an even greater problem. Spot prothrombin times indicate that 33–50% of anticoagulated patients have prothrombin times outside the therapeutic range (1,11,12) (Fig. 1). In anticoagulated patients with prosthetic heart valves, nearly one-third of all prothrombin times measured are outside the therapeutic range. When surveillance is increased, the incidence of aberrant prothrombin times and thromboembolic and bleeding complications decreases (13). The introduction of self-surveillance using home prothrombin time tests may improve warfarin regulation; pilot studies are encouraging (14).

Low prothrombin times, defined as prothrombin times below the therapeutic range 25% or more of the time, increase the risk of thromboembolic complications two to six times (1,15). Excessive warfarin above 5.0 INR units increases the risk of bleeding two to six times (1,9,11,16). Bleeding complications most frequently involve the gastrointestinal tract and increase with age (1,11). Prior history of bleeding also increases the risk (11).

Aspirin prolongs bleeding times by inhibiting platelet cyclooxygenase and synthesis of thromboxane A2 (17). Since platelets lack nuclei, cyclooxygenase is not replaced and the loss of platelet function is permanent for the life of the platelet (8 to 12 days). Thus aspirin given every 2 or 3 days inhibits platelets as effectively as aspirin given daily (19,20) (Fig. 2). Aspirin also inhibits endothelial cell cyclooxygenase and the production of prostacyclin, a platelet inhibitor and vasodilator. There is evidence that low-dose aspirin (100 mg daily) is as effective in suppressing thromboxane A2 synthesis as high-dose (1 g daily) aspirin (Fig. 3) (18–20), and that up to 40% of normal prostacyclin production continues at either a low or high dose (17,20,21). Complications of aspirin therapy (principally

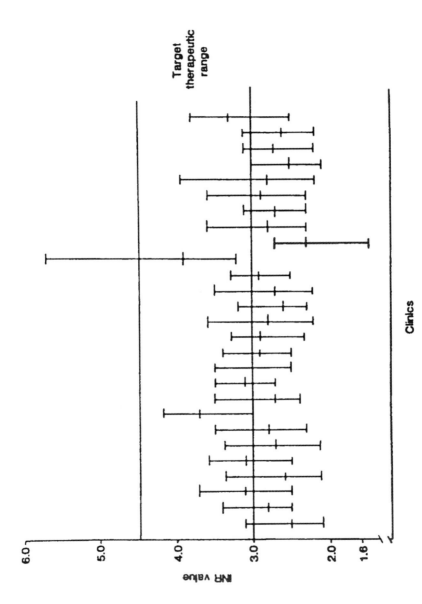

Figure 1 Variability in median prothrombin times ± standard deviation of different anticoagulation clinics in 1 year. The target range is 3.0–4.5 INR units. (Reproduced with permission from Ref. 12.)

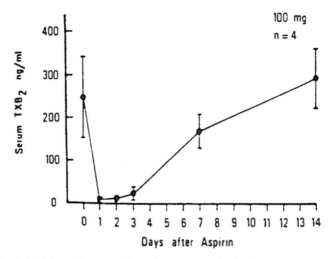

Figure 2 Inhibition of serum thromboxane synthesis by a single oral dose of aspirin of 100 mg in four subjects. Bars represent one standard deviation from the mean. (Reproduced with permission from Ref. 18.)

gastric ulcer and gastrointestinal bleeding) are less with low-dose aspirin or enteric-coated aspirin, and can be further reduced with cimetidine (21). Aspirin is rapidly absorbed and has a half-life in plasma of about 15 min.

Dipyridamole and sulfinpyrazone are weak platelet inhibitors at doses that can be tolerated by patients (400 mg and 800 mg/day, respectively) (1). Neither drug prolongs bleeding time. Absorption of dipyridamole is highly variable, and plasma concentrations do not reach the 10-μmol concentrations required to inhibit platelets (22). Sulfinpyrazone reversibly inhibits cyclooxygenase, but its action in vivo is so minimal that it is not approved as an antithrombotic drug in the United States. However, both drugs do increase platelet survival in patients with prosthetic heart valves, but the relevance of this observation to thromboembolism is not clear. At the present time, neither drug has been shown to reduce the incidence of thromboembolism in patients with prosthetic heart valves (1,22).

Combinations of aspirin and dipyridamole have been recommended, but there is no evidence of a synergistic effect of dipyridamole on aspirin (21). Dipyridamole in combination with warfarin may reduce thromboembolism in patients with prosthetic heart valves without increasing bleeding, but the data are not strong (1,21). Low-dose aspirin (100 mg/day) with high-dose warfarin (3.0–4.5 INR units) reduces thromboembolic compli-

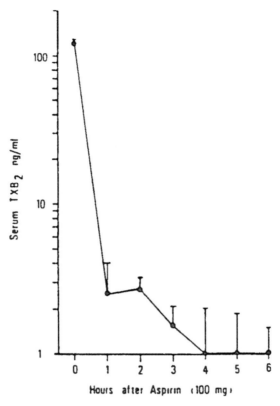

Figure 3 Effect of a single 100-mg dose of aspirin on thromboxane synthesis in a healthy woman. Values are means and one standard deviation of triplicate measurements. (Reproduced with permission from Ref. 18.)

cations in patients with prosthetic heart valves (23) and does not increase major bleeding over warfarin alone (23). High-dose aspirin (1000 mg/day) with warfarin greatly increases bleeding (21). No trials to date have tested low-dose aspirin with low-dose warfarin (2.5–3.5 INR units).

IV. INCIDENCE OF THROMBOEMBOLISM AND BLEEDING

The incidence of thromboembolism as defined by published guidelines (8) for porcine heterograft tissue valves is approximately 1% per patient-year (1,9,24) (Fig. 4). There is no significant difference between Hancock and Carpentier-Edwards prostheses, and the range of different reported series varies between 0.1% and 3.3% (1,24). The incidence of valve thrombosis

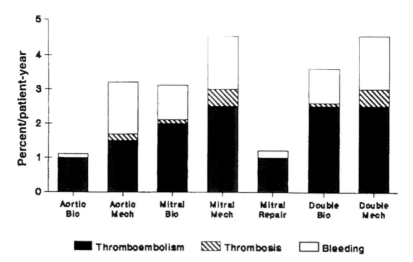

Figure 4 The approximate incidence (percent/patient-year) of thromboemboli, thrombotic, and serious bleeding complication for bioprosthetic (Bio) and mechanical (Mech) valves in different locations.

ranges between 0 and 0.2% per patient-year (1,24); the mean incidence is close to zero. Although most surgeons do not anticoagulate patients with aortic heterograft valves, some prescribe coumadin for the first 3 months after operation (1,9,24). This policy has caused rare serious anticoagulant-related hemorrhages (1).

The incidence of thromboembolism in anticoagulated patients with St. Jude, Bjork-Shiley, or Medtronic-Hall aortic prostheses is approximately 1.5% per patient-year, with a range of 0.4 to 3.0% (Fig. 4) (1,24,25). The incidence of valve thrombosis ranges from zero (12) to 0.7% with a mean near 0.2%. The incidence of anticoagulant-related serious bleeding is about 1.5% per patient-year and ranges between 0.5 and 3.0% (1,25). There are no significant differences in these figures among these three valves.

At 5 years, approximately 95% of patients with porcine heterograft aortic valves are free of valve-related thromboembolism, thrombosis, and bleeding. For the three popular low-profile mechanical aortic prostheses, approximately 90% are free of bleeding, thrombosis, or thromboembolism.

The incidence of thromboembolism for Starr-Edwards (model 1260) aortic prostheses is slightly higher than for the low-profile valves (1,9,24,25), and may be due to earlier placement of the majority of these valves (1). The incidence of valve thrombosis and anticoagulant bleeding is the same.

Porcine heterograft mitral prostheses have a higher incidence of thromboembolic complications than aortic heterografts, with an average incidence of approximately 2.0% (1,9,24,25) (Fig. 4). The incidence in reported series ranges between 0.8 and 3.6%/patient-year. The incidence of valve thrombosis is low but slightly higher at 0.1% than the nearly zero for aortic heterograft valves. Because approximately half of patients with mitral bioprostheses are anticoagulated with warfarin or similar coumaric acid derivatives, the incidence of anticoagulant-related bleeding is approximately 1.0% or slightly less.

Mechanical mitral prostheses have the highest incidence of thromboembolic, thrombotic, and bleeding complications of all left-sided valves (1,9,24,25). For Bjork-Shiley, St. Jude, and Medtronic-Hall valves, the mean incidence of thromboembolism is approximately 2.5%/patient-year (Fig. 4) (1,24,25). The range varies between 1.3 and 5.0% (1,24–27). The incidence of valve thrombosis is about 0.5%, and the incidence of anticoagulant-related bleeding is approximately 1.5%. The total incidence of thromboembolism, thrombosis, and serious bleeding is approximately 4.5%/patient-year. Again, the incidence of thromboembolic complications may be slightly higher with the Starr-Edwards ball valve, but the incidence of valve thrombosis and serious bleeding is essentially the same as for low-profile mechanical mitral prostheses. At 5 years, 80–85% of patients with mitral mechanical valves are free of thromboembolism, thrombosis, and serious anticoagulant-related bleeding.

Repair of mitral valve disease reduces the incidence of thromboembolism to a range from zero (28) to 2.5% (2,28–31) and averages approximately 1%. The incidence of anticoagulant-related bleeding ranges from zero to 0.9% (2,28,29). Repaired valve thrombosis has not been reported. Although the incidence of thromboembolism is only somewhat reduced by repair as compared to mitral valve replacement with a mechanical valve and is roughly similar to that observed with heterograft valves, most patients who are in sinus rhythm are anticoagulated for only 3 months (25,28,31,32).

The experience with simultaneous aortic and mitral valve replacement is much less than with isolated aortic or mitral valve replacement. When heterografts are used for both aortic and mitral valves, the incidence of thromboembolism is roughly 2.5%/patient-year (1) (Fig.4). Valve thrombosis is rare (1), but because many of these patients are anticoagulated, the incidence of serious bleeding is about 1.0%.

When low-profile mechanical prostheses are used to replace both mitral and aortic valves, the incidence of thromboembolism ranges between 1.3 and 4.8%/patient-year and averages about 2.5% (1,25,27). The valve thrombosis rate is approximately 0.5%. The incidence of anticoagulant-related bleeding is about 1.5%, although one substantial series reported no serious bleeding in patients with two St. Jude valves (33). Freedom from all thromboembolic, thrombotic, and serious bleeding complications at 5 years is about 85% (33,34).

For bioprosthetic aortic, mitral, or aortic and mitral prostheses, approximately 15% of all thromboembolic events are fatal. Approximately 18% of thromboembolic events are fatal in patients with mechanical aortic valves (1). The percentage increases to 25% if a mechanical mitral is involved. Roughly 15–20% of serious bleeding episodes are fatal (1,9).

V. RISK FACTORS FOR THROMBOEMBOLISM

The first 3 months after operation, atrial fibrillation, prosthetic valve endocarditis, left atrial thrombus, previous embolus, and operation before the mid-1970s are the most frequently cited additive risk factors for thromboembolism (1,9,24). Large left atrium, low cardiac output, age over 60, previous cardiac operation, and concomitant mitral disease in patients with aortic prostheses are less clearly established additive risk factors (1,9).

Recently, low-dose warfarin (2.0–3.0 INR units) has been recommended for all patients with atrial fibrillation, including those with normal valves (35). For patients with aortic bioprostheses, long-term warfarin anticoagulation is also recommended in patients who have had thromboembolism and possibly in those who have had an event prior to valve replacement (9). For patients with a mitral bioprosthesis, long-term warfarin is recommended for patients with a left atrial thrombus or previous emboli before or after implantation of a prosthesis (1,9). Patients with mechanical prostheses all need warfarin anticoagulant, but the level of anticoagulation and the use of platelet inhibitors are variables that are addressed below.

About 80% of patients with fungal prosthetic endocarditis develop thromboemboli, and perhaps 50–60% of those with bacterial prosthetic endocarditis do (1). The type of valve (bioprosthetic or mechanical) and location does not seem to affect the incidence of endocarditis. These patients primarily need antibiotics (36) and often early operation. The decision to anticoagulate (with heparin) is difficult because of increased cerebral bleeding. Patients with small cerebral infarcts are usually anticoagulated 2 days after the event in patients with mechanical valves. Anticoagulation is delayed longer if the stroke is large (36).

VI. WARFARIN AND PLATELET INHIBITORS: RECOMMENDATIONS

Despite a few clinical trials demonstrating reduced thromboembolism with a combination of warfarin and dipyridamole (9,25,37), these drugs together are not recommended in patients with prosthetic heart valves. Dipyridamole in the doses that patients can tolerate as a weak platelet inhibitor, and the relevance of increased platelet survival to the problem of thromboembolism remains unclear.

The incidence of thromboembolism is higher during the first 3 months after operation (1,9). On the basis of this fact, warfarin anticoagulation has been prescribed for this period in patients with bioprosthetic valves who otherwise are not candidates for long-term warfarin anticoagulation. Although the prescription of warfarin for 3 months after operation is eminently logical, only one report indicates that the incidence of thromboemboli is reduced (38).

The increasing acceptance of INR units to report results of prothrombin times has produced an illusion of better control of warfarin anticoagulation and introduced the concept of low-intensity (2.0–3.0 INR units) and high-intensity (3.0–4.5 INR units) anticoagulation (37). Although the target windows of the two anticoagulant schemes differ, cardiologists and surgeons must be aware of the unresolved difficulties and poor success of maintaining patients within targeted ranges (1,12). For bioprosthetic valves, one study (38) shows that low-intensity anticoagulation prevents thromboembolism as well as high-intensity anticoagulation and is associated with fewer episodes of serious bleeding. Since all of the emboli occurred in patients with bioprosthetic mitral valves, the study does not establish the need to anticoagulate patients with aortic tissue valves. Two other recent studies document the efficacy of low-intensity anticoagulation in patients with mechanical prostheses (one also used aspirin and dipyridamole) and showed a similar decrease in serious bleeding complications (17,39).

Aspirin is an effective platelet inhibitor, but when used with warfarin it increases the incidence of serious bleeding complications, which usually involve the stomach (1,9,21,39–41). Bleeding complications and subjective side effects are dose-related and can be reduced by antiacids, cimetidine, and enteric coating (21). Most of the clinical trials of warfarin-aspirin combinations have used aspirin doses above 660 mg/day. This huge dose is unnecessary to inhibit platelets permanently. Oral aspirin (100 mg) effectively inhibits platelet thromboxane A2 synthesis, and moreover only partially inhibits prostacyclin synthesis by endothelial cells (17,20,21). Oral aspirin at 200 mg once every 3 days effectively stops platelet thromboxane synthesis (18). Thus 100 mg of enteric-coated aspirin given every 2 days with an antacid and cimetidine is unlikely to cause serious or chronic gastrointestinal bleeding even if given with low-intensity warfarin. The low, infrequent dose of aspirin inhibits platelets very effectively, and more frequent, higher doses are not needed. However, it is difficult to take a pill every other day.

Based on the above information and mindful of published clinical trials and recommendations (25), this surgeon recommends the following scheme for suppressing thromboembolism and thrombosis in patients with prosthetic heart valves: for aortic bioprostheses, nothing; if an embolus occurs, start low-dose (100 mg) aspirin daily or even 2 days; if an embolus recurs (which has not happened in my experience), add low-intensity warfarin (2.0–3.0 INR units).

For mitral or aortic/mitral bioprostheses that have added risk factors, use low-intensity warfarin and 100 mg of enteric-coated aspirin every 2 days with an ounce of antacid and 200 mg of cimetidine 1 h before the aspirin. The same regimen is recommended for all patients with mechanical aortic valves. Although low-intensity warfarin and low-dose, infrequent aspirin may be effective for patients with mechanical mitral or aortic and mitral valves, the higher incidence of thromboembolism argues for increasing the intensity of warfarin anticoagulation to the range of 3.5–4.5 INR units. For intelligent patients who can afford the machine, a program of home self-surveillance is highly recommended, with prothrombin times measured at least twice per week.

VII. SPECIAL PROBLEMS

The incidence of thromboemboli from tricuspid valve prostheses is unknown, since nearly all emboli are undetected. Both heterograft and mechanical tricuspid valves thrombose; the incidence is higher with mechanical valves. Warfarin anticoagulation is recommended for all patients with tricuspid prostheses, but the intensity of anticoagulation probably can be lower with tissue valves. Thrombolytic agents can be used if valve thrombosis occurs and often may be preferable to reoperation (1).

Thrombolytic therapy has also been used to treat thrombosed left-sided valve prostheses (42). The incidence of systemic emboli is approximately 18%, and mortality is 15% (42). However, except in unusual circumstances, where operation is contraindicated, reoperation is recommended. Mortality varies between 11% for those who have prompt reoperation (43) to 31% for those who fail thrombolytic therapy (42).

The presence of a prosthetic heart valve causes serious complications for mother and fetus during pregnancy. Pregnancy accelerates deterioration of heterograft prostheses. Coumadin anticoagulation reduces the chance of a live healthy infant by 25–30% (1). Heparin anticoagulation also reduces the chance of a healthy infant by about one-third and increases the chance of a serious bleeding complication in the mother to approximately 15% (1). There are little data regarding schemes to use aspirin and low-intensity warfarin; intermittent warfarin and heparin timed to prevent warfarin embryopathy; and aspirin alone. In young women, repair of diseased valves or insertion of homograft aortic valves have high priority; otherwise, a bioprosthesis may be advised with a recommendation to proceed forthwith with reproduction if children are desired. This valve will likely need replacement after the family is produced. None of the options available are very attractive, and careful review of the choices with the patient and her husband is strongly recommended.

A prosthetic heart valve imposes a serious handicap on a child. Because of accelerated deterioration, porcine heterograft valves cannot be used. Although mechanical valves have been used in children without warfarin, this writer cannot recommend the practice. Serious bleeding complications in children due to coumadin are infrequent, but thrombotic complications and strokes are often catastrophic if warfarin is omitted (1). There is no question that warfarin is very difficult to monitor in children, who universally abhor needles; nonetheless, the child's future depends on avoiding a catastrophic stroke. Compromises are not in the child's long-term interest.

Thromboembolism, thrombosis, and anticoagulant bleeding remain the most common and perhaps the most difficult complications of prosthetic heart valves. Nevertheless, small, incremental improvements in valve design and construction and in the management of warfarin and aspirin have steadily, albeit slowly, reduced the problem and improved the quality of life for prosthetic valve recipients. Improved therapeutic anticoagulant regimens, home surveillance of prothrombin times, more durable bioprosthetic valves, and discovery of a new, effective oral anticoagulant that is more easily managed than coumaric acid derivatives offer promise for even better control of this serious problem.

REFERENCES

1. Edmunds LH Jr. Thrombotic and bleeding complications of prosthetic heart valves. Ann Thorac Surg 1987; 44:430–45.
2. Deloche A, Jebara VA, Relland JYM, et al. Valve repair with Carpentier techniques. J Thorac Cardiovasc Surg 1990; 99:990–1002.

3. Edmunds LH Jr. The sangreal. J Thorac Cardiovasc Surg 1985; 90:4–6.
4. O'Brien MF, Stafford EG, Gardner MAH, Pohlner PG, McGiffin DC. A comparison of aortic valve replacement with viable cryopreserved and fresh allograft valves with a note on chromosomal studies. J Thorac Cardiovasc Surg 1987; 94:812–23.
5. Kirklin JW, Barratt-Boyes BG. Cardiac Surgery. New York: Wiley, 1986; 409–12.
6. Pumphrey CW, Dawes J. The platelet release reaction in cardiovascular disease: evaluation of plasma beta thromboglobulin as a marker of a prothrombotic state. Eur Heart J 1984; 5(suppl D):7.
7. Prengo V, Peruzzi P, Baca M, et al. The optimal therapeutic range for all anticoagulant treatment as suggested by fibrinopeptide A (FpA) levels in patients with heart valve prostheses. Eur J Clin Invest 1989; 19:181–4.
8. Edmunds LH Jr, Clark RE, Cohn LH, Miller DC, Weisel RD. Guidelines for reporting morbidity and mortality after cardiac valvular operations. J Thorac Cardiovasc Surg 1988; 96:351–3.
9. Fuster V, Badimon L, Badimon JJ, Cehseboro J. Prevention of thromboembolism induced by prosthetic heart valves. Sem Thromb Hemost 1988; 14: 50–65.
10. Hirsch J, Dalen JE, Deykin D, Poller L. Oral anticoagulants: mechanism of action, clinical effectiveness and optimal therapeutic range. Chest 1992; 102: 312S–26S.
11. Levine MN, Raskob G, Hirsh J. Hemorrhagic complications of long-term anticoagulant therapy. Chest 1986; 89:16S–25S.
12. Butchart EG, Lewis PA, Grunkemeier GL, Kulatilake N, Breckenridge IM. Low risk of thrombosis and serious embolic events despite low-intensity anticoagulation; experience with 1004 Medtronic-Hall valves. Circulation 1988; 78:I-66–77.
13. Thulin LI, Olin CL. Intiation and long-term anticoagulation after heart valve replacements. Arg Bras Cardiol 1987; 49:265–8.
14. White RH, McCurdy SA, von Marensdorff H, Woodruff DE Jr, Leftgoff L. Home prothrombin time monitoring after the initiation of warfarin therapy. Ann Intern Med 1989; 111:730–7.
15. Myers ML, Lawrie GM, Crawford ES, et al. The St. Jude valve prosthesis: analysis and clinical results in 815 implants and the need for systemic anticoagulation. J Am Coll Cardiol 1989; 13:57–62.
16. Saour JN, Sieck JO, Mamo LAR, Gallus AS. Trial of different intensities of anticoagulation in patients with prosthetic heart valves. N Engl J Med 190; 322:428–32.
17. Pedersen AK, Fitzgerald GA. Dose-related kinetics of aspirin. N Engl J Med 1984; 311:1206–11.
18. Patrono C, Ciabattoni G, Pinca E, et al. Low dose aspirin inhibition of thromboxane B2 production in healthy subjects. Thromb Res 1980; 17:317.
19. Patrignani P, Filabozzi P, Patrono C. Selective cumulative inhibition of platelet thromboxane production by low-dose aspirin in healthy subjects. J Clin Invest 1982; 69:1366–72.

20. FitzGerald GA, Oates JA, Hawiger J, et al. Endogenous biosynthesis of prostacyclin and thromboxane and platelets function during chronic administration of aspirin in man. J Clin Invest 1983; 71:676–88.

21. Hirsh J, Dalen JE, Fuster V, Hanker LB, Salzman EW. Aspirin and other platelet-active drugs; the relationship between dose, effectiveness and side effects. Chest 1992; 102:327S–36S.

22. Fitzgerald GA. Dipyridamole. N Engl J Med 1987; 316:1247–57.

23. Turpie AGG, Gent M, Laupacis A, et al. Reduction in mortality by adding aspirin (100 mg) to oral anticoagulants in patients with heart valve replacement. J Am Coll Cardiol 1992; 19:103A.

24. Grunkemeier GL, Rahintoola SH. Artificial heart valves. Ann Rev Med 1990; 41:251–63.

25. Stein PD, Alpert JS, Copeland J, Dalen JE, Goldman S, Turpie AGG. Antithrombotic therapy in patients with mechanical and biological prosthetic heart valves. Chest 1992; 102:445S–55S.

26. Lindblom D. Long-term clinical results after mitral valve replacement with the Bjork-Shiley prosthesis. J Thorac Cardiovasc Surg 1988; 95:321–33.

27. Nitter-Hauge S, Abdelnoor M. Ten-year experience with the Medtronic-Hall valvular prosthesis; a study of 1104 patients. Circulation 1989; 80:I-43–48.

28. Cohn LH, Kowalker W, Bhatia S, et al. Comparative morbidity of mitral valve repair versus replacement for mitral regurgitation with and without coronary artery disease. Ann Thorac Surg 1988; 45:284–90.

29. Angell WW, Oury JH. A comparison of replacement and reconstruction in patients with mitral regurgitation. J Thorac Cardiovasc Surg 1987; 93:665–74.

30. Orszulak TA, Schaff HV, Danielson GK, et al. Mitral regurgitation due to ruptured chordae tendineae. J Thorac Cardiovasc Surg 1985; 89:491–8.

31. Duran CG, Revuelta JM, Gaite L, Alonso C, Fleitas MG. Stability of mitral reconstructive surgery at 10–12 years for predominantly rheumatic valvular disease. Circulation 1988; 78:I-91–6.

32. Galloway AC, Colvin SB, Baumann FG, et al. Long-term results of mitral valve reconstruction with Carpentier techniques in 148 patients with mitral insufficiency. Circulation 1988; 78:I-97–105.

33. Arom AV, Nicoloff DM, Kersten TE, Northrup WF III, Lindsay WG, Emergy RW. Ten-year follow-up study of patients who had double valve replacement with the St. Jude medical prosthesis. J Thorac Cardiovasc Surg 1989; 98:1008–16.

34. Armenti F, Stephenson LW, Edmunds LH Jr. Simultaneous implantation of St. Jude medical aortic and mitral prostheses. J Thorac Cardiovasc Surg 1987; 94:733–9.

35. Ezekowitz MD, Bridgers SL, James KE, et al. (VASP in NAFI). Warfarin in the prevention of stroke associated with nonrheumatic atrial fibrillation. N Engl J Med 1992; 327:1406–12.

36. Levine HJ, Pauker SG, Salzman EW, Eckman MH. Antithrombotic therapy in valvular heart disease. Chest 1992; 102:434S–445S.

37. Chesbro JH, Fuster V, Elveback LR, et al. Trial of combined warfarin plus dipyrimadole or aspirin therapy in prosthetic heart valve replacement: danger of aspirin compared with dipyrimadole. Am J Cardiol 1983; 51:1537.
38. Turpie AGG, Gunstensen J, Hirsh J, Nelson H, Gent M. Randomized comparison of two intensities of anticoagulant therapy after tissue heart valve replacement. Lancet 1988; 1:1242–5.
39. Altman R, Rouvier J, Gurfinkel E, et al. Comparison of two levels of anticoagulant therapy in patients with substitute heart valves. J Thorac Cardiovasc Surg 1991; 101:427–31.
40. Altman R, Boullon F, Rouvier J, et al. Aspirin and prophylaxis of thromboembolic complications in patients with substitute heart valves. J Thorac Cardiovasc Surg 1976; 72:127.
41. Dale J, Myhre E, Storstein O, et al. Prevention of arterial thromboembolism with acetyl salicytic acid: a controlled clinical study in patients with aortic ball valves. Am Heart J 1977; 94:101–11.
42. Graver LM, Gelber PM, Tyras DH. The risks and benefits of thrombolytic therapy in acute aortic and mitral valve dysfunction: report of a case and review of the literature. Ann Thorac Surg 1988; 46:85–8.
43. Kontos GJ Jr, Schaff HV, Orszulak TA, Puga FJ, Pluth JR, Danielson GK. Thrombotic obstruction of disk valves: clinical recognition and surgical management. Ann Thorac Surg 1989; 48:60–5.

23

The Valve Clinic

Begonia Gometza, Elias Saad, and Carlos M. G. Duran
King Faisal Specialist Hospital, Riyadh, Saudi Arabia

Two elements are needed to form a truth—a fact and an abstraction.

Remy de Gourmont, 1890

I. INTRODUCTION

Valve surgery has a long history of failed attempts and successes that speak for the inventiveness, persistence, and courage of the cardiac surgeons. The number of valve substitutes and surgical techniques is staggering. Most of them undergo a fairly standard pattern of initial excitement promoted by its creators, increasing popularity due to the encouraging reports of other groups, and, eventually, universal acceptance. The appearance of negative facts, secondary to a wider and longer experience, casts doubt on the procedure, which eventually is abandoned and a new device takes over. This process is not circular, i.e., returning to the point of origin, but rather spiral, because it starts each time at a higher level of knowledge.

It is interesting that, as in other fields of human endeavor, the proponents of a particular new solution are inclined to see it as unquestionable, universal, and definitive. It is also surprising that usually their results tend to be superior to others or even to those of its followers. Although the first and easy explanation is to doubt the objectivity of such favorable reports, it is more likely to be due to careful patient selection and to better and meticulous surgical technique. There is nothing wrong with this lack of detachment, which is what gives dynamism to science (1). However, scientific acceptance of a fact requires it to be reproducible by anyone under similar circumstances.

Objective evaluation of any technique at the personal, local, or general level needs a conscious and continuous effort, often started but seldom attained. This evaluation is hampered by (1) the subjective impact on the surgeon's short memory by his or her latest results, (2) the very large discordance in patient population in terms of age, etiology, and functional status, (3) the often unconscious differences in attitude and technique introduced by the individual surgeon, (4) the frequent variability in the definition and acquisition of negative events, (5) the absence of a complete and objective follow-up, (6) the difficulty of a good data retrieval system, and (7) the lack of a uniform method for reporting the results.

The basis of this chapter is to describe an attempt at obtaining an objective methodology for the evaluation of the results of the invasive treatment of valvular disease. It is our contention that this can be achieved only through a dedicated "valve clinic," where all valvular patients are continuously followed by a motivated group of physicians, who conform vigorously to preestablished questionnaires and definitions.

II. OBJECTIVES OF THE VALVE CLINIC

1. Improvement in patient care: Besides the obvious advantages for future patients derived from the continuous flow of information on every procedure, the clinic should offer definite advantages to the individual patient already operated upon. It ensures a uniform management and drug therapy, which is particularly essential in those patients under anticoagulation. It offers an occasion for continuous patient education and reinforces his or her compliance. It facilitates the earlier detection of valvular dysfunction and its prompt treatment.

2. Evaluation of the results: The valve clinic should provide continuous, permanent, and immediate feedback on the invasive treatment of all valve patients. It should avoid changes in technique based on often very subjective, personal impressions and provide an excellent method for quality control of the unit's activity.

3. The valve clinic's specialization can provide a very valuable platform for intensive education on valvular disease for physicians, surgeons, nurses, and related health personnel.

4. A well-organized clinic should provide a reliable and uniformly collected database for statistical analysis and generation of clinical research, reports, and publications.

III. ORGANIZATION

A. Personnel

Ideally, the clinic should be governed by a single physician, so as to reduce, or at least homogenize, the variability in the collection and recording of the data. This person can be a surgeon, a cardiologist, or, even better, a well-trained general practioner. His or her wider range of knowledge and interest make him or her ideally suited to deal with the many, even if often unimportant, problems that arise during the long-term follow-up of the valvular patient.

This ideal situation is not always possible, either because of the large volume of patients or their inability to return regularly to the clinic because of geographic or economic problems. In this last case the referring physician should be enlisted to perform this task, provided he or she understands and is prepared to follow the guidelines of the valve clinic. Regular communication and meetings, where the importance of this data collection is stressed and demonstrated, should maintain their collaboration.

A nurse clinician, social worker, or equivalent person should be recruited for this clinic. His or her specialized knowledge, interest, and frequent contact with the patient before surgery, during the hospital stay, and after discharge ensures an absolutely essential personal relation.

A secretary or data-entry clerk should form part of the group as a full- or part-time employee, according to the patient volume.

B. When and Where

As pointed out above, the valvular patient should enter the system even before admission, when the modality of treatment is proposed. Its advantages, complications, and consequences are explained and discussed, together with the need for a permanent follow-up. All the demographic data of the patient must be checked, and in particular his or her address and telephone number and that of the contact relative and referring physician. Once the patient is admitted, a member of the team must maintain regular contact and before discharge ensure the completeness of the pre- and immediate postoperative data. The degree of understanding and reliability of the patient, in terms of compliance to treatment and attendance to the follow-up clinics, must also be evaluated at that time.

A precise calendar of follow-up visits cannot be universally recommended. It is generally accepted that the patient should be seen in the center a few weeks after discharge and then at regular intervals of several months. Although this pattern must be designed according to local conditions, once decided, it must be followed very rigidly. Failure to attend a clinic should be immediately detected, and no effort should be spared until the patient is contacted and the reason for the absence established and recorded. In our case, given that our patients come from a very large area, we require them to attend the clinic at 6 weeks and 6 months after surgery, and then once a year if no problems are detected. The patient is followed by his or her local physician or hospital at more frequent intervals.

C. Questionnaires

Although a well-completed chart includes all the relevant information of a patient, often obvious and essential data are missing or difficult to find. Furthermore, at some stage the data must be entered into a computerized database and, unless a totally computerized system is available in the hospital, a questionnaire for each patient must be extracted from his or her chart. It is far easier to design a series of questionnaires that make sure that all essential data are collected at key moments of the patient's evolution. The responsibility for filling each of them lies initially in the hands of each physician who treats the patient, although a method for checking their completeness must be established. In our case we have designed four separate questionnaires. The first one includes all the demographics of the patient, clinical data, echo, and hemodynamic findings (Table 1). The software should be a very flexible program that allows one to enter any number of answers to any given question and also to add new questions thought to be useful at any stage. The clinical data should include diagnosis according to valve site, lesion (stenotic and/or regurgitant), etiology (congenital, rheumatic, degenerative, infective, other), acute or chronic, previous surgery, and the very important functional class. Although many important facts can be recorded on the electrocardiogram and chest X-ray, we record only whether the patient is in sinus rhythm or not and the cardiothoracic index. This questionnaire is completed on the ward. A second questionnaire (Table 2) covers all the operative data and is completed by the surgeon. It should include the surgical diagnosis and its etiology, since these do not necessarily coincide with the preoperative one. The surgical findings must be recorded carefully. We specify them at each level of the valve complex, i.e., annulus, leaflets, commissures, subvalvular. The intraoperative echocardiographic findings must be included. The third one is completed on the ward at the time of discharge from hospital, including postoperative complications, days of stay in intensive care and ward, discharge rhythm, echocardiographic data, and medication (Table 3). The fourth questionnaire is completed at each follow-up clinic, recording patient and valve status, medications, and possible unwarranted events (Table 4).

Table 1 Preoperative Data

Demographic data	Clinical data	Echocardiographic data	Hemodynamic data
Name	Diagnosis	LA dimension	PA pressure
Sex	Probable etiology	LVID systolic	Wedge pressure
Date of birth	Relevant symptoms/signs	LVID diastolic	LVED pressure
Nationality	Previous embolic history	Percent shortening	Cardiac index
Address	Previous cardiac surgery: Valvular	LV function = EF	Coronary artery disease
	Congenital Ischemic Other		Pulmonary resistance
Telephone	Functional class	Valvular area	Valvular area
Referring cardiologist	Chest X-ray	Valvular gradient	Valvular gradient
Referring hospital	EKG	Grade of regurgitation	Grade of regurgitation

All positive questions are entered into a software program and filed [Patient Analysis and Tracking System (PATS), Dendrite Systems, Inc., Portland, Oregon]. The program selected should not only be able to retrieve the information of any patient, it should also extract groups of patients according to whatever characteristics are chosen. It should provide ranges, means, medians, mode, and standard deviation as well as incidence of events (% patient-year), actuarial curves, and significant values. A very useful capacity is the possibility of forming lists of patients who have failed to be followed after a predetermined length of time.

Although they should be easy to fill out, the questionnaires must have a set of instructions in order to achieve unity of interpretation. Definitions must be established by a consensus of all the members of the team. The adoption of a single method for defining and reporting negative events is essential to achieving consistency in the analysis of the results. This task has been greatly simplified by the excellent set of "guidelines for reporting morbidity and mortality after cardiac valve operations" issued by the Ad Hoc Liaison Committee for Standardizing of Prosthetic Heart Valve Morbidity of the American Association for Thoracic Surgery and the Society of Thoracic Surgeons (2). The completed questionnaires must be checked by a single person, who makes sure that newcomers do not intro-

Table 2 Surgical Data

Date of surgery	No. of valves:			
Valve site		A[a]	M[a]	T[a]
Surgical diagnosis	1 = regurgitation 3 = mixed diseases 2 = stenosis			
Etiology	1 = rheumatic 5 = congenital 10 = other 2 = ischemic 6 = endocarditis 0 = unknown 3 = degenerative 7 = prosthesis dysfunction 4 = functional 8 = repair dysfunction			
Surgical findings	1 = annulus 6 = degeneration 2 = leaflets 7 = vegetations 3 = commissures 8 = abscess 4 = subvalv apparatus 9 = thrombosis 5 = calcium 10 = dehiscence 11 = others			
Explanted prosthesis	1 = biological 3 = ring 2 = mechanical 4 = trade name			
Surgical procedure	1 = repair 4 = homograft 10 = others 2 = biophosthesis 5 = attempt repair 3 = mechanical 6 = redo			
Implanted prosthesis	Trade names:			
Prosthesis size				
Postoperative echo	1 = normal 6 = moderate stenosis 2 = mild regurgitation 7 = severe stenosis 3 = moderate regurgitation 4 = severe regurgitation 5 = mild stenosis			
Right/left ventricular function	1 = good 3 = moderate dysfunction 2 = mild dysfunction 4 = severe dysfunction			
Bypass time				
Ischemic time				
Concurrent procedures	1 = LA thrombectomy 3 = CABG 2 = congenital 10 = others			
Perioperative complications	1 = bleeding 4 = IABP 2 = annulus rupture 5 = AMI 3 = low cardiac output 10 = others			
Surgeons				

[a] A = aortic, M = mitral, T = tricuspid.

Table 3 Postoperative Data

Complications	1 = low cardiac output 2 = renal 3 = respiratory 4 = neurological	5 = arrhythmias 6 = pericardial 7 = infection 8 = hemolysis 10 = others			
Reoperation (cause)	1 = bleeding 2 = dysfunction 3 = severe hemolysis	4 = sternal dehiscence 5 = wound infection 10 = others			
Discharge rhythm	1 = sinus rhythm 2 = atrial fibrillation/flutter	3 = pacemaker			
Discharge echo	1 = normal 2 = mild regurgitation 3 = moderate regurgitation 4 = severe regurgitation 5 = mild stenosis	6 = moderate stenosis 7 = severe stenosis	A	M	T
Discharge medication	1 = digoxin 2 = diuretics 3 = ace inhibitors 4 = Beta blockers	5 = antiarrhythmics 6 = rheumatic prophylaxis 7 = anticoagulation 8 = antiaggregants 10 = others			
Stay (days)	1 ICU ...... days 2 Ward ...... days				
Patient status	1 = alive 2 = operative death	3 = hospital death			
Cause of death					
Comments					

duce errors into the system. It is often surprising to discover that questions which seem to have a single interpretation can be read very differently.

D. Protocols

At each visit the patient should undergo a preestablished set of investigations, such as weight, blood pressure, heart and respiratory rate, temperature, chest X-ray, electrocardiogram, and echocardiogram. Laboratory tests include blood cell count, ESR, liver and renal profiles, streptozyme, ASO, DNase B, C reactive protein, and prothrombin time or INR. Standard protocols for anticoagulation and prophylaxis for infective endocarditis and rheumatic fever must be given when applicable to each patient

The importance of prophylaxis of infective endocarditis, cannot be stressed sufficiently. All valvular patients should be clearly and graphically made aware of the value of dental hygiene and the need for antimicrobial coverage. Poor dental hygiene and periodontal infections may produce bacteremia. Dental procedures and instrumentation involving mucosal surfaces commonly cause transient bacteremia, which rarely persists for more than 15 min. Given that alpha-hemolytic (viridans) streptococci are the most common causes of endocarditis following dental procedures, the prophylaxis should be directed against this organism (4). Although several protocols were suggested in the past, we adhere to the latest proposed by the American Heart Association (4). which has been simplified by accepting the use of amoxicillin orally for dental, oral, and upper respiratory tract procedures and a parenteral regimen for genitourinary and gastrointestinal procedures (Table 6).

Young patients with rheumatic valvular disease are at risk of recurrence. This situation rarely presents in the developed countries, but is unfortunately still prevalent in many areas of the world and probably represents the main problem that valvular surgery faces at the present

Table 6   Prophylaxis for Infective Endocarditis

Dental, Oral, Upper Respiratory Tract Procedures	
Amoxicillin	3 g orally 1 h before procedure, then 1.5 g 6 h after initial dose
Amoxicillin/penicillin-allergic patients:	
Erythromycin stearate	1 g orally 2 h before procedure, then half-dose 6 h after initial dose
Genitourinary and Gastrointestinal Procedures	
Ampicillin	2 g IV or IM,
plus	
Gentamycin	1.5 mg/kg (not to exceed 80 mg) IM or IV 30 min before procedure
followed by	
Amoxicillin	1.5 g orally 6 h after initial dose
Ampicillin/amoxicillin/penicillin-allergic patients:	
Vancomycin	1 g IV over 1 h
plus	
Gentamycin	1.5 mg/kg (not to exceed 80 mg) IM or IV 1 h before procedure

Source: Ref. 4.

Table 7 Prophylaxis for Rheumatic Fever Recurrences

Rheumatic recurrences	Benzathine penicillin or	1.2 MU IM every 4 weeks
	Penicillin V	250 mg twice daily orally
	If allergic to penicillin:	
	Erythromycin stearate	250 mg twice daily orally

Source: From Ref. 6.

moment. Because of the young age of these patients, frequent pregnancies, difficulty of anticoagulation, and poor compliance, mechanical prostheses are not the solution. Bioprostheses, because of their very limited durability in the young, are not a satisfactory alternative. Valve repair tends to deteriorate early due to the ongoing rheumatic process or recurrent reactivations (5). A prophylaxis for recurrence of rheumatic fever must be followed strictly until the patient is at least 30 years of age (6) (Table 7).

E. Educational Material

The concentration of a group of professionals with a common goal, unified methodology, and continuous feedback is an exciting experience that results in a better quality of care. This experience generates very valuable educational material, not only for the health-care personnel, but also for the patients. Instructional videos, patient books, and pamphlets can be prepared that adapt the general knowledge on valve disease to the specific needs of the local population. A reference valve library with the locally most relevant literature can be made available to the whole team and particularly to newcomers to the program.

IV. RESULTS

It is outside the scope of this chapter to report the results of the valvular surgery performed in this center. However, as an indication of the type of work that can be done by a valve clinic, between July 1988, when the clinic commenced, and July 1991, 1036 valves were operated upon in 714 patients. The basic information that can be obtained immediately is shown in Tables 8–11. A rapid analysis of our valvular population (Table 8) shows that there are very young (mean age 33 years), mostly rheumatic (72%), and very evolved (88% in functional class III-IV). Over half of the valves were repaired (60%). The hospital mortality (Table 9) shows a rather low

Table 8 Valvular Patients Entered into the "Valve Clinic" Database, July 1988–July 1991

	Mitral n = 514	Aortic n = 349	Tricuspid n = 173	Total valves = 1036 Pts = 714
Age: Range	1–77	2–90	1–75	1–90
Mean	31.8	32.3	33.7	32.9
Median	30	27	33	30
Sex: Male	232 (45.1%)	251 (71.9%)	59 (34.1%)	373 (52.2%)
Female	282 (54.9%)	98 (28.1%)	114 (65.9%)	341 (47.8%)
Etiology:				
Rheumatic	455 (88.5%)	235 (67.3%)	60 (34.7%)	750 (72.4%)
Degenerative	18 (3.5%)	52 (14.9%)	—	70 (6.8%)
Congenital	17 (3.3%)	55 (15.8%)	4 (2.3%)	76 (7.3%)
Endocarditis	22 (4.3%)	22 (6.3%)	5 (2.9%)	49 (4.7%)
Functional	7 (1.4%)	—	103 (59.5%)	112 (10.8%)
Ischemic	10 (1.9%)	—	—	10 (1.0%)
Other	3 (0.6%)	2 (0.6%)	4 (2.3%)	9 (0.9%)
Functional class:				
I–II	43 (8.4%)	55 (15.7%)	10 (5.8%)	84 (11.8%)
III–IV	471 (91.6%)	294 (84.3%)	163 (94.2%)	630 (88.2%)
Surgery:				
Repairs	299 (58.2%)	158 (45.3%)	164 (94.8%)	621 (59.9%)
Replacements	215 (41.8%)	191 (54.7%)	9 (5.2%)	415 (40.1%)
Biological	112 (52%)	88 (46%)	8 (88.9%)	208 (50%)
Mechanical	103 (48%)	103 (54%)	1 (11.1%)	207 (50%)

Table 9 Hospital Mortality—Valvular Surgery (July 1988–July 1991)

Surgery, n = 714		Hospital mortality, n = 27 (3.8%)
Isolated:	437 (61.2%)	Isolated n = 19 (4.3%)
Mitral:	239	
Aortic:	182	
Tricuspid:	16	
Double valve:	232 (32.5%)	Double valve n = 5 (2.2%)
Mitral + aortic:	120	
Mitral + tricuspid:	110	
Aortic + tricuspid:	2	
Triple valve:	45 (6.3%)	Triple n = 3 (6.7%)

Table 10 Actuarial Analysis (Maximum Follow-up 40 Months)[a]

	Repair $n = 347$	Prosth. $n = 243$	Mixed $n = 124$	Total $n = 714$
Percent actuarial survival (total)	94.45 ± 1.99	86.27 ± 3.09	74.79 ± 6.90	88.75 ± 1.80
Percent actuarial survival (ex. hospital deaths)	96.14 ± 1.90	92.38 ± 2.91	77.95 ± 7.04	92.05 ± 1.80
Freedom from embolism	98.23 ± 0.79	96.10 ± 1.66	93.48 ± 2.86	96.78 ± 0.82
Freedom from reoperation	77.21 ± 5.15	98.55 ± 0.83	94.75 ± 2.37	86.27 ± 3.10
Pt-years follow-up	523.03	321.69	162.46	1007.19

[a] Repair = one or all valves repaired. Prosth. = one or all valves replaced. Mixed = combination of replacement and repair.

incidence, probably due to the young age of the patients. The long-term or follow-up figures (Table 10) show a significantly higher overall survival of the patients with repair than with replacement (94% versus 86%), and higher freedom from thromboembolic events (98% versus 96%). The relationship between nationality of the patients and probability of continuous long-term follow-up is shown in Table 11. A follow-up of 98% at 3.5 years for our Saudi population is in our opinion the best indication of the efficiency and usefulness of the valve clinic.

Table 11 Follow-up Compliance According to Nationality

	Saudi	Yemeni	Other Nat.	Total
Patients at risk	569	61	57	687
Follow-up entries:				
Personal	1224	91	103	1418
Letter	2	—	—	2
Phone	93	37	15	145
Indirect	70	20	15	205
Total entries	1489	148	133	1770
Patient status:				
Alive	535	28	52	615
Late deaths	22	2	1	25
Lost to follow-up	12 (2.1%)	31 (50.8%)	4 (7%)	47 (6.8%)

It is well understood that local conditions vary greatly among centers
and that many of our suggestions in this chapter might be irrelevant. It is
our conviction, however, that an objective, unified, and careful recording
of the evolution of our valvular patients can only lead to a better understanding of their problems and bring us closer to the still unattainable
ideal situation.

REFERENCES

1. Walpert L, Richard A. Pasion for science. Oxford: Oxford Univ Press, 1988:
    206.
2. Edmunds LH, Clark RE, Cohn LH, Miller DC, Weisel DR. Guidance for
    reporting morbidity and mortality after cardiac valvular operations. J Thorac
    Cardiovasc Surg 1988; 96:351–3.
3. Saour JN, Sieck JO, Memo LAR, Gallus AS. Trial of different intensities of
    anticoagulation in patients with prosthetic heart valves. N Engl J Med 1990;
    322:438–32.
4. Dajani AS, Bisno AL, Kyung JC, et al. Prevention of bacterial endocarditis.
    Recommendations by the American Heart Association. JAMA 1990; 264:
    2919–22.
5. Duran CMG, Gometza B, DeVol EB. Valve repair in rheumatic mitral disease.
    Circulation 1991; 84(suppl III):125–31.
6. Dajani AS, Bisno AL, Chung KJ, et al. Prevention of rheumatic fever. A
    statement for health professionals by the committee on rheumatic fever, endo-
    carditis and Kawasaki disease of the council on cardiovascular disease in the
    young. Circulation 1988; 78(4):1082–6.

APPENDIX

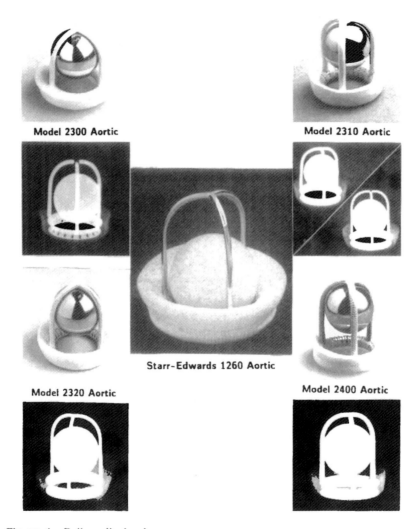

Model 2300 Aortic

Model 2310 Aortic

Starr-Edwards 1260 Aortic

Model 2320 Aortic

Model 2400 Aortic

Figure 1 Ball medical valves.

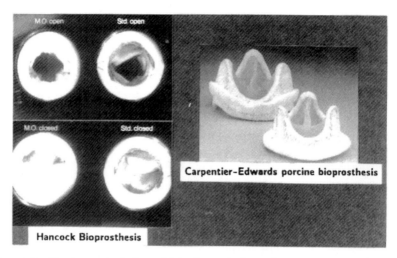

Figure 2 Stent-mounted glutaraldehyde-treated porcine aortic valves (Carpentier-Edwards and Hancock).

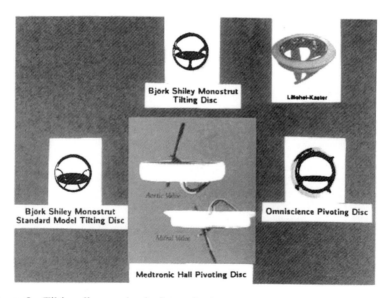

Figure 3 Tilting disc mechanical prosthesis.

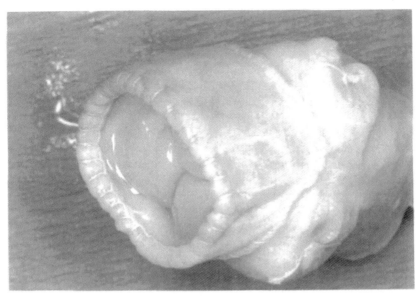

(A)

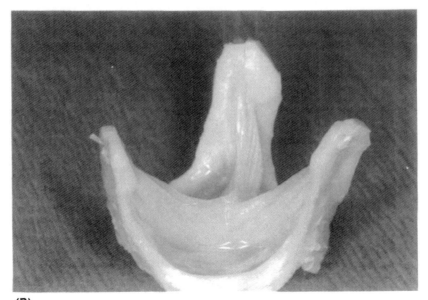

(B)

Figure 4   "Free-hand" glutaraldehyde-treated procine aortic valve. (A) root, (B) composite scalloped. (O'Brien)

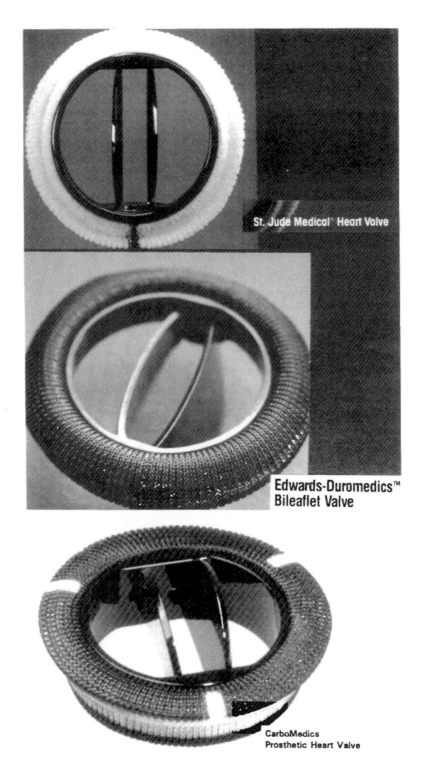

Figure 5 Bileaflet mechanical valves.

Index